NORTH AMERICAN FOLK HEALING

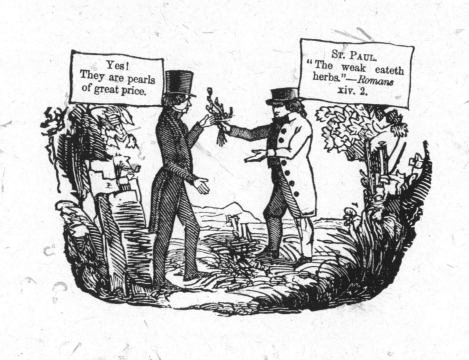

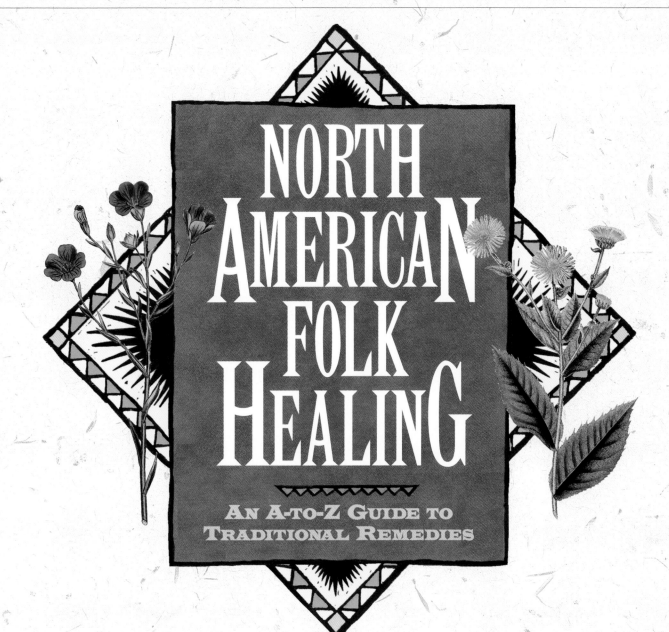

NORTH AMERICAN FOLK HEALING

AN A-TO-Z GUIDE TO TRADITIONAL REMEDIES

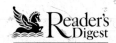

Reader's Digest

The Reader's Digest Association, Inc.
Pleasantville, New York / Montreal

The credits and acknowledgments that appear on
pages 407–408 are hereby made a part of this copyright page.

Address any comments about
NORTH AMERICAN FOLK HEALING to
Editor, Books and Home Entertainment, c/o Customer Service,
Reader's Digest, 215 Redfern Avenue, Westmount, Quebec H3Z 2V9.

For information on this and other Reader's Digest products
or to request a catalogue, please call our 24-hour Customer Service
hotline at 1–800–465–0780.

You can also visit us on the World Wide Web at http://www.readersdigest.ca

Printed in the United States of America

97 98 99 / 5 4 3 2 1

Canadian Cataloguing in Publication Data

Main entry under title:
    Reader's Digest North American folk healing: an a-to-z guide to traditional remedies.

Includes index.
ISBN 0-88850-613-9

    1. Herbs—Therapeutic use. 2. Traditional medicine.
I. Reader's Digest Association (Canada). II. Title: North American folk healing.
    RM666.H33R42 1998   615.8'82   C97-900890-5

NORTH AMERICAN FOLK HEALING

CANADIAN STAFF

EDITORIAL
PROJECT EDITOR
Enza Micheletti

ASSOCIATE EDITOR
Anita Winterberg

COPY EDITOR
Gilles Humbert

ART
ART DIRECTOR
John McGuffie

DESIGNER
Manon Gauthier

PRODUCTION
PRODUCTION MANAGER
Holger Lorenzen

PRODUCTION COORDINATOR
Susan Wong

READER'S DIGEST BOOKS AND HOME ENTERTAINMENT

EDITORIAL DIRECTOR
Deirdre Gilbert

MANAGING EDITOR
Philomena Rutherford

U.S. STAFF

EDITORIAL
PROJECT EDITOR
Fred DuBose

SENIOR ASSOCIATE EDITOR
Marianne Wait

ASSOCIATE EDITOR
David Egner

ASSISTANT EDITOR
Nancy Berrian-Dixon

ART
PROJECT ART EDITOR
Susan Welt

ASSOCIATE ART EDITORS
Bruce R. McKillip
Jason Peterson

With special assistance from
DESIGN DIRECTOR
Perri DeFino

RESEARCH
PROJECT RESEARCH EDITOR
Susan Biederman

TEXT AND ART RESEARCH EDITOR
Sandra Streepey

CONTRIBUTORS

PRINCIPAL CONSULTANTS

Thomas Kurt, MD, MPH
Clinical Professor, Department of Internal Medicine, University of Texas Southwest Medical Center

Ara Der Marderosian, PhD
Professor of Pharmacognosy and Medicinal Chemistry, Philadelphia College of Pharmacy and Science

Edward M. Croom, Jr., PhD
Coordinator, Phytomedicine Program, National Center for the Development of Natural Products, University of Mississippi

Don Yoder, PhD
Professor of Folklife Studies, University of Pennsylvania

David J. Hufford, PhD
Professor of Humanities, Pennsylvania State University College of Medicine

Steven Foster
Steven Foster Group, LLC

Mark Blumenthal
Director, American Botanical Council

SPECIAL FEATURE CONSULTANTS

Michelle Benoit
James A. Duke, PhD
Joe S. Graham, PhD
June Gutmanis
Kelly Kindscher
Carl Lindahl, PhD
Theodore H. Mala, PhD
Daniel Moerman, PhD
Aviva J. Romm
Holly H. Shimizu
Loudell H. Snow, PhD

WRITERS

Peter Ainslie
Joanne Barkan
Jean Callahan
Jim Dwyer
Matthew X. Kiernan
Lisa Light
Cathy Sears
Carol Weeg
Scott Weidensaul

SPECIAL FEATURE WRITERS

James J. Cassidy, Jr.
Rosemary G. Rennicke
Henry Wiencek

RESEARCHERS

Melanie Kindrachuk
Cathy Sears

COPY EDITOR
Gina Grant

PROOFREADER
Judy Yelon

PICTURE RESEARCHER
Steven Diamond

COMMISSIONED PHOTOGRAPHY
Colin Cooke

SPECIAL FEATURE ILLUSTRATIONS
Tom Edgerton

ABOUT THIS BOOK

Within these pages you will learn of the ways our great-grandparents and their forebears made extensive use of folk remedies. These remedies were based largely on herbs—some so medically effective that they became the source of modern drugs, others that proved to be dangerous, and still others that eventually fell from use.

In a browsable A-to-Z format, NORTH AMERICAN FOLK HEALING intermixes articles featuring 89 ailments and 105 medicinals. But before you delve in, take note: Just as anyone using herbal products should be an informed consumer, so should you understand how to use this book.

The Ailments Articles

These describe ailments and how our ancestors used folk medicine to remedy them, whether wisely or not. Within each article, certain remedies—all of them generally regarded as safe—are set off in a separate section. Most of these, such as garlic and slippery elm, are botanicals that have a long history of use. Others, like eucalyptus and gotu kola, are new to North American folk medicine. Still others are nonmedicinal self-treatments—exercises or dietary changes, for example.

Before trying a featured botanical for a particular ailment—licorice for asthma, for example—check the index to see if the botanical is covered in either the book's A-to-Z section (pp. 18–359) or the Addendum (pp. 360–373). If it is, look it up: the more you know about a botanical, the more you'll be able to make an informed decision about using it. If it receives no further coverage in the book, follow the guidelines in the Buyer's Guide (pp. 386–387) before trying it.

The Medicinal Articles

Each of the medicinal articles—most featuring botanicals, others highlighting such animal or mineral products as honey or salt—includes an information box that

appears on the article's first page. This box lists the herb's active parts, uses, and any cautions that pertain to using it. Take note, however, that the inclusion of an ailment in the "uses" portion of this box does not suggest that the medicinal is necessarily efficacious for the specified ailment, but that it is generally regarded as safe when used properly. Also note that a number of these medicinals should be used only after consulting your doctor.

The Foldout Features

Found throughout the A-to-Z section are 12 foldout features that focus on the healing traditions of various ethnic groups, periods, and regions. These spotlight the folk practices of groups as culturally diverse as the early settlers and the pre-Western Hawaiians, as geographically wide-ranging as the mountain dwellers of Appalachia and the Inuit of Alaska and the Canadian North. Each foldout contains a large illustration that portrays a certain ceremony, ritual, or moment in time.

Back of the Book

Following the A-to-Z section is an Addendum that describes 52 more botanicals, some of which played no part historically in North American folk medicine but are popular today—tea tree and cat's claw, for example. Also included are herbs that were once a part of North American folk medicine but have fallen out of favor; even these, however, are still available.

A 12-page Preparing Herbal Remedies section (pp. 374–385) shows you how to go back to basics and concoct your own syrups and tinctures, poultices, balms, infused oils, and more. Rounding out the book are a two-page Buyer's Guide, which offers important advice and tips to consumers, and a helpful Glossary of terms.

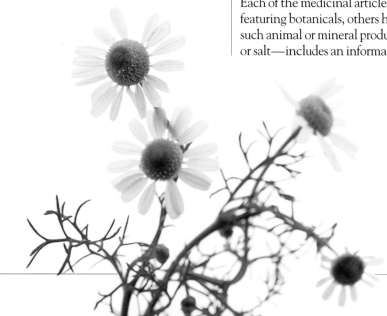

CONTENTS

A New Joining Together

As we enter the new millennium, the many fields of health care are joining together to include more alternatives, both new and old. I foresee an incorporation of all forms of health care, including herbal medicine and folk healing, into a broad but selective approach. This will usher in a new era of the eclecticism that existed in a different way in the 19th century. NORTH AMERICAN FOLK HEALING accepts this challenge in today's world, providing a practical guide that describes the use of herbal medicines both past and present.

North American physicians and pharmacists have not learned how to prescribe and dispense herbs for 50 years, a result of the gradual elimination of herbal medicines from national pharmacopeias. This is in contrast to medicine in Europe, where the use of herbs is taught as pharmacognosy and where herbal medicines comprise one-quarter of the drug market. With serious adverse drug reactions and interactions frightening the public, the appeal of natural products adds to the rapidly growing use of herbs as single-choice therapeutic agents, such as ginger for nausea and motion sickness.

When a buyer purchases any product, a certain degree of caution is advised, following the old adage, "Let the buyer beware!" This applies in any medical marketplace. Purchase products from a reliable manufacturer and look to self-policing organizations, such as the American Herbal Products Association, for information.

NORTH AMERICAN FOLK HEALING approaches the use of herbs in an historical context. It describes, extensively and on an easy-to-read basis, botanicals and treatments that have been in use in North America for more than four centuries.

Thomas L. Kurt

Thomas L. Kurt, MD, MPH
Clinical Professor of Internal Medicine,
University of Texas Southwestern
Medical Center at Dallas
Scientific Advisory Board,
American Herbal Products Association

A Brief History of Herbs

Herbs have woven their way through North American medicine from the beginning—first as part of the healing arsenal of the native peoples, next as alternatives to the harsh treatments administered by colonial physicians, and later as the source of patent medicines that promised miracle cures. In the early 1900s, these plants were for the most part replaced by more powerful, faster-acting synthetic drugs. Yet today they have returned, this time as part of the new "integrative" medicine that many see as the wave of the future—a blend of conventional medicine, herbal remedies, exercise, and sound nutrition.

The Power of Plants

Botanists classify herbs as seed-producing plants that have little woody tissue and die down at the end of the growing season. However, in phytomedicine (the term for plant-based medicine), "herb" refers to any plant part that is used medicinally, whether the root of the ginseng plant or the flowers of chamomile. Furthermore, animal and mineral substances, such as honey and salt, are recognized as a part of the natural medicine repertoire.

The use of medicinal plants stretches back to the earliest civilizations. Many botanicals were employed in the healing rituals of ancient cultures for their emetic, purgative, and hallucinogenic effects; in Egypt, Greece, Mexico, and Europe, these plants were even cultivated in guarded botanical gardens. Specific medicinal uses for plants were etched in stone and drawn on scrolls. In China, the *Pen Tsao*, written c. 2900 B.C., listed more than 300 herbs. In India, medicinal plants were mentioned in the religious poems known as Vedas, written several centuries before the birth of Christ.

Many of the healing plants of China and India eventually made their way to Greece, where medical botany was studied by such scholars as Hippocrates and Aristotle. In the first century, Dioscorides, a Greek surgeon who served in Nero's Roman Army, wrote *De Materia Medica*, which served as the standard catalog of botanical drugs for 15 centuries. Around the same time, Pliny the Elder (A.D. 23–79) published *Historia Naturalis*—a 37-volume anthology written by Greek and Roman scholars and counting medicine and botany among its nearly 2,000 articles. In the next century, the Roman physician Galen developed an elaborate system of classifying healing plants as either hot or cold, dry or moist, and related their use to the Hellenistic theory of the body's four humors. The works of these men remained highly influential in Europe and the New World for centuries, an indication of the close alliance between medicine and botany that would exist up to the 20th century.

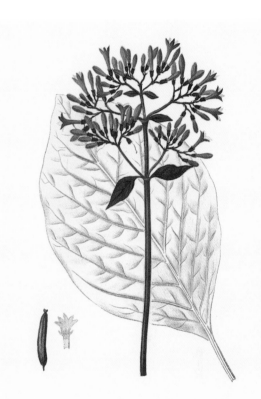

Quinquina pubescent.

The foundations of modern pharmacology are based largely on knowledge gained about the active principles isolated from plants. Peruvian bark (above), of the Cinchona genus, was used medically for centuries in the Andes before it was tapped as the source of the drug quinine. Likewise, yew yields a new drug, taxol, to treat ovarian and breast cancers.

Although plants have now largely been replaced by synthetic drugs, especially in Canada and the United States, they are—and will continue to be—the source of important new medicines. In fact, some 25 percent of prescription drugs are derived from plants, and well over half of over-the-counter drugs come in some way from natural sources.

Herbs in North America

To early North Americans, herbal medicine was not so much a choice as a necessity. The few formally trained doctors that practiced between the 1600s and early 1800s usually resided in large cities. Moreover, many people were reluctant to consult doctors because of their practice of so-called "heroic" medicine—the bleeding of patients and the administering of such "mineral poisons" as mercury and arsenic. Not surprisingly, many in the population turned to home remedies.

Household gardens were planted not only with food plants but with such medicinal herbs as feverfew and pot marigold, which were transformed into poultices, tonics, and syrups. In cities and towns, apothecaries sold herbal-remedy ingredients and packaged medicines, both imported and domestic. In the countryside, itinerant drug peddlers, sometimes

called botanical doctors, hawked their wares from farm to farm, door to door.

Guiding the early use of home remedies were medical books and herbals. In fact, the settlement of the New World coincided with the so-called golden age of herbals, a flood of books born of the popular interest in the medicinal herbs that were being imported to Europe and the New World from Asia and India. Among popular English-language works that early North Americans relied on were John Gerard's *The Herball* (1597)

and Nicholas Culpeper's *Complete Herbal and English Physician* (1652), the latter an amalgam of plants, medicine, and astrology. Also trusted by the settlers was John Wesley's *Primitive Physic(k)*, which was updated numerous times from 1745 to the late 18th century.

In time, North Americans could consult a variety of homegrown texts. *Domestic Medicine: or, Poor Man's Friend* (1830) was written by the Tennessee physician John Gunn. In 1857, Dr. Gunn published what would become the most popular medical book of its time: the revised and enlarged *New Domestic Medicine or Family Physician*. Gunn's books, along with Charles Millspaugh's *American Medicinal Plants* (1852), lessened the reliance on English herbals and covered native medicinal plants as well as Indian practices.

Many pioneer women kept record of their medicinal recipes, including Catharine Parr Traill, who wrote of "the use of native plants" in *The Canadian Settler's Guide* (1855) and *Studies of Plant-Life in Canada* (1885). In New France, some convent women sent correspondence of their herbal cures to physicians in France.

The 19th Century

Herbal medicine reached its peak in North America in the 19th century, starting with an "every man his own doctor" movement led by the New England herbalist Samuel Thomson, progressing to the Eclectic movement (of

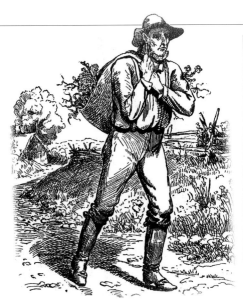

Itinerant herbalists *like the one in this 18th-century engraving peddled their wares to country folk well into the 19th century.*

which herbs were an integral part), and culminating in a shameful era of quackery.

The Thomsonian era began with a rebellion against the medical establishment. Angered by the successful early 1800s campaign of educated physicians to create licensing requirements, Thomson denounced so-called regular doctors as "learned quacks." In his *New Guide to Health: or, Botanic Family Physician* (1822) the onetime farmer argued that folks could more easily heal themselves.

Thomson's patented system of botanic medicine held that all diseases stemmed from a lack of body heat, caused by the body's failure to properly digest food. His remedies involved generating heat with steam baths and clearing "obstructions" with the use of lobelia, a violent emetic. The movement declined in the late 1830s, defeated by a growing faction of Thomsonians who demanded stricter rules and more formal schooling.

In the mid-1800s, many Thomsonians joined forces with the Eclectics, who claimed to cull worthy practices from any school of thought—hence their label. They were led by a New Yorker named Wooster Beach. Like the Thomsonians, the Eclectics campaigned against doctors' use of mineral poisons and the bleeding of patients. One member, John King, precipitated the advent of laboratory-made drugs by developing what he called "concentrated" medicines, made with the hydroalcoholic extracts of plants. King also published the *American Dispensatory,* the bible of the Eclectic movement.

By the turn of the 20th century, regular doctors had regained much of the respect they had lost in the Thomsonian era. Moreover, their ready incorporation of scientific advances in medicine soon rendered the Eclectic system obsolete.

The Age of Quackery

The 19th century also saw the culmination of a North American indulgence in patent medicines, which had begun as soon as the first English settlers landed. The origin of these medicines, many of which achieved a status that would rival that of the most popular over-the-counter drugs today, was fairly modest. The earliest settlers had brought with them such nostrums as John Hooper's Female Pills. Soon afterward, ads for other English medicines, such as Daffy's Elixir (for "colic and griping"), appeared in newspapers.

However, by the early 19th century many such products had come to resemble witches' brews, containing everything from popular herbs to the skins of rare snakes. Many nostrums pretended to draw on Indian wisdom: the Kickapoo Indian Medicine Company—named for an Oklahoma tribe but based in Connecticut—offered Indian Cough Cure, Indian Salve, and Worm Killer. Many patent medicines also contained substantial amounts of alcohol, morphine, or cocaine—additives whose

Samuel Thomson was scorned by regular doctors, and the healers who practiced his system were denounced as "puke doctors and steamers" or "lobelia doctors." Nevertheless, Thomsonian books and almanacs were bestsellers until the mid-19th century.

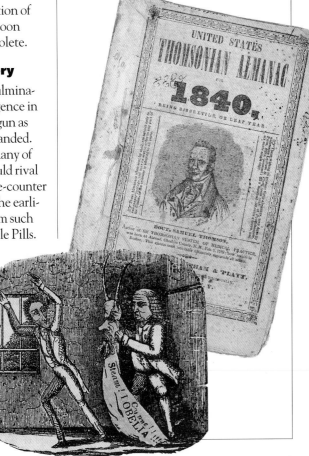

effects served primarily to convince the patient that some sort of healing was taking place. Examples included Gin Pills for the Kidneys, sold by the National Drug and Chemical Co. of Canada.

At a time when small-time hucksters were common, "medicine shows" took selling to another level. Featuring pitchmen, magicians, and circus animals, these colorful caravans toured far and wide, their performers cloaking themselves in the trappings of tradition by dressing as Indians, Quakers (perceived as trustworthy), and healers from the Far East. Around the turn of the century, the shows were a major source of medicine, particularly in rural areas.

Legitimate Use

Despite the popularity of patent medicines, crude botanical drugs were still widely used at the turn of the century. The old-time North American apothecary displayed jars of roots, leaves, powders, and tinctures. In New York State, the Shakers were gaining renown worldwide for their herbal formulations, which were

shipped overseas. Many of the herbs sold today, like feverfew and peppermint, were marketed by the leading pharmaceutical firms of the time, and every pharmacist and physician was trained in their use.

Moreover, standards for herbal drugs were set in 1820, when 11 physicians met in Washington, D.C., to establish the first United States Pharmacopeia (USP). At its inception, the USP's publication, also called the *United States Pharmacopeia,* included formulas for the preparation of drugs and drug products. Now in its 23rd revision, the USP sets standards of identification, strength, quality, purity, packaging, and labeling for more than 3,200 drug products. In 1980, the USP incorporated a similar body: the National Formulary. Its publication, which carries the same name, was conceived in 1883 as a guide for pharmacists in New York and was later distributed across the United States.

New Regulations

While a modicum of standards existed for herbal medicines in the early 20th century, quackery was still rife. As a result, the

federal governments in Canada and the United States launched campaigns to outlaw questionable manufacturing practices and eliminate the inclusion of such narcotics as morphine and cocaine in medicines.

In Canada, the federal government passed the Act to Prevent the Adulteration of Food, Drink, and Drugs in 1875. The statute was superseded by the Food and Drugs Act in 1920. Intended to protect consumers from health hazards and fraudulent claims, the act classifies any product used to heal or prevent disease as a drug. For an herbal remedy to be sold as a therapeutic product in Canada, the manufacturer must provide proof of its efficacy and safety to Health Canada. Products that meet requirements are issued a Drug Identification Number (DIN) by Health Canada (see p. 387).

In the United States, the Pure Food and Drug Act (1906) outlawed false claims on labels and required the disclosure of a product's drug and alcohol content. Still more regulations were enacted in the Food, Drug, and Cosmetic Act (1938). Also established early in the century was the Food and Drug Administration (FDA), which today protects U.S. consumers in part by requiring the ingredients of a drug to be stated truthfully on the package label. The 1994 Dietary Supplement Health & Education Act (DSHEA) now allows herbal products to be marketed so long as they meet certain labeling requirements.

Apart from governments, a number of organizations promulgate standards for herbal products and provide information to the public. Among them are the American Botanical Council, the Herb Research Foundation, the American Herbal Products Association, and the Canadian Health Food Association.

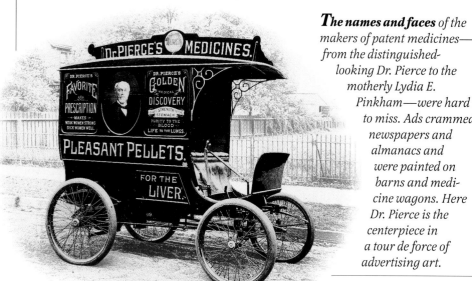

The names and faces of the makers of patent medicines— from the distinguished- looking Dr. Pierce to the motherly Lydia E. Pinkham—were hard to miss. Ads crammed newspapers and almanacs and were painted on barns and medicine wagons. Here Dr. Pierce is the centerpiece in a tour de force of advertising art.

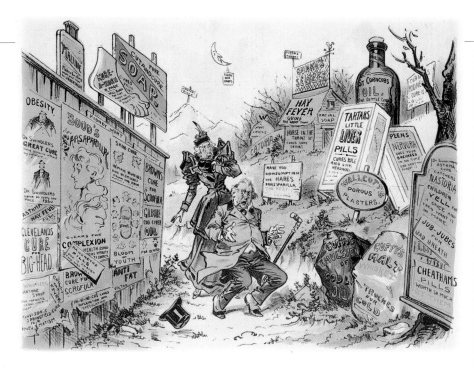

An 1875 cartoon satirizing the claims made for patent medicines foreshadowed the tactics of some herbal-products manufacturers today. As knowledge of herbs increases, such bombast may become a relic of the past.

It is important to realize that self-medication with herbs is not a replacement for conventional medicine. There are many times when the patient should at least seek a diagnosis from a conventional physician. Depending on the diagnosis, the patient and physician can discuss a potential alternative treatment—including, whenever appropriate, the use of well-researched herbs.

Also remember that "natural" does not equal "safe." Because even herbs that are generally recognized as safe can be dangerous when improperly used, consumers should become knowledgeable about herbs before trying them (see pp. 386–387).

Today North Americans are taking a greater role in their own health care—eating healthier foods, exercising more, and exploring alternative treatments. As a result, herbal medicines have assumed a new importance. Yet the fact that herbs are beginning to coexist comfortably with conventional medicine should hardly be surprising: the use of these plants to combat illness is as old as mankind.

Herbal Medicine Today

In the 1990s, herbs have become the focus of enormous interest, with sales of herbal products on the rise. Ironically, this phenomenon results in part from advances in science: modern pharmacognosy and chemistry are now able to analyze plants more accurately. Moreover, there is a better understanding of how herbs work compared to regular drugs.

Most studies on herbs take place not in North America but in Western Europe and Asia, where herbal medicine is an accepted part of medical care. In the forefront is Germany, whose government in 1978 established the Commission E. This body has prepared more than 300 monographs on herbs and herbal combination products and is seen as the world's leading authority on the efficacy and safety of herbs.

So what has science found? In short, a better understanding of how herbs work in comparison to synthetic drugs. Chemists have known since the early 1800s that plants have chemical constituents with medicinal properties. Examples of these so-called active principles are glycosides (one being digitoxin, from foxglove) and alkaloids (such as caffeine, from coffee). When isolated and used as the basis for regular drugs, these principles produce rapid, often immediate results. Conversely, crude or "whole plant" drugs, with their many secondary compounds, generally act more slowly and at a lower level, possibly in a synergistic biochemical way. In addition, both conventional drugs and crude herbal drugs have proved to sometimes produce a placebo effect—a physiological improvement brought on by a psychological mechanism.

Modern scientific research has validated the historical use of dozens of medicinal herbs—now sold in pills instead of apothecary jars. Future research will no doubt continue to explain the benefits of nature's own medicines.

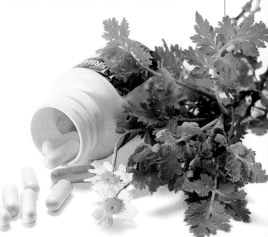

HERBAL REMEDIES A TO Z

The next 342 pages paint a fascinating picture of the ways our ancestors treated illness and maintained health by using herbs. Some 105 medicinals—botanicals and such folk standbys as honey, salt, and vinegar—appear alphabetically, intermixed with 89 common ailments. Each medicinal article is accompanied by an information box that lists the plant's active parts, its uses, and any necessary cautions. Within the ailment articles appear folk remedies, set off in a separate box. The herbs used in most of these were part of our forebears' materia medica, while others are

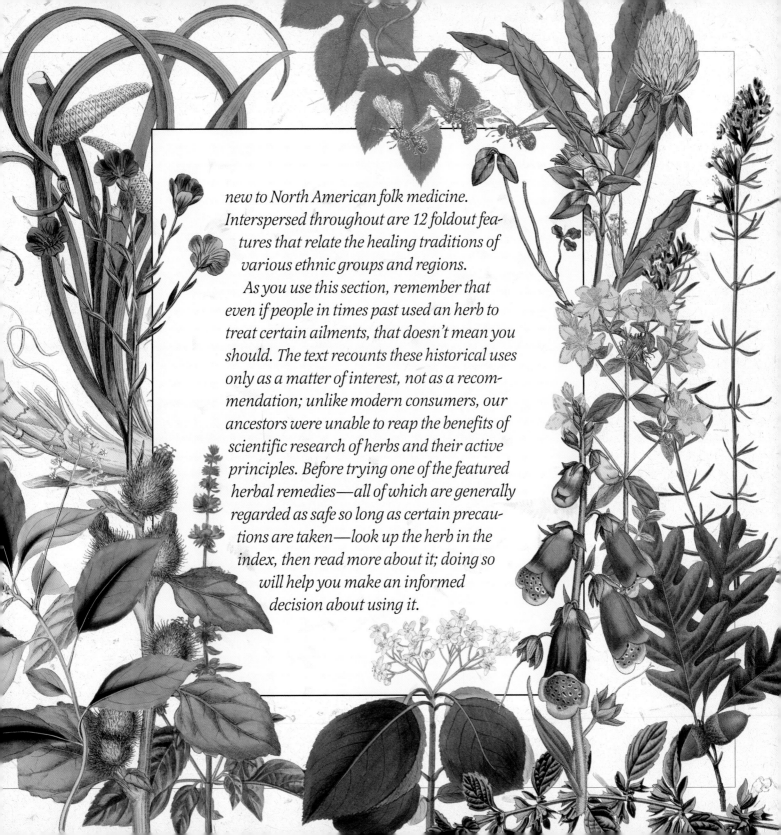

new to North American folk medicine. Interspersed throughout are 12 foldout features that relate the healing traditions of various ethnic groups and regions.

As you use this section, remember that even if people in times past used an herb to treat certain ailments, that doesn't mean you should. The text recounts these historical uses only as a matter of interest, not as a recommendation; unlike modern consumers, our ancestors were unable to reap the benefits of scientific research of herbs and their active principles. Before trying one of the featured herbal remedies—all of which are generally regarded as safe so long as certain precautions are taken—look up the herb in the index, then read more about it; doing so will help you make an informed decision about using it.

ABDOMINAL PAIN

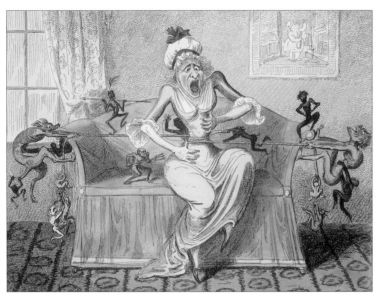

Gluttony and its punishment *were so common in the 19th century that they were often satirized, as in this 1819 etching.*

Abdominal pain can signal a dizzying array of ailments. Sometimes the cause is as simple as too much food or alcohol. Stress can also trigger stomach pain. So can a case of nerves. (In the 19th century, if you had stomach pain due to nervousness, you had the "collywobbles"—from *colic* and *wobbles*—and were probably advised to drink a cup of chamomile tea.) The symptoms are often relieved by taking an antacid medication or by drinking ½ tablespoon of baking soda in half a glass of water.

Certain medications, notably aspirin and ibuprofen, can cause stomach pain. So can milk products among those who have difficulty digesting lactose. Occasionally, abdominal pain is a sign of a more serious problem, such as a disorder of the appendix, intestines, gallbladder, liver, kidneys, pancreas, spleen, stomach, or reproductive system. If the pain is severe or persistent, consult a doctor.

Old-time Stomachache Cures

Homegrown cures for stomachache have changed little over the years. Mothers still send ailing children to bed with a heating pad, a glass of "flat" ginger ale, or a warm cup of milk. Before the advent of heating pads, some used a warm compress of chamomile tea. Another remedy called for a rag soaked in kerosene to be placed over the lower-right quadrant of the abdomen, in which the appendix lies; it was then covered with a towel and a hot-water bottle. It was also suggested that "flannels dipped in hot water and wrung out, then placed over the abdomen, relieve the pain." Heat indeed helps relax cramps and improve blood flow. Undoubtedly less effective was the following advice: "To cure cramps, put a pan of water under your bed."

Before the invention of ginger ale, ginger tea was a surefire succor. Ginger is still trusted to settle the stomach and prevent vomiting and nausea. Milk has also been long used to soothe the stomach, but although some still swear by it, research shows that milk actually increases the production of stomach acid. It therefore probably does more harm than good, at least in cases of acid indigestion.

Still another cure for abdominal pain was to chew and swallow a teaspoon of flaxseed. The seeds have a thick coating of mucilage cells, which helps shield the lining of the stomach and intestines from irritants. They also act as a bulk laxative.

Tonics and Teas

For every aching belly there was a tea or an infusion "guaranteed" to bring relief. Many were made from herbs that are still valued today, such as chamomile, peppermint, anise, cinnamon, sage, thyme, nutmeg, ginseng, and caraway seed. Most of these are carminatives, which help expel gas and increase stomach secretions and bile flow, thus improving digestion. Some, such as chamomile, are also anti-inflammatories, which help soothe an inflamed stomach.

Another remedy, parsley tea, was favored for stomach cramps and believed to cure gallbladder ailments; in truth, the tea was probably no more than a diuretic. Teas made from wild strawberry leaves were thought to cure stomachaches, diarrhea, and bladder and kidney ailments; the mildly astringent leaves may indeed have been of some use against diarrhea, but they were probably not effective otherwise. Licorice root and marsh mallow root teas were also taken to calm gastritis, most likely to some effect. Licorice is still recommended today by some herbalists for treating gastric and duodenal ulcers, although long-term use can produce unwanted side effects.

Wild onions sautéed with garlic were thought to aid digestion and relieve stomach pains, as were garlic teas and tinctures. One remedy for stomachache prescribed boiling a sliced onion in a cup of milk. "It sounds awful and probably is," read the recipe, "but it's an old home remedy that may work." Garlic and onion do indeed stimulate the secretion of gastric enzymes and so may relieve flatulence—but too much may cause indigestion instead of curing it. The Indians nibbled native calamus root for stomachaches; the North American variety probably provided some relief, but the Asian variety of calamus that was introduced later has proved to be toxic.

Other remedies were not only ineffective but also utterly unappetizing—and sometimes dangerous. It was claimed that teas made from sheep droppings were good for all varieties of stomach ailments. The inside of a chicken's gizzard, dried and powdered, was also said to cure certain stomach complaints.

A Bitter Drink to Swallow

Bitter-tasting teas made of such herbs as gentian and wormwood, known as bitters, were drunk to promote the production of bile by the liver and therefore cure gallstones, which are caused by insufficient bile production or blockage of the bile duct. Bitter tonics were also believed to improve the appetite and aid digestion if ingested before meals. The bitter taste does in fact stimulate the taste buds at the back of the tongue and increases the flow of saliva and gastric juices.

Boneset tea, which is extremely bitter, was therefore extremely popular. However, it is now known that boneset can cause indigestion and even liver problems. Many other once-popular bitter tonics—including comfrey, angelica root, sweet woodruff, and absinthium extracts—are now considered ineffective or unsafe. But others, most notably gentian root, are still sometimes used.

Much to the disgust of children everywhere, when all else failed—and sometimes even before anything else was tried—a spoonful of castor oil, often mixed with orange juice to disguise the taste, was taken to purge the system.

A Guide to Symptoms

◆ General abdominal pain, sometimes accompanied by chronic burning or colic-like pain in the upper abdomen, loss of appetite, nausea, and vomiting, can signal gastritis, an inflammation of the stomach lining. It is the result of excess stomach acid and is often stress induced. Gastritis can also be brought on by such drugs as aspirin and some antibiotics, and by alcohol abuse.

◆ A gnawing ache or burning sensation that is relieved by antacids might stem from an ulcer. If the pain is provoked by eating, a biopsy should be done to rule out stomach cancer.

◆ Pain that occurs very low in the abdomen might indicate a bladder infection or, if it extends to the side, a kidney infection or stone.

◆ If abdominal pain starts in the small of your back and moves to the groin, and is accompanied by a fever, you may have a prostate infection.

◆ Intermittent abdominal cramps, abdominal swelling, flatulence, and altered bowel habits (including constipation, diarrhea, or both) may result from irritable bowel syndrome (IBS).

◆ Wavelike pain, accompanied by recurring episodes of diarrhea or constipation, flatulence, fever, and weight loss, may signal inflammatory bowel disease, a general term for diseases that include ulcerative colitis and Crohn's disease.

◆ Wavelike pain can also indicate a blockage of the gallbladder, bile duct, or urinary tract, usually by a stone. A diet high in saturated fats encourages cholesterol buildup and the formation of gallstones. Attacks may occur after fatty meals. An inflamed gallbladder with or without gallstones can cause nausea, loss of appetite, gas, and pain in the upper-right abdomen.

◆ Abdominal cramps can signal a bout of food poisoning, especially if accompanied by fever and either diarrhea or vomiting.

◆ Moderate to severe abdominal pain in women may result from gynecological disorders, such as endometriosis, an ectopic pregnancy, fibroids, ovarian cysts, or a sexually transmitted disease. If these trigger severe pain during ovulation, see a doctor at once.

◆ Appendicitis pain begins in the area of the abdomen around the navel and may move to the lower right or it may subside. The pain eventually worsens and is exacerbated by movement. See a doctor immediately.

PEPPERMINT The leaves or oil of peppermint have traditionally been used to treat indigestion, nausea, and abdominal cramps. An antispasmodic, peppermint relieves discomfort caused by spasms in the digestive tract. It also stimulates bile flow and gastric secretions. To make a tea, pour 1 cup boiling water over 1 to 2 teaspoons finely chopped leaves. Let steep for 5 to 10 minutes, then strain.

CHAMOMILE Both German and Roman chamomile oils lessen the production of intestinal gas and calm inflammation. To make a tea, pour 1 cup boiling water over 1 to 2 teaspoons finely chopped flowers. Let steep for 5 to 10 minutes, then strain. Those allergic to ragweed pollens should avoid chamomile.

ANISE Anise's carminative effects help ease the painful bloated feeling caused by gas. Grind 1 teaspoon of the seeds, called aniseed, and combine with 1 cup boiling water to make a tea. Let steep for a few minutes, then strain. Drink the tea slowly.

FENNEL This common garden herb is a traditional folk remedy for digestive problems. Make a tea with 1 teaspoon crushed seeds and 1 cup boiling water. Let steep for 10 minutes, then strain and drink. Avoid fennel oil, which can cause respiratory problems and seizures.

GINGER Dried gingerroot has been used for thousands of years in China to treat stomachache, diarrhea, and nausea. Today it is found in some over-the-counter digestive, laxative, and antacid preparations. To prepare a tea, peel and mince enough root to make 1/3 to 1/2 teaspoon. Add 1 cup boiling water and let steep, then strain. Alternately, add a few drops of fluid extract to hot water and drink. Ginger is also available in capsule form.

TURMERIC A commonly used spice in Indian cuisine, turmeric is a member of the ginger family. Science has confirmed its many benefits: it increases the flow of bile, protects the lining of the stomach and intestines, reduces the formation of intestinal gas, and protects the liver cells. Take 1/4 to 1/2 teaspoon powdered root several times a day between meals. Or sprinkle the spice on food as a seasoning. Turmeric tea is rarely made because the active principles are not water-soluble. Taking too much can result in gastric disturbances. People with gallstones should avoid turmeric as well as curry powder, which contains turmeric.

LICORICE Licorice root is known to soothe a stomachache. It contains an acid that increases mucous secretions and calms the membranes that line the digestive tract. To make a tea, pour 1 cup boiling water over 1/3 to 1/2 teaspoon minced or powdered root. Let steep, then strain. Licorice should not be taken in large amounts or for long periods of time because it can cause serious side effects. Extracts of various strengths are available for instant teas, as are licorice candies and throat lozenges.

CINNAMON Cinnamon bark has been used throughout the ages for gastrointestinal upset of all sorts, including chronic diarrhea, kidney troubles, and cramps. It has antidiarrheal and pain-relieving properties. It is usually mixed in small amounts with regular tea. Or you can make a tea using at least 1/2 to 1 teaspoon of powdered cinnamon per cup of boiling water. Drink three cups a day. Cinnamon oil is also available. A few drops will make a tea.

Ginger ranks as one of the most popular remedies for stomach upset. Its forms are many, including ginger ale, ginger tea, and candied ginger.

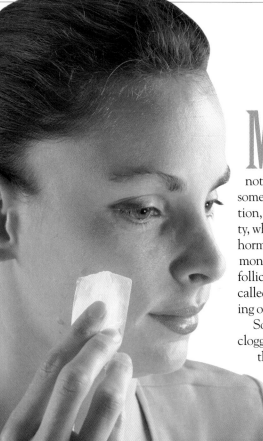

ACNE

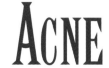

Many of the trials teens face today were unknown to their counterparts of a century ago. But there is one plight the earlier youth did not escape: acne. Most teenagers—and some adults—suffer from this skin condition, which typically begins during puberty, when the body produces more hormones called androgens. These hormones stimulate the oil glands of the hair follicles to produce a fatty substance called sebum, which travels to the opening of the follicle and produces oily skin.

Sometimes the hair follicle becomes clogged with sebum and dead cells from the follicle walls. When this mixture reaches the skin's surface, blackheads develop; these are colored by their exposure to air, not by dirt. If the follicle becomes closed off, whiteheads form. Bacteria may develop if the follicle becomes too full and the sebum mixture invades the surrounding skin layers.

Despite what you may have heard, acne is not caused by dirt or by eating chocolate or greasy foods. In fact, it is often hereditary. It can be aggravated by stress and by hot, humid weather.

Early North Americans had many "cures" for acne. Some swore by poultices made from chamomile or red-clover flowers. Others put stock in milkweed, stump water, or watermelon juice. None of these are especially effective, although rainwater that collects in old tree stumps does tend to contain astringent tannins.

Endless numbers of other astringents were concocted, including mixtures of garlic or strawberry juice and vinegar and a paste made of onions and honey. To banish blackheads, lemons were rubbed on the face before bedtime. Many insisted that fresh urine, or an infant's wet diaper, would clear up pimples. Thankfully, that practice fell by the wayside. On the other hand, cucumber juice had some success at calming irritated skin, and oatmeal paste certainly dried out oily skin.

Washing your face regularly will help keep your skin free of oil, but too much scrubbing can irritate the skin and create new blemishes. For best results, wash your face in cool water with your hands instead of a washcloth, since washcloths can harbor bacteria. And use an astringent several times a day.

To make a blemish less noticeable, *apply an ice cube for a minute to relieve inflammation.*

WITCH HAZEL The leaf and bark of this plant contain astringent tannins. Ironically, some commercial products are prepared by steam distillation, which eliminates the tannins. Wet your finger with the witch hazel and dab your tongue. If it doesn't taste astringent, it isn't. To make a tea, boil ½ to 1 teaspoon bark or leaf in ½ cup water. Strain, then apply.

ELDER FLOWER For centuries people have used elder-flower water as a gentle astringent, although it is faster to make an infusion. To do so, steep 1 teaspoon crushed flowers in 1 cup hot water. Strain, then apply. Those with extreme sensitivity to pollen might experience an allergic reaction.

BURDOCK Burdock root contains the carbohydrate inulin, which forms a protective layer on the skin. Use the dampened root or leaves as a poultice. Or steep ½ teaspoon chopped root in 1 cup hot water. Strain, then apply.

TEA TREE Tea-tree oil has long been used as a topical antiseptic. Apply to acne lesions three to four times a day.

ALCOHOL

On the battlefields desperate surgeons sometimes used alcohol topically to disinfect wounds and internally to relieve pain.

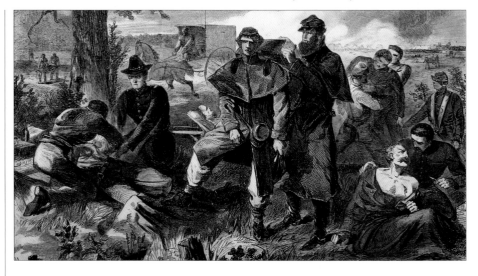

Ethyl alcohol is the active ingredient in alcoholic drinks, such as beer, wine, and liquor. Although the exact origins of its consumption are unclear, it is known that ancient cultures in Asia and Arabia drank alcoholic beverages and used wine as a tonic and topical wound cleanser. In Europe it was known as *aqua vitae*, or "water of life." When the Irish first distilled whiskey 600 years ago, it was revered for its ability to warm the body and lift the spirits.

The Pilgrims brought this reverence with them to North America: Puritan preacher Increase Mather called alcohol a "good creature of God." The drink was used to treat the most common ailments: cold and cough, fatigue, and indigestion. Today alcohol is served at social gatherings and during the modern-day "happy hour" to promote relaxation. However, its social and medicinal values have been hotly debated since the 19th century.

The Hot Toddy

By temporarily widening blood vessels in the face, chest, and skin, alcohol loosens mucus in the nose, sinuses, throat, and lungs and produces a feeling of warmth. For this reason, it was widely used to treat the common cold. However, when the blood vessels and mucous membranes return to normal, congestion also returns. Flushed skin also causes the body to lose heat faster. Furthermore, because it is a diuretic, alcohol dehydrates the body and can make any cold worse.

Nevertheless, alcoholic cold remedies were used throughout North America.

Many, like the "hot toddy" recipe that called for whiskey, honey, and lemon juice, combined hard liquor with a sweetener to make the drink more palatable, especially to women and children. Tonic wines, made with elderberry, elecampane, or dandelion, were drunk to ward off colds. A "nightcap," a small drink before bedtime, was taken to ensure rest (alcohol, a depressant, promotes sleep, but too much can disturb it). Today alcohol remains an ingredient in many over-the-counter cold and cough remedies.

An Age-old Antiseptic

Although alcohol was used by pioneers to treat open wounds, it can damage raw tissue. Alcohol can, however, help to disinfect, soothe, and harden the skin's surface. This effect helps prevent bedsores, protect the soles of the feet before a long walk, and relieve sore muscles.

Uses Common cold, loss of appetite, insomnia, minor cuts and scrapes
Cautions Alcohol impairs short-term concentration, memory, and coordination. Do not drive an automobile after drinking or taking medication that contains alcohol. Binge drinking may cause intoxication, reckless behavior, nausea, unconsciousness, and death. Chronic drinking increases the following risks: alcohol dependence, obesity, osteoporosis, and disorders of the brain, nerves, pancreas, stomach, liver, and heart. Pregnant women who drink risk giving birth to a child with fetal alcohol syndrome. Nursing mothers who drink can adversely affect their child's motor development. Used externally, alcohol may cause skin irritation. Alcohol is flammable; keep away from open flame.

Doctors and nurses commonly apply isopropyl, or rubbing, alcohol on the skin before administering an injection. Rubbing alcohol and denatured ethyl alcohol—common ingredients in skin applications—are toxic and should not be taken internally.

Hit-and-miss Treatments

Alcohol, in modest amounts, has been used to treat digestive ailments, and it does aid digestion and stimulate appetite. A 1995 study showed that polyphenols in red and white wine may also fight the bacteria that cause traveler's diarrhea.

Although alcohol was once used to alleviate morning sickness, low breast milk, snakebite, and pain during surgery, these uses have proved ineffective, even harmful. In fact, pregnant and nursing women should abstain from alcohol in any form. It is not an antidote for snake venom, and using it internally or externally can worsen the effects of a snakebite. Finally, the amount of alcohol needed to anesthetize is dangerously high.

Moderation Versus Abuse

Moderate consumption is an average of one to two drinks per day. ("One drink" is defined as 30 ml of 80 proof liquor, 125 ml of wine, or 375 ml of beer.) Studies point to the health benefits of moderation: higher levels of "good" cholesterol and a reduced risk of clogged coronary arteries. Alcohol, however, is a drug, and its use should be monitored.

The immediate and long-term dangers of alcohol are many. Light drinking impairs motor function and causes dehydration. Excessive drinking causes drunkenness and hangover—an aftereffect marked by fatigue, thirst, and headache. Extreme amounts consumed at one time can cause alcohol poisoning and death.

The "Hidden" Ingredient

Patent medicines—elixirs of herbs and alcohol—were popular from the early 18th century until the mid-20th century. These potions were said to have the power to cure all sorts of ailments, such as cancer and undefined "female complaints," and their alcoholic content was often kept secret because of emerging concerns over alcohol abuse. Although the Puritans of New England embraced alcohol, they also rued the "abuse of drink." Indians were devastated by the white man's "firewater." In the 1800s the Protestant-led temperance movement sought to protect families from the dangers of drinking. Eventually, political pressure for alcohol legislation resulted in many local regulations and, ultimately, in the short-lived period of Prohibition in the United States (1920-33) and Canada (1918-19).

Still, alcohol was a staple of folk medicine. Often mixed with small doses of herbs and sweeteners, alcohol and its dramatic effects were thought to heal. Patent medicines walked a fine line, espousing potency while appealing to the proper ladies of the temperance movement. Dr. Bateman's Pectoral Drops for "rheumatism, afflictions of the stone, gravel, agues, and hysterics" contained mainly opium and alcohol and was sold for more than 100 years in the United States. A Canadian cure-all, Pelletier's Syrup, contained alcohol, tar, and codeine. The National Drug and Chemical Co. of Canada manufactured Gin Pills for the Kidneys. The fabled Lydia E. Pinkham's Vegetable Compound, which consisted of many herbal ingredients and 19 percent alcohol, was also common in households for more than 50 years. (It is still sold today in the United States, but without the alcohol.)

Sadly, the association of such quack patent medicine with North America's herbal tradition damaged the credibility of folk medicine at a time when modern medicine began to emerge.

Lydia Pinkham's motherly face, used to promote her alcohol-laced compound, was one of the most recognized products in the late 19th century.

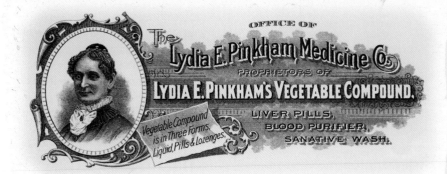

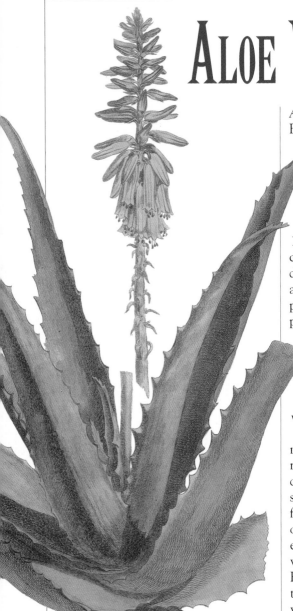

ALOE VERA

Aloe barbadensis
BARBADOS ALOE, CURAÇAO ALOE,
JELLY LEEK

A loe vera made its way from Africa to North America by way of the West Indies, where it was widely cultivated in the 17th and 18th centuries. It later became a common ornamental plant. From earliest days, the wound-soothing properties of aloe vera's gel made it known as the "burn plant" and "first aid plant." A second plant product, the yellow sap, was widely used as a laxative—a practice we now know should be used only with caution. Today aloe vera's extracts are among the most commonly used folk medicines, with potted aloes occupying windowsills from sea to shining sea.

Although aloe vera has been used medicinally since the time of the pharaohs, the proof of its efficacy is still in question. Studies published in 1994 in the scientific periodical *Phytotherapy Journal* found that the gel could speed the healing of some forms of frostbite in humans and experimental animals. But beyond aloe vera's efficacy as a soothing emollient, Health Canada only recognizes its laxative properties when ingested. In aloe vera's case, centuries of use rather than scientific proof may serve as the test of its healing powers.

North American use of aloe vera began more than two centuries ago in the herb gardens of Mexican grandmothers in the Rio Grande Valley. Some 90 cm (3 ft) tall in this ideal climate, the plants were big enough to flay for their gel, which was rubbed on the skin as an emollient or to heal kitchen burns. Word of mouth soon spread northward, and folks were quick to make use of the easy-to-grow houseplant that was said to heal burns. In the 1930s doctors began to use the gel to treat X-ray and radium burns. But it was not until the early 1960s that the aloe vera "boom" began, capturing the popular imagination so effectively that the labels of scores of cosmetic products—from shaving creams to deodorants—trumpet its inclusion.

The Two Extracts

Many consumers believe that the gel and sap (also called latex) of aloe vera are one and the same—a common confusion. In fact, each of these extracts has its own

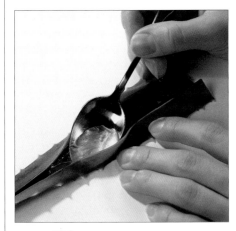

When scooping out gel, *avoid scraping the rind, which can adulterate the gel with unwanted laxative anthraquinones.*

Active plant parts Leaf gel and rind
Uses Wounds, burns, and skin conditions
Cautions Products containing the dried sap of aloe leaf, called aloin, have a laxative effect and should be avoided by women during pregnancy or lactation.

chemical composition and therapeutic properties. The first, the internal gel, is the clear, jellylike substance obtained from the tissues of the center portion of the plant's stiff leaves. It can be applied externally to aid wound healing or used as a tonic. The second, the plant's yellow sap, comes from the leaf's rind. In its dried form, called aloin, the bitter sap is a potent cathartic. It has a tendency to produce more griping and irritation than do other purgative herbs—including cascara sagrada and senna—and an overdose can result in abdominal pain, hemorrhagic gastritis, and bloody diarrhea.

Although the anti-inflammatory activity of aloe vera gel has been explored by numerous researchers in the U.S. and the Far East, its many active compounds remain something of a mystery. Some scientists believe that a substance called glucomannan is the most important active principle. Others hypothesize the presence of certain "biogenic stimulators," or wound-healing hormones that accelerate the rate at which cells recover from injury. A certainty, however, is the fresh gel's abundance of malic acid—a desirable alpha hydroxy acid renowned for its anti-wrinkle effect. Despite this confusion of beneficial agents, all scientists agree that the efficacy of aloe vera is based upon a synergistic cooperation among its biologically active molecules.

Aloe Tonics

Besides valuing aloe vera for its skin-soothing properties, the Mexican grandmothers of the Rio Grande Valley stirred the gel into a cup of tea, believing that it made a healthful tonic. Decades later, numerous claims are made for the benefits of aloe vera ampoules sold in health food stores. Evidence shows, however, that the ampoules' only advantage may be in helping superficial stomach ulcers to heal. In any case, those taking aloe vera juice internally should limit use to one teaspoon after meals so as not to risk a laxative effect. And beware: an industry-sponsored study in the mid-1990s found that a high percentage of aloe products were mislabeled, misrepresented, or adulterated. Worse still, some unscrupulous suppliers were discovered to be substituting cornstarch for aloe vera.

Fortunately, aloe vera is one of the few herbal products that can be certified: look on the label for the International Aloe Science Council (IASC) seal of approval. This watchdog organization is one of the few that have been formed to establish quality and ethical standards for the methods used to market and promote herbal products. Another way to know if an aloe vera product is the real thing is the slight and temporary tingling sensation you will feel in the stomach; if you don't, you may be drinking cornstarch instead.

Growing Your Own

Because the active principles in extracts and dried aloe in some over-the-counter products may diminish over time, you may want to grow your own aloe. The plant grows best in a subtropical climate like that of the Southwest, Florida, and Hawaii. You can plant your aloe in a pot and keep it indoors, where it will flourish; aloe vera won't survive temperatures below 4°C (40°F).

For a healthy plant, use a moist, porous potting mixture of 2 parts soil, 2

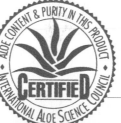

The International Aloe Science Council *certifies trustworthy aloe products with a seal of approval.*

Not to be confused with ...

Aloe vera is native to Africa and should not be confused with the similar-looking century plant (*Agave americana*), which is often called American aloe. Another "aloe" is referred to in both the Old and the New Testaments, yet is an entirely different plant: *Aquilaria achallocha*. Commonly called lignaloe or eaglewood, the biblical aloe is a tall tree native to southern Asia. The fragrant resin of its heartwood was probably the source of the spice used to perfume garments in Psalms 45:7-8 and the Song of Solomon 4:14. It was also used to anoint the body of Christ:

And there came also Nicodemus, which at the first came to Jesus by night, and brought a mixture of myrrh and aloes.... Then took they the body of Jesus, and wound it in linen clothes with the spices.... (John 19:39)

parts coarse sand, ¼ part bone meal, and ½ part dehydrated cow manure. Place the plant in full sun and bring it indoors in winter, keeping the surrounding temperature at 15°C (59°F) to 26°C (79°F). To obtain the gel, cut off a leaf at the fleshy base and split it open with a knife or razor blade. Then gently scrape out the internal gel with a spoon, taking care not to rupture the green rind, which contains the aloe's laxative anthraquinones. Apply the gel directly to the skin with your fingers, but be careful not to get it on your clothes; it can leave an ugly stain.

Medical Care & Folk Cures in

Pioneer Days

*L*ife is fragile, *"like a bubble, or the brittle glass," mused the wife of a colonial governor in the 1600s. Indeed, until the early 19th century, epidemics ran rampant in pioneer settlements, professional medical care was scarce, and many remedies were not only ineffective but often more dangerous than the ailments themselves.*

Folk medicine was not a choice in early North America but a necessity. What few doctors there were between the 1600s and early 1800s clustered mainly in cities and towns, leaving frontier settlers to fend for themselves. Besides being unaffordable, many "doctors" were inadequately trained, having learned primarily through apprenticeship. Even physicians with credentials— from European or North American medical schools— had little to offer, given the historically slow pace of medical advancement.

The prevailing theory maintained that illness was caused by an imbalance of the body's four "humors": blood, phlegm, black bile, and yellow bile. Doctors spared no means— whether bloodletting, blistering, or toxic purgatives—to restore balance. Little wonder that physicians were often distrusted: more often than not, their treatments increased suffering and hastened death.

A New World

So were the settlers forced to make do, handling ailments both familiar and unexpected. For although the New World was deemed a promised land, free from the pollution and plagues that afflicted Europe, it offered a host of hazards. Clearing virgin country for settlement

*A **proponent of herbal cures,** Samuel Thomson (above) published his "New Guide to Health" in 1822. Feverfew (left) was commonly recommended for headaches.*

brought injuries, Indian and animal attacks resulted in wounds, and poor sanitation practices led to the spread of infectious diseases. Indeed, yellow fever, diphtheria, smallpox, and similar epidemics raged frequently, some outbreaks killing thousands in months.

The first line of defense against all ills was women, and their principal weapon was plants from the family garden and the wild. Relying on recipes and techniques from their homelands, women turned such common herbs as mint, lavender, and sage into healing "pultices," tonics, and syrups. When circumstances dictated, they included more exotic materials in their armamentarium. One ointment used on sprains, for example, called for boiled toads, whereas the main ingredient in a 1710 sciatica liniment was earthworms.

Everyday Healers

Women were complemented by lay practitioners—both self-taught, like slaves and midwives, and learned, like governors and plantation owners. Religious leaders, especially, were respected healers. Their ministrations were twofold: since many settlers believed that God punished sin with illness, clergy could care for soul and body. They also used the pulpit to proselytize. When a crude—and controversial—smallpox vaccine became available in the 1720s, preachers pro and con voiced their prejudice in their sermons. At very least, a parson's prayers helped parishioners cope with

The Shaker Way

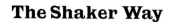

The Shakers, a utopian sect that established itself in New York in 1774, believed in separation from the "World," eventually founding 19 self-contained communes from Maine to Kentucky. Pragmatic and innovative in all their endeavors, they were especially progressive in medical care. Shakers were "careful of our health"—keeping quarters scrupulously clean, taking in fresh air, and enjoying nutritious meals from the bounty of their farms— so they would be fit to carry out God's work. When illness struck, patients were confined to a "Nurse Shop" and treated with remedies that designated members prepared in an on-site pharmacy from herbs raised in carefully tended gardens. Considering it a sacred obligation to help others, these respected healers began selling medicinal herbs and proprietary remedies worldwide—to great acclaim—around 1820, launching a pharmaceutical industry that would prosper for the next 100 years.

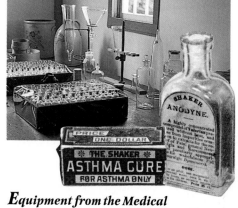

Equipment from the Medical Department *at the Mt. Lebanon, N.Y., Shaker community (top) was used in producing patent medicines from the 19th century into the 1920s. Among the group's noted cures were Shaker Anodyne, a compound of valerian prescribed to relieve various pains, and a remedy for asthma (above).*

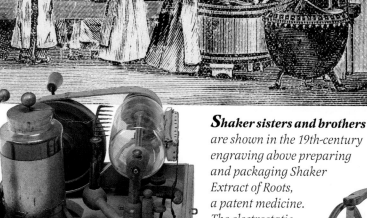

Shaker sisters and brothers *are shown in the 19th-century engraving above preparing and packaging Shaker Extract of Roots, a patent medicine. The electrostatic generator (left) was developed in 1810 by a Shaker brother and produced a mild current useful in treating various joint illnesses.*

A maple rocker *(left), its spare lines typical of all Shaker furniture, was ingeniously converted into a wheelchair. The wheels were later outfitted with rubber tires.*

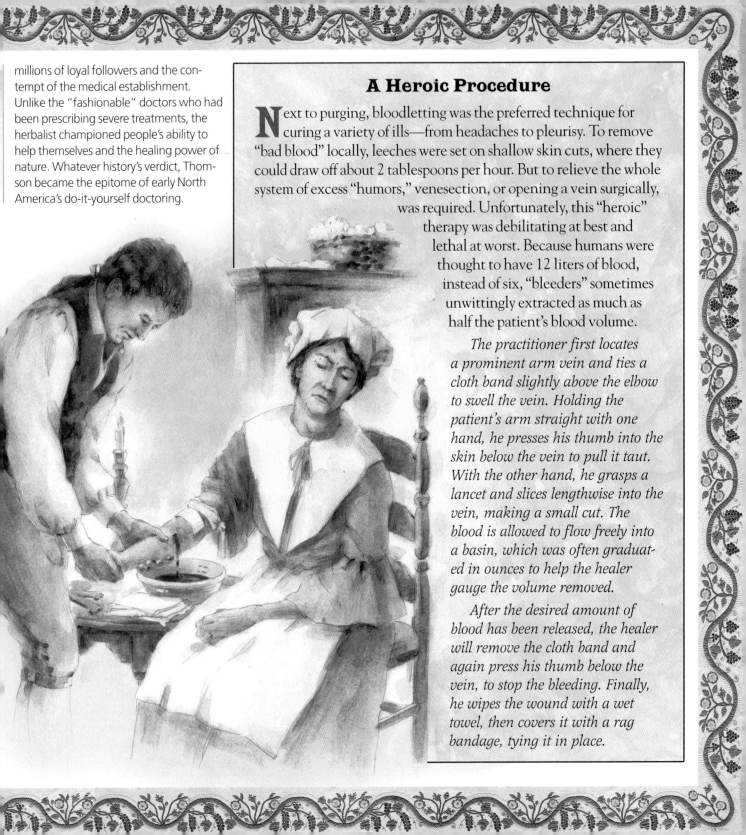

millions of loyal followers and the contempt of the medical establishment. Unlike the "fashionable" doctors who had been prescribing severe treatments, the herbalist championed people's ability to help themselves and the healing power of nature. Whatever history's verdict, Thomson became the epitome of early North America's do-it-yourself doctoring.

A Heroic Procedure

Next to purging, bloodletting was the preferred technique for curing a variety of ills—from headaches to pleurisy. To remove "bad blood" locally, leeches were set on shallow skin cuts, where they could draw off about 2 tablespoons per hour. But to relieve the whole system of excess "humors," venesection, or opening a vein surgically, was required. Unfortunately, this "heroic" therapy was debilitating at best and lethal at worst. Because humans were thought to have 12 liters of blood, instead of six, "bleeders" sometimes unwittingly extracted as much as half the patient's blood volume.

The practitioner first locates a prominent arm vein and ties a cloth band slightly above the elbow to swell the vein. Holding the patient's arm straight with one hand, he presses his thumb into the skin below the vein to pull it taut. With the other hand, he grasps a lancet and slices lengthwise into the vein, making a small cut. The blood is allowed to flow freely into a basin, which was often graduated in ounces to help the healer gauge the volume removed.

After the desired amount of blood has been released, the healer will remove the cloth band and again press his thumb below the vein, to stop the bleeding. Finally, he wipes the wound with a wet towel, then covers it with a rag bandage, tying it in place.

Best-selling home medical guides among *the early settlers were William Buchan's "Domestic Medicine" and John Wesley's "Primitive Physic."*

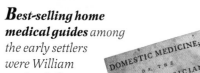

chronic suffering that might linger for years.

Tradespeople fulfilled medical needs as well. Barbers performed surgery, setting bones and treating wounds, but so did wigmakers, millers, tailors, and others with mechanical skill. Metalsmiths extracted teeth and repaired dentures. Apothecaries, found in most towns, sold "chymical" and herbal remedy ingredients, as well as imported and domestic packaged cures. And as the rigors of travel eased, itinerant drug peddlers began riding the circuit, hawking herbs along with patent nostrums that often contained nothing more "medicinal" than alcohol.

Sources of Knowledge

Healers gathered information from sources originating on both sides of the Atlantic. Among the most accessible were newspapers and almanacs, which carried the latest cures and oft florid advertisements for patent remedies. Ben Franklin, for example, offered techniques—such as dissolving kidney stones with lemon juice—in his *Poor Richard's Almanack* and promoted his mother-in-law's anti-itch salve in a 1731 edition of his *Pennsylvania Gazette*.

European books on medicine were imported to North America from the early 1600s onward and supplemented with an increasing number of volumes printed domestically. While some were for professionals, others were for common folk. The Scots physician William Buchan called his *Domestic Medicine* of 1769 "an attempt To render Medical Art more useful by shewing People what is in their own Power with respect to the Prevention and Cure of Diseases." These guides provided not only cure "receipts," but also advice on exercise, diet, and hygiene. John Wesley, who established the Methodist Church, filled his *Primitive Physic* of 1747 with "plain, easy rules" on everything from rejecting the "slow poison [of] spiritous liquors" to taming injurious "passions" through piety. His moralizing was followed by a list of 300 ailments, each teamed with several remedies.

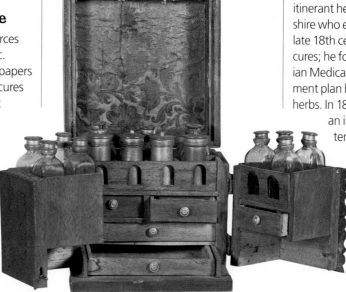

Settlers who forged friendly relations with North American Indians—as Pennsylvania Quakers did with the Leni-Lenape and French fur traders did with the Huron—admired their robust health and adopted their healing traditions. The Indians revealed how to steam away "foulness" in sweat lodges and soothe aches with petroleum skimmed from ponds. They also introduced newcomers to indigenous flora used in medicine, especially tobacco, sassafras, and snakeroot. For example, in the winter of 1535-36, when Jacques Cartier's men suffered from scurvy, the natives of Hochelaga cured them with conifer tea—which was high in vitamin C. Natives were such renowned healers that some settlers billed themselves as "Indian doctors," claiming knowledge of "medicine man" techniques. "Indian" patent medicines were big sellers beginning in the early 1700s.

A Natural Salesman

Perhaps the era's most vocal—and controversial—advocate for folk medicine was Samuel Thomson, an itinerant herbalist from New Hampshire who earned a reputation in the late 18th century for his botanical cures; he formulated the Thomsonian Medical System, a simple treatment plan based on steam baths and herbs. In 1806 Thomson began selling an instruction guide to his system—"so that every family should practice for itself"—and won

Drug chests, *like the 18th-century example at left, were usually equipped with remedies, a scale for weighing medicines, a lancet, and an instruction booklet on drug use.*

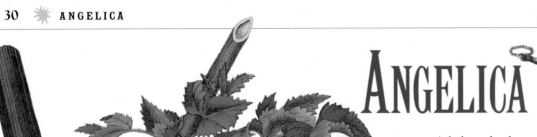

ANGELICA

Angelica atropurpurea
GREAT ANGELICA, ALEXANDERS,
MASTERWORT

According to legend, the tall, fragrant angelica plant was revealed to humans by an angel as a cure for the plague—hence its name. (In the 17th century angelica was widely employed to combat the plague.) A host of powers has been ascribed to this herb. European peasants, using the species *Angelica archangelica*, which grows throughout Europe, made necklaces of the leaves to ward off illness and evil spirits. The juice from the crushed root was used to make "Carmelite water," which was believed to bestow long life and guard against poisons and evil spells. Adding a bit of dried root to a glass of wine was thought to quell desires of the flesh. Angelica was even said to neutralize the bite of mad dogs.

Herb of 1,000 Uses

Here in North America, the Ute Indians of the Rocky Mountains used the native angelica species, *Angelica atropurpurea*, to treat tuberculosis and to induce vomiting and as an expectorant. They made teas from the root and drank them as tonics for general health and to boost strength after an illness. The Arkansas Indians mixed the root with their tobacco for extra flavor.

When the pioneers began harvesting angelica, they tried using it in large doses to induce abortion, which we now know is ineffective. Many settlers took the word of 17th-century British herbalist Nicholas Culpeper, who declared that angelica root resisted the plague "and all epidemical diseases," provided the patient was "laid to sweat in his bed" after ingesting it. Culpeper also claimed that angelica fought off pleurisy and "other diseases of the lungs and breast," and "helps pains of the cholic, the strangury [slow, painful urine discharge] and stoppage of the urine, procureth women's courses, and expelleth the after-birth." He recommended putting the juice of the root into hollow teeth to ease tooth pain and eating the candied stalks to "warm and comfort a cold stomach."

Active plant parts Leaves, roots, seeds
Uses Coughs, digestive complaints
Cautions Angelica contains suspected carcinogens. Research indicates that angelica may increase red blood cell counts and encourage blood clotting. Anyone at risk for heart disease should avoid this herb, since increased blood clotting can lead to decreased blood flow to the heart and possibly trigger a heart attack. If angelica causes any problems, such as diarrhea, discontinue its use. Do not try to collect wild angelica, which is easy to confuse with the highly toxic water hemlock (*Cicuta maculata*).

In the 19th century North American doctors recommended angelica for everything from heartburn and indigestion to bronchitis and even malaria and typhoid. The herb was also used to treat rheumatism and nervous headaches, to cure insomnia, and to promote menstrual flow (as a diuretic and an emmenagogue).

Teas made from angelica root were dropped into the eyes and the ears to cure "dimness of sight" and deafness. When applied to old ulcers, the teas were said to cleanse and heal them. The root tea was also believed to cure stomach cancer. As recently as 1918, people chewed on the root to guard themselves from the worldwide influenza epidemic.

Aside from its role in folk medicine, angelica, which tastes and smells somewhat like juniper, is also used to flavor alcoholic beverages, especially gin. The stalk is traditionally candied or crystallized, and it is also used as a flavoring for candies and desserts. The essential oil—derived from the roots, leaves, and seeds— is added to soaps and perfumes. Infusions of angelica root were once used to dispel unpleasant scents in the home.

Dubious Virtues

Most of the claims made about angelica appear untrue in the light of scientific studies. Still, the herb continues to be used today as a digestive remedy, an appetite stimulant, and as an expectorant—uses for which there is some scientific support.

The plant belongs to the group of bitters (herbs that stimulate the secretion of saliva and gastric juices), and this may account for its soothing effects on the stomach. Furthermore, it is known to relax the smooth muscle of the intestine

Dong Quai: The Chinese Angelica

American angelica (*Angelica atropurpurea*) is a different plant from *Angelica sinensis*, the scientific name for dong quai (also spelled tang kwei or danggui), pictured here as it appeared in a 17th-century Tibetan medical textbook. Dong quai, sometimes called Chinese angelica, is one of the most popular herbs in China, second perhaps only to ginseng. Decoctions of the root have been used throughout the ages for treating menstrual cramps, premenstrual syndrome, hot flashes, and irregular menses.

Dong quai is sometimes called "female ginseng." Like ginseng, it is given as a general tonic and energy booster. It has also been used to treat allergies, hypertension, rheumatism, anemia, and constipation. Today dong quai is available in the United States and Canada as extract capsules.

Studies performed on dong quai have found substances that calm muscular spasms and stimulate the central nervous system. The plant also contains phytoestrogens, which may help diminish the symptoms of menopause. However, like American angelica, dong quai contains psoralens, which can cause increased sensitivity to light and may be carcinogenic. For this reason, many herbalists advise against taking it, although some see the risk as small. In any case, it should never be taken during pregnancy.

and uterus, helping to soothe cramps. It is also a mild anti-inflammatory, which may explain its traditional use against arthritis. Finally, research indicates that angelica may have the ability to lower blood pressure by dilating the blood vessels.

Safety Concerns

Although for centuries angelica has been regarded as safe for consumption, recent studies suggest that the herb may be a carcinogen because it contains certain psoralens, including bergapten, a substance which is also found in bergamot. These substances may induce photosensitivity and increase the risk of skin cancer. Therefore, many experts believe that unnecessary exposure to angelica should be avoided. When applied topically, or even when taken internally, the plant may cause a rash upon exposure to sunlight. Severe poisoning has resulted from large doses of angelica root taken in an attempt to induce abortion.

ANXIETY

Although anxiety may be associated with modern living, it is a common condition as old as mankind itself. English settlers—unfamiliar with stress as it is defined today—knew anxiety by a variety of names, including "nerves," "hysteria," and "the vapors." Its sufferers were "worrywarts" and "nervous Nellies."

Anxiety is rooted in our fight-or-flight response to a real or perceived threat of danger. The body tenses up and produces adrenaline and other hormones, causing the uneasiness known as anxiety.

The condition takes many forms, from mild worrying, stage fright, and distress to severe panic attacks. It can occur at any time, but it is more likely in difficult times, such as changing jobs or waiting up for a child who is late coming home.

Usually, anxiety is temporary. Severe or chronic cases, as when getting a divorce or working for a difficult boss, can lead to depression and fatigue.

Anxiety can cause a host of symptoms, including a pounding heart, muscle tension, higher blood pressure, sweaty palms, trembling, palpitations, diarrhea, confusion, shortness of breath, nail biting, male erectile dysfunction, and insomnia. In a different light, mild anxiety can be beneficial, prompting caution or heightening our senses in dangerous situations. It also pushes us to help ourselves or others.

Myth Versus Reality

Many generations wrongly believed that anxiety was a disorder suffered solely by women. The word *hysteria*, coined in 1801, comes from the Greek *hystera* (meaning "womb") and reflects the belief that women suffered mentally from disturbances of the womb. Until the early 20th century, many patent medicines pandered to this misconception. One such miracle remedy, a mild aloe-based laxative, boasted the ability to cure "all hypocondriac, hysterick or vaporish disorders." Similar patent medicines were marketed to women upset by their insensitive

A relaxing cup of herbal tea can help defuse mild anxiety and provide daily calm.

VALERIAN To make a relaxing and sedative tea, pour boiling water over ½ to 1 teaspoon fresh roots, steep, then strain. Drink two to three times a day and once before bedtime. Capsules, extracts, and tinctures are also available.

PASSION FLOWER Take 4 to 8 grams a day in capsule form or make a mildly sedative tea. Pour boiling water over 1 to 2 teaspoons minced herb, steep, then strain. Drink two to three times a day and once before bedtime. Extracts are also available.

CHAMOMILE To make a relaxing tea, pour boiling water over ½ to 1 teaspoon minced flowers, steep, then strain. Extracts and tinctures are also available. Flowers may cause an allergic reaction in people sensitive to pollen.

CATNIP To make an aromatic and mildly sedative tea, pour boiling water over 1 to 2 teaspoons dried leaves, steep, then strain.

SKULLCAP Take 2 to 6 grams in capsule form or 1 teaspoon minced herb (the whole plant except the root) raw

doctors. According to several studies, today anxiety is only slightly more common in women than in men. It is also particularly common in adolescents and the elderly. Inactivity, isolation, and boredom, in both sexes, are major contributors to anxiety.

Teas and Baths

Folk and orthodox treatments primarily take one of two roads: lessen the excited state or release the bottled-up tension through some form of physical therapy.

Although valerian is not related to Valium, a popular prescription tranquilizer, it is a legendary folk treatment and a proven sedative. Skullcap got its nickname, mad-dog skullcap, from its use in calming the hyperactivity of rabies victims, although it is not a cure for rabies. Passionflower and the fresh milky juice of wild lettuce leaves, often called lettuce opium, are also mild sedatives.

In many regions, in city and country alike, people took a warm bath (with or without Epsom salts) in the evening to relieve daily tension or applied a cold compress to the forehead or neck to calm down. A variety of teas, particularly those

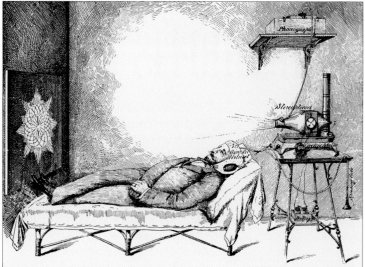

Music and moving color images have long been used to soothe emotions. In 1899 Dr. J. Leonard Corning used an acoustic hood, a phonograph, and a projector to induce mild hypnosis, sleep, and sweet dreams.

made with catnip, chamomile, or lemon balm, were used as calmatives and sleep aids. Perhaps the simple act of enjoying a cup of tea induced some sense of peace. Although raw onions, lavender, and vervain can be mildly sedative, the folk use of motherwort, hops, sage, celery, and garlic has yet to be validated.

Conventional treatment often consists of antianxiety drugs, such as Valium and other commercial tranquilizers. Self-care includes getting more rest, avoiding caffeine, exercising, talking with friends, keeping a journal, and meditating.

Severe attacks or a constant feeling of anxiety are forms of a more serious condition. Anxiety disorders include generalized anxiety disorder (GAD), adjustment disorder with anxious mood, panic attacks, phobias, and obsessive-compulsive disorder. Folk remedies should not be used alone in these more serious cases.

or in a tea—two to three times a day. Skullcap, a former treatment for nervous disorders, contains the sedative and antispasmodic principle scutellarin.

VERVAIN To make a mildly sedative and analgesic tea, pour boiling water over 1 teaspoon minced herb (the whole plant), steep, then strain. May induce sweating. Capsules and extracts are also readily available.

KAVA This Pacific Islands relative of black pepper is sold in capsule form in health food stores, usually under the name of kava kava. The pulverized rootstock is traditionally mixed with water and imbibed by islanders as a social and ceremonial drink. It has a mild sedative effect. Excessive use of kava can result in muscle weakness, sensitivity to light, and double vision.

EPSOM SALTS BATH Pour 2 cups Epsom salts (magnesium sulfate) into a warm-water bath. Bathe for no more than 30 minutes. The salts cleanse and tone the skin and may lower blood pressure. A regular warm-water bath also soothes the body and mind.

See a doctor if...

Chronic anxiety may be a sign of hormonal imbalance or hyperthyroidism, both of which require a doctor's supervision. Also consult a doctor if you suffer from any of the following conditions:
◆ Hyperventilation
◆ Post-trauma anxiety
◆ Chronic insomnia
◆ Extended depression

ARTHRITIS

Arthritis is nothing new: even dinosaurs had it. So did primitive man. The Latin word *arthritis* means "inflammation of the joint" but actually refers to many different forms of the disease. Osteoarthritis (also called degenerative arthritis), the most common type, usually results either from injury or from normal wear and tear on the cartilage of frequently used joints; almost everyone over 40 suffers to some degree from this kind of arthritis. The condition called rheumatoid arthritis is an autoimmune disease and is more severe.

Early pioneers called any disorder involving pain and stiffness in the joints rheumatism. Many firmly believed it could be cured by carrying horse chestnuts in one's pockets. If the nut eventually cracked, it was thrown away and replaced. Wearing a copper bracelet was also widely believed to fend off the ailment.

Aching joints were often rubbed with warm chicken fat, goose grease, or skunk oil, sometimes mixed with wintergreen oil, which is still prescribed today for its pain-relieving properties. Kerosene and turpentine were also used as rubs, but they are no longer recommended.

Natives had many remedies for arthritis, including wintergreen and boneset, both of which are considered unsafe today for internal use. Chaparral was used by the Indians of the American Southwest, who boiled the leaves and branches and applied them as poultices for bruises and rheumatism. They also drank it as a tea. Today the plant's safety has been called

RED PEPPER Also called capsicum or cayenne pepper, red pepper has recently gained popularity as an arthritis remedy. It contains a substance called capsaicin, which reduces the levels of a chemical compound that transmits pain signals to the brain. Mix a few dashes of the ground pepper with 2 to 3 teaspoons olive oil. Apply with gauze several times a day. Allow a week or more of continued use for the desensitization to take place. The first few doses will cause a mild burning sensation. Alternatively, capsaicin ointment is available commercially. It is also an ingredient in several over-the-counter products. Cayenne is highly irritating. Keep it away from the mouth, eyes, and other mucous membranes, and avoid direct contact with the pepper's seeds.

WINTERGREEN The oil from wintergreen leaves contains methyl salicylate, a close relative of aspirin. Modern-day folk healers prescribe wintergreen oil in external preparations to reduce joint and muscle inflammation and pain. The number of applications should not exceed five per day. Wintergreen oil is toxic if taken internally.

DANDELION Studies in the 1980s found that dandelion root has moderate anti-inflammatory properties. The powdered root extract is available in capsule form. Liquid root extracts are also sold. To make tea from a plant, add 3 tablespoons finely chopped dandelion root and leaves to 2 cups cold water. Boil for 3

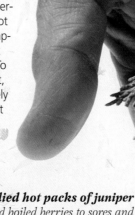

Indians applied hot packs of juniper twigs and boiled berries to sores and aches. Contemporary herbalists recommend using juniper externally for arthritis.

into question. In the 19th century many physicians recommended drinking tinctures of ripe pokeberries for arthritis, but the berries faded from use in the 20th century without ever having been studied. Poke, particularly the roots, is now known to be poisonous.

Diet and Exercise

A small percentage of those with arthritis suffer from food allergies to milk products. They can find significant relief by avoiding milk and anything made with milk. One group of arthritis sufferers experienced a notable improvement after consuming increased amounts of oily saltwater fish, such as salmon and sardines, which are rich in omega-3 fatty acids. These chemicals are believed to inhibit inflammation.

Non-weight-bearing exercise is an important component of combating arthritis. When one is in pain, there is a natural tendency to minimize movement, but inactivity only weakens the muscles that stabilize the joints. Specialized stretching and strengthening exercises can help maintain flexibility. Swimming (preferably in a heated pool) and walking, as opposed to high-impact sports like tennis and running, are good ways to maintain overall fitness.

minutes. Let sit for about 10 minutes before straining. Drink three times a day. Some people may have allergic reactions after handling dandelion.

JUNIPER Apply an alcohol extract of juniper after heat treatments or massage, when the joints are warm. Or make an infusion using 1 teaspoon crushed dried juniper berries in ½ cup hot water. Steep for five minutes, then strain and apply. Do not use juniper for more than a few weeks, because the essential oil can cause kidney irritation when absorbed. Juniper may cause an allergic reaction in people with hay fever.

NETTLE This weed's leaves are noted for their stinging needles, which cause irritation when handled. Nettle juice or tea has been used both internally and externally to treat arthritis. Research has shown it to be effective but has not yet identified its active principles. Add 2 teaspoons dried leaves to 1 cup boiling water. Steep for five minutes, then strain. Drink the tea three times a day.

CHAMOMILE This herb has long been used as a tea for digestive upset. More recently, it has been used as an external compress for arthritis because of its anti-inflammatory properties. Brew a strong infusion using 2 tablespoons dried flowers in ½ cup hot water. Steep, then strain. Soak a clean cloth in the liquid and apply. People allergic to pollen may experience an allergic reaction.

EVENING PRIMROSE The cis-gamma-linolenic acid (GLA) found in the oil of the seeds of evening primrose, a common wildflower, were shown in scientific tests performed in the 1990s to have a significant effect on both rheumatoid arthritis and morning stiffness. The oil is available in both capsule and extract form.

See a doctor if...

Arthritis is most easily treated when it is discovered early. See a doctor if you experience any of the following symptoms.

◆ Persistent early-morning pain and stiffness in the joints
◆ Swelling
◆ Recurrent pain in any joint, especially joints on both sides of the body
◆ Loss of strength in association with joint pain
◆ Unexplained weight loss, fatigue, and fever accompanied by joint pain

ASTHMA

The word *asthma* comes from the ancient Greek word meaning "to pant." During an asthma attack, the bronchial tubes, which distribute air to the lungs, constrict, making it difficult to breathe. Mucus blocks the smaller tubes, compounding the problem.

Emotional distress was once believed to be a major cause of asthma. It was commonly thought that the disease occurred in nervous children of overprotective parents. Although anxiety can contribute to the severity of an asthma attack, we now know that asthma is basically an allergic response.

The disease is usually caused by an allergy to pollen, mold spores, animal dander, or dust mites. Some cases are triggered by food allergies, often to the sulfites sometimes added to fruits and vegetables, wine, beer, dried fruits, and some shellfish. It is most common in children, people of African descent, and certain families. Many children outgrow it during adolescence. Asthma can be aggravated by respiratory infections, exercise, air pollution, and anti-inflammatory drugs—including aspirin. Cold, dry air can worsen the symptoms, so it's better to exercise indoors during the winter. If you have asthma, breathe through your nose in cold weather to warm and humidify the air that enters your lungs. Severe asthma attacks can be dangerous, and anyone with asthma should be under a doctor's care.

Homegrown Remedies

Throughout the centuries, people have tried countless cures for asthma, with limited success. Burning powders were especially popular. In the early 1900s people burned the leaves of jimsonweed and inhaled the smoke; a chemical called atropine contained in the herb increases the heart rate, thereby dilating the blood vessels and opening the bronchial tubes. Today inhaling smoke is not advised because it is irritating and may worsen asthma over the long term.

Asthma sufferers discovered long ago that a strong cup of coffee can provide quick relief from an asthma attack. The caffeine in coffee is converted by the body into a substance called theophylline, which helps relax and open the airways.

A host of other so-called remedies were no doubt less effective. One dubious prescription was to "live a fortnight on boiled carrots only." More promising was the following advice: "Cut an ounce of stick licorice into slices, steep this in a quart of water four and twenty hours and use it when you are worse than usual, as a common drink." The use of licorice was probably justified: licorice root has been shown to have antispasmodic and expectorant properties.

In the 19th century people concocted "asthma lozenges" on the stove at home. A common ingredient was extract of

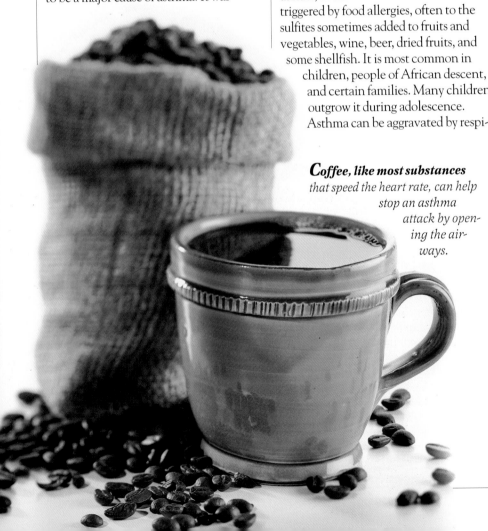

Coffee, like most substances that speed the heart rate, can help stop an asthma attack by opening the airways.

elecampane, now found in some drug-store expectorants and cough remedies.

Another popular herb used to combat asthma is ephedra. Chinese ephedra, called ma huang, has been used in China for at least 5,000 years. It contains an alkaloid called ephedrine, a highly effective bronchodilator. Recently, Health Canada has warned against the use of products containing ma huang, unless the label carries a Drug Identification Number (DIN). The ephedra species that grows in North America—*Ephedra nevadensis*, known as Mormon tea—was also used against asthma, but it appears to be devoid of ephedrine. If Mormon tea works for asthma, no one knows why.

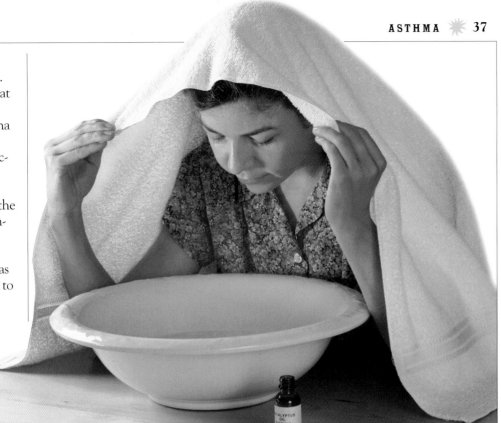

Steam inhalations *of eucalyptus oil are easily made by adding 5 to 10 drops of oil to a basin of steaming water.*

LICORICE The root of licorice has been used for centuries to treat coughs. Its anti-inflammatory properties may provide added relief from asthma. To make a tea, pour ½ cup boiling water over ½ to 1 teaspoon minced or powdered root. Steep for five minutes, then strain. Don't take licorice for more than four to six weeks; long-term use can cause serious side effects.

EUCALYPTUS Eucalyptus oil is commonly used in nasal inhalers and sprays. Steam inhalations of the vapors can easily be made at home. Or try adding the oil to your bathwater. Ointments applied to the chest are also popular. To make a tea, pour 1 cup boiling water over 1 to 2 teaspoons dried leaves. Strain, then drink. Long-term internal use is not recommended.

HOREHOUND This pleasant-tasting herb has a long tradition as a mild expectorant. To make a tea, pour 1 cup boiling water over 1 to 2 teaspoons minced herb. Steep for five minutes, then strain. You can safely drink three to five cups a day. Horehound candy and lozenges are also available.

ELECAMPANE This herb's roots were once boiled in sugar water to make cough drops and asthma lozenges. They have been shown to work against asthma, although their active principles have not been identified. To make a tea, pour 1 cup boiling water over 2 teaspoons chopped root. Steep, then strain and drink; a spoonful of honey will help mask the bitter taste. Side effects can include allergic reactions, diarrhea, cramps, and vomiting.

MULLEIN Smoking dried mullein leaves was once a folk remedy for asthma. Inhaling any form of smoke is no longer recommended for asthma sufferers, but mullein leaves and flowers are still made into teas to quell coughs and soothe throat irritation. To make a tea, pour ½ cup boiling water over 3 to 4 teaspoons minced herb. Steep for five minutes, then strain.

SENECA ROOT Used as an expectorant because of its saponin content, seneca root *(Polygala senega)* is said to be especially effective against asthma and bronchitis. To make a tea, pour 1 cup water over a scant ¼ teaspoon chopped or powdered root. Steep for five minutes, then strain. You may drink 3 or 4 cups a day. Too much will cause stomach upset.

ATHLETE'S FOOT

The term *athlete's foot* did not come into use until the 20th century, but this common condition has long been the target of folk treatments. Athlete's foot is a fungus infection of the moist skin between the toes. The resulting redness, discomfort, and occasional cracks in the skin are similar to the effects of ringworm. In fact, athlete's foot was known to some as "ringworm of the feet," and many of the same antifungal remedies are used for both.

The irritating fungus thrives in warm, moist, and dark places, such as poorly ventilated shoes, shower floors, and locker rooms. Redness, itching, burning, and scaling are common. Severe cases can produce weeping blisters and infect the toenails. In such cases, and if the condition worsens with over-the-counter or folk treatment, consult your physician.

When using either a folk remedy or an over-the-counter medication, take certain measures. Air your feet often and

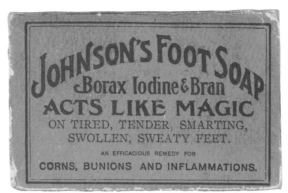

*A **popular product** from the early 1900s used simple ingredients to soothe the feet.*

keep them as clean and dry as possible— in general, sprays, powders, and washes are preferable to ointments. Keep your socks and shoes clean and dry as well, and disinfect any surfaces that could harbor or transmit the fungus. To prevent a recurrence, continue treatment for one week after the infection is no longer visible.

The most practical folk remedies are those with antiseptic and antifungal properties that are applied directly to the affected skin. Garlic, clove oil, and calendula are efficacious home remedies. Some people believed, wrongly, that garlic in one's diet cleansed the blood and cleared up any skin malady. However, its external use has shown real results; its antifungal agents are activated when the garlic clove is crushed.

The use of foot baths often included a healing herb or salt, although the cleansing of the feet was the most helpful effect. In the American South, folks soaked their feet in a bath of persimmon bark tea. Other bath additives were boric acid, Epsom salts, sulfur, bleach, oatmeal, vinegar, cornstarch, and red clover. Natives used heated balsamic juice of sweet gum, as well as poke root tea, castor oil, and sorrel juice, against fungal infections. Indiana Hoosiers are reported to have let their dogs lick their feet for relief.

Other folk remedies include honey, soaking the socks in vinegar, aloe vera gel, whale oil, baking soda, the juice of jewelweed, urine, and walking through fresh manure (which could actually worsen the infection). Today, Australian tea tree oil is a popular, effective, and highly recommended herbal treatment.

KEEP THE SKIN CLEAN To disinfect the skin and keep it dry, wash feet with alcohol or vinegar applied with a cloth or added to a foot bath. Sprinkle unscented powder and baking soda on washed feet or into clean socks to keep moisture off the skin. Repeat often.

GARLIC Crush a raw garlic clove and apply the pulp directly to the skin. If irritation occurs, rinse the skin with cold water and place a cloth on the affected area before reapplying.

TEA TREE OIL Steam the leaves to distill the antifungal pale yellow oil. Apply two or three times a day. If you use commercial tea tree oil, make sure the label says "pure." Ointments with a reduced concentration are available.

WALNUT LEAF The tannins in walnut leaf have antibiotic properties. Make a tea with 6 teaspoons powdered leaf (available at some health food stores) to 1 cup water and apply to the feet with a cotton ball.

CLOVE OIL To make clove oil, soak whole cloves in olive oil. Apply directly to the affected skin. Commercial tinctures, containing 15 percent clove, are available. Higher concentrations and the pure oil are likely to irritate the skin.

CALENDULA Add 2 teaspoons chopped flowers to 1 cup boiling water to make a topical infusion. Steep, then strain. Make an ointment by adding crushed calendula flowers to olive oil. Commercial ointments are available.

BACK PAIN

An aching back is the most common type of work injury reported in Canada. This nagging ailment encompasses numerous variations, including shooting pains, pinched nerves, strained muscles, and herniated disks. The most commonly affected areas are the lumbar vertebrae and muscles of the lower back. In fact, back pain was once known as "lumbago."

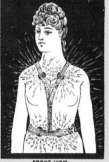
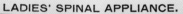
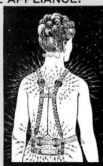
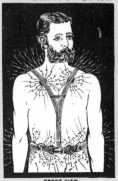
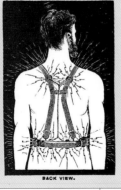

LADIES' SPINAL APPLIANCE.

FRONT VIEW. BACK VIEW.

GENTS' SPINAL APPLIANCE.

FRONT VIEW. BACK VIEW.

*The **wondrous devices** that delivered electric shocks proved that back pain sufferers would try anything.*

Folk remedies include analgesic teas, herbal liniments, hot plasters, and the motherly advice to "Sit up straight!"

Good Posture Is Key

A basic cause of back pain—chronic low back pain in particular—is a misaligned spine. This can result from abnormal spinal development, poor abdominal and back muscle tone, obesity, emotional stress, or the degeneration of arthritic vertebrae. A major factor in spinal misalignment and chronic back pain is poor posture.

Standing or sitting up straight uses muscles in the abdomen, shoulders, and upper and lower back to pull the spine into its normal, slightly S-shaped curve. Muscles weakened by poor posture put pressure on the spine and are more susceptible to strain. They are ill-equipped to provide sufficient support when the back is stressed, for example, while sitting, standing, or driving for long periods of time. Strengthening these muscles, reducing body weight, and practicing good posture can prevent and alleviate most chronic back pain.

Poor posture and weak lower back muscles can exaggerate the spine's normal curve, causing kyphosis (rounded shoulders and a caved-in appearance) or lordosis (also called swayback, in which both the abdomen and the buttocks protrude). Pregnant women are particularly susceptible to lordosis. Back pain can even be caused

See a doctor if...

Any of the following may signal a serious condition.
- Pain after a fall or a car accident
- Pain that persists, is severe, or keeps you from sleeping
- Pain that does not improve after two days of bed rest, lying flat
- Pain, numbness, or tingling that travels down an arm or a leg
- Pain associated with weakness in a leg or bladder-control problems
- Pain associated with vomiting, fever, or skin rash
- Any kind of backache in a pregnant woman, an elderly person, or a child

by a spine lacking enough of a curve—a back that is too straight. Poor posture can also increase the risk of a herniated disk, the bulging of fibrous disk material between vertebrae that often pinches nerves against the bone of the spine.

Sudden, acute pain from muscle strain or a herniated disk is commonly caused by lifting a heavy load, sleeping in a bad position, sneezing violently, wearing high heels, or any quick, twisting movement. Severe pain, especially sciatica, which travels into one buttock or both or down the back of the leg to the knee or foot, often accompanies a herniated disk.

For muscle strain, ice is standard first aid, applied 10 to 20 minutes at a time. Other treatments include aspirin, prescription drugs, heat, acupuncture, spinal manipulation, massage, and yoga. Bed rest is no longer a standard recommendation, but strenuous activity should be avoided for five days. If the pain persists or worsens, consult a physician. Back pain can be an emergency, as in the case of meningitis or a spinal abscess. Serious conditions, such as scoliosis, sciatica, or a prolapsed disk, require a doctor's supervision and should not be treated with folk remedies. Surgery or a back brace may be options.

Herbal Heat

Many folk remedies for back pain are heat-producing applications, the most effective of which are counterirritants. These substances increase local circulation, produce redness, warmth, and minor irritation, and bring temporary relief of muscle pain close to the skin's surface.

Wintergreen, mustard, turpentine, and red pepper were formerly popular counterirritants. Wintergreen oil is almost 98 percent methyl salicylate, the synthetic variety of which is commonly used today in commercial muscle ointments. The Penobscot, Sioux, Nez Percé, and other Indian tribes drank wintergreen tea and made poultices of crushed wintergreen leaves to ease sore muscles and back pain.

Mustard plasters (made with the powdered seed) and turpentine oil (made from pine-tree sap) are also proven counterirritants. Menthol (from mint) and camphor have also been used; rather than heat, they produce a cool feeling.

The Chippewa used a decoction of carrion-flower root to treat back pain. The root was kept in a bag made of bear's claws and carried only by those men of high rank in the *midewiwin*, an esteemed healing society. The Catawba drank a root decoction of broomsedge. Other ingredients in Indian remedies were cup plant, ground ivy, chaparral, white-pine resin, pipsissewa, and large bellwort. Poultices included belladonna, fennel, gelsemium, myrrh, chamomile, coconut oil, turtle oil, lavender, red pepper, and rubbing alcohol. A pioneer recipe for "Back Health Wash" called for mixing clary sage, wormwood, pennyroyal, strawberry leaf, and white-willow bark into a hot bath. Studies on the efficacy of these remedies have been inconclusive.

Tough-acting Teas

Some teas, like that made from valerian root, were taken to relieve spasms and promote rest; others acted as mild painkillers. Meadowsweet tea may have been the most effective pain reliever. Its flowers contain aspirinlike salicylates, and a tea made from the flowers was used both internally and topically. Similarly, tea made with white-willow bark contains small amounts of salicin, another chemical relative of aspirin, and was used to relieve muscle pain and fight headaches.

Many other remedies were employed. Users of sevenbark claimed that it contained a "vegetable cortisone." Teas with horsemint, clary sage, pepper vinegar, pennyroyal, beech, chamomile, and boiled grapevine were also taken.

Belief-based remedies also existed. Wearing red flannel as you slept or worked was believed to cure all types of pain. Another curious remedy was this: "When the whippoorwill calls, lie down and roll over three times."

SWEET BIRCH OIL Massage oil, diluted with alcohol, into the skin. Do not apply more than four times a day, before or after vigorous exercise, or while using a heating pad. Do not apply to abrasions or sensitive skin. The pure oil can irritate the skin; it contains a high concentration of methyl salicylate, a mild counterirritant and analgesic. The oil is highly toxic if taken internally. Keep away from children.

WINTERGREEN TEA The herb wintergreen contains methyl salicylate. To make a tea, add 1 teaspoon chopped fresh leaves to 1 cup boiling water. Steep, then strain. The tea is safe in low doses, but do not consume the oil—it is highly toxic.

MUSTARD To make a plaster, mix equal parts powdered mustard seed and flour and slowly add water. Spread on a cloth and apply to the skin for a short period of time. Use no more than three or four times a day. The plaster can blister the skin if it is left on too long. The oil can also be used, but only in concentrations of less than 5 percent.

HEAT OR COLD For acute muscle strain, apply a cold pack for 15 minutes every couple of hours. After swelling has subsided (24 to 48 hours after injury) and for muscle stiffness, apply a heat pack for 15 minutes every couple of hours for the next two to five days as needed, to promote healing. Discontinue use if either is uncomfortable.

MEADOWSWEET To make a tea, pour boiling water over 3 to 4 teaspoons of dried flowers, steep, then strain. Drink the tea or use as a rub. The flowers contain salicylate compounds, which can be toxic if ingested in large doses. The flowers and oil can also be added to baths and are used in topical pharmaceutical products.

WILLOW BARK White willow bark contains analgesic salicin but in highly variable amounts. Even though this folk remedy has a long history, it may be inadequate as a pain-reliever when taken as regular doses of willow bark tea or the commercially available capsules. At safe doses, the salicin level of the bark may be no more effective than a baby aspirin.

Practicing Correct Posture

Extreme measures to correct rounded shoulders are hardly necessary.

Because chronic back pain is difficult to treat, prevention—namely, correct posture—is the most important consideration. Follow these basic steps to maintain correct posture 24 hours a day. Keep it simple: exaggerated movements can do more harm than good.

◆ **Standing** Stand tall, hands at your side, neck and pelvis straight. Hold chin and abdomen in. Do not push your chest out and pin your shoulders back; this can worsen swayback. Shift your weight from foot to foot. Do not stand too long in one position.

◆ **Sitting** Keep your shoulders level, head centered, abdomen in. Do not hunch or slide down in the chair. Keep your hips slightly higher than your knees and your feet flat on the floor or on a footstool. Your chair should not exaggerate the curve in your lower back.

◆ **Lifting** Do not bend over at the waist. Squat, with your back straight and knees bent. As you rise, let your leg muscles do the work.

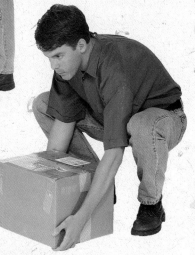

◆ **Sleeping** Use a firm mattress and stay warm. Sleep on your side or back, using only one small pillow for your head and neck. On your back, place a pillow under your knees. On your side, bend your knees at right angles. Sleeping on your stomach can worsen swayback.

BAD BREATH

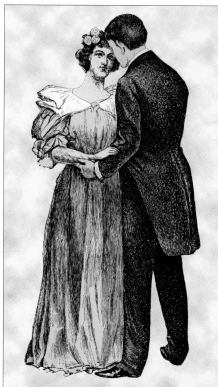

FACE TO FACE.

The pleasure of a confidential chat is doubled by the sweet breath that goes with a well-ordered system. And that is always insured by

Ripans Tabules.

For thousands of years human beings have been searching for a remedy for bad breath—which came to be called "halitosis" after the makers of Listerine coined the Latin-derived word in the 1920s. The Greeks tried chewing gum mastic, or tree resin. So did early North American settlers, who were partial to the rubbery sap of the white spruce.

Anyone can have temporary bad breath resulting from smoking, drinking alcoholic beverages, or eating onions or garlic. It can also be caused by poor oral hygiene. To find out what your breath smells like, lick the back of your hand and wait several seconds before taking a sniff.

In most cases, preventing bad breath is as simple as brushing your teeth twice a day and flossing daily. And don't forget to

Not even fine clothes and good breeding could stave off the worrisome threat of unpleasant breath.

brush your tongue, scrubbing as far back as you can: germs in the pits and crevices of the tongue's surface, marked by a white coating in the morning, are key causes. The Cherokee used a foamflower mouthwash to fight the "white-coated tongue."

However, brushing thoroughly isn't the whole solution. A good flow of saliva is necessary for sweet-smelling breath, since the oxygen in saliva kills bacteria. Saliva flow is decreased when you sleep—the reason people wake up with "morning mouth." Some medications also dry the mouth, and it naturally becomes drier with age. Stimulate saliva flow by chewing sugarless gum or eating raw vegetables. Drink at least eight glasses of water or other fluids a day, but avoid coffee, tea, and alcohol, which dry the mouth.

If bad breath persists, consult your dentist; the problem may be the result of gum disease. If it isn't, your doctor should investigate a possible medical cause.

BAKING SODA AND PEROXIDE Baking soda is an alkalinizing agent valuable for its mild antiseptic and deodorizing properties. To make a gargle, combine 1 tablespoon baking soda with 1 cup hydrogen peroxide (2 to 3 percent), which releases baking soda's nascent oxygen. The resulting foam has a powerful oxidizing effect that destroys odor-causing bacteria.

SAGE Bad breath caused by oral infections is discouraged by the anti-inflammatory and antiseptic action of thujone, one of the active principles in common sage. To make a tea, pour 1 cup boiling water over 1 tablespoon of chopped fresh sage leaves (1 to 2 teaspoons dried), let steep, then strain. Drink the tea slowly for maximum effect.

MYRRH An antiseptic, myrrh kills oral bacteria. Make a mouthwash by stirring 5 to 10 drops of myrrh tincture into a glass of water. Mixing the tincture with mint or rosemary tea will enhance its breath-freshening effect and mask myrrh's disagreeable taste.

FENNEL SEED Lovers of Asian food may be familiar with fennel seeds, which are often offered as an after-dinner treat at Indian restaurants. Chewing a small handful will help freshen the breath. Look for the seeds in the spice section of a grocery store.

PEPPERMINT The menthol in peppermint can mask bad breath temporarily. Steep 2 tablespoons chopped leaves and flowering tops (or 1 teaspoon dried peppermint) in 1 cup boiling water for 10 minutes. Strain, then drink.

SODItext SMALL CAPS Sodium bicarbonate
Bicarbonate of soda, Saleratus

BAKING SODA

In the early 1800s North Americans thought of the opaque white, odorless, crystalline bicarbonate of soda primarily as a leavening agent for baking. It was imported from Europe—at considerable cost—until 1839, when one Dr. Austin Church began manufacturing "saleratus," as the powder was then called, in a factory in Rochester, New York. Today we use it to calm an upset stomach, soothe a bee sting, get rid of bad breath, prevent razor burns and oily skin, and soften a callus. It also moves happily from the medicine cabinet to the refrigerator, where it absorbs unwanted odors. Still, baking soda's most extensive consumer use worldwide is as an antacid.

How Does It Work?

Baking soda is a mildly alkaline salt that reacts easily with acids, releasing carbon dioxide and creating effervescence. The compound is also quite stable, so it has an almost limitless shelf life.

Most baking soda—that is, sodium bicarbonate—is derived from soda ash, which is actually sodium carbonate. When Dr. Church started his business, he used the LeBlanc process, which was created by a French scientist, to produce soda ash. The enterprising doctor then chemically converted this substance into baking soda. In the late 1800s manufacturers switched to the Solvay method, which yields crude sodium bicarbonate directly. This product is still converted into soda ash and then refined into baking soda that meets the purity standards of the U. S. Pharmacopeia. Soda ash also occurs naturally as an ore called trona, which is mined in only one place in North America—the Green River Basin in Wyoming. (A local county is named Natrona—a pairing of "Na," the chemical symbol for soda, with "trona.") The basin has enough trona to meet the needs of North American consumers for several centuries.

Uses Aplenty

Today, a survey would certainly turn up at least one box of baking soda in almost every North American household. It is used not only to cure minor ills but also to

The yellow-and-red box of *Arm & Hammer baking soda became a common fixture in North American homes.*

clean and deodorize almost anything imaginable— from the litter box to the kitchen sink to our own bodies. Mixed with a little water to form a paste, baking soda has functioned as an alternative to toothpaste for generations, and it has the advantage of being less abrasive than most toothpastes. The paste will also help fight acne: rubbing a blackhead gently with the paste for two to three minutes will loosen it. A dusting of baking soda under the arms or on the feet serves as an inexpensive deodorant.

Baking soda has yet another nonmedicinal application: it can smother grease, electrical, and chemical fires. As such, manufacturers use it as a main ingredient in commercial dry chemical fire extinguishers. Even when poured straight from the box, it will put out a small kitchen fire. Just be sure to allow extinguished materials time to cool before handling.

Uses Upset stomach, bad breath, skin rashes and irritations, insect bites, and calluses
Cautions Baking soda is generally considered a safe food additive and can be used freely, with two critical exceptions. First, anyone on a sodium-restricted diet should consult a physician before taking it internally. Second, because baking soda contains sodium, repeated ingestion by those with high blood pressure or heart failure is not advised.

Balm of Gilead

Populus balsamifera var. *candicans*
BALSAM POPLAR, COTTONWOOD, HACKMATACK, TACAMAHAC, BLACK POPLAR, BLACK COTTONWOOD

Known for its aroma and healing powers, balm of Gilead is a safe and effective remedy long used in folk medicine. North America's native peoples drank tea made from the leaves and buds as an expectorant to help loosen chest congestion—a use that has been proven to work. Also effective was the external application of the infusion or salve (the Cherokee and Potawatomi used the infusion to relieve rheumatism and tooth pain, and the salve for eczema). The Menominee and the Ojibwa mixed boiled buds with lard to rub on wounds and placed the buds in their nostrils to relieve head colds and chest congestion. Many early settlers followed suit, using balm of Gilead for ailments as wide-ranging as headaches, burns, eye infections, frostbite, and piles.

Many of these popular folk remedies simply consisted of a handful of fresh or properly dried leaf buds in a tincture or salve: the resin found in the leaf buds contains salicin, an aspirin-like ingredient that relieves sore muscles and joints. The resin also contains anti-inflammato-

The Biblical Balm?

The settlers were so fond of the native poplar that they named it after the balm of Gilead found in the Bible (Jeremiah 8:22), which was known for its healing resin. The original may be the Arabian balsam tree (named *Commiphora gileadensis,* although it never grew in Gilead), believed to be the Queen of Sheba's gift to Solomon. Or it could be the mastic tree (*Pistachia lentiscus*), an evergreen that may have grown on Mount Gilead. Gilead may also have been a point of sale along a caravan route to Egypt (Genesis 37:25).

Go up to Gilead,
and take balm.... In vain you
have taken many medicines;
there is no healing for you.
(Jeremiah 46:11)

ry bisabolol, bearing out its use for joint pain and burns. However, homemade remedies with concentrations higher than 20 to 30 percent of the resin can irritate the skin.

A Plethora of Poplars

The balm of Gilead tree that is native to North America is actually a poplar. But because poplars interbreed easily, many Populus species that grow in the same range have shared this venerable name. Among them are the cottonwood (*P. deltoides*), black poplar (*P. nigra*), and the balsam poplar or hackmatack (classified as both *P. balsamifera* and *P. tacamahacca*). All of these species have medicinal properties similar to those of *P. balsamifera* var. *candicans*, considered the "true" balm of Gilead of North American folklore.

Active plant parts Leaf buds, bark, leaves
Uses Congestion, muscle and joint soreness, throat and skin inflammation
Cautions External use of the resin may irritate the skin or cause an allergic skin reaction. Because the herb contains salicin, it should not be given to children.

BASIL

Ocimum basilicum
SWEET BASIL, GARDEN BASIL,
COMMON BASIL, ST. JOSEPHWORT

This "king of herbs" is one of the most widely used herbs in the world. Known best for its aroma and its culinary use, basil has also earned a considerable medicinal and symbolic reputation, particularly in Europe and Asia. For Italians it has symbolized love, for the Greeks hate, for the French royalty. In Jewish lore the herb provided strength during fasts, and in India it was considered sacred. Some ancient herbalists warned that basil caused internal damage, blindness, insanity, coma, worms, and lice, yet more than 50 different uses for the herb have been passed down through the years.

Dating back to its origins in ancient China, basil has been used to treat stomach problems. Settlers drank basil tea or ate the leaves to alleviate gas, nausea, and headache, and to stimulate the appetite. The tea was also used as a gargle to soothe sore throat. Other folk uses included lifting the spirits, fighting dental plaque, regulating menstruation, calming the nerves, and reducing fever.

Although little evidence exists to support many of basil's applications, studies have confirmed effectiveness for its most common use: the relief of flatulence. Scientists have also found that basil oil is slightly antiseptic and may soothe insect bites. Basil may also inhibit the organisms that cause dysentery. At one time, nursing mothers took basil tea to increase lactation and help expel gas in their infant. Today, however, doctors recommend that children and women who are pregnant or nursing refrain from taking the herb's volatile oil medicinally; the estragole present in the oil has been found to cause tumors in laboratory mice. Still, the popular use of the herb in cooking is considered safe.

Perfect for the Garden

Basil, an annual herb, is easy to grow, and its minty licorice fragrance perks up any garden. The plant is usually green but can range from yellow-green to dark green. Its bushy stems reach up to 60 cm (2 ft) high and sprout small white or purple flowers. The leaves are ovate, sometimes toothed, and often have a purplish hue.

To grow your own, use a starter mix of 85 percent peat or a ratio of one part compost to one part sand. Sow the seeds 6 mm (¼ in.) deep in rows 30 cm (12 in.) apart. Because it prefers heat, basil is best started indoors, then transplanted. To encourage healthier leaves, pinch back the buds before they bloom. As a companion plant, basil is said to improve the growth and flavor of tomatoes and ward off pesky insects.

Active plant parts Leaves
Uses Flatulence, depressed appetite, cuts and scrapes
Cautions Children, pregnant women, and nursing mothers should not take volatile oil.

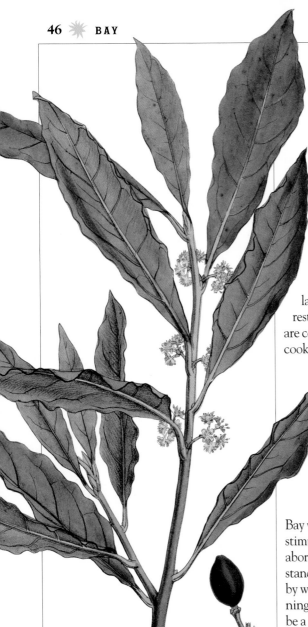

BAY

Laurus nobilis
LAUREL, SWEET BAY, BAY LAUREL

This aromatic evergreen is the laurel whose branches symbolized victory to the Greeks and Romans. The tree has even influenced the English language: lauded poets are known as laureates, and others are said to be resting on their laurels. Dried bay leaves are commonly used as a seasoning in cooking. Their essential oil, produced by steam distillation, is used in traditional medicine. The tree is native to the Mediterranean, where it grows as tall as 18 m (60 ft). The species that grows in North America is more shrublike, and it is often grown in a large pot.

Fragrant Medicine

Bay was used for thousands of years to stimulate menstruation and to induce abortion. It was once believed that a man standing near a bay tree could not be hurt by witches, the devil, thunder, or lightning. The death of the tree was thought to be a bad omen. A bay leaf placed under one's pillow was said to ensure pleasant dreams. Bay was also used to treat a variety of afflictions ranging from indigestion to colic and hysteria. Natives and early settlers used bay to bring on labor and menstruation and to treat stomachache, urinary problems, insect bites and stings, and skin wounds.

Stomach Soother?

The late Appalachian folk healer Tommie Bass wrote: "I have made several gallons of bay-leaf tea for some men who say it's the finest thing they can get for the nerves; they drink it like drinking water. It settles their nerves and it does their stomach good." One family drank bay-leaf tea as a favorite remedy for indigestion; they believed it had the power to neutralize stomach acid.

Bay leaves were also scattered around the house to keep fleas away, and women put them in their flour canisters to repel cockroaches. We now know that bay contains a chemical called cineole, which does indeed repel insects.

By the 19th century, however, bay had fallen out of favor. There is still no proof that bay leaf settles the stomach or relieves gas, and research has failed to discover any anti-inflammatory action. Today bay is not often used as a remedy internally because of its narcotic properties. But studies show that its essential oil kills some bacteria and fungi, possibly justifying the use of freshly crushed leaves on minor cuts and scrapes. If nothing else, some people find that adding a few crushed bay leaves to their bath water makes for a relaxing bath.

Active plant parts Leaves
Uses Cuts, scrapes, indigestion
Cautions Don't confuse this laurel with mountain laurel, which has poisonous leaves. Bay should not be used during pregnancy and should be taken internally only in moderation because of its narcotic properties. Using bay externally may cause an allergic reaction.

BEDSORES

Bedsores—also known as decubitus ulcers, trophic ulcers, and pressure sores—develop where the skin endures unrelieved external pressure. Those who are paralyzed, unconscious, or immobile and anyone confined to a bed or wheelchair for long periods of time are most susceptible. In folk medicine, herbal remedies with anti-inflammatory properties are effective against these "old sores" and "surface ulcers."

The sores occur most commonly on the buttocks, as well as on the shoulders, elbows, lower back, hips, knees, ankles, and heels. They begin as red, tender patches of skin that slowly thicken and swell. Blisters and openings in the skin are common. Ongoing pressure prevents the sores from healing and invites infection. Severe bedsores, which always require medical attention, can expose the bone and may require surgery and skin grafting.

Because bedsores are difficult to treat, prevention is the best medicine. To minimize pressure in any one place, the patient's position should be changed every two hours. Pressure areas should be washed and dried carefully—sponge gently and use a small amount of soap. (Wet skin, especially if caused by incontinence, is prone to infection.) Prevention also involves the use of protective barrier creams, sheepskin pads, cushions, pillows,

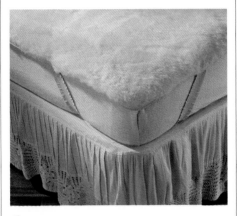

***A**dding a wool mattress pad, like this one made of lambswool, is a simple, age-old measure for preventing bedsores.*

and special mattresses. Other measures include foot and leg exercises, gentle massage, and a vitamin-fortified diet.

Natural Applications

The best folk remedies contained plant elements that are now known to have healing properties: myrrh, aloe vera, witch hazel, arnica, calendula, echinacea, plantain, and balm of Gilead. These medicinals were used for many skin conditions similar to bedsores because of their well-known healing efficacy. Many of these plants are included in widely available over-the-counter preparations.

Some lesser-known folk cures were simple poultices made with powdered herbs, bark, or leaves. These preparations utilized many different ingredients, such as sugar, honey, bread, milk, cucumber juice, charcoal powder, egg whites, wine, crushed garlic cloves, elder stalks, powdered alum, slippery elm, chickweed, and mashed carrots. Of these substances, only honey, garlic, alum, and the alcohol in wine are known to be mildly antiseptic.

The time-tested practice of padding beds with wool blankets can help relieve pressure. Cornstarch and talcum powder —often sprinkled on damp skin and open sores—can help keep skin dry.

MYRRH To make an astringent and antiseptic tincture, mix 1 part resin of the myrrh shrub with 5 parts 90 percent isopropyl rubbing alcohol. Test on healthy skin first to make sure further irritation does not occur. Never apply tincture to an open sore.

ALOE VERA GEL Carefully slice along the center of the aloe leaf, peel back the edges, and scrape out the gel. The gel is available in most stores, but the anti-inflammatory and antibacterial effect of the fresh gel is much greater.

WITCH HAZEL To prepare a cooling antiseptic wash, steam the leaves and recently cut twigs, save the water, and add 1 part alcohol to 4 parts water. To make a compress, add 2 to 3 teaspoons chopped leaves and twigs to 1 cup boiling water. Let cool, strain, and apply with a cloth. Commercial products are also available.

ARNICA The anti-inflammatory and antiseptic qualities of the flower heads are captured in commercial tinctures and ointments. Apply with a cloth or add to a poultice. Long-term use may cause dermatitis. Do not take internally.

CALENDULA Use 1 to 2 teaspoons flowers to make a standard tea (for external use), tincture, or ointment. Apply the steeped tea with a clean cloth. Or use a commercial ointment.

Bedwetting

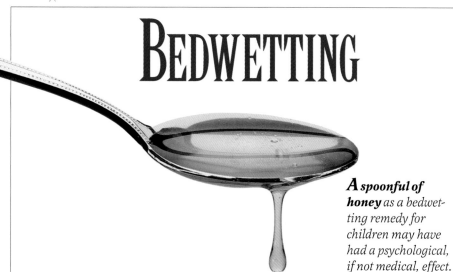

A spoonful of honey as a bedwetting remedy for children may have had a psychological, if not medical, effect.

Folk treatments for bedwetting, or enuresis, were many. Children were given a soothing spoonful of honey at bedtime or a tea made from corn silk, wintergreen, or prince's pine. Chronic bedwetters were doused in cold morning baths or told to sleep only on their sides or stomach. Some Indians chewed the red berries of the wing-rib sumac bush. One old-time cure even called for the child to eat a fried mouse!

Some folk practitioners believed that bedwetting could be prevented at birth: "When the navel cord is removed bring it over the child's head, down behind the back and out between the legs and the child will never wet the bed." Today, some herbalists recommend bearberry, or uva ursi, which is claimed to strengthen the urinary tract and help control bedwetting when taken in small doses.

Still, bedwetting is as common among young children today as it was in the past. At the age of five, about 10 percent of youngsters still wet the bed. Slightly more boys than girls have the problem, which usually runs in families.

Modern science, however, may have come to the rescue. A posterior pituitary hormone called DDAVP (desmospressin acetate), when taken as a nasal inhalant, has been found to effectively control bedwetting in 85 to 90 percent of cases.

Parental Help

Bedwetting usually occurs because the nervous-system functions that control the bladder are slow in maturing. Sometimes it is caused by stress resulting from the arrival of a new baby or the start of school.

Nearly all children stop wetting the bed before adolescence. In the meantime, however, the condition can be the source of acute embarrassment. Parents can help by understanding that the child cannot control bedwetting and should never be scolded for accidents. It often helps to wake the child to go to the bathroom a few hours after he or she goes to sleep. And be sure to praise the child for any dry nights.

A bedwetting alarm, sold at baby-supply stores, works well for about two-thirds of children over the age of seven. When it detects moisture, it rings and wakes the child, who can then get to the toilet. Eventually, the child is conditioned to awaken before starting to urinate.

If a bedwetting child suffers from excessive thirst and urinates more often than usual, it may signal diabetes, while a stinging pain on urination may indicate a urinary tract infection. If either of these symptoms appears, consult a doctor.

SAW PALMETTO Although bedwetting is usually associated with children, adult males with BPH (benign prostatic hypertrophy, or enlarged prostate) may also have the problem. An extract of the berries of saw palmetto has proven in German studies to help control frequent nocturnal urination in men with BPH. The extract's antiandrogenic and anti-inflammatory properties account for its beneficial effects. Look for extracts in capsule form.

PARSLEY The Amish still brew parsley tea to stop bedwetting, although its effectiveness has not been proven. Steep 1 teaspoon of dried parsley leaves in 2 cups of boiling water. Avoid stems and seeds. Parsley may cause photosensitivity in people with fair skin.

FENNEL This herb has a long history as a folk remedy for bedwetting but little clinical verification. Steep a tea made from 1 cup boiling water and 1 teaspoon ground seeds for 10 minutes; strain, then drink. Consult a doctor or pharmacist before taking fennel for longer than a few weeks. Avoid fennel oil, which can cause respiratory problems and seizures.

BELCHING

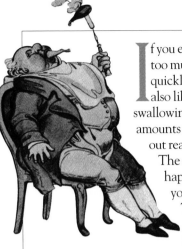

If you eat or drink too much too quickly, you are also likely to be swallowing large amounts of air without realizing it. The same thing happens when you chew gum. To relieve the resulting uncomfortable feeling of fullness, you belch.

Early settlers treated this discomfiting problem with herbal digestive aids, making leaf teas from angelica, fennel, peppermint, dill, parsley, chamomile, caraway, and cow parsnip (also known as masterwort). The Chippewa made a decoction from the root of big bluestem grass for indigestion, and doctors recommended the Indian practice of drinking wild bergamot tea to alleviate gas. All of these herbs contain volatile oils that act as carminatives—that is, they soothe the digestive tract and relieve excess gas. Studies show that the teas may work partly as placebos, but because many people who suffer from indigestion seem to feel better after drinking them, the teas continue to be used today.

Easy Does It

To prevent belching, make mealtime as relaxing as possible. Try to eat and drink slowly, which will give your digestive system time to work; some doctors recommend waiting a minute between bites. Cut down on or eliminate beer, soda, sparkling wine, and hard cider, and do not chew gum. In some cases, excessive belching is caused by an enzyme deficiency—usually of lactase (the enzyme that metabolizes lactose); the problem can be corrected with enzyme-replacement drops, sold at pharmacies.

Certain foods, such as beans, cabbage, and broccoli, are notorious gas producers. Still, they are good sources of vitamins and fiber. Instead of eliminating them, try cooking them with an exotic spice that helps prevent gas, such as cuminseed, ginger, turmeric, and coriander.

Chronic belching can sometimes signal a stomach ulcer or gallbladder disease. If belching is excessive or you have abdominal pain, consult a doctor.

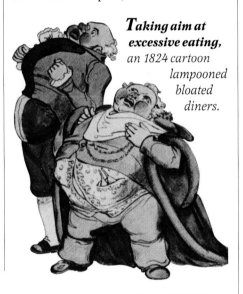

Taking aim at excessive eating, an 1824 cartoon lampooned bloated diners.

GINGER Ginger is a traditional tonic for the intestinal muscles. Stir a few slices of fresh ginger into a cup of boiling water and add honey if desired. Drink after meals to relieve gas. Or, for a delicious treat, eat candied or crystallized ginger, which is also effective. People with gallstones should avoid using ginger, and it should be used only for short periods during pregnancy.

ANISE In folk tradition, anise was used as protection against the evil eye. Today its widest uses are as a flavoring and a carminative, or gas reliever. To control belching, drink a cup of anise tea after a meal. To prepare it, steep 1 teaspoon of ground aniseed in 1 cup of boiling water. Let steep for a few minutes, then strain. Drink the tea slowly.

CHAMOMILE Chamomile is an old folk standby for treating digestive problems. Both the German and the Roman species are effective. If you grow chamomile in your herb garden, use the just-picked flowers to prepare a tea. Mince a few flowers, place 1 to 2 teaspoons in a cup, and add 1 cup boiling water. Let steep for 5 to 10 minutes, then strain. Alternatively, use store-bought chamomile tea bags.

CINNAMON This spice is a common and flavorful folk remedy for indigestion. To make a tea, steep 1 teaspoon or less of the ground inner bark in 1 cup of boiling water for 10 minutes, then strain. Drink with meals. Cinnamon preparations should not be used in large amounts by pregnant women or people with stomach ulcers.

BITES & STINGS

A dog may be man's best friend, but the affection doesn't necessarily extend to children. More than half of the dog-bite victims in North America each year are kids, and three out of four bites are unprovoked. And although dog bites are far more common than cat bites, a feline attack is more likely to result in infection. Rarely, however, are animal bites fatal. More North Americans die each year from the sting of a wasp, a bee, or a fire ant than from the bite of an animal—including snakebites. Those most at risk are the small percentage of people who suffer anaphylactic shock, an allergic reaction to the formic acid in a bee, wasp, or fire ant sting. It can result in death unless treated promptly.

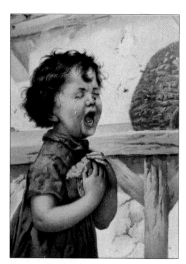

A bee-stung lass *expresses her anguish in this 1893 depiction by an unknown artist.*

No Dog Licks

Folklore says to let the dog that bites you lick the wound, for it will speed up the healing process. Wrong advice. Dogs have rough tongues, which are more likely to irritate than soothe, and the bacteria in a dog's mouth can actually cause an infection. If the skin is torn, wash the bite with soap and water and hold it under running water for a few minutes to wash out any saliva. Then see a doctor, who will clean the wound and start antibiotic treatment.

To treat superficial bites, wash with soap and water and apply an antiseptic, such as hydrogen peroxide or an antibiotic cream.

Treating Stings

For bee stings and insect bites, folk healers recommend applying everything from baking soda or a wad of chewed tobacco to a slice of raw onion or honey from the hive of the bee that stung. This last remedy, if it doesn't provoke more stings, no doubt is based on the same principle as the one that calls for applying the leaves of three different field weeds to the sting: by the time the materials are rounded up, the sting has lost most of its bite! Mud, another popular poultice for stings and bites, may be somewhat easier to find—or to create, mixing dirt with a bit of saliva. Not only does it soothe the wound, but the stinger is likely to come out when the dried mud is removed. Still, common sense holds that it is better to remove the stinger first to prevent additional toxin from being pumped into the skin. In fact, the faster you extract the stinger, the better: gently flick it with a credit card or the side of a knife instead of grasping it with your fingernails or tweezers, which can actually release more venom.

PAPAIN Commercial meat tenderizers are the most readily available source of papain, an enzyme derived from papaya skin's milky juice. To treat an insect bite, moisten a teaspoon of meat tenderizer with a little water and rub it immediately into the skin; papain's protein-digestive properties will help decompose the venom. Papain may induce allergic reactions in sensitive people. Meat tenderizers may also contain monosodium glutamate (MSG), to which some people show sensitivity.

ECHINACEA When applied topically, echinacea may be helpful in treating animal bites and insect stings because of its immune-system-boosting and anti-inflammatory properties. Use a commercial echinacea product containing at least 15 percent of the pressed juice of the plant.

PLANTAIN Not to be confused with the banana variety of the same name, plantain (*Plantago major*) is a weed that grows in most parts of the world and is valued for its wound-healing properties. To treat bites or stings, apply a poultice made from crushed fresh leaves. Or use a commercial plantain extract.

ALOE VERA A time-tested wound soother and emollient, aloe vera is one of the most widely used herbal folk remedies in the U.S. and Canada. Apply it to a bite or sting, using fresh gel scooped from the leaf. Fresh gel is more effective than many of the aloe products found in stores.

BLACK HAW

Viburnum prunifolium
AMERICAN SLOE, CRAMP BARK,
STAGBUSH

Black haw, native to the eastern U.S. from Connecticut to Florida and west to Michigan and Texas, is a spreading deciduous shrub or small tree growing up to 5 m (15 ft) tall. The tree's bark has a long history as a "ladies' medicine." *The American Family Physician*, published in 1857, described the boiled bark as a "uterine tonic," used to affect the muscles of the uterus during childbirth. Nineteenth-century doctors often prescribed an extract made from black haw bark to prevent miscarriage and relieve painful menstruation and the discomfort following childbirth. It was also used to treat morning sickness and complaints related to menopause, and was sometimes employed as a contraceptive. This female-friendly botanical was so popular that its bark was listed in the U.S. Pharmacopeia from 1882 to 1926.

Yet there was also a sinister side to black haw's past: it was used by American slave owners, who often impregnated black women to increase the number of slaves, to prevent the women from terminating their pregnancies with an abortifacient tonic made from cotton root. The 1898 edition of the Eclectic medical book *King's American Dispensatory* stated, "It was customary for planters to compel female slaves to drink an infusion of black haw daily whilst pregnant to prevent abortion from taking the cotton root."

Scientific studies have shown that black haw may in fact prevent miscarriage and abortion: the bark contains scopoletin, which relaxes the muscles of the uterus. But it also contains salicin, an aspirin-like chemical. Because aspirin has been linked to birth defects, black haw is no longer recommended for use by pregnant women. It is still used to relieve menstrual cramps, however, because of both the uterine relaxant scopoletin and the pain-relieving salicin. The salicin in black haw may also relieve the pain of headache and arthritis and reduce fever. But it should never be given to children under age 16: salicin can cause Reye's syndrome, a rare but sometimes fatal childhood disease. This also makes black haw off-limits to nursing mothers.

A Cup of Haw

Black-haw products are sold commercially. Or if you can obtain bark from a black-haw tree, make your own decoction or tea. Dry the bark in the shade (branch bark is collected in summer; trunk bark in fall). For a decoction, boil 2 teaspoons dried bark in 1 cup water for 10 minutes. For a tea, steep 1 teaspoon finely chopped bark in 1 cup of boiling water for 10 minutes. Strain, then drink either preparation two or three times a day. To disguise the bark's bitter taste, add honey or mint.

Active plant parts Bark
Uses Uterine sedative, antispasmodic
Cautions The Indiana poet James Whitcomb Riley rhapsodized, "What is sweeter, after all, than black haws, in early fall?" In truth, the sweet berries may produce nausea and should be avoided. Black haw should not be used by pregnant women, nursing mothers, or children under the age of 16. Large doses can produce nausea or ringing in the ears. Consult your doctor before using.

BLADDER PROBLEMS

When our ancestors complained of bladder problems, folk practitioners recommended cream of tartar stirred into a glass of water, elder flower tea, or regular shots of juniper berry gin. Other traditional remedies were asparagus, pumpkin seeds, and teas made from golden-thread cypress or mullein. North American Indians used echinacea, or purple coneflower, to treat bladder complaints. Toward the end of the 19th century, some doctors were prescribing potash and saltpeter for urinary tract conditions. Although today's treatment of bladder problems has changed dramatically and relies on few of the old-time standbys, the most common causes remain the same: bladder stones, tumors, infections, and old age.

Incontinence

Incontinence, or involuntary urination, is a common problem for older people—especially women—because the sphincter muscles that surround the urethra become gradually weaker with age. Most sufferers can be helped, but because

Your health teacher was right. The admonition to drink eight glasses of water a day still holds true.

there are different kinds of incontinence, it is important to have a doctor investigate the cause. Many drugs can contribute to the problem, so be sure to tell your doctor about any prescription or over-the-counter medication you are taking.

Stress incontinence is the leakage of a bit of urine when you cough, laugh, lift something heavy, or run. It is common in women—especially after childbirth, when the circular muscles of the opening of the bladder are stretched. Kegel exercises (a series of contractions and releases) can help strengthen the muscles of the pelvic floor, which control the bladder's opening and closing.

Urge incontinence is the sudden need to empty the bladder, followed by urinating before you can reach a toilet. Causes include stress, drinking too much coffee or tea, or a sudden move to a cold environment. Inflammatory bladder problems (such as infections), restricted flow from an enlarged prostate gland, or a weakening of the bladder-controlling detrusor muscle also lower the urination threshold. Working on holding the detrusor muscle may help to strengthen control.

If you are overweight, losing weight will give you more bladder control. Constipation can also interfere with bladder control, so try to have regular bowel movements. Make sure you empty your bladder completely when you urinate.

Tumors and Stones

Bladder tumors occur most frequently in men and women over 50 and can be either benign or malignant. The main symptom is blood in the urine, without pain, although tumors located near the urethra can make it difficult to urinate.

Tumors are diagnosed with a cystoscope, a thin viewing tube that is passed through the urethra into the bladder.

Small tumors are usually burned away with an instrument that destroys the cells. Large tumors may require abdominal surgery. You can reduce your risk of developing bladder tumors by not smoking.

Bladder stones are usually bigger than kidney stones and therefore more difficult to pass. They cause a need to urinate frequently, painful urination, and blood in the urine. Treatment depends on the size and the number of stones. Small stones can be extracted with a small basket in the cystoscope; larger ones must be broken up with lasers or ultrasound, or may require surgical removal.

Prostate Troubles

The prostate gland encircles part of the urethra, the tube leading from the bladder, like a small doughnut. Bacteria can travel up the urethra to the gland, infecting it—a condition call prostatitis. This results in fever, lower back and groin pain, and frequent, painful urination. Careful hygiene reduces the risk of a recurrence.

In men over 50, the prostate gland typically enlarges, squeezing the urethra and thereby obstructing the flow of urine from the bladder. Usual symptoms are difficulty when beginning to urinate, frequent urination, waking during the night to urinate (nocturia), and dribbling a little urine after you have stopped.

Except for prostatitis, prostate problems are rare in men under the age of 30. Cancer of the prostate is common in old age and may cause symptoms similar to those that occur with enlarged prostate.

Women's Concerns

Cystitis, an infection of the bladder, is much more common in women than in men. This is because the female urethra—the tube that carries urine from the bladder to outside the body—is only a few

See a doctor if ...

Changes in frequency of urination or the urine itself are indications of a bladder problem. In men, they may indicate a prostate condition. Below are symptoms to take seriously.

◆ Frequent and painful urination. In women, this may be a sign of cystitis. In men, it may signal prostate infection or enlargement.

◆ Blood in the urine may indicate bladder stones.

◆ Blood in the urine, without pain, may signal a bladder tumor.

◆ Voiding more than 2 liters of urine a day may indicate one of these conditions: diabetes mellitus, kidney disease, or a pituitary gland disorder.

centimeters long, giving undesirable bacteria easy entry into the bladder.

Cystitis can have many causes; for example, "honeymoon cystitis" is due to frequent sexual intercourse. Rarely, vaginal infections and yeast can be contributors. By far the most common agent, however, is *Escherichia coli* (*E. coli*), a bacterium that exists naturally in the colon and rectum but is a troublemaker in the bladder. Symptoms of cystitis are a frequent urge to urinate, a burning or stinging sensation when urinating, cloudy and occasionally bloody urine, and sometimes pain in the lower abdomen.

A doctor can perform a urine culture to determine which bacterium is responsible for your cystitis. Antibiotics are the usual treatment for this condition. Drinking eight glasses of water per day and acidifying the urine by eating citrus and other fruits can be preventive.

CRANBERRY Because it keeps bacteria from adhering to the walls of the urinary tract, cranberry juice is valuable for preventing and treating urinary tract infections. As a preventive, drink 80 ml of juice per day; to treat infections, drink 375 ml to 1 liter each day. Capsules of dried cranberry powder are also available; six capsules equal approximately 80 ml of juice.

LOVAGE Even though the Shakers grew and sold this herb as a gas-reliever, modern studies have found that lovage's volatile oils contain a host of anti-inflammatory and antiseptic constituents that can sooth inflammation of the urinary tract. To make a tea, pour 1 cup boiling water over 1 teaspoon minced dried lovage root. Steep for 10 minutes, then strain and drink. The tea should not be taken by people with kidney problems.

One of nature's gifts to those plagued with bladder problems is the cranberry.

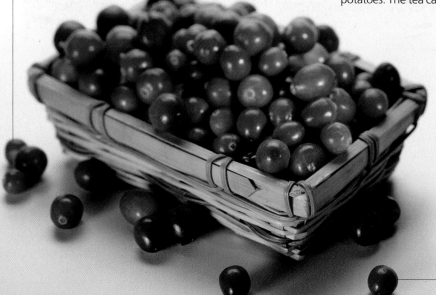

PARSLEY Parsley leaves and roots contain varying amounts of a volatile oil with diuretic properties. A parsley tea may be useful for mild bladder problems, to reduce urinary tract inflammation, and to facilitate the passage of small kidney stones. Add 1 teaspoon of minced leaves to 1 cup boiling water. Avoid the seeds and oil, which can be toxic in large doses. People with kidney disease should consult a doctor before using parsley. Photosensitivity may develop with excessive ingestion.

UVA URSI Before the discovery of sulfa drugs, the herb uva ursi (traditionally known as bearberry) was used as an antiseptic to treat urinary tract infections. Tea bags and extracts are now widely available. The leaves' antiseptic effect results from the metabolic breaking down of the herb's glycosides into an antibacterial substance known as hydroquinone. For this breakdown to happen, the urine must remain alkaline for three to four hours after drinking the tea. To alkalinize the urine, take the tea with a teaspoon of baking soda or with tomatoes, fruit, milk, or potatoes. The tea can be drunk three or four times a day. The taste is bitter and may cause nausea in children and those with sensitive stomachs. Pregnant women should avoid the herb entirely. Others should use it only for a few days at a time: hydroquinone can be toxic with overuse.

BUCHU Buchu leaves, from a South African shrub, have been used as a disinfectant and diuretic for mild urinary tract inflammations. Diosphenol in the leaves accounts for the antibacterial effect, and flavonoids for the diuretic effect. Pour 1 cup boiling water over 1 teaspoon dried buchu leaves, cover and let stand for 10 minutes, then strain. The tea can be drunk several times a day.

ECHINACEA Echinacea helps stimulate the body's immune system and has been approved for use with antibiotics to support the treatment of urinary tract infections. It is also used to treat the vaginal yeast infections that can cause bladder infections. Echinacea should not be used by those with systemic illnesses, such as tuberculosis and multiple sclerosis. It should not be taken for longer than eight weeks in a row.

SAW PALMETTO Today an extract of this palm is the premiere herbal remedy for infection and enlargement of the prostate. If you are taking long-term medication for prostate problems, continue as directed and consult your doctor before taking saw palmetto.

NETTLE The root of the stinging nettle has been shown to be mildly effective in treating enlarged prostate, while the dried leaves have a diuretic effect. To make a tea, add 3 to 4 teaspoons crushed nettle leaves to 1 cup boiling water. Steep, then strain. The tea can be drunk three or four times daily.

BLISTERS

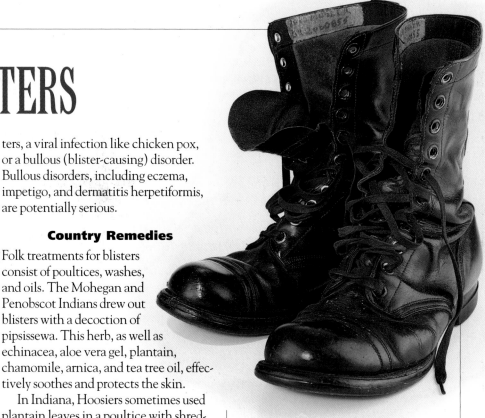

Friction, like that caused by new or ill-fitting shoes, is the main cause of blisters. Heat and skin diseases can also raise these bubbles on the skin's surface. The often painful bubbles, formed when clear liquid serum leaks from the damaged blood vessels underneath the skin, act as a form of protection.

The first treatment choice is to leave a blister alone: new skin will form under it, absorbing the fluid, and the outer layer of skin will eventually fall away. Puncturing a blister can invite infection, but it can also make a blister on the heel, hand, or fingers more comfortable. Make a hole near the blister's edge with a needle that has been sterilized in a flame for a few seconds. Gently squeeze out the liquid without removing the top layer of skin and keep the area clean, dry, and protected with a nonslip bandage.

Consult a physician for especially large or troublesome blisters, a rash with blis-ters, a viral infection like chicken pox, or a bullous (blister-causing) disorder. Bullous disorders, including eczema, impetigo, and dermatitis herpetiformis, are potentially serious.

Country Remedies

Folk treatments for blisters consist of poultices, washes, and oils. The Mohegan and Penobscot Indians drew out blisters with a decoction of pipsissewa. This herb, as well as echinacea, aloe vera gel, plantain, chamomile, arnica, and tea tree oil, effectively soothes and protects the skin.

In Indiana, Hoosiers sometimes used plantain leaves in a poultice with shredded carrots or applied boiled oak bark, containing helpful tannins, to blisters. Elsewhere, comfrey was commonly used; today, however, the herb is no longer recommended for use on broken skin.

ECHINACEA The polysaccharides in echinacea are anti-inflammatory and promote healing. To make a tincture, add 3 tablespoons chopped roots to 1 cup ethyl alcohol. Strain, then apply. Extracts and ointments are available.

PIPSISSEWA This wildflower contains traces of helpful glycosides, resins, antiseptic methyl salicylate, and astringent tannins. Apply a poultice of fresh leaves, a decoction of dried leaves, or the leaf extract to tender, blistered skin.

ALOE VERA The gel of the aloe leaf is the most widely used herbal treatment for skin conditions. The gel coats and protects the blister, while its antibacterial polysaccharides promote healing.

PLANTAIN The freshly pressed juice of plantain leaves contains the antibacterial glycoside called aucubin as well as helpful mucilages and tannins. Apply a poultice of fresh crushed leaves, a decoction of steeped leaves, or the fresh sap-like juice to a blister. Commercial extracts are also available.

Thoreau's Troublesome Shoe

Before shoes were sized, they were custom-made at home or by a cobbler. A shoe's fit, like that of a wig or eyeglasses, involved a personal relationship between the maker and the wearer. In 1846 such a kinship brought Henry David Thoreau out of seclusion at Walden Pond to Concord, Massachusetts, to have his shoe repaired. While in town, he was asked to pay his poll tax, but refused. Accordingly, he spent the night in jail, where he wrote his most famous essay, "Civil Disobedience." Could this abiding treatise have been born of an ill-fitting shoe?

THE HEALING TRADITIONS OF
THE IROQUOIS

The empire of the Iroquois once stretched from the Hudson River to the Niagara, across a woodland wilderness of beauty and bounty alive with powerful spirit forces—many of them intent on causing harm. In response, the people devised a comprehensive system of rituals and remedies to counter all ills.

The world of the Iroquois revolved around health—or, rather, around the pervasive supernatural forces that could affect health. They had rituals to protect it, ceremonies to maintain it, and, when it failed, medicines and healers to restore it. Even today, among traditional Iroquois, health and its treatment remains a centerpiece of their culture.

Ancient Roots

Such preoccupation is rooted in ancient Iroquois beliefs. The Creator, as legend told, endowed the earth with everything good: the dense forests that provided wood for the longhouses, the fertile soil that supported their crops, the plentiful game that yielded meat and hides. Indeed, the Iroquois homeland in present-day New York State—which the five nations of the Seneca, Mohawk, Oneida, Onondaga, and Cayuga had occupied since the 1300s—was one of the richest in native North America.

The Creator's Evil Twin, however, tainted all his brother's works and rivaled his power by producing monsters and vermin, wind and ice, disease and death. Thus did the spirits of good and evil come to reside in all things. It would be the never-ending task of the Iroquois to propitiate the good spirits and not provoke the evil ones in order to achieve a harmonious balance.

Sources of Sickness

Any number of factors could upset that balance and spell illness. Prime among them were violating a taboo, coming in contact with evil, and being bewitched, whereby harmful objects like hair balls and bear teeth would be implanted in the body. Even ailments that seemed to arise from "natural" causes were traced to the supernatural: wounds sustained in battle, for instance, were attributed to spirits of war.

Perhaps the most prevalent cause of disease—and death—was failure to fulfill desires expressed in dreams. The Iroquois put much stock in dreams, during which the soul wandered the spirit world, and spared no effort to satisfy the soul's wishes, either symbolically or literally. Wrote a Jesuit in the 1600s, "The Iroquois have … only a single Divinity, the dream … and [they] follow all its orders with the utmost exactness."

One group of ills was blamed not on spirits but on man: the "secret poison" of epidemic diseases introduced

Rattles and drums often accompanied healing chants. The tone of the water drum (left) depended on the water level inside. The head and neck of the turtle rattle (above) are reinforced to make a handhold.

Faces of the Spirits

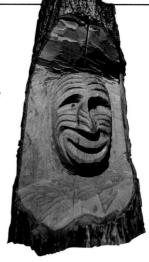

Several Iroquois medicine societies, including the Company of Mystic Animals, the False Face Society, and the Husk Face Society, employed masks in their rituals. Made by society members themselves or designated craftsmen, the representative masks were possessed by spirits, who conferred their curative powers upon the wearer. Masks had to be cared for properly to appease the spirits and encourage their healing forces: they were rubbed with sunflower oil, were "fed" cornmeal mush or popcorn, and had tobacco burned for them, its smoke intended as a gift to the spirits. While the origins of medicine masks are unknown, their use was first recorded by a Dutch traveler in 1634.

__M__asks of the False Face Society were carved from a living tree—as was the one above, made by a contemporary Iroquois artist for display. A mask with flared lips (above left) was used for blowing ashes in a ritual, whereas one with a grotesque visage (above right) represented the Evil Twin, whose face was distorted in a battle with the Creator. A Cayuga healer on a Canadian reserve (left) wears a mask in 1907.

__M__asks of the Husk Face Society, like this Seneca mask (right), represented agricultural spirits and were crafted by women from husks of corn, often braided and sewn together. A sheathed corncob served as the nose, and loose husk ends formed a fringe of hair.

A False Face Curing Ceremony

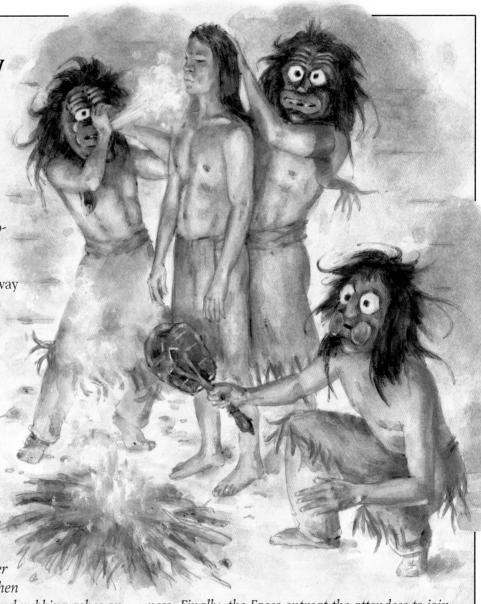

The False Face Society was—and continues to be—among the most prominent of the Iroquois medicine societies. It proved especially effective in healing ailments of the head, shoulders, and joints. Their ceremony, which comprised several sequential rituals, would be enacted essentially the same way regardless of the symptoms, as the entire ceremony was considered "medicine."

After tobacco is burned to invoke the spirits, the patient stands before an open fire in the longhouse, while family and guests gather around. Society members, wearing their distinctive masks, scoop up hot embers in their bare hands—the spirits of the masks protecting them from being burned. The False Faces scatter ashes throughout the room, then treat the patient by blowing and rubbing ashes on his head, shoulders, elbows, and knees.

Concurrently, other members dance around the room to the accompaniment of a singer and turtle rattles, the rhythmic music helping to drive out illness. Finally, the Faces entreat the attendees to join in a dance, lest they, too, court misfortune. The ceremony concludes with a feast of cornmeal mixed with maple sugar and the presentation of tobacco to society members by the patient's grateful family.

by Europeans that, the Iroquois learned, would "eat the life from their blood and crumble their bones." As the Indians increased contact with Dutch and French colonizers in the 1600s and 1700s, they fell prey to measles, smallpox, and typhus, against which they had no immunity. In the 1630s alone, epidemics reduced the Iroquois population of 20,000 by half.

Diagnosis and Treatment

While the cause and treatment of some ailments were obvious or suggested in dreams, a proper diagnosis often required the aid of a clairvoyant, who was adept at communicating with spirits. This shaman divined the source of illness through tea leaves or trances and interpreted the meaning of dreams, then prescribed the appropriate therapy.

Anything or anyone might be medicinal, provided that its spirit force was properly invoked, and the Iroquois had a choice of treatments. Mild ailments were treated at home. Nearly everyone knew a few botanical remedies; Iroquois used some 450 plants, most of them native but some introduced by Europeans. An individual could also undertake preventive procedures, such as purging with herbs or steaming in the sweat lodge.

If self-treatment failed, the patient sought a herbalist, who was expert in exploiting the power of plants. In cases of witchery, shamans were called to massage affected body parts or suck out implanted objects or poison.

The Medicine Societies

Severe or persistent ailments required the intervention of specialized healers, who were organized into medicine societies that acted as intermediaries between the spirit world and the sick. The Iroquois had nine such societies, and their services were available to anyone who had dreamed of the group or been recommended by a clairvoyant; those cured later became members.

Each society had its own rituals, dances, and songs. The rites of the Company of Mystic Animals—which encompassed the Bear, Buffalo, Eagle, and Otter societies—included dances in which members imitated the various animals.

While some groups used special paraphernalia, such as masks and musical instruments, others possessed secret medicines. The Little Water Society maintained a blend of powdered animal parts, which was mixed in minute amounts with water and applied to a wound or consumed by the patient.

The societies convened according to their own schedules. Many took part in community events, such as the nine-day Midwinter Ceremony, when they treated new patients and repeated cures at the request of former patients. Groups also met periodically to "renew" their powers or to perform preventive rituals, like visiting every house in their village to exorcise disease. Most often, however, a society was invited to a patient's home to conduct a private cure.

Contemporary Curing

The Iroquois no longer roam the realm of their ancestors—they have lived mainly on reservations in New York and on reserves in Canada since the late 1700s—but their healing traditions have endured, against all odds. Christian missionaries often sought to replace "Old Heathenish practices" with prayers. In the early 1800s, an Iroquois reformer condemned the medicine societies as covens of witches. And in modern times, it is "white man's medicine" that encroaches on the Iroquois heritage. Yet, in many of the communities, the population perpetuates ancient beliefs and performs the age-old rituals—evidence that the spirit of Iroquois healing remains alive, as dynamic as the spirits that inhabit their world.

***M**edicinal plants revered by the Iroquois include (left to right) yarrow, to reduce fever; catnip, for headache; and cardinal flower, used against epilepsy in women.*

BODY ODOR

Truth be told, for much of human history, body odor simply did not cause much alarm. Although people did not live in filth, the daily shower or bath was extremely rare. When it was time to get clean, various folk treatments were tried.

Most remedies for body odor strive to mask odor, limit sweating, and pro-

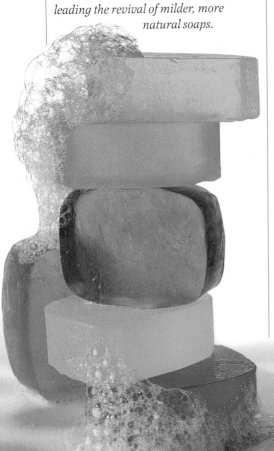

Transparent glycerine soaps, in use since the late 18th century, are leading the revival of milder, more natural soaps.

tect the skin from bacteria-friendly moisture. Although sweat itself does not smell, sweat produced by the apocrine glands—located in the armpits and the breast and genital areas—emits protein and fatty materials that foster odor-causing bacteria.

Washing with deodorant soaps removes nearly all bacteria from the skin. Antiperspirants and deodorants are effective, too, but can irritate the underarms. Like bacteria, food can affect your scent: avoid garlic, onions, and fish and eat more leafy greens and foods that contain zinc. Excessive sweating, chemical imbalances, and serious internal diseases can also produce body odor. If you suspect an odor-causing disorder, see your doctor.

Washes, Powders, Soaps

Folk remedies sought to clean the skin or limit perspiration. A wash or a daily cup of sage tea was believed to reduce

sweating, and antibacterial sage oil was applied to the underarms. Antiseptic washes included ammonia, alcohol, white-wine vinegar, yarrow tea, witch hazel, and turnip juice. Among useful modern antiseptics are rubbing alcohol, tea tree oil, and green tea extracts.

Powders that form a protective, absorbent layer on the skin were also common. Smoothed onto the skin, baking soda absorbs odor and neutralizes the fatty acids that nurture bacteria. The Eclectics used cornstarch to "take up acrid secretions from the external surface." The powdered root of skunk cabbage was also used, despite its name and its toxicity if ingested.

Although soap was once used primarily on clothes, it eventually became a bathing staple. Soapmaking was a common pursuit for early pioneers, and the three basic ingredients remain the same today: animal fat, lye, and water. Popular bath additives included peppermint, basil, and thyme. A tomato juice bath was considered first aid for encounters with skunks.

Today soaps often contain traditional complements, such as oatmeal, sand, glycerine, baking soda, and herbs.

SAGE This herb has both antibacterial and perspiration-reducing properties. Sage oil, tincture, and tea bags are available. Apply the tincture or diluted oil directly to sweaty areas, except the face and genitals. You can also drink the tea or use it as a wash. Pregnant women should not take the tea or tincture internally.

TEA TREE OIL This cinnamon-scented oil comes from *Melaleuca alternifolia,* an Australian tree. Apply directly to the offending areas. The oil

is mildly antiseptic and deodorizing but may cause dermatitis.

BAKING SODA OR CORNSTARCH Dust on the offending areas. Both powders absorb moisture, but neither is an antiperspirant. Baking soda is mildly antiseptic and fights odor.

TOMATO JUICE BATH Add 2 or 3 cups tomato juice to bathwater. Soak for 15 minutes. The effectiveness of this historical and harmless treatment has never been scientifically verified.

BOILS

Over the years folk practitioners have unleashed enough food products into the battle against boils to feed a good-sized church picnic. Eating a dozen oranges or grapefruits a day was said to cure boils, as was consuming quantities of nutmeg or cornmeal. Poultices for external application have been made from mashed egg whites or honey and breadcrumbs. Covering the boil with mashed cranberries, the inside of banana peels, a slice of raw onion or potato or lemon, a piece of fatty meat, and as the Bible suggests (Isaiah 38:21), a raw fig, have also been widely tried.

A painful sore that can occur almost anywhere on the body, the boil begins as an inflamed red lump. (Much less common is the carbuncle—an extremely large boil or, in some cases, a number of boils joined under the skin.) Boils occur when bacteria penetrate oil glands or hair follicles and cause infection, often in sweaty areas of the body where skin bacteria multiply. As the boil

fills with pus, it begins to swell and ache, eventually forming a white or yellow head. When the pressure is sufficient, usually within two weeks, the boil bursts and begins to drain, relieving the pain and beginning the healing process. Doctors sometimes hasten the process by lancing the boil and prescribing antibiotics to stop the infection.

Common Compresses

Some still swear by the folk remedy for boils that calls for applying a poultice of stale bread

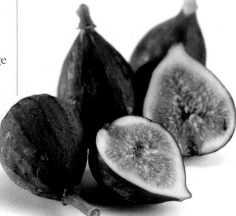

Raw figs were once used to draw out boils.

soaked in hot milk and covering it with a cloth overnight. While such a cure may seem farfetched, there is no question that our forebears were on the right track. All of the remedies for boils that have stood the test of time involve a warm, moist compress, regularly applied (even the ancient fig treatment may work if the fig is warmed first). Just make sure that the compress is as germ-free as possible or it may introduce new infection.

However a boil is treated, wash your hands after touching it: the bacteria can cause food poisoning if you then touch warm food. And note that showers rather than baths will help prevent a boil from spreading to another part of the body.

See a doctor if ...

◆ The boil is large and very painful or is on the face, groin, armpit, or the breasts of a nursing woman.
◆ You have recurrent boils. They can be a symptom of a staph infection, diabetes mellitus, or an immunosuppressant disease.
◆ You see red lines on the skin emanating from the boil.
◆ You have fever, chills, or swelling in other parts of your body or you are diabetic and have a boil.

HONEY AND COD LIVER OIL Mix honey with an equal amount of cod liver oil (or use honey alone) and apply directly to the boil. Cover with a sterile bandage and replace three times a day.

GARLIC Mix finely grated garlic with olive oil, apply the mixture to the boil,

then cover with a sterile bandage. Repeat several times a day.

SLIPPERY ELM The powdered bark of the slippery elm is available commercially. Mix it with lard or petroleum jelly until it forms a paste, then apply to the boil with a cotton ball. When the paste dries, replace with fresh paste until

the boil is drawn out. You can also make an infusion using dried bark.

GOLDENSEAL The antibacterial effect of goldenseal can help heal boils. Make a strong infusion with 2 teaspoons of commercial powdered goldenseal root and 1 cup hot water. Apply repeatedly with a cotton ball.

BONESET

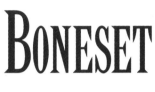

Eupatorium perfoliatum
THOROUGHWORT, EUPATORIUM,
SWEATING PLANT, INDIAN SAGE,
AGUEWEED, FEVERWORT, CROSSWORT,
VEGETABLE ANTIMONY

Native to North America, boneset got its name from its use as a treatment for "breakbone," or dengue fever, a prevalent condition in the American South in the 19th century. This illness, very rare today, caused muscle pain so severe that one felt as if the bones were breaking. Because it promotes sweating, boneset tea gained a reputation for reducing a variety of fevers. Today, however, its traditional use as an emetic and purgative is not recommended, and its effectiveness against fever has been called into question.

The "Sweating Plant"

Indians used boneset tea to treat all fever-producing illnesses, including influenza, cholera, malaria (intermittent fever), and typhus (lake fever). They used the herb for other ailments, too, with various tribes taking it for different reasons: the Menomini, Iroquois, and Mohegan, for fever and colds; the Alabama, for upset stomach; and the Creek, for body pain and sprained joints. All of these uses, as well as those for constipation and loss of appetite, were passed on to the settlers.

Settlers were easily convinced of boneset's power to treat colds and the flu, as well as coughs, rheumatism, headache, snakebite, gout, and "James River ringworm." The leaves were also applied as a poultice for tumors. For malaria, boneset tea rivaled Peruvian bark, the source of quinine. During the American Civil War, soldiers drank the tea for fever and as a "strength tonic." Boneset tea was even used to fight the great flu epidemics of the 19th and 20th centuries.

Active plant parts Dried upper leaves and flower tops
Uses Fever, constipation
Cautions Boneset may cause nausea and vomiting, especially in young children. Large amounts of tea or extract can result in severe diarrhea. Pyrrolizidine alkaloids (found in most species of Eupatorium) are known to cause long-term indigestion and liver impairment. Because these alkaloids may be found in boneset, doctors urge caution when ingesting this plant. Anyone with a history of alcoholism or liver disease should be particularly careful. Do not exceed recommended doses or use for more than two weeks at a time. Do not eat the fresh herb: it contains tremerol, a toxic chemical that causes nausea, vomiting, muscle tremors, and increased rate of respiration. Use by pregnant women and nursing mothers is strongly discouraged.

Not to be confused with ...

Comfrey (*Symphytum officinale*) was also known in some parts as boneset. Like boneset, it contains pyrrolizidine alkaloids—known to cause long-term indigestion and liver impairment—but at dangerously toxic levels. Although the herb is still recommended by many herbalists, only the limited external use of cosmetic products containing comfrey is deemed safe—and then only on unbroken skin.

Unparalleled Popularity

Part of boneset's appeal, from country cabins to city hospitals, may have been its nauseatingly bitter taste. A widespread folk belief stated that the worse a remedy tasted, the better it worked, and few remedies tasted worse than boneset. Proffering this home remedy, women often prompted their reluctant children and husbands, "Drink this boneset. It'll do you good." Because of the plant's bitterness and powerful effect on the body, the dosage was commonly limited to a mere teaspoonful or no more than a half cup.

The public's long-held respect for the herb was understandable: boneset affects the body in extreme ways. Taken warm and in moderate doses, the tea causes sweating, which may help reduce a fever. Taken hot and in larger doses, it induces vomiting (as well as sweating) and quickly loosens the bowels. By prompting such dramatic effects, the tea was thought to clean out the system and put one squarely on the road to recovery. It was also believed to aid the uterus, act as a diuretic, and "assist in raising phlegm from the lungs." For these reasons, boneset was also used for "female disorders," bladder ailments, and chest congestion.

The popularity of boneset was noted by Dr. C. F. Millspaugh in his 1892 book, *American Medicinal Plants*: "There is probably no plant in American domestic practice that has more extensive or frequent use than this. The attic, or woodshed, of almost every country farmhouse, has bunches of the dried herb hanging tops downward from the rafters during the whole year, ready for immediate use should some family member or neighbor be taken with a cold." The herb was regarded as a virtual cure-all, but its folk use declined steadily after aspirin gained predominance in the early 1900s.

Joe-Pye Weed: Boneset's Mysterious Cousin

A species closely related to boneset, *Eupatorium purpureum*, may have been named Joe-Pye weed after a traveling Indian medicine man who used the herb to treat typhoid fever throughout New England in the late 18th century. Two other common species were also called Joe-Pye weed: *E. fistulosum* (hollow Joe-Pye weed) and *E. maculatum* (spotted Joe-Pye weed).

Although Joe Pye's reputation as an Indian medicine man spread far and wide, there is little evidence of his existence apart from the record of a purchase of a quart of rum from a Stockbridge, Massachusetts, tavern in 1775. Adding to the mystery are two other explanations for the plant's name. First, the plant was also known as "jopi weed," from *jopi*, an Indian word for typhus; the word could have been misunderstood as "Joe Pye," a person's name. Second, Joe Pye has been said by some to be a white man who promoted the root at traveling medicine shows, during which fraud and deceit were common. The "Joe Pye" Indian persona, it is thought, could have been cleverly invented and used as a selling device.

Regardless of the plant name's origin, the bitter tea was used by Indians and settlers alike to treat typhoid and other fevers, colds, coughs, loss of appetite, kidney problems, and nervousness. One Indian notion even held that a young man could win a maiden's heart if he tucked a piece of Joe-Pye weed leaf under his tongue.

Joe-Pye weed, the magenta-flowered relative of boneset, was also used to treat fever.

Benefits Are Questioned

Despite boneset's popularity, its many folk uses have received little scientific support. Most significant, no direct evidence has been found to confirm its use as a fever reducer. Still, boneset may have some medicinal value. Limited research has shown that it may have mild anti-inflammatory and immunity-boosting properties, possibly validating its topical use for arthritis and for colds. In small doses, it may act as a mild diuretic and laxative.

Use caution, for boneset can be toxic if taken in excessive doses. The herb may be dangerous because of the presence of pyrrolizidine alkaloids—known to cause long-term indigestion and liver impairment—in the *Eupatorium* genus, even though they have not been found in the boneset species of traditional use.

BRUISES

The ways our ancestors dealt with a bruise ranged from the simple to the exceedingly odd. One old-time cure called for a live frog: "Catch a toad-frog and hold the stomach to the bruise until it dies. The fever from the bruise will go into the frog and kill it." While this so-called remedy was clearly based on folklore, many others have scientific merit and are still used today.

Bruises are the black-and-blue splotches that form when a bump or scrape ruptures capillaries just beneath the skin, leaking blood into the surrounding tissues and causing swelling. They can occur from impact anywhere on the body, including the head, shin, and eye area—the telltale "black eye." Initially, the skin appears blue or black; then the breakdown of hemoglobin in the pooled blood turns the bruise yellow. This minor internal bleeding causes no permanent harm:

the body's natural defenses soon intervene and repair the damaged tissue. A normal bruise will fade away without any treatment within 10 to 14 days. A bruise that won't go away or reappears, however, should be checked out by a doctor: it may be a symptom of a bleeding disorder.

Cool Compresses

Early settlers had the right idea when they relied on medicated compresses to treat a bruise. They dipped rags into a cool herbal infusion or decoction and used them to cover the affected area. Happily, the herbs used for compresses—from arnica to yarrow, from chamomile to thyme—contained one or more compounds with

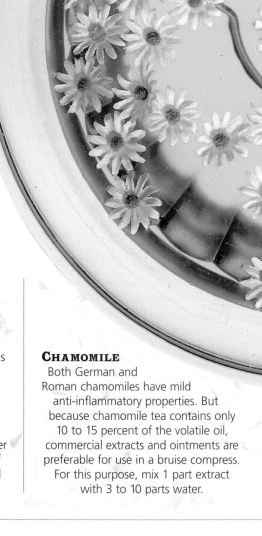

CALENDULA Even though the active principles of calendula, or pot marigold, have not been identified, preparations containing the herb have been shown to inhibit inflammation and help promote wound healing. The plant was used extensively to treat topical wounds and is a common ingredient in commercial skin preparations. To make a compress for a bruise, pour 1 cup boiling water over 1 to 2 teaspoons of the chopped dried flower heads. Soak a cloth with the cooled liquid, wring it out, fold, and apply to the bruise. Change the compress several times a

day. Allergic reactions, although rare, may occur in some people.

ARNICA Natives and early settlers used arnica for a number of ailments, including bruises. Two isomeric alcohols contained in the herb, called arnidol and foradiol, have proven counterirritant properties, while the compound helenalin reduces inflammation and swelling. For bruises, mix 1 part commercial tincture with 3 to 10 parts water and use in a compress. Internal use of arnica is toxic, and prolonged external use can cause dermatitis.

CHAMOMILE Both German and Roman chamomiles have mild anti-inflammatory properties. But because chamomile tea contains only 10 to 15 percent of the volatile oil, commercial extracts and ointments are preferable for use in a bruise compress. For this purpose, mix 1 part extract with 3 to 10 parts water.

modest antiseptic, analgesic, and anti-inflammatory properties.

Today compresses remain an effective treatment for bruises. They ease the pain and reduce swelling by helping to constrict the ruptured tiny blood vessels.

Before applying a compress to a bruise, first check to see if the skin is broken. If so, gently cleanse it with soap and water or an antiseptic, such as hydrogen peroxide, to remove debris, which could lead to infection. To make the compress, dip a clean dish towel or wash-cloth in an herbal infusion or decoction, wring it out, fold it, and place it over the bruise. Then secure the compress with a surgical bandage

The dainty flowers of **chamomile** *are the source of its bruise-soothing qualities, which have long been recognized.*

and change it every few hours.

Instead of using compresses, many early settlers simply mashed mullein, plantain, St. Johnswort, or peach-tree leaves directly against a bruise, then bound the wound with a cloth to "draw out infection." (Folk healers in Europe continue to use plantain and peach-tree leaves in a similar fashion today.) They also made herbal salves and poultices with beeswax, cornmeal, or mutton suet.

Bruise Lore

Despite its traditional use, a cold slab of steak pressed against a black eye is little more than an unsanitary and expensive "cold pack." (One variation advised placing a thin slice of ice-cold raw veal over the eye and covering it with a lettuce leaf.) Also dubious was the advice from an 1843 medical book, which advised one to "bathe the part with warm vinegar, to which a little brandy or rum may occasionally be added." Still, one old-time cure remains: the practice of using leeches to draw out the dried blood of a bruise is currently used by some plastic surgeons to reduce swelling and bruising after surgery.

PLANTAIN Known among native tribes as "Englishman's foot" because it spread from pioneer settlements, plantain remains a popular folk remedy for inflamed skin: its mucilage and iridoid glycosides are known to have antibacterial properties. A bruise can gain a modest benefit from the anti-inflammatory and wound-healing properties of the crushed leaves. Pour boiling water over 2 teaspoons of the chopped herb; steep for 10 minutes and press through a strainer. Apply to the bruise and secure with a clean cloth.

YARROW Yarrow's antiseptic and anti-inflammatory properties are due to chamazulene—one of many sesquiterpene, lactone-derived compounds in the volatile oil. To use in a bruise compress, pour 1 cup hot water over 2 teaspoons dried yarrow leaves, available commercially. Steep for 10 minutes, strain, then dampen a clean cloth with the liquid and apply to a bruise. Itching and inflammation signal yarrow dermatitis; if these symptoms occur, discontinue use of yarrow immediately.

WITCH HAZEL An infusion made from the leaves or powdered bark of witch hazel may have a concentration of anti-inflammatory tannins stronger than that of commercial witch hazel products. To make an infusion, pour 1 cup hot water over 2 to 4 teaspoons dried leaves or bark and let sit for 10 minutes before using in a bruise-soothing compress.

BURDOCK

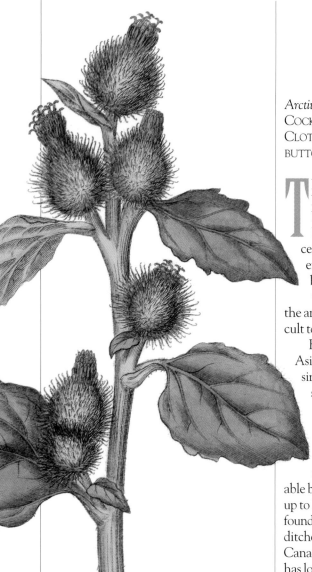

Arctium lappa
COCKLE-BUR, BARDANE, GOBO, CLOTBUR, STICK BUTTON, BEGGAR'S BUTTONS, TURKEY BURRSEED, HAREBURR

The weed called burdock is familiar to hikers: its clusters of small, bristly burrs cling to their socks and pant legs and tangle their pets' coats. For centuries, the weed has been the pesky enemy of farmers and shepherds because it is often found in pastures where sheep graze. The burrs snarl the animals' fleece, making it more difficult to prepare for spinning.

Burdock originated in Europe and Asia and has been used medicinally since the Middle Ages. Early European settlers brought it to North America when the burrs, with seeds inside, hitched a ride on their clothing and the hides of their livestock.

In spite of persistent efforts to root out this hardy plant—recognizable by its tall, dull green stalks and leaves up to 30 cm (12 in.) long—it can be found today in fields, along roads, and in ditches throughout much of the U.S. and Canada. Yet what is a nuisance to farmers has long been prized by herbalists the world over, who have prescribed burdock's use against everything from leprosy to hysteria—and even the common cold.

Nature's Cure-all?

Despite the extravagant claims that have been made for burdock, no real evidence exists for its therapeutic effects. In fact, Germany's Commission E, recognized as the most accurate body of knowledge on herb safety and efficacy in the world, has declared that burdock is not only medicinally useless but "obsolete."

Still, burdock's extensive folk use is of historical interest. As far back as the Middle Ages, a mixture of pounded burdock leaves and wine was taken by Europeans for edema, or dropsy, and the leaves were made into poultices to treat gout. The plant was also used to make a remedy for syphilis and was said to have cured France's King Henry III of that disease in the 16th century. In his book published in 1640, the English surgeon Parkinson claimed that "the juice of the leaves given to drink with old wine doth wonderfully help the biting of any serpents."

Indians, too, learned to use the weed. The Cherokee gave a tea made from burdock roots or seeds to "weakly females" and mixed equal portions of burdock, dandelion, and white-oak bark into a tea for treating varicose veins.

In the 19th century, burdock was a popular "spring cleaning" tonic, used to "purify the blood" by acting as a diuretic and a mild laxative. Some folk practitioners believed that the plant had a magnet-like effect on women in labor: if the leaves and seeds were applied to the soles of the woman's feet, the baby would be drawn downward; if they were put on her navel, a premature baby would stay in place.

Active plant parts Roots, seeds
Uses Constipation, gastrointestinal disorders, arthritis, rheumatism, skin conditions
Cautions The rough hairs of the growing plant may cause contact dermatitis.

Native Hawaiians, introduced to the herb in the 19th century by the Japanese, believed that eating burdock would increase their strength and stamina.

Today many herbalists use a medicine made from dried or roasted burdock seeds to treat fevers, colds, coughs, tonsillitis, and measles. (Burdock has been used as a folk treatment for cancer in Indiana, where a decoction made from the root has been said to shrink tumors of the intestine, breast, knee, liver, tongue, and uterus—claims that are dubious at best.) A root extract is available, and is taken by mixing a few drops into a glass of water.

An Herb for Skin

Burdock has a long history as a skin cleanser. In 1888 the U.S. Dispensatory recommended its use for psoriasis, eczema, and other chronic skin diseases, which were treated with a tea made by boiling the root in water. It noted, however, "To prove effectual, its administration must be long continued." It is still used for this purpose, and lotions made from crushed burdock leaves are applied externally to burns, acne eruptions, warts, and ringworm. Burdock root has indeed been proven in scientific studies to be an effective antiseptic—but only when it is fresh; the efficacy of commercially available dried products has not been proved.

Some even claim that burdock prevents baldness—a belief that stems from the Doctrine of Signatures, which holds that whatever gives the plant such a dense growth of hair would do the same for people. Enthusiasts soak fresh leaves in hot water and massage the mixture into the scalp twice

a day. A preparation believed to keep the scalp healthy is made from equal parts pounded burdock root, fresh burdock leaves, and wine vinegar, then applied to the scalp. Like most other claims made for burdock, these have yet to be verified.

Despite its effectiveness as an antiseptic, burdock's most important contribution to good health may be its high nutrient content: it is a rich source of vitamins A, B, C, and E, as well as iron, calcium, potassium, and fiber.

As food, the weed takes many forms. Our ancestors candied the stalks and made a cordial from the root. The first-year roots can also be boiled and eaten buttered or with a sauce—a culinary use the Japanese prize. Called gobo at the Japanese markets found in many North American cities, sliced or whole burdock root is available in refrigerated packets.

Young burdock stalks, too, are edible. Chefs cut them before they flower, peel off the coarse brown skin, and boil them like asparagus. The taste is pleasantly earthy, if slightly fibrous. Peeled stalks and young leaves can also be tossed into salads and added to soups.

A Recent Lesson

Since the 1970s, several cases of poisoning resulting from commercially packaged burdock root tea in the United States and Europe have served to highlight the dangers that can arise as a result of insufficient quality control of herbal preparations. At first these poisonings were attributed to the burdock root itself, but more recent investigators have blamed them on accidental contamination of burdock supplies with belladonna. Belladonna roots look similar to burdock roots but contain dangerously high levels of a substance called atropine. Cases such as these are important reminders of the care consumers must take when choosing and using herbal products.

Burdock stalks are peeled to reveal a white inner core. The roots are sold either sliced or whole—sometimes artificially colored, as at left.

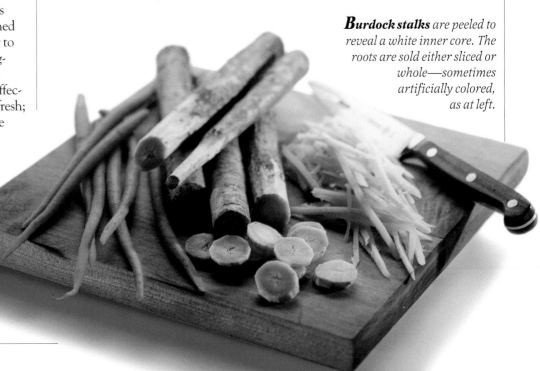

BURNS

Minor burns are usually treated at home, and folk medicine enlists dozens of remedies to soothe and protect slightly burned skin. Burns range from minor sunburns, scalds, and rope burns to blisters and charred skin. The level of seriousness is classified by degrees and can be determined within 30 minutes of being burned. The usual effects of a first-degree burn are pain, discomfort, and a reddening of the skin's surface; a typical sunburn is an example. The skin heals quickly, with the damaged top layer peeling away after a day or two. Second-degree burns are characterized by blisters, sharper pain, deeper redness, and swelling. Third-degree burns destroy all the layers of the skin, sometimes turning the area white or charred black. The nerve endings may also be damaged, so that little or no pain is felt after the excruciating initial pain.

Folk remedies should be used only for first-degree burns and small second-degree burns. Anyone with second-degree burns affecting the hands, feet, or genitals or with blisters more than 2.5 cm (1 in.) across should consult a physician immediately. Serious burns over more than 10 percent of the body may cause shock.

All third-degree burns are considered medical emergencies, since muscle and bone may be exposed and the risk of infection is high. Electrical burns may also require a doctor's evaluation; they can penetrate muscle and damage the heart and other internal organs with only minimal marking of the skin.

Cold Water

For first- and second-degree burns, no first aid is better than cold water. However, water that is too cold, as well as ice, may irritate the tender skin. Holding the affected area in a container of cold water or under a running tap for at least 5 to 10 minutes can reduce the potential degree of the burn. Folk wisdom put faith in the

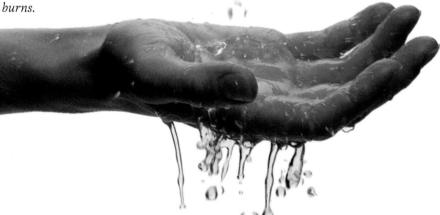

Clean, cold water *is the best first aid for all types of burns.*

ALOE VERA To extract the anti-inflammatory gel directly from the plant, carefully slice along the center of the leaf, peel back the leaf edges, and scrape the gel from the inner portion of the leaf. Avoid scraping the rind, which can adulterate the gel with laxative anthraquinones. Apply the gel directly to sunburn and other minor burns; as it dries, it will form a protective layer on the skin and promote healing. The fresh gel is generally more effective than store-bought lotions, which often have insufficient amounts of aloe.

CALENDULA To make a mildly antiseptic compress, add 1 to 2 teaspoons flower heads to 1 cup boiling water. Steep, strain, and let cool. Apply with a clean cloth. To make a lotion, add freshly crushed calendula flowers to olive oil and let stand overnight. Apply to minor burns only. Commercial lotions containing calendula are also available.

RED CLOVER To make a soothing compress, pour 1 cup boiling water over 1 to 2 teaspoons flowers. Steep, strain, and let cool. Apply with a clean cloth. Red clover's antiseptic properties have not been identified, and its healing potential may be as limited as that of other mild herbs and honey.

efficacy of cold water, though sometimes for dubious reasons. One healer considered it a "vital force," explaining that "the water itself is taken up and passed into the dry, burned, cooked, and roasted places where the blood has been congested."

Chemical burns in particular need to be washed with water for at least 15 minutes. For extensive burns, douse the area with water and then wrap the victim in a blanket. Any exposed burned skin should be covered with a dry, clean cloth that will not stick to or "shed" on the open wound. Additional treatment for a minor burn is simply to take a mild analgesic and apply a light antibacterial dressing, which allows exposure to the air while disinfecting, protecting, and preventing dryness. Many folk remedies have similar aims, but only a few are recommended.

Herbs and Rituals

A seemingly endless variety of herbs and plants have been used to treat burns. Poultices and teas made from herbs that contain tannins or other mild anti-inflammatory substances—lavender, peppermint, St. Johnswort, witch hazel, plantain, white oak bark, ginger, and balm of Gilead—may help. However, many herbal burn remedies have not been adequately tested, and any use is strongly discouraged. These include pekoe, sweet gum, goldenseal, pennyroyal, slippery elm, fireweed root, red raspberry, and the leaves of beriberi, blackberry, and jewelweed. Other remedies that have been applied externally are toxic internally: stoneroot leaves, wild hydrangea root, bracken fern root, and bittersweet bark.

Besides herbs, unusual treatments were tried. The lores of European and African descendants included "talking out fire" through prayer and rituals that involved blowing on the affected area. Some Indi-

Butters, Oils, and Lotions

All across North America, butter, lard, animal fat, and a variety of oils were used to treat burns. The greasy substances were applied directly to the burn or used to thicken the consistency of herbal burn salves. Today these folk remedies are not recommended for burn first aid: once applied, they trap heat in the skin and increase the risk of infection.

Butter was thought to soothe burn pain and protect the damaged skin. Over time, the salt in butter was often found to irritate the wound, and many folk remedies soon called for unsalted butter or lard. Chicken fat, hog suet, and "fatty meat" were also employed. Linseed oil and olive oil enjoyed great popularity, as did cod liver oil, garlic oil, sesame oil, castor oil, and whale oil. Even axle grease was used.

The only potential value in using herbal oils (as well as modern ointments and lotions) for minor burns comes after the skin has already started to heal. If the substance forms an antiseptic coating, is anti-inflammatory and antibacterial, and keeps the skin moist, it can promote healing without scarring. One such substance is calamine, a pinkish mixture of zinc oxide with a small amount of ferric oxide; it is readily available in pharmacies. Oils and lotions made from lavender and peppermint are also effective for minor burns, preferably after cool water has been applied.

ans believed that cold water was the worst treatment for burns and that burns should not be cooled too quickly. Another folk remedy called for placing a minor burn near a fire to draw out the pain.

Kitchen Remedies

Because burns commonly occur in the kitchen, many folk remedies are found there. The best, aloe vera, grows comfortably on any kitchen windowsill. Other home remedies include a poultice of cabbage leaves or a raw potato or onion slice that is gently rubbed on the burn. Also on the list are honey, milk, apple cider vinegar, table mustard, yogurt, oatmeal, egg whites, pumpkin rinds, cornmeal, baking soda, piecrust without salt, a ripe banana peel, and—for a burned tongue—vanilla extract. Tar, cool wax, mud, and charcoal have also been used, possibly for their ability to absorb

heat. For the most part, these remedies merely relieve burn pain; only aloe vera and honey have shown any healing potential. Butter, once a very common burn ointment, actually interferes with healing and should be avoided.

Compresses made from calendula, a common garden plant, and red clover, which grows in pastures across North America, may help comfort and heal minor burns. Both plants are mildly antiseptic.

The spiny leaves of aloe vera contain its soothing gel.

CALAMUS

Acorus calamus
SWEET FLAG, FLAGROOT,
SWEET MYRTLE, SWEET-
ROOT, SWEET RUSH

The perennial yellow-flowering calamus resembles the iris and thrives in swamps and marshlands across North America. Long considered a cure-all in Indian and folk medicine, the native variety was used for everything from tobacco addiction and asthma to digestive disorders and childhood colic. It was also the source of tonics or aromatic bitters, flavoring products ranging from tooth powders to liqueurs to beer. Children once chewed calamus root as candy.

The rootstock was boiled in teas to relieve fevers and dyspepsia and was applied topically in poultices to heal burns and boils. When chewed, it was said to aid digestion, soothe irritated throats, and sweeten the breath. In powdered form, calamus root was used as a spice in food. Even Brer Rabbit sang its praises in relation to good down-home cooking: "I done got so now dat I can't eat no chicken 'ceppin she's seasoned up wid calamus root."

Calamus even acted as a kind of makeshift room deodorizer. European settlers scattered the plant's fragrant leaves across the floors of their homes to mask the stench of inadequate sanitation and ventilation. It was believed as well that the herb kept away household pests, such as bedbugs and fleas.

A Foreign Invader

Botanists have classified *Acorus calamus* as four separate varieties that grow in different locations worldwide: it was the American variety that was the "wonder drug" of yore. Not until the Asian variety, imported from the Indian subcontinent in the 19th century, became naturalized in North America did calamus's suitability for medicinal use become inadvisable.

Studies have shown that the Asian calamus contains a high percentage of beta asarone, which has caused cancerous tumors in animals. Accordingly, in an effort to avoid the risk of one calamus variety being confused with another, the U.S. FDA in 1968 declared all calamus unsafe. Despite the prohibition, calamus is still seen on the American market, usually sold as a root extract.

In Canada, calamus products intended for internal use are not approved for sale. Concerns about the herb led Health Canada to issue a strong warning about *Acorus calamus*—particularly after four cases of severe liver toxicity, and two deaths in New Zealand, were reported.

Active plant parts Root
Uses Digestive disorders, colic, and fever
Cautions Regardless of claims made by manufacturers, calamus products may be extracted from the Asian variety, which has caused cancerous tumors in laboratory animals.

CAMPHOR

Cinnamomum camphora
GUM CAMPHOR, LAUREL CAMPHOR

The pungent scent of camphor is known to anyone who uses mothballs: the vaporous, crystalline resin has been used for centuries to repel insects. This Asian relative of cinnamon has long been advocated as a medical cure-all as well, used to ward off a number of ills ranging from rheumatism to lung congestion. In fact, during the American Civil War the demand for camphor was so great that the United States contracted with the island of Formosa for its entire output of camphor oil. Camphor derivatives were so highly valued at the time that the U.S. even made an effort to purchase Formosa from the Chinese in order to monopolize the camphor trade.

Camphor's volatile oil is distilled from the leaves, roots, and wood of the camphor tree. The tree was introduced into South and Central America in the early 19th century and ultimately made its way into parts of Florida, Texas, and California. By the late 18th century, the oil was commonly available and affordable enough to be prescribed medicinally to both rich and poor—unlike the more prized fragrant wood, which is used to make expensive luxuries like shipping chests and armoires to this day.

Folk healers, who often mixed camphor with goose fat or skunk grease, favored it as a preventive against influenza and colds. Pioneers mixed it with whiskey and melted it with pork fat as a chest rub to clear congestion.

At the turn of the century, it was a nearly universal practice to wear a small bag of crystal lumps of camphor gum around the neck during winter. Enthusiasts believed that the fumes from the bags destroyed germs; others subscribed to the idea that the sharp odor simply kept other people (and their germs) away. In truth, camphor's aromatic oil, 2-bornanone, works somewhat as an external antiseptic to help the body fight off viral intruders.

Over-the-Counter Only

Although science has confirmed camphor's antiseptic, analgesic, and counterirritant properties, it has also declared that prolonged exposure to the fumes can cause poisoning. Ingestion of camphor can have an extremely toxic effect, and its topical use among small children, especially when applied directly under the nose, is strongly discouraged. Health Canada does not recommend ingesting camphor oil, nor does it allow the sale of camphor products intended for internal use. However, topical preparations with low percentages of oil are still considered safe; they remain available in some over-the-counter remedies.

Active plant parts Wood, leaves, roots
Uses Commercial topical salves, usually for loosening congestion
Cautions Never ingest camphor oil or any camphor product.

CANKER SORES

Canker sores, the usual name for recurrent aphthous ulcers of the mouth, were a common complaint among early settlers. Just about everyone had a remedy for "sore mouth," as the painful oral blisters were called, from an echinacea "chaw" to goldenseal root mouth rinses to soothing baking soda pastes. Still another method was bizarre: dabbing the canker with a wet diaper.

Settlers also relied on mouth rinses made of oak and pine bark, which contain astringent compounds (tannins) that shrink cankers. Folk healers continue to recommend oak bark extract today for this very purpose.

What Are They?

Canker sores are little crater-like ulcers that appear alone or in clus-

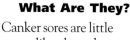

Canker sore soothers *include tea bags, baking soda, hydrogen peroxide, and salt.*

ters on the inside of the mouth and cheek or on the tongue, and may be caused by a localized immune reaction, usually to stress or minor abrasions inside the mouth. They may also be due to allergies or menstruation. The sores usually heal by themselves within a week or two. Current treatments include anesthetic mouth rinses and over-the-counter oral analgesic gels; antibiotic rinses and steroid ointments are also prescribed.

Some of today's self-treatments are actually favorite old-time folk remedies: antibacterial table salt rinses and alkaline baking soda mouthwashes, which neutralize the acid secretions produced by the bacteria coating a canker. Other alkaline therapies include dabbing the canker with hydrogen peroxide or a tea bag, or dissolving an antacid in the mouth. Reducing stress and avoiding spicy or citrus foods can help, too. Many people also swear by *Lactobacillus acidophilus* capsules, while applicator sticks dipped in silver nitrate provide topical relief.

TABLE SALT MOUTH RINSE
Mix ½ teaspoon salt with ½ cup warm water. Swish in the mouth and spit out. Repeat several times a day.

GOLDENSEAL The gold-colored root of goldenseal has modest antiseptic and anti-inflammatory properties. To make a strong tea, use 6 teaspoons powdered root, available in bulk and capsule form. Add to 1 cup boiling water, stir well, and let cool. Swish the tea in your mouth three to four times daily. (Do not drink; the safety of goldenseal taken internally has not been determined.) Some herbalists recommend a mixture of ½ teaspoon goldenseal powder and ¼ teaspoon salt in 1 cup warm water. But don't overdo it: too many applications or extended use can cause severe ulceration of the skin as well as other side effects.

MYRRH Prescribed by early North American and modern German doctors for topical treatment of moderate inflammation of oral tissue, this imported gum resin contains astringent and antimicrobial compounds. Dab undiluted tincture of myrrh on the sore two to three times daily, or make a mouth rinse with 5 to 10 drops in a glass of water.

SAGE As a mouth rinse—not tea—use 2 teaspoons of the herb in 1 cup boiling water. Because of the high content of thujone in the volatile oil, drinking sage tea frequently is considered unsafe and is strongly discouraged.

CALENDULA This herb, also known as pot marigold, has been found to promote wound healing when applied topically. To make a mouthwash, add 1 teaspoon chopped leaves to 1 cup boiling water. Alternatively, add 1 teaspoon calendula tincture to 1 cup water.

CASCARA SAGRADA

Rhamnus purshiana
CASCARA, CHITTAM BARK, WAHOO,
CALIFORNIA BUCKTHORN, SACRED BARK

Traditionally, the bark of the cascara sagrada tree was one of the most effective and widely used laxatives that folk medicine had to offer. Seventeenth-century Spanish and Mexican explorers gave this member of the buckthorn family its name, which means "sacred bark"— perhaps because it was so highly valued by the Indians they encountered. The Cherokee used cascara sagrada and other members of the *Rhamnus* genus not only as a treatment for stomach upset and constipation but also as a remedy for itching and eye infections. Early settlers followed their example, drinking a cold tea as a tonic and boiling the bark to make a laxative. The bark was popular among North American herbalists throughout the 19th century, and in 1877 it came to the attention of doctors. In 1890 cascara sagrada was listed in the U.S. Pharmacopeia.

Today cascara sagrada is gathered in the forests of the Pacific Northwest and is marketed as liquids, pills, and powder; its bitter taste is masked by licorice and other flavorings. In some parts of California, the flowers of this plant are the source of a honey, which has a slightly laxative effect.

Cascara is effective because of two active ingredients: free anthraquinone, which speeds up movement in the large intestine, and various sugar derivatives, which signal a nerve center in the large intestine to stimulate a bowel movement. For this reason, the herb is classified as a stimulant laxative. When taking it for constipation, wait at least two hours before taking any other medications, since cascara can lessen their effects. Cascara preparations are typically taken at night, to be effective the next morning.

Like all stimulant laxatives, cascara sagrada should be used only occasionally and for short periods of time. Recent scientific studies indicate a possible link between chronic use of the herb and cancers of the colon and rectum. Moreover, prolonged use can also trigger chronic diarrhea and potassium deficiency, and may even damage the nerves and muscles of the intestines, creating dependency on the herb or another laxative— or even enemas—for evacuation.

Active plant parts Bark
Uses Constipation
Cautions Do not use for more than a week without a doctor's supervision. Cascara sagrada should be avoided by pregnant women, nursing mothers, children under age six, and people with stomach ulcers or irritable bowel syndrome. Prolonged use of cascara-like laxatives can make a person dependent on this stimulation for a bowel movement, while withdrawal can result in constipation and bloating.

CASTOR OIL

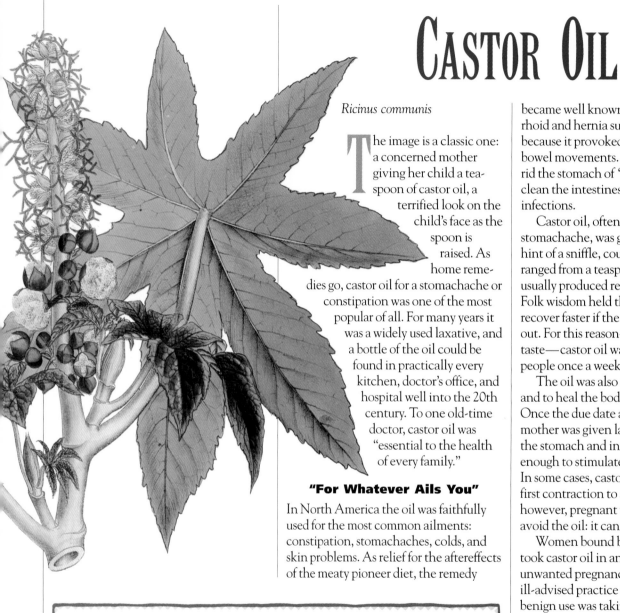

Ricinus communis

The image is a classic one: a concerned mother giving her child a teaspoon of castor oil, a terrified look on the child's face as the spoon is raised. As home remedies go, castor oil for a stomachache or constipation was one of the most popular of all. For many years it was a widely used laxative, and a bottle of the oil could be found in practically every kitchen, doctor's office, and hospital well into the 20th century. To one old-time doctor, castor oil was "essential to the health of every family."

"For Whatever Ails You"

In North America the oil was faithfully used for the most common ailments: constipation, stomachaches, colds, and skin problems. As relief for the aftereffects of the meaty pioneer diet, the remedy became well known as a laxative. Hemorrhoid and hernia sufferers also took the oil because it provoked quicker and easier bowel movements. It was also believed to rid the stomach of "black bile" and to clean the intestines of diarrhea-causing infections.

Castor oil, often used to treat colds and stomachache, was given at the slightest hint of a sniffle, cough, or cramp. Doses ranged from a teaspoon to a half ladle and usually produced results within hours. Folk wisdom held that the body would recover faster if the system was cleaned out. For this reason—and despite its awful taste—castor oil was taken by some people once a week for good health.

The oil was also used to induce labor and to heal the body after childbirth. Once the due date arrived, the expectant mother was given large doses: the jolt to the stomach and intestines was often enough to stimulate uterine contractions. In some cases, castor oil was given at the first contraction to speed delivery. Today, however, pregnant women are advised to avoid the oil: it can cause miscarriage.

Women bound by slavery sometimes took castor oil in an attempt to terminate unwanted pregnancies, a dangerous and ill-advised practice then as now. A more benign use was taking the oil as a spring tonic to purify the blood and to "lubricate the joints" that had stiffened over the winter months.

A Magic Skin Healer?

Applying the oil to the skin was also common. In cases of burns, ringworm,

---

Uses Constipation (internally), skin problems (topically)
Cautions Castor seeds contain ricin, one of the deadliest natural substances known, and should never be eaten; a single seed may be fatal to a child. Poisoning is a medical emergency and is characterized by burning of the mouth and throat, severe stomach pains, and dulled vision. The leaves may also induce poisoning. Only proper steam treatment of the pressed seed cake can denature the poison. The processed oil is not poisonous but may induce vomiting, miscarriage, or allergic reactions; pregnant women should avoid it.

and rashes, it soothed and softened the skin. Devotees of the oil claimed that it could eradicate warts, moles, and liver spots in a matter of weeks. Bruises, frostbite, dandruff, earache, and diaper rash were also treated topically, and the oil made an odorless, skin-friendly soap. Pioneers applied it to thinning hair, eye irritations, hemorrhoids, corns, calluses, and sore feet (in many parts of the continent, it was brushed on the skin with a feather). The oil was also used by nursing mothers to soothe sore breasts and increase the flow of breast milk.

A castor oil "pack"—flannel or another fabric soaked in the oil and heated with a hot towel or heating pad—was placed on the chest to relieve congestion or on the joints to relieve pain. When applied to the abdomen, the pack was said to act as a mild laxative and to improve the health of the internal organs, regulate metabolism, and cure infections.

Castor oil does contain properties that soften the skin and soothe the eyes, and it is a common ingredient in cosmetics.

Dangerous Seeds

Castor seeds contain ricin, a dangerous poison, and ingestion of the seeds is a medical emergency. Castor oil is extracted by means of cold compression—pressing the small, tough seeds with great force—and steam treatment. In this process, it is denatured and becomes safe to use.

The ricinoleic acid in the oil stimulates the intestinal walls and can provoke a bowel movement within two to eight hours. The usual dose is 1 to 3 teaspoons; larger amounts may cause vomiting or abdominal pain. Since the oil results in evacuation of the bowels, for general use, doctors recommend laxatives that are less potent. Furthermore, laxatives should not be given to children under six years of age.

Lasting Childhood Memories

Castor oil's harsh taste and pungent smell made it hard to forget, and many older folks can clearly remember the fear and queasiness it provoked when taking it as children. There were many reasons for giving the oil to youngsters: stomachaches, colds, and as a means of getting them to pass accidentally swallowed objects. It was even used to deter pouting and misbehaving and as a punishment: those who got out of school early by feigning sickness were likely to face a large dose of castor oil when they got home. To avoid the dread dose, children muffled coughs with their own pillows and gladly went off to school when not feeling well. When administering the oil, a mindful mother would sometimes hold the child's nose to make it more bearable. The oil could induce gagging and was known to cause adults to vomit and faint.

Measures were taken to make the oil taste better. It might be chilled in the refrigerator and added to a full glass of orange juice. It was also taken with coffee or flavored with lemon, sassafras, or peppermint. Molasses was sometimes added, but this only made more of the stuff to finish—without improving the flavor. Sophisticates prepared a mixture with milk, sugar, and cinnamon.

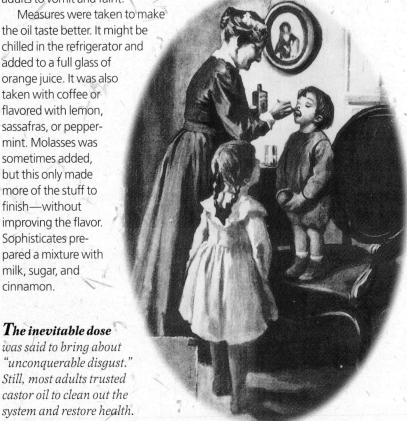

The inevitable dose was said to bring about "unconquerable disgust." Still, most adults trusted castor oil to clean out the system and restore health.

CATNIP

Nepeta cataria
CATMINT, CAT'S PLAY, CATNEP,
CATSWORT, FIELD BALM

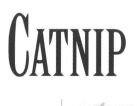

European colonists introduced catnip to North America, where it quickly naturalized and was adopted by Indians as a folk remedy. Beginning in the 1830s, Shakers promoted the sale of the herb. Though widely recognized as a home remedy for a variety of ailments, this member of the mint family has been little used in professional medicine. As a stomach soother, however, it found a place in the U.S. Pharmacopeia for 40 years (1842 to 1882) and in the U.S. National Formulary from 1916 to 1950.

An Herb of Many Uses

Early settlers chewed, boiled, or smoked the leaves to relieve toothaches, bronchitis, asthma, barrenness, and gas. In some parts, catnip tea is still favored for colds, hives, and stomach ailments.

Today catnip leaves and flowers are commonly used to make a mild lemon- or mint-flavored tea. Adults drink the tea to relieve gas pains, as a stimulant for menstrual flow, and to bring on sweats and reduce fever. The tea is given to infants as a digestive aid and to relieve colic.

Catnip's active principle, nepetalactone, is found in the flowers and leaves and is released when they are crushed, chewed, or infused in boiling water. Yet despite its reputation, there is little scientific evidence to support the many claims made for the herb. It does appear to act as a mild sedative similar to valerian, even though the chemical compounds responsible for this action remain unidentified.

Feline Euphoria

Nepetalactone, the same ingredient that may act as a mild sedative on humans, makes cats euphoric. But don't worry if your pet is indifferent—only about two-thirds of cats react ecstatically to catnip. Catnip euphoria is inherited, and your pet may not demonstrate this trait.

Although cats may get high from catnip, you won't. An article in the *Journal of the American Medical Association* in 1969 suggested a similar reaction in humans when catnip and marijuana were smoked. The article created a sensation and caused a run on catnip in pet stores. Nevertheless, later studies failed to find any evidence of any marijuana-like effects from this garden herb.

Active plant parts Flowering tops, dried leaves
Uses Anxiety, fever, gas, infant colic
Cautions Although tests of catnip have shown no significant toxicity and no severe side effects, some people experience mild headache, malaise, or upset stomach after drinking catnip tea. The herb may increase menstrual flow. Pregnant women should exercise caution when using catnip. Consult a doctor if any side effects occur.

CELANDINE

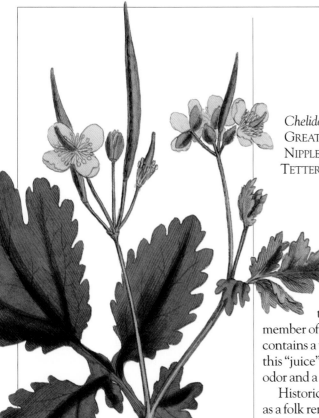

Chelidonium majus
GREATER CELANDINE, CHELIDONIUM,
NIPPLEWORT, SWALLOWWORT,
TETTERWORT

The weed celandine, introduced to North America by Europeans, is a common sight along fences and in vacant lots throughout most of the Northern Hemisphere. A member of the poppy family, the plant contains a yellow-orange resin in its stem; this "juice" has a peculiar, unpleasant odor and a bitter, pungent taste.

Historically, celandine has been used as a folk remedy for a lengthy list of skin ailments. The plant's juice was applied not only to get rid of warts, corns, and calluses but also to soothe rashes caused by eczema, ringworm, and poison ivy. It was also rubbed on burns to prevent scarring. Mixed with sulfur (called brimstone by early settlers), celandine was even supposed to fade summer freckles.

The herb's many uses were hardly confined to the skin. Celandine was thought to cure hemorrhoids and jaundice, while crushed roots mixed with chamomile oil were taken for stomach pain. Celandine tea was said to stimulate the gallbladder and liver. An ointment made by simmering the herb in olive oil or mother's milk was used for sore eyes.

Active Principles

If celandine is an effective treatment for warts and calluses, it is because of the skin-irritant properties of the alkaloids sanguinarine and chelerythrine (warts are thought to be caused by a virus, which celandine juice may inhibit or kill). It is also known that chelidonine, celandine's primary active principle, stimulates bile flow in the liver and gallbladder. There is evidence, too, that celandine has an antispasmodic effect on the upper digestive tract, and may be effective in treating high blood pressure and muscle rigidity.

The level of chelidonine in celandine varies widely, and fresh plants are a better source of the ingredient than commercial preparations, which may have little effect. Because celandine is a common weed, it may be easy to collect in the wild. Wash the roots and leaves thoroughly before putting them through a juicer (if the plant is in flower, add the flowers too). To treat skin problems, allow the juice to dry on the problem area and leave on as long as possible. Repeat daily. To make a tea (best drunk between meals), add 2 teaspoons minced leaves, roots, and flowers to 1 cup boiling water and steep for 10 minutes. For an eyewash, simmer 2 tablespoons fresh leaves and flowers in 2 cups boiling water for 15 minutes. Strain through cheesecloth before bathing the eyes.

Active plant parts Stems, leaves, and flowers
Uses Skin conditions, gallbladder and liver ailments, sore eyes
Cautions Side effects are unlikely if used in moderation. Handling the juice and crushed plant parts may cause skin irritation. The undiluted juice may cause severe irritation of mucous membranes and is a central nervous system depressant. Because of the presence of chelerythrine, the juice may cause paralysis; it is potentially toxic in large doses.

CHAMOMILE

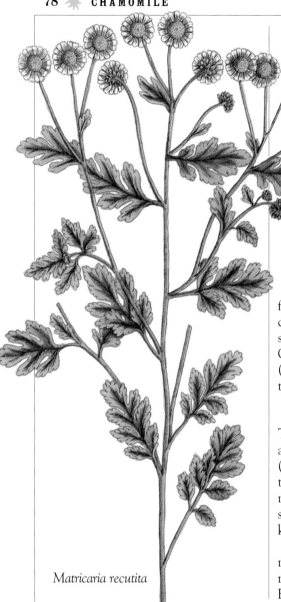

Matricaria recutita

Matricaria recutita
(GERMAN CHAMOMILE)
Chamaemelum nobile
(ROMAN CHAMOMILE)

The same chamomile tea that was used in early North American history—and for thousands of years in ancient Greece, India, and Europe—has become one of the most acclaimed of all herbal remedies for restlessness and indigestion. Many of chamomile's folk uses have received scientific backing, and in present-day Germany, the herb—called *alles zutraut* ("capable of anything")—is used in more than 90 officially licensed preparations.

One Name, Many Plants

The Greeks named chamomile "ground apple," from *chamos* ("ground") and *melos* ("apple"). There are numerous forms, but the German and Roman species are the most prominent. Both plants have a sweet scent, grow low to the ground, and are known by a variety of common names.

The German species was the chamomile of choice on the European continent, and remains so today in both Europe and North America. German immigrants introduced it here, where it has naturalized. A branching annual, it grows 80 cm (2½ ft) high and is sometimes called Hungarian chamomile, wild chamomile, or sweet false chamomile.

The Roman species, on the other hand, was used primarily in England and its colonies, where it was called English chamomile. At one time it was scientifically classified *Anthemis nobilis*, and it has also gone by the names of manzanilla and garden chamomile. Unlike its German cousin, this plant is a creeping perennial that grows no higher than 30 cm (1 ft).

Although the two chamomiles are fairly similar and have been used to treat many of the same ailments, their chemical compounds differ. In the United States and Canada, German chamomile has been considered more efficacious and is used more often than the Roman type.

Inside and Out

German chamomile was historically made into a tea for both internal and external use. Cold-related symptoms, stomach and gastrointestinal problems, toothaches, convulsions, and insomnia were all said to be relieved by a cup of tea. Typically, children suffering from the same ailments were given a teaspoonful of the soothing beverage.

Centuries ago, Egyptians drank the tea to treat colds, malarial chills, and agitation. More recently, the Pennsylvania Dutch used it for upset stomach, diarrhea, and anxiety and to calm fussy babies.

Active plant parts Flower heads
Uses Indigestion, peptic ulcers, nervousness, menstrual cramps, sore throat, burns and skin inflammations, vaginal infections
Cautions Chamomile may cause an allergic reaction among those sensitive to ragweed and other members of the aster family: the flowers contain pollen and may cause dermatitis, although allergic skin reactions are rare. Chamomile can irritate the eyes and sensitive skin. It may also cause nausea when taken in large doses.

It was believed that the best results could be achieved by taking the tea between meals on an empty stomach.

A clean cloth soaked in a hot chamomile infusion and applied externally made a soothing treatment for back pain, gout, earaches, skin inflammations, bruises, and arthritis. The infusion was also added to poultices and used as a gargle or antiseptic wash. Inhaling the infusion's steam for 10 minutes or longer was believed to reduce congestion and clear up irritations throughout the respiratory tract.

Fabled Use

Roman chamomile was best known as a pleasant-tasting tea, although it was also used to treat many of the same conditions —indigestion and frazzled nerves, in particular—as the German herb.

The tea's virtue was immortalized in Beatrix Potter's famous children's story, *The Tale of Peter Rabbit*, treasured by children for nearly 100 years. Against his mother's wishes, Peter sneaks into Mr. McGregor's garden, eats too much, is chased by Mr. McGregor, and catches a chill while hiding in a watering can. When Peter arrives home, he doesn't feel well. His mother puts him to bed early with a dose of chamomile tea—"one tablespoonful to be taken at bedtime"— still a common remedy for ailing and anxious children.

In the United States and Canada, the same tea made from Roman chamomile was taken to calm an upset stomach. Dr. John Gunn, a 19th-century physician from Knoxville, Tennessee, who became famous for his herbal remedies, held the herb's medicinal use in high regard. He cited its ability to quell "green sickness" (either irregular menses or morning sickness), calm menstrual and other cramps, and relieve "nervous weakness" and "hysteric complaints" in women. He was also aware that large doses of the tea could induce nausea and vomiting.

Exhaustive Research

German chamomile has received considerable attention from the scientific community. Yet despite its extensive folk applications and continued use today, the herb's healing potential has not been completely

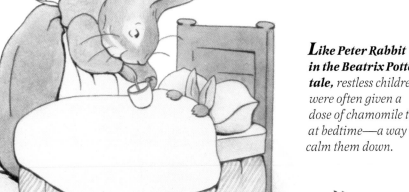

Like Peter Rabbit in the Beatrix Potter tale, *restless children were often given a dose of chamomile tea at bedtime—a way to calm them down.*

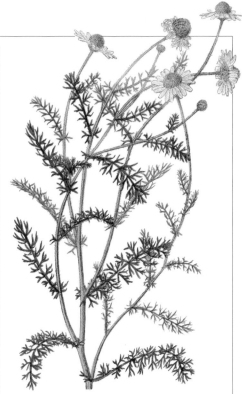

R*oman chamomile, used by early settlers, has been superceded by the German species.*

verified. Studies have identified numerous healing compounds, but the strength of these constituents in chamomile's most common form of use — tea — has been questioned. Because only 10 to 15 percent of the volatile oil is present in chamomile tea, the medicinal effect when the tea is taken for the short term is minimal at best. Researchers believe that real benefits are possible only after weeks or months of continuous use.

Nevertheless, scientists have confirmed two major healing components in German chamomile: chamazulene and alpha-bisabolol. Chamazulene, formed during the heating of the tea or extract, makes up 5 percent of the volatile oil and has proven anti-inflammatory activity. Alpha-bisabolol is antibacterial, antifungal, and anti-inflammatory and can promote the healing of burns and eczema. When ingested, it has shown the ability to protect against peptic ulcers, reduce fever, and exert a mild depressant effect.

German chamomile has also shown the ability to prevent muscle spasms and relax the smooth muscles that line the internal organs, such as the stomach and the uterus. It can also act as a carminative, expelling gas from the stomach and the intestines. These effects support the use of chamomile for stomach upset and menstrual cramps, as well as for general anxiety and mild insomnia.

Difficulties associated with pregnancy and childbirth were historically treated with the tea as well. Today, despite reservations that chamomile's known effect on the muscles of the uterus could stimulate uterine contractions, the tea is generally considered safe for pregnant women.

Even though chamomile flowers contain pollen and may cause an allergic reaction when ingested or applied externally, researchers have found that both the German and the Roman species may have antiallergenic properties. The potential effect is attributed to the as yet unconfirmed histamine-blocking action of chemical compounds called azulenes.

Chamomile Today

Many chamomile products are available today. In Germany, the herb is so popular that physicians prescribe a variety of extracts and derivatives for conditions ranging from ulcers to dental problems.

Around the world, tea continues to be the most widely used form — an estimated 1 million cups are drunk each day. If you buy tea bags, make sure that they are made with the flowers. If you are making your own from scratch, start with fresh

A Choice Herb for Women

For centuries, women have turned to chamomile tea to ease anxiety, menstrual cramps, and morning sickness. To a lesser extent, women have used chamomile cosmetically. Cleopatra used crushed chamomile flowers to protect her skin against dryness. European and North American folklore holds that the mashed flowers were mixed into beaten egg whites to make a softening and cleansing facial mask.

Such folk wisdom was put to the test in the early 1990s by Dr. H. W. Kreysel, director of the Dermatologic Clinic at the University of Bonn in Germany. Studying women aged 22 to 62, whose healthy skin had been made rough by ultraviolet radiation, Dr. Kreysel found that a chamomile cream restored skin health and smoothed out fine lines and wrinkles. These benefits were attributed to its ability to buffer the skin's acidity. The result is a nourishing and moisturizing effect.

Chamomile flowers, tea, and oil are added to baths to tone the body, while shampoos and hair rinses are also made

Chamomile's blue oil can restore health to dry skin.

with the tea (it is said to enhance the hair's blond highlights). Today countless cosmetic products—wrinkle creams, soaps, shampoos, and skin lotions—contain chamomile extracts. The oil is also used in aromatherapy, where it is dabbed on the skin or inhaled in a steam vapor to treat indigestion, anxiety, headaches, fatigue, and menstrual cramps.

or dried flower heads (avoid the pulverized or powdered herb). Pour boiling water over a heaped tablespoon of minced flowers, steep for 10 minutes, then strain. Traditionally, the recommended medicinal dosage calls for drinking a cup three or four times a day. However, for long-term benefits, a daily cup will do.

Chamomile oil, which is stronger than the tea, is also used for its soothing effect on irritated skin and in the digestive tract. But beware: the oil—blue when fresh—is often adulterated by unscrupulous manufacturers with cheaper blue-colored compounds. Buy only from a company with a reputation for quality products.

Chaparral

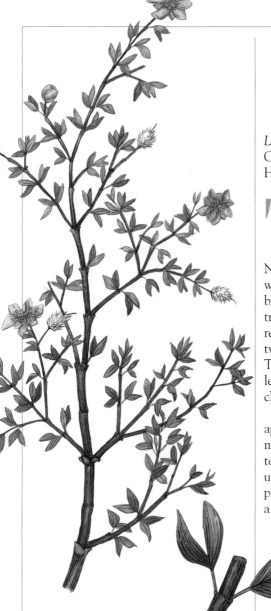

Larrea tridentata
CREOSOTE BUSH, GREASEWOOD,
HEDIONDILLA, STINKWEED

The chaparral, native to the Southwestern desert, gives off such a foul odor that its Mexican name—*hediondilla*—means "little stinker." Nevertheless, the creosote-like smell—which comes from a waxy resin secreted by the leaves—did not keep local Indian tribes from using it. The Pima rubbed the resin on sores and burns and they heated twigs and applied them to painful teeth. They also drank a tea made from the leaves and twigs as a remedy for snakebite, chicken pox, arthritis, and bronchitis.

Pioneers in the American Southwest applied the plant's resin to wounds and made a poultice for rheumatism. They took chaparral internally for stomach upset, diarrhea, tuberculosis, menstrual problems, and venereal disease. It was also a popular folk treatment for cancers of the stomach, liver, and kidneys. From 1842 to 1942, the herb was listed in the U.S. Pharmacopeia as an expectorant and a bronchial antiseptic. More recent claims for the herb—that it will make your hair grow or help you lose weight—are questionable at best. Still, there is scientific evidence to back up some of its other uses. Chaparral's active principle is the chemical nordihydroguaiaretic acid (NDGA), which kills bacteria and other microorganisms. NDGA is a powerful antioxidant, especially for fats, but Health Canada does not permit its use as a preservative in lard and animal shortenings.

The Safety Factor

The U.S. FDA took chaparral off its "Generally Recognized as Safe" list in 1968 as a result of tests showing that laboratory animals fed large doses for long periods developed lesions in their lymph nodes and kidneys. In several reported cases, people who took chaparral for periods of six weeks to three months developed liver abnormalities. Accordingly, the American Herbal Products Association (AHPA) issued a warning about the herb in 1992. It then rescinded the warning three years later, concluding that the liver disease was the result of an individual idiosyncratic reaction.

In Canada, chaparral products are not authorized to be sold for internal use. Health Canada has serious concerns about the ingestion of chaparral, since it has been reported to cause severe liver toxicity and kidney lesions in people. Chaparral is allowed, however, for use in topical products. It makes a good ointment for skin wounds and burns and may help rheumatism. To prepare a homemade salve, mix 4 tablespoons of fresh leaves and twigs in a liter of vegetable oil, steep for a week, then strain before using.

Active plant parts Twigs, leaves
Uses Burns, cuts, abrasions, rheumatism
Cautions People who have had liver problems should never take chaparral internally. Pregnant women and nursing mothers should avoid the herb entirely.

CHAPPED HANDS & LIPS

Like most pharmaceutical products used for chapping, folk remedies contain animal or vegetable fats and oils that create a moisture barrier on the hands and lips. Healing herbs and other substances are often added as well. Nineteenth-century folk also washed their skin with vinegar and applied equal parts of honey and petroleum jelly, used glycerin and rose water, and rubbed the skin with a lotion made from cooked-down persimmon bark and milk. Other old-time remedies ranged from the curious (washing your hands in the first snow of winter) to the unappetizing (washing your hands in fresh urine and letting them air dry). A more common folk treatment, however, undoubtedly soothed chapped skin: farmers simply ran their hands through the lanolin-rich wool of a sheep. Likewise, knowledgeable knitters have used unscoured or lightly processed wool to soften their hands while working.

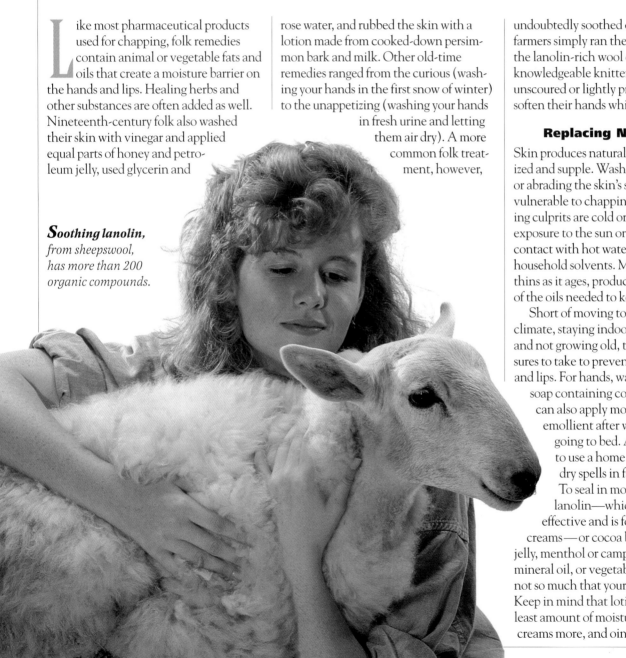

Soothing lanolin, *from sheepswool, has more than 200 organic compounds.*

Replacing Natural Oils

Skin produces natural oils to stay moisturized and supple. Washing these oils away or abrading the skin's surface leaves skin vulnerable to chapping. Other oil-depleting culprits are cold or dry air, prolonged exposure to the sun or water, and lengthy contact with hot water, detergents, and household solvents. Moreover, the skin thins as it ages, producing lesser amounts of the oils needed to keep skin supple.

Short of moving to a warm, moist climate, staying indoors, rarely washing, and not growing old, there are easy measures to take to prevent chapped hands and lips. For hands, washing with a mild soap containing cold cream helps. You can also apply moisturizer or a topical emollient after washing and before going to bed. Another measure is to use a home humidifier during dry spells in fall and winter.

To seal in moisture, apply a little lanolin—which is particularly effective and is found in many hand creams—or cocoa butter, petroleum jelly, menthol or camphor ointment, mineral oil, or vegetable shortening—but not so much that your hands feel greasy. Keep in mind that lotions provide the least amount of moisture to your hands, creams more, and ointments the most.

An increasingly popular remedy is the petroleum-based product known as bag balm. Formulated to soften cows' udders, it is available in farm-supply stores and some natural products stores.

Soothing Chapped Lips

Dehydration and exposure to the elements are the primary causes of dry, sore, cracked lips. Glaring sunlight, drying winds, extremes of cold and heat—all can deprive lips of the oils that keep them soft and supple. Weather, however, is not the only cause. Most people tend to lick their lips to relieve the dryness, but shouldn't: digestive enzymes in saliva actually promote dryness, and licking makes chapping worse. Even toothpastes and mouthwashes can cause chapping, and tartar-control toothpastes are especially drying. If your lips dry out frequently after brushing, try changing your toothpaste.

Some folk remedies for chapped lips are simplicity itself—such as rubbing your finger along your nose or behind your ear, then over the lips (the oil from the sweat glands helps keep lips moist). Some Indians used an ointment made from slippery elm. Sheep farmers often rub lanolin on their lips and have also tried warm mutton tallow mixed with camphor. Aloe vera gel, although not very palatable, can be applied directly to cracked lips to relieve soreness.

The best way to prevent chapped lips is to drink plenty of water—especially during cold, dry weather—to help maintain a proper level of moisture in the skin.

Beneficial Balms

The most common remedies for chapped lips are lip balms, which act as a barrier between your lips and the air to keep moisture and natural oils from evaporating. Balms containing beeswax and phenol are particularly effective.

Commercial lip balms can also protect against harmful rays of the sun. Look for an SPF (sun protection factor) of 15 or higher. Because lips tend not to hold balms well, frequent application is necessary. Creamy lipsticks also block the sun while keeping in moisture. Menthol and camphor ointments help lips retain moisture and soothe them when sore. If your lips are severely chapped or cracked, you may want to apply an antibiotic ointment to prevent infection. And make sure your diet includes sufficient B-complex vitamins and iron, which help make lips less vulnerable to chapping.

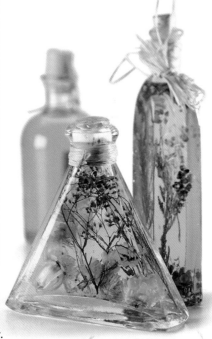

ALOE VERA MOISTURIZER Make a homemade moisturizing cream by melting 1 teaspoon white beeswax and 2 tablespoons lanolin (available at natural products stores and pharmacies) in a double boiler. Stir in ⅓ cup olive oil, 1 tablespoon fresh aloe vera gel, and 2 tablespoons rose water. Let cool before applying to hands or lips.

OATS The gluten and mucilaginous material in oats make them effective in treating dry, itchy skin. Oat extracts are used in emollients and in many bath soaps and gels. Refined oat powder is preferred for baths. Some people may experience contact dermatitis when handling oat flour.

Essential oils and tinctures *can be added to skin lotions.*

SLIPPERY ELM Combine the powdered inner bark with a little water and apply the resulting gummy substance as a lotion. Slippery elm is generally safe, though the pollen is allergenic and may cause contact dermatitis.

COCOA BUTTER & CALENDULA Also known as theobroma oil, cocoa butter is widely used as a base in commercial ointments and lotions. To increase its effectiveness on chapped skin, buy it in stick form, melt it in a double boiler, and mix in 2 teaspoons powdered calendula flowers or 1 teaspoon calendula extract. Let cool before applying to lips or hands. Although cocoa butter is generally considered harmless, some people may develop a skin allergy.

ROSE WATER LOTION Once a common household item, rose water can be bought in pharmacies. To make it yourself, combine 1 teaspoon rose oil and ½ cup distilled water. For a fragrant homemade hand lotion, mix ¼ cup of glycerin with ½ cup of rose water.

CHARCOAL

Charred wood *is the source of activated charcoal—ready for the taking in capsules.*

GAS BLACK, LAMPBLACK

Today most of us think of charcoal as the briquettes we pile on outdoor grills, but this material has had medicinal uses for hundreds of years. *Kings American Dispensatory*, published in 1898, recommended powdered charcoal made from animal bones to treat "scrofulous and cancerous affections, goitre, [and] obstinate and chronic glandular indurations [hardened masses]." It was also used in cases of "digestive derange-ments" resulting in upset stomach, vomiting, gas, and diarrhea. A lump of charcoal placed on a burn was said to draw the pain away, and charcoal poultices were used to prevent gangrene. The respected *Domestic Encyclopaedia* of 1804 declared that "charcoal prepared from maple wood, and finely powdered, makes a simple, efficacious, and safe toothpowder, and ought to be preferred to any other."

Charcoal's most important use was as an emergency antidote to poison. People who had swallowed poison were fed powdered charcoal to keep their bodies from absorbing the toxins. This works because charcoal has a large surface area relative to its weight, enabling it to attract a variety of complex chemicals and keep them from entering the bloodstream.

The Modern Form

Charcoal is still effective in reducing the impact of most poisons. Today, however, we use it in the form of activated charcoal, made from wood or vegetable matter that has been steamed and air-heated to remove impurities. It is usually given along with a laxative to speed the poison's trip out of the body. Although no prescription is needed for activated charcoal, be sure to get advice from a poison control center before taking it as an antidote.

Activated charcoal will not neutralize all poisons, nor will it work with alcohols, caustics, iron, or lithium. And take note: if you are told to take both the charcoal and ipecac syrup, do not take them at the same time. Instead, take the syrup first to induce vomiting; then take the activated charcoal after the vomiting has stopped—usually after about 30 minutes.

Cholesterol Fighter?

Interestingly, recent studies indicate that charcoal may have the same effect on blood cholesterol molecules that it does on poisons—that is, attract them and usher them out of the body. In one study, 7 grams of activated charcoal taken three times a day for four weeks lowered total cholesterol while raising the beneficial HDL and lowering harmful LDL.

What's more, charcoal is still used to relieve stomach pain, gas, and diarrhea. If you are taking any prescription or over-the-counter medication, wait at least two hours after taking activated charcoal, which can prevent another medicine from being absorbed. And do not be tempted to use charcoal as a topping for ice cream: doing so may lessen its effect. If stomach discomfort has not improved after a week—or diarrhea after two days—check with your doctor.

Uses Chemical poisoning, upset stomach, gas, diarrhea
Cautions If poison is swallowed, call a poison control center, your doctor, or a hospital emergency room before taking charcoal or any other antidote. For gas and diarrhea, babies and children under three should be given charcoal only for short periods; otherwise it may interfere with their absorption of nutrients. Do not use charcoal if you have ever had an allergic reaction to it, if you are on a special diet, or if you are allergic to any food or food additive. Charcoal should also be avoided by pregnant or nursing women.

CHICKEN POX

Thankfully, one obscure folk treatment for chicken pox—spreading chicken manure on a child's body to "bring out the rash"—has fallen by the wayside. Today a preventive vaccine, approved in 1995 in the U.S., may result in significantly fewer cases. However, it is not approved for use in Canada. Many people still look upon this childhood disease as inevitable—usually non-threatening, but a nuisance.

Caused by the varicella zoster virus, the illness's symptoms run through a predictable sequence: first comes a gener-al malaise, often accompanied by fever and swollen lymph glands. Then follows a rash of small, itchy red spots, sometimes everywhere on the body; the spots rapidly transform into itchy fluid-filled blisters. Finally, the blisters dry and scab over. All symptoms should disappear over the course of one or two weeks.

Itching and Fever

Faced with this lengthy process and an uncomfortable child, adults have adopted the same general approach to treatment for generations: relieve the itching, reduce the fever, and keep the patient rested and hydrated. To relieve itching, some folk practitioners bathed patients several times a day in lukewarm water to which they added cornstarch, baking soda, finely ground oatmeal, or ginger. To reduce a fever or induce sleep, patients drank hot teas made from boneset, sage, catnip, raspberry, calendula, or ginger.

A simple aid is a baking soda-and-water paste dabbed onto the blisters. And gargling with salt water lessens discomfort. Aspirin, however, is off limits: never give it to a child whose fever might be caused by chicken pox. Aspirin increases the risk of Reye's syndrome.

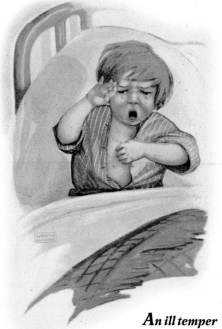

An ill temper
is another manifestation of chicken pox's effect on children, as shown in this 19th-century lithograph.

Chicken pox is a highly contagious illness. If you hear of a neighborhood child who is infected, watch your own children for symptoms. The virus's incubation period lasts from 11 to 21 days. Relatively few adults get the disease, but those who do often suffer more severe symptoms, longer recovery periods, and even a slight risk of complications, such as pneumonia or encephalitis.

See a doctor if ...

Any chicken pox-infected adult, newborn, pregnant woman, or child with the following symptoms should see a doctor.
◆ Blisters on an eye
◆ A fever higher than 39°C (102°F) for more than two days
◆ Uncontrollable itching
◆ Severe headache or persistent vomiting

YELLOW DOCK The tannin-rich root of yellow dock (*Rumex crispus*) relieves itching and helps to cleanse and heal sores. Boil 125 grams minced fresh root—not leaves—in 2 cups water (yellow dock leaves can be toxic). Apply the decoction to affected skin or drink ¼ cup several times a day. An extract of yellow dock is also available.

YARROW Early settlers used this plant to reduce inflammation, kill bacteria, and speed up the healing of wounds. Pour 1 cup hot water over 1 to 2 teapoons of the dried flower heads. Let steep for 10 minutes. You can either drink the infusion or apply it externally to affected areas of skin. Yarrow extracts are also available. Some individuals are allergic to yarrow. At the first sign of dermatitis, stop using this herb.

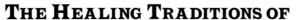

THE PENNSYLVANIA DUTCH

For centuries the Pennsylvania Dutch have believed what modern medicine is just now coming to terms with: *"Der Dokter wees net alles"—"The doctor doesn't know everything."* Believing that diseases can have spiritual as well as physical causes, these practical people employ a range of remedies and judge each by one simple standard: does it work?

Industrious, insular, and conservative, the Pennsylvania Dutch have been tending to their own medical needs since first immigrating to the fertile farmlands around Philadelphia in the 1680s. Their tradition of self-reliance, strong family ties, and effective, time-tested remedies have helped folk healing continue to survive alongside modern medicine to this day.

A Resourceful Folk

The Pennsylvania Dutch came to North America from the German-speaking regions of central Europe; the term "Dutch" refers not to their country of origin but to the word for the German dialect they speak: *Deitsch*.

Not only language but also beliefs and geography separated the Dutch from their "English" neighbors. While most of them belonged to recognized Protestant churches, the community also comprised such conservative sects as the Amish and the

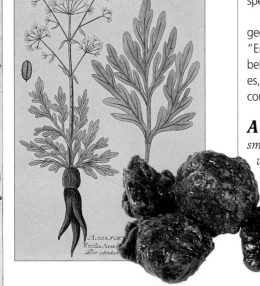

A mass of asafetida, *a foul-smelling resin derived from plants, was worn in a bag around the neck to protect against smallpox, flu, arthritis, and other ills. Also called "devil's dung," it was supposed to ward off the disease and absorb it at the same time.*

Mennonites, who are often called the Plain People because of their simplicity in customs and dress. These groups and others had fled Europe in part to escape persecution and brought with them a wariness of outsiders—including doctors. Settling in the countryside far from Philadelphia's physicians and apothecary shops, the Dutch had no choice but to rely on themselves when illness or an accident struck.

Cures were passed down orally through the generations and were recommended to friends. Families recorded proven recipes in the back of the Bible or a hymnal. Remedies were also printed in almanacs, pamphlets, and other publications.

Their materia medica was gathered largely from the gardens and woods outside their doors. Cultivated herbs, wild plants, and minerals were all employed in household remedies. Even common objects found around the farm—from horseshoe nails to straw—could become therapeutic agents.

Astrology and Theology

Both Christian and pre-Christian beliefs played a role in Pennsylvania Dutch medicine. Certain treatments, for instance, were governed by the heavens: the phase of the moon might determine when to shave off a corn or massage a sprain.

While some diseases were traced to natural causes or were inherited "in the blood," others were thought to be inflicted by God, either as a punishment or simply as part of one's fate. Likewise, faith and reli-

Magic or Medicine?

The religion of the Pennsylvania Dutch included numerous ancient traditional folk beliefs brought from Europe, such as assigning magical significance to numbers and looking to the stars, moon, and planets for guidance. Their beliefs were incorporated into their approach to healing and influenced how particular medicinal plants were raised and used or when a treatment might be undertaken. Such medical folklore was widely known in Pennsylvania Dutch communities and was recorded in numerous publications—written in German and English—beginning in the 1700s.

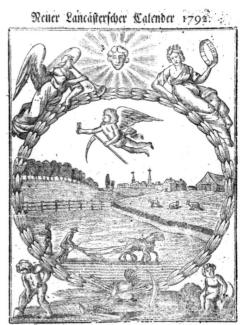

Neuer Lancästerscher Calender 1792

Almanacs like the 1792 volume at far right offered both medical and astrological information and were indispensable for those who healed by the heavens. While they contained such "rational" remedies as treating rheumatism with a rub of wintergreen and olive oil, they also featured the "almanac man" (near right). Such woodcuts showed which zodiac signs governed the health or treatment of which body parts—Leo ruled the heart, for instance—especially in regard to bloodletting and cupping, used to purify "bad" blood.

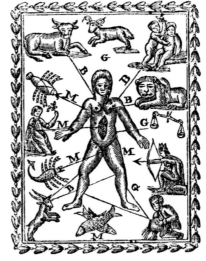

Herbs from the home garden and wild plants from the woods and fields were the mainstays of the Pennsylvania Dutch medicine chest—and their effects were thought to be enhanced by how and when the plants were handled. For example, to be potent as "wound wood," which helped staunch bleeding and heal cuts, a branch from an ash tree (far left) had to be cut in three strokes on Good Friday before the sun rose. The root of a white peony (center), which was believed to combat epilepsy, was at its most powerful if harvested when the sun was in the sign of Leo. And the leaves of the herb boneset (near left) had to be picked perpendicular to the stalk if they were to be effective against colds, picked upward if they were to induce vomiting, and picked downward if they were to be used as a laxative.

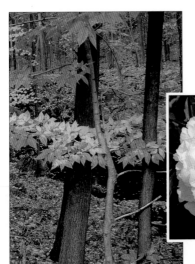

fact, healers were known for their faith in God, whom they credited as the source of their power. Treatments often entailed making the sign of the cross or invocations to the Holy Trinity.

Nonetheless, astrology might also come into play, dictating when to perform rituals. A visitor to the Pennsylvania Dutch in 1891 wrote that one powwower was "most powerful on Friday of a new moon, and that, on one such evening of the summer [when] I called upon him, he had three hundred patients."

Present-day Practice

Although folk-healing practices, especially powwowing, began to decline in popularity in the early 20th century, many Pennsyl-

vania Dutch remain true to their roots. Their reliance on tradition continues to reflect the experience of one doctor in the 1920s whose new patients always asked him, *"Kannscht du Deitsch?"*—"Do you speak Pennsylvania Dutch?" Acknowledging that his patients would not turn their backs on centuries of folk medicine, he remarked, "They can't be sick in English."

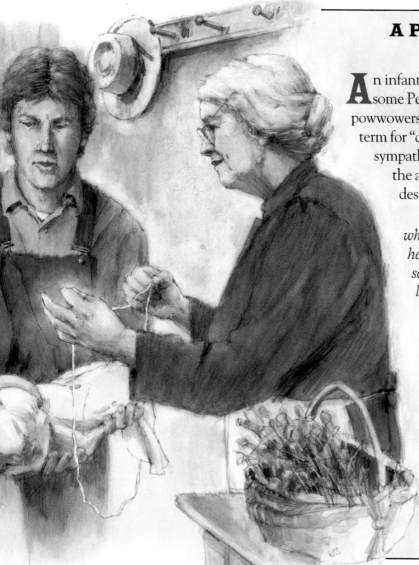

A Pennsylvania-Dutch Powwowing

An infant's failure to thrive is terrifying, and some Pennsylvania Dutch parents turned to powwowers for help. The cure for *abnemmes*, the term for "decline" or "wasting away," was often sympathetic—that is, the healer "captured" the ailment in an object, which was then destroyed, taking the illness with it.

In this case, the powwower uses a white thread, measuring the baby from head to heel, then measuring the foot seven times. She will tie the string in a large loop and pass the child through the middle—symbolic of rebirth or "stripping off" the disease—saying the baby's full name three times and invoking the name of the Father, the Son, and the Holy Ghost while making the sign of the cross.

The powwower will later wind the thread into a small ring and instruct the parents to place it inside a hinge on their barn door. As the thread is worn away and eventually disappears due to the action of the hinge, so will the disease.

gious symbolism were brought to bear in the cures for these ailments. A dose of a baby's baptismal water, for example, was prescribed for curing colic and croup.

Other illnesses might be caused by evil spirits or induced by witches and sorcerers, who were called *Hexe*. These evildoers were believed to have the power to cast a spell merely by talking with or touching someone or through the dreaded evil eye. When ailments were caused by the supernatural, only supernatural remedies could effect a cure.

Powwowing

A unique form of healing among the Pennsylvania Dutch involved a blend of folk medicine, magic, and faith healing known as *Brauche*. The word can be translated as "trying," "sympathy healing," or "calling a blessing"—but it is more widely known in English as "powwowing," from the Algonquian word *powwow*, meaning "medicine man." Powwow healers, or *Braucher*, included both men and women. Indeed, it was

tradition that the art be learned from an older person of the opposite sex, although practitioners could also be born with the gift.

To bring about a cure, the powwower conducted rituals using amulets, strings, herbs, and other objects and recited verses, prayers, or charms. There was a special ritual for each ailment, and techniques and incantations were documented in books. Sometimes the words were secret, and the healer said them silently; more often the healer said them aloud, and the patient repeated them. While sufferers did not necessarily need to be present during the recitation, they did need to believe in the realness of *Brauche*.

Cures were not always immediate. A powwower might "try" many times and still fail—a sign that faith was lacking, in either the practitioner or the patient.

When the ritual was successful, the *Braucher* might feel a chill surging along the spine. In cases where the cure had been exceptionally difficult, the powwower could be left drained and exhausted, as if the healer's strength had flowed into the patient's body.

While powwowing involved the use of incantations and could be employed to counteract sorcery, it was not witchcraft. In

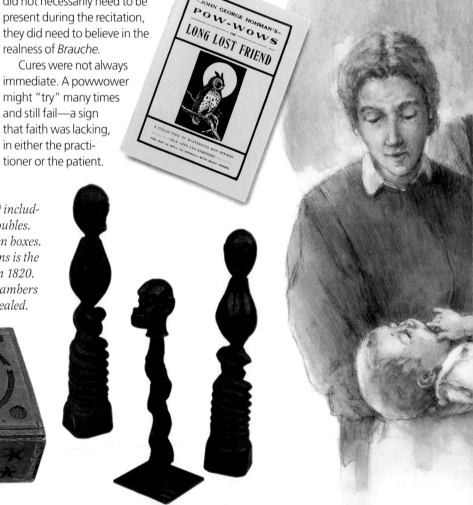

JOHN GEORGE HOHMAN'S
POW-WOWS
OR
LONG LOST FRIEND

A COLLECTION OF MYSTERIOUS AND INVALU-
ABLE ARTS AND REMEDIES
FOR MAN AS WELL AS ANIMALS—WITH MANY PROOFS

***P**owwowing aids (clockwise from bottom left) included linked hearts, which helped treat marital troubles. Powwowers often kept their materials in wooden boxes. The best-known collection of powwowers' charms is the* Long Lost Friend, *first published in German in 1820. Figurines carved from bedposts have hidden chambers to hold the hair or clothing of the person to be healed.*

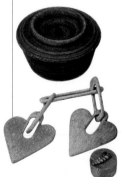

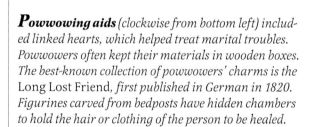

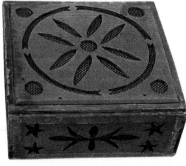

CINNAMON

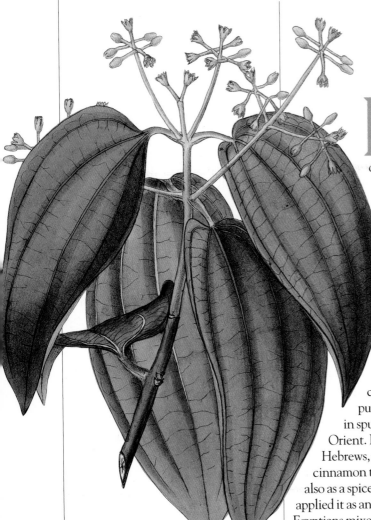

It may come as a surprise to learn that the simple act of sprinkling cinnamon on a piece of toast represents the continuation of culinary and medical traditions that reach back 3,000 years. The spice's long history is every bit as rich as the flavor it has imparted across the ages in cuisines around the world. In fact, securing a steady supply of cinnamon for culinary and medical purposes was a key factor in spurring trade with the Orient. Biblical Greeks, Hebrews, and Romans used cinnamon to treat indigestion and also as a spice in perfume. Moses applied it as an anointing oil. The Egyptians mixed it with other ingredients to embalm bodies. By the 19th century many Eclectic physicians were prescribing cinnamon for stomach cramps, flatulence, nausea, vomiting, diarrhea, infant colic, and uterine hemorrhaging.

More recently, cinnamon's standing as a medicinal plant has been questioned by the medical community, although recent studies may bring it into favor once again. An indication of cinnamon's reputation as a mere spice is the fact that a maker of a leading "natural" toothpaste lists cinnamon as an ingredient in the product but says that its purpose is simply to provide flavor. This is contrary to strong supporting evidence that cinnamon kills the bacteria that cause tooth decay.

The Spice of Life?

Cinnamon's role as one of the world's oldest folk remedies—in both Eastern and Western cultures—has been well documented. It was mentioned as early as 2700 B.C. as a treatment for fever, diarrhea, and menstrual problems. Ancient Greek, Latin, and Chinese texts contain references to the relief cinnamon provides for stomach cramps and diarrhea. Historically, the spice has also been prescribed for everything from kidney trouble, bedwetting, morning sickness, rheumatism, heart pain, warts, and toothaches (apply oil of cinnamon to the affected tooth).

Even an ancient Druid formula that was said to stimulate a hearty sexual appetite has been unearthed and updated by modern sex therapists. It calls for mixing 2 tablespoons skim milk powder

Active plant parts Leaves, roots, stems, bark, flowers
Uses Flatulence, mild cramping, gastrointestinal disorders, cuts and abrasions
Cautions Occasional allergic reactions to cinnamon may occur in some people, but the amounts of powdered cinnamon used in cooking are generally considered safe. Do not ingest large quantities of the oil or bark. Cinnamon oil can cause redness and burning when it comes in contact with the skin; taken internally, it can cause nausea, vomiting, and kidney damage. Pregnant women and people with stomach or intestinal ulcers should not use cinnamon medicinally in large quantities.

and water in a blender, adding ¼ teaspoon powdered ginger, ⅛ teaspoon powdered cinnamon, 4 tablespoons raw honey, and a dash of lemon juice. You can also add fresh fruit juice, if you like.

Although science has yet to prove that cinnamon is a sexual stimulant, many of cinnamon's medical applications have withstood the rigors of scientific testing. For example, recent studies have demonstrated its ability to stimulate the gastrointestinal tract, lending support to folk healers' long-held notion that the spice is an effective remedy for gas, nausea, vomiting, and other forms of gastrointestinal distress.

Recent Findings

That cinnamon is also a powerful antiseptic is no longer simply a matter of folk wisdom. A Japanese study has demonstrated its ability to kill fungi, bacteria, and other microorganisms, including the

A Valued Import

Cinnamon is native to a variety of the world's tropical climates, including Sri Lanka, the West Indies, southeastern India, and Central and South America. It is grown commercially in many of these countries. From the leaves, bark, stems, roots, and flowers of the tree come cinnamon oil, which is used as a flavoring for food and gum as well as in incense and perfumes. Cinnamon "sticks" are simply pieces of bark that have been stripped from young trees and that curl as they are dried. Pulverizing the dried bark produces cinnamon powder.

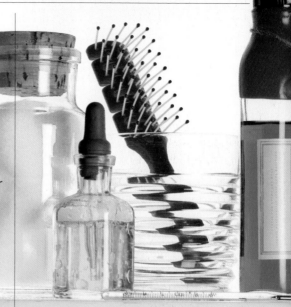

Cinnamon sticks are right at home in the medicine cabinet.

bacteria that cause botulism and staph infections. Furthermore, researchers in India have discovered that extracts from the leaf of the cinnamon plant attack the bacteria that cause tuberculosis. With solid scientific evidence to support cinnamon's germ-killing characteristics, the folk remedy that calls for sprinkling powdered cinnamon on minor cuts and scrapes after they've been thoroughly washed takes on a new credibility.

Another recent study of cinnamon's antiseptic properties, by German researchers, came to the conclusion that impregnating toilet paper with cinnamon "suppresses completely" the cause of most urinary tract infections and the fungus responsible for vaginal yeast infections. The researchers went on to argue that urinary tract infections in women could be eliminated worldwide if such a product was made available globally.

Even more promising are the findings of the United States Department of Agriculture, which foresees a role for cinnamon in the treatment of Type II, or non-insulin-dependent, diabetes. In Type II diabetes, the pancreas produces insulin, but the body is unable to use it efficiently to metabolize carbohydrates. According to the American ethnobotanist James A. Duke, ⅛ to ¼ teaspoon of ground cinnamon taken at mealtime may triple the body's insulin efficiency.

In addition to the cinnamon sold at grocery stores as a spice, cinnamon extracts and oil are available. Just be sure to follow the directions on the label: in large doses, cinnamon can cause gastrointestinal problems and kidney damage.

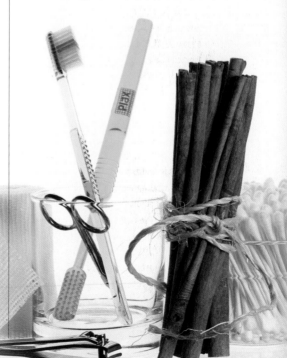

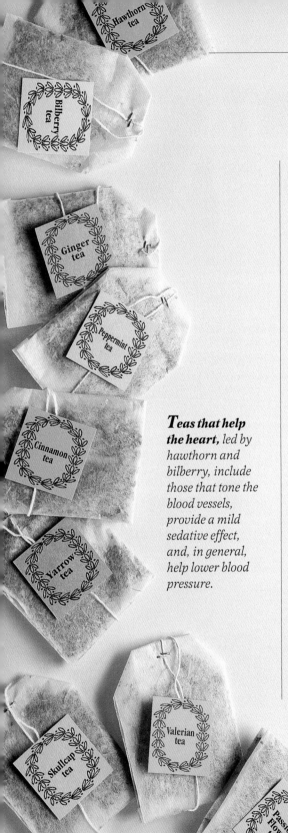

CIRCULATORY PROBLEMS

Folk medicine's teas and extracts have long been used to cleanse the blood, strengthen arteries, and normalize blood pressure. Nevertheless, the best treatment for such disorders is simply a healthier diet and lifestyle.

The circulatory system encompasses the heart and the complex group of arteries, veins, and capillaries that transport blood throughout the body. One of the greatest threats to the system is hypertension, or high blood pressure—a major factor in a number of more serious conditions, including atherosclerosis (arteries hardened by cholesterol-laden plaques). Cardiovascular disease is the leading cause of death in Canada.

Diet and Exercise

Smoking, stress, a fatty diet, alcohol abuse, and a lack of exercise are the major risk factors that raise blood pressure and imperil the heart. It makes sense, therefore, that the best treatment for improving circulatory health is a lifestyle that consists of regular aerobic exercise (at least 20 to 30 minutes at a time, three times a week), weight control, giving up smoking, averaging two or fewer alcoholic drinks per day, and adopting a diet lower in fat, cholesterol, and sodium. Diet and exercise become even more important for those with risk factors that cannot be controlled: pregnancy, old age, and a family history of high blood pressure.

Males in general are more at risk. In all cases, folk remedies can augment but cannot replace the benefits that lifestyle changes offer.

Furthermore, many circulatory problems—including aneurysms (bulging arteries), embolisms (life-threatening artery blockages), thrombosis (blood clot), arrhythmia (irregular heartbeat), and shock (inadequate blood flow to major organs)—are too serious to be treated with folk medicine alone. For these conditions, treatments include anti-coagulants (blood thinners), vasodilators (artery dilators), cholesterol-reducing drugs, and coronary artery bypass surgery.

Help for the Heart

Many old-time remedies sought to treat "poor circulation," although the underlying condition may have been fatigue, exposure to cold, low blood pressure, anemia, or weak or hardening arteries. In

Teas that help the heart, led by hawthorn and bilberry, include those that tone the blood vessels, provide a mild sedative effect, and, in general, help lower blood pressure.

See a doctor if ...

All circulatory problems are serious conditions and should be monitored by a doctor. If you suspect high blood pressure, see a doctor and have a proper reading. Any of following symptoms are possible signs of a circulatory disorder and should be evaluated immediately by a doctor.
◆ Pain in your calf while walking
◆ Excessive leg cramping
◆ Abnormal swellings in the legs
◆ Weakness and pallor
◆ Breathlessness and dizziness
◆ Heart palpitations

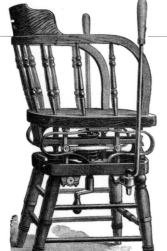

The Health Jolting Chair, promised by its makers to "increase the force of the whole circulation," was advertised at the turn of the century as "the most important health mechanism ever produced."

truth, there are only a few circulatory conditions that folk medicine can help treat. These include hypertension (high blood pressure), hypotension (low blood pressure), chilblains (swellings due to exposure to cold) and anemia (low concentrations of hemoglobin).

Two folk favorites are teas made from hawthorn and bilberry, both of which have been found to expand large blood vessels and reduce blood pressure. The minor vasodilating and anticlotting effects of yarrow, ginger, cinnamon, and peppermint teas help improve circulation to the extremities. Sedative teas, such as valerian, passion flower, skullcap, and goldenseal can lower blood pressure by inducing calm. Infusions made from nettle, gentian, and prickly ash may also have a relaxing effect.

Horse chestnut extract and witch hazel tincture were once popular rubs used to stimulate peripheral circulation. Invigorating powders and oils—added to baths and topical ointments—included rosemary, clove, lavender, calendula, mustard, cayenne pepper, coriander, arnica, lemon balm, and horseradish. For chilblains, poultices made from turnips, rotten apples, and white-oak leaves, and compresses of garlic, alum, ammonia, brandy, and vinegar soothed cold limbs. A highly original Louisiana remedy for hypertension suggested walking around with Spanish moss in one's shoes.

An effective modern herbal treatment is ginkgo. Taken orally, extracts of ginkgo tone blood vessels and improve circulation to the brain and extremities. Eating cholesterol-fighting foods, such as garlic, oat bran, apples, and raw onions can also help reduce high blood pressure.

Blood Tonics

Oftentimes fatigue, poor circulation, and such common ailments as colds and rheumatism were blamed on the blood itself. Patients drank blood tonics—usually teas made of dandelion, sassafras, corn silk, or red clover blossoms—to tone and cleanse the blood. Taken daily or every spring, tonics invariably failed to affect the blood, but they may have invigorated the body in some way.

Now—as then—very few home remedies may be able to help blood disorders. Iron-rich herbs, including hawthorn, burdock, yellow-dock root, vervain, skullcap, raspberry leaves, apricot, nettle, and hops may help anemia without treating the underlying cause. The common weed loosestrife, as well as hops, birch, sweet bay leaves, bearberry, alfalfa, and dandelion, may boost insulin activity, reduce blood sugar, and help control diabetes; however, studies on these herbs are inconclusive.

GINKGO Standardized ginkgo biloba extract is available in tablet form. The usual dose is 40 milligrams taken three times a day with meals. Glycosides and related compounds have proven effective against peripheral vascular disease and sluggish circulation in the brain.

HAWTHORN To make a tea, pour 1 cup boiling water over 1 to 2 teaspoons finely chopped leaves and flowers. Steep, then strain. Procyanidins and flavonoids dilate the smooth muscles of the coronary blood vessels, increasing blood flow. Do not use hawthorn medicinally without a doctor's supervision.

BILBERRY Flavonoids contained in bilberry may relieve diabetic circulatory disorders. To make a tea, add 1 cup boiling water to 1 to 2 teaspoons dried and powdered leaf. Steep, then strain. Or boil 1 tablespoon dried berries for 10 minutes, then strain. Large doses or chronic consumption of the tea are potentially toxic and are not advised.

WITCH HAZEL Applied topically, homemade or commercial preparations containing the extracts of witch hazel leaves, stems, or bark can help tone veins near the skin's surface and soothe hemorrhoids and varicose veins. A decoction made from 10 or more teaspoons chopped leaves in 1 cup boiling water can also be mildly effective when applied externally. The common distillate form does not contain the beneficial tannins and, as a result, has a weaker effect than the extracts.

CLOVE

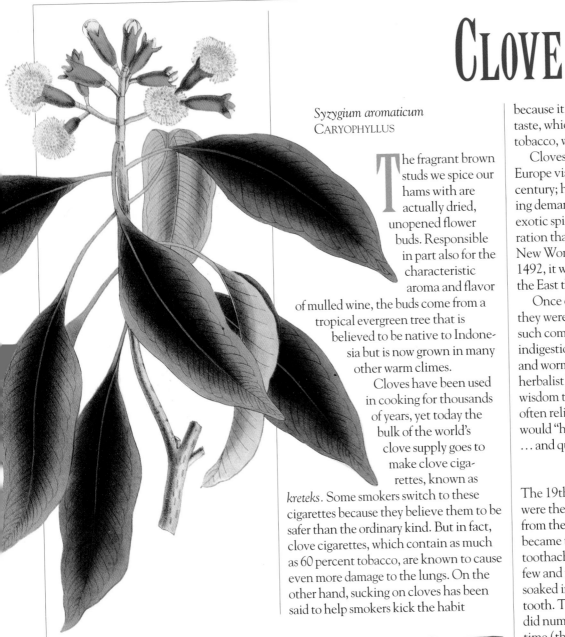

Syzygium aromaticum
CARYOPHYLLUS

The fragrant brown studs we spice our hams with are actually dried, unopened flower buds. Responsible in part also for the characteristic aroma and flavor of mulled wine, the buds come from a tropical evergreen tree that is believed to be native to Indonesia but is now grown in many other warm climes.

Cloves have been used in cooking for thousands of years, yet today the bulk of the world's clove supply goes to make clove cigarettes, known as *kreteks*. Some smokers switch to these cigarettes because they believe them to be safer than the ordinary kind. But in fact, clove cigarettes, which contain as much as 60 percent tobacco, are known to cause even more damage to the lungs. On the other hand, sucking on cloves has been said to help smokers kick the habit because it replaces nicotine's lingering taste, which increases the craving for tobacco, with the piquant taste of cloves.

Cloves had made their way into Europe via overland caravans by the 4th century; hundreds of years later, increasing demand for the tiny buds and other exotic spices helped inspire the exploration that led to the discovery of the New World. When Columbus set sail in 1492, it was a route to the spice lands of the East that he sought.

Once cloves became readily available, they were put to use as folk remedies for such complaints as nausea, vomiting, indigestion, diarrhea, toothache, warts, and worms. The 17th-century British herbalist Nicholas Culpeper, whose wisdom the early North American settlers often relied upon, advised that cloves would "help digestion, stop looseness … and quicken the sight."

Toothache Relief

The 19th-century Eclectic physicians were the first to extract the volatile oil from the clove bud. In turn, the oil became the foremost folk remedy for toothache. In the days when dentists were few and far between, a cotton ball was soaked in the oil and applied to an aching tooth. The oil had a fearful sting, but it did numb the ache—at least for a short time (the main component of clove oil is eugenol, which acts as a local anesthetic). In the absence of clove oil, you can bruise a clove or dip it in warm honey to release the volatile oil, then roll it in your mouth near the afflicted tooth to dull the pain.

Active plant parts Unopened flower bud and its oil
Uses Toothache, sore throat, mouth inflammations
Cautions Pure clove oil can irritate the skin. It is too concentrated for internal use, except for local application against toothache pain or as a gargle for sore throat.

Clove oil is not only an effective painkiller but also a potent antiseptic. Dentists use it to disinfect root canals and, mixed with zinc oxide, for temporary fillings. In the past, cloves were used also for the treatment of corns and calluses, infected wounds, and insect stings. Some people still recommend dipping a cut into powdered cloves to ease the pain and speed the healing process.

Clove oil was dropped into the ear to relieve earaches. Some preferred liniments made with equal parts oil of clove, hemlock, cedar, juniper, and wintergreen to relieve earache, toothache, and facial neuralgia. These mixtures were less irritating than pure clove oil.

Morning Sickness Medicine?

Clove tea was once drunk to relieve nausea and indigestion. A few drops of clove oil in water is still said to alleviate vomiting, and some herbalists recommend clove tea to help relieve morning sickness. However, clinical trials have yielded mixed results. If nothing else,

cloves help disguise the taste of bitter teas drunk to aid digestion.

For unknown reasons, the scent of cloves was thought to aid the memory. So was drinking a cup of sage tea to which four cloves were added. Cloves were also believed to improve the eyesight. The distinctive smell of cloves was thought by some to relieve depression and aid sleep. On a more intriguing note, eating cloves was rumored to "stir up bodily lust."

What Scientists Say

Clove oil has been shown to possess a number of medicinal properties, although more research is needed to confirm some of its most promising uses. In addition to its painkilling and antiseptic actions, clove oil kills intestinal parasites and a wide range of bacteria, supporting its traditional use against diarrhea and intestinal worms. Tinctures of clove are effective when used externally against ringworm infections, such as athlete's foot. Take note that the oil is irritating and should not be taken internally, unless diluted in another liquid.

Clove oil has been found to be effective against the herpes simplex virus. It may also function as an anti-inflammato-

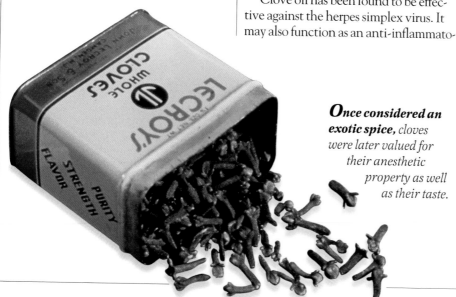

Once considered an exotic spice, cloves were later valued for their anesthetic property as well as their taste.

A Natural Mouth Freshener

For centuries, cloves were used to counter bad breath. During the Han dynasty in China, those fortunate enough to win an audience with the emperor were expected to hold a clove in their mouths as a sort of breath mint. Today clove oil is a common ingredient in mouthwashes and gargles because of its antiseptic properties. It may also help numb a sore throat. Preliminary research indicates that the oil may even suppress the formation of dental plaque.

To make a pleasant tasting mouthwash or sore-throat gargle, steep 2 tablespoons of bruised cloves and 1 tablespoon of bruised cinnamon bark (also a powerful antiseptic) in a half-liter of sherry or light wine. After a week, strain and bottle. When you're ready to use, add 1 to 3 teaspoons of the tincture to a glass of water.

ry, which would justify the historic use of cloves against rheumatism and lumbago. What's more, clove extract has been shown to be a powerful antioxidant, and may help heal stomach ulcers.

Clove oil can be purchased in most pharmacies. To make your own, bruise a handful of cloves, then place them in a jar and cover them with olive oil. Strain after a week, then add new cloves and wait another week before straining again.

Cloves can also be used to make pomanders. Once thought to ward off disease, these are good for scenting rooms and also for repelling insects and moths.

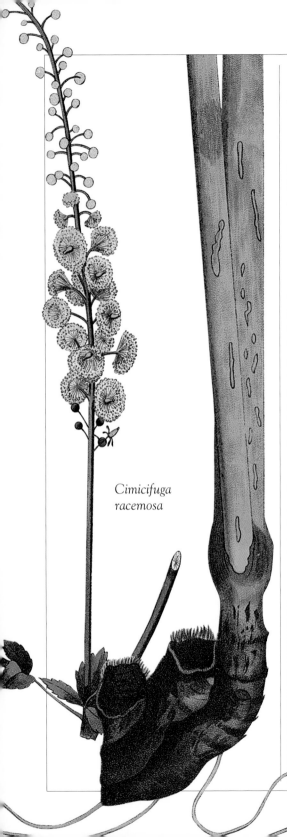

Cimicifuga racemosa

COHOSH

Cimicifuga racemosa (BLACK COHOSH)
Caulophyllum thalictroides (BLUE COHOSH)
Actaea alba (WHITE COHOSH)

Native to eastern North America, the cohoshes are three entirely different species yet were used by the Indians and the settlers for many of the same medicinal purposes. The word *cohosh* comes from an Algonquian word meaning "rough" and describes the texture of the rhizome, the medicinal part of the plants. The black and blue varieties were extremely popular—particularly among women—and, despite their potential dangers, are still sold today. White cohosh was also used, though less often; it is now known to be toxic.

Black Cohosh

Cimicifuga racemosa is a perennial that grows up to 2.5 m (8 ft) high, mostly across Canada and the eastern United States, as far south as Florida. Its black rhizome and white flowers are its identifying characteristics.

Four of the plant's common names—bugbane, black snakeroot, rattle root, and squawroot—reflect its uses and characteristics. Its genus, *Cimicifuga*, is Latin for "bug repellent"—hence bugbane. (Rubbing the foul-smelling flower on the skin can indeed ward off insects.) Once the flower heads form pods with loose seeds inside, they rattle in the wind, sounding like a rattlesnake; this helps to explain the root's use as a snakebite remedy and the common names of rattle root and snakeroot. Squawroot refers to one of its most common uses: relieving menstrual pain.

Feminine Relief

The Algonquins used black cohosh for irregular menstruation, menstrual cramps, labor pain, and the symptoms of menopause. The plant was also a principal ingredient in Lydia E. Pinkham's Vegetable Compound, which was marketed specifically to women to treat a host of physical and psychological ills. Belief in black cohosh tea's ability to affect the uterus was so strong that it was taken to

---

Active plant parts Rhizomes
Uses Menstrual irregularity and irritability, menopausal symptoms, estrogen deficiency
Cautions Black cohosh should be used only in therapeutic doses: large doses can cause nausea, vomiting, diarrhea, liver problems, abnormal blood clotting, dizziness, dimness of sight, headache, tremors, joint pain, reduced pulse rate, and increased perspiration; overuse may also increase the risk of breast cancer. Blue cohosh has still higher risks. Even therapeutic doses of blue cohosh may irritate gastrointestinal conditions and cause severe stomach pain; excessive doses can raise blood pressure and blood sugar levels. The herb's raw blue berries are poisonous and potentially fatal in children. Anyone with heart disease, high blood pressure, diabetes, glaucoma, or a history of stroke should not use black or blue cohosh. Avoid both black and blue cohosh during pregnancy; large doses or prolonged use can provoke miscarriage or premature labor and irritate the uterus.

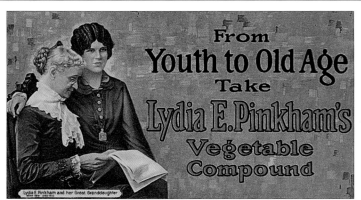

From
Youth to Old Age
Take
Lydia E. Pinkham's
Vegetable
Compound

Lydia E. Pinkham and her Great Granddaughter

One of the primary "vegetables" in Mrs. Pinkham's fabled compound, black cohosh may actually relieve the symptoms of menopause.

stimulate delayed menstruation, regulate labor contractions, and strengthen the whole female reproductive system.

More recently, a German study of menopausal women reported that 40 drops of black cohosh tincture taken twice daily relieved symptoms (hot flashes, profuse sweating, headaches, dizziness, sleeplessness, mood swings, heart palpitations, and ringing in the ears) after only four weeks of use and without long-term side effects. Although these results have been repeated, the limited scope of the study renders them inconclusive. A drug used to treat hot flashes and made from a derivative of black cohosh, remifemin, is available in Germany and Switzerland.

Folk Wisdom...

Natives used the root tea for rheumatism, upset stomach, kidney ailments, and sore throat. The tea was also taken as a tonic for the blood, heart, and nerves and—although ineffective—as a treatment for smallpox symptoms: fever, rash, and kidney pain. The herb was given if one was too "up" (insomnia and nervousness) or too "down" (fatigue and depression). The colonists used the same rhizome tea or tincture as an expectorant for respiratory problems, including bronchitis and whooping cough. Like the Indians, they

took the tea to treat fever, as well as for diarrhea and muscle spasms—from a crick in the neck to epileptic seizures. The powdered root was applied externally for "the itch" (eczema), snake and insect bites, swellings, and tumors.

... Meets Science

Black cohosh tea has been found to be mildly sedative and can lower blood sugar levels. In Russia, it is even prescribed as a calming "nerve tonic" to relieve high blood pressure. Furthermore, anti-inflammatory salicylates in the powdered root can help relieve external sores and rashes.

Despite these hints of efficacy and the wide support from Shakers, Eclectics, and orthodox doctors that lasted into the early 20th century, many risks are associated with black cohosh. It can cause abdominal pain, vomiting, and diarrhea. Large doses can cause dizziness, headache, and joint pain. Long-term dangers include liver problems and abnormal blood clotting. Counter to its traditional use by women, black cohosh can provoke premature labor, irritate the uterus, and increase the risk of breast cancer. Pregnant women should avoid it.

Even though its therapeutic value and side effects have not been fully investigated, black cohosh is recommended by

some herbalists for rheumatoid arthritis, skin inflammations, insomnia, and delayed menstruation, and as an expectorant for chest congestion. Whatever its application, black cohosh should not be taken for a period longer than six months.

Blue Cohosh

The bluish leaves, yellow-green or purple-brown flowers, dark blue berries, and shorter growth of *Caulophyllum thalictroides*, or blue cohosh, differentiate it from black cohosh—yet they have many parallels. Both plants are perennials and grow predominantly in eastern North America, and their dark-colored rhizomes were revered by Indians and settlers alike for their medicinal value. For their similar

White Cohosh: The Toxic One

Actaea alba, also known as *Actaea pachypoda*, is a tall perennial with small white flowers and reddish berries. It belongs to a different genus from the black and blue cohoshes, even if two of its common names—baneberry and snakeberry—sound similar. Shaker communities peddled the herb for its supposed efficacy against eczema, rheumatism, flatulence, and nervous irritability. Although many of its uses also matched those of the black and blue cohoshes, white cohosh was used less often than these: it was not as abundant in the wild. Another reason for its lesser reputation is its severe toxicity. All parts of the plant are highly dangerous (especially the berries) and should never be used.

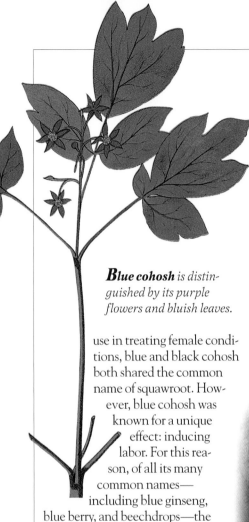

Blue cohosh *is distinguished by its purple flowers and bluish leaves.*

use in treating female conditions, blue and black cohosh both shared the common name of squawroot. However, blue cohosh was known for a unique effect: inducing labor. For this reason, of all its many common names—including blue ginseng, blue berry, and beechdrops—the most telling is papooseroot.

Use by Indian Women

Like its black counterpart, blue cohosh is reported to be one of the first native plants used for medicinal purposes. Employed by the Indians for a variety of ailments, its primary uses were to relieve menstrual problems and induce childbirth. The Indians also believed that the herb could induce abortion. The Ojibwa, Menominee, Mesquakie, and Potawatomi found it useful for pain, cramps, irritability, and breast soreness related to men-

struation. The tea was also taken internally and applied externally for vaginal infections. The Chippewa used a strong decoction as a contraceptive, and a tea made from blue cohosh and pennyroyal was said to regulate the menstrual cycle.

Like those made with black cohosh, these Indian remedies had some merit. Science has found that blue cohosh can boost estrogen production, provoke uterine contractions, and soothe inflamed tissue. It may also have immune-boosting and contraceptive potential.

"For Quick Delivery"

After blue cohosh was introduced to the pioneers—sometimes by the white "Indian herb doctors" who traveled the byways

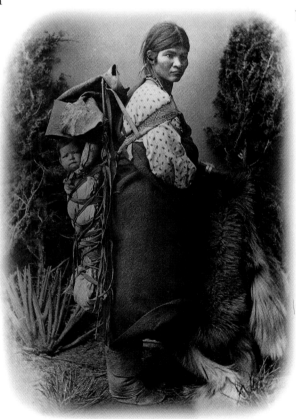

to peddle their wares—its uses multiplied to include the treatment of arthritis, back pain, colic, hiccups, hysteria, and intestinal worms. Still, as the Indians well knew, its primary use was as an aid to pregnancy and childbirth. A tea made from the rhizome was drunk for a week or two to ensure birth on the scheduled due date or to remedy a late pregnancy. In a practice still used today, midwives administered the tea once contractions had started in order to speed delivery, especially if the mother was fatigued. One ingredient, caulosaponin, can indeed trigger uterine spasms, but its unpredictable and potentially harmful effect on the heart prohibits physicians from recommending blue cohosh to pregnant women today.

Settlers and African slaves drank blue cohosh tea to treat gonorrhea, gout, and breathing difficulties. Larger amounts of the tea were taken to promote sweating and even induce vomiting. The powdered root of the herb was included in poultices for sores and rashes, as well as an old cancer remedy.

In contrast to its multiple uses, blue cohosh can produce many adverse reactions. Most significant, the blue berries can be poisonous, even fatal, if ingested by children. Due to blue cohosh's high methylcytisine content, large doses and prolonged use of the tea can raise blood pressure and cause long-term narrowing of the arteries. The tea can also raise blood sugar levels and should be avoided by diabetics.

Papooseroot is another name *for blue cohosh, traditionally used by Indian women to induce labor. Pictured here is a Navajo.*

COLD SORES

Also called fever blisters, cold sores usually appear in the mouth and on the lips, often in clusters. Although children are generally more susceptible to them, they are a recurrent problem for many adults as well.

Our ancestors, too, were plagued by these annoying blisters. Both Indians and white settlers found that powdered goldenseal or the thick gum of slippery elm bark were effective remedies. The fresh gel of aloe vera leaves was dripped onto the blisters, too. Some folk healers recommended dusting cold sores with powdered alum, even though its taste was said to be so disagreeable that it "curls the tongue to the top of the head."

Other practitioners advised rubbing a clove of raw garlic over the sores. A more unusual practice was to smear the sores with one's own earwax. (Some folklorists believe that this treatment originated with the *curanderos*, or folk healers, in Mexico and South America before it eventually spread northward.)

Herpes Virus

Cold sores are caused by the herpes simplex type 1 virus (HSV1), which usually affects the lips, mouth, and face. (It is not related to genital herpes, called herpes simplex type 2 virus, or HSV2.) When the virus first takes hold, the sufferer may experience flu-like symptoms and swollen glands; the virus then lives harmlessly in the nerve cells until another cold or fever occurs or when the person is under stress, run down, or exposed to sun or wind. Women are more susceptible during the menstrual phase of their cycles.

Eruption of a cold sore is often preceded by a tingling of the lips. The blisters usually last from one to three weeks, and may be itchy and painful. The virus stays dormant in cranial nerve ganglia and pops out in cold sores when immune resistance is decreased. Rarely, the virus may infect the fingers, causing an eruption of painful blisters. In people who have preexisting dermatitis or have undergone cancer chemotherapy, HSV1 may create a large area of blisters—a condition called herpeticum. Treatment of sores anywhere on the body involves soothing the pain of the blisters and forcing the virus to go dormant. Gargling with salt water or an analgesic mouthwash will also help.

If you have frequent outbreaks of cold sores, your physician can prescribe acyclovir, an antiviral compound that has been successful in suppressing the herpes simplex virus. Occasional outbreaks may be treated with herbal remedies. Among the choices are a topical application of infusions or decoctions of lemon balm, myrrh, goldenseal root, and hyssop.

LEMON BALM This herb is widely used in European over-the-counter products used to treat both HSV1 and HSV2; its volatile oil contains monoterpenes and sesquiterpenes, which have been shown to inhibit these viruses. To make an infusion, combine 2 to 3 teaspoons minced leaves with ½ cup hot water. Soak a cotton ball in the solution and apply it to the blisters several times a day. Lemon balm tea bags are also available.

MYRRH An ingredient in many commercial lip ointments, this gum resin is widely used to treat infections in and around the mouth. Tinctures are also available, and are dabbed on cold sores with a cotton ball. Alternatively, make an infusion by pouring 1 cup boiling water over 1 to 2 teaspoons powdered myrrh; let steep for 10 to 15 minutes. Apply to cold sores several times a day.

GOLDENSEAL Indians used a decoction of goldenseal root to treat skin conditions. The dried rhizome of the plant has been shown to have cytotoxic activity, making it useful against viruses, including herpes simplex. To treat cold sores, make a strong tea by pouring 1 cup boiling water over 2 teaspoons powdered root. Let steep for 5 to 10 minutes, then apply to cold sores several times a day. Products containing goldenseal are also available.

HYSSOP The tannins and polysaccharides contained in hyssop leaves account for the herb's antiviral and antibacterial properties. Infusions, tinctures, and extracts can be applied liberally to a cold sore. The volatile oil, however, should be diluted before being applied. To prepare, mix 1 part hyssop oil with 2 parts corn oil or safflower oil.

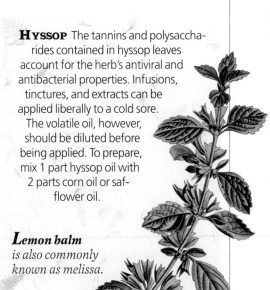

Lemon balm is also commonly known as melissa.

COLDS & FLU

It may be known as the common cold, but the misery it causes is nothing to sneeze at. For centuries man has battled this dreaded scourge, to no avail. The hard truth is that there is not one but hundreds of different cold viruses. What's worse, many of them routinely alter themselves, posing new threats at every turn. With no cure in sight, the same remedies administered by our forebears remain our first line of defense: chicken soup, hot lemonade, tea with honey.

None of these will cure a cold, but anything that eases the agony even temporarily is just what the doctor ordered.

In isolated communities, colds were relatively uncommon because most people developed immunity to the few strains of the virus in circulation. The appearance of a stranger in town, however, could literally make people sick. Today the average adult gets 2.4 colds a year; children, who have developed fewer immunities, often suffer many more. Bouts of influenza are less common.

Over the years the basic advice to cold and flu sufferers has not changed: Stay home in a warm (but not overheated) room, increase the moisture in the air with a humidifier if it makes you feel better (it will not help you get better faster), drink plenty of fluids, and get lots of rest. To relieve a sore throat, gargle with a solution of one teaspoon salt in a glass of warm water. Doing so will also inhibit the growth of bacteria, which can lead to strep throat. To keep a cold from spreading, cover your mouth when you sneeze or cough, and wash your hands frequently.

Feed a Cold ... ?

Feed a cold, starve a fever? Or is it the reverse? This dilemma has bedeviled folks for generations. Actually, the original saying was "Feed a cold, stave a fever," "stave" meaning "to prevent." Even with fever, the body needs nourishment; fasting will only make you weaker. Enter the world's most popular cold remedy: chicken soup, also known as Jewish penicillin. A steaming bowl of chicken soup, especially if made by a loved one, is often palatable even when little else may be. But does it offer any real medical benefits? Most likely. Studies show that, for some reason, hot chicken

Chicken soup not only comforts, it may also help cure what ails you.

soup is more effective at clearing nasal passages than other hot liquids are. It also has been shown to inhibit the movement of white blood cells, which contributes to inflammation of the lining of the respiratory tract. And, of course, the soup offers plenty of nutrition and fluids.

Many of the other standard cold remedies have their benefits, too. Hot lemonade, like any hot drink, decreases congestion (although the effect is short-lived), and it also provides a healthy dose of vitamin C, believed by many to help fight off colds and lessen their severity. Tea with honey also helps break up congestion and soothes a sore throat. Steam inhalations, to which camphor or eucalyptus may be added, help the lungs by loosening the mucus in the respiratory tract. The warm steam also serves to kill viruses in the nasal passages.

Skunk Oil, Anyone?

In addition to tasty tonics like tea and hot lemonade, there were countless other remedies, some far less appealing. At the top of the list was skunk oil, which was often taken with a spoonful of sugar. (Many people were convinced that this was the quickest way to cure a cold.) One country doctor advised patients who were suffering from a bad cold to "mix a little kerosene on sugar and eat it." In fact, a spoonful of kerosene, or even turpentine, was considered a remedy for sore throats, colds, and croup. Both highly dangerous, these substances can cause a chemical form of pneumonia if inhaled.

Second only to skunk oil were onions, perhaps because their pungent taste and odor were thought to overpower the virus. There were numerous ways to administer them. Many advocated eating them raw. Some people pressed an onion half between two plates and drank the juice

that ran out. More than one kitchen cupboard held a jar of raw chopped onions in honey or sugar, to be taken by the tablespoon every few hours to cure coughs. Because they are irritants, onions actually do act as an expectorant. To cure a cold or the flu overnight, some determined patients slept with sliced onions in the bottom of their socks to "draw out" the infection. Onions have indeed been shown to have mild antibacterial and antiviral properties, although wearing them in one's socks undoubtedly had more effect on the feet than on the cold.

Garlic was also used to fight viruses. Eating raw cloves was thought to break up congestion—that is, if one could manage to get them chewed and swallowed: doing so was likened to eating a fireball. Garlic "necklaces" were worn to ward off colds, and might have been successful, too, since they probably kept people with viruses—and everyone else—far away.

Recently, garlic has become widely popular as an immune-system stimulant, although its effects are still being studied. In addition to being an irritant, it has definite antibacterial and antiviral properties, especially when eaten raw.

Tea and Sympathy

Not surprisingly, teas were standard ammunition against colds and flu. Some Indians drank boneset tea (now considered unsafe) as a fever remedy. In the Smoky Mountains people drank catnip tea for colds, while in the mountains of the southern U.S., Indians made teas from wild cherry bark, as did the Pennsylvania Dutch. Western Indians used willow bark tea to induce sweating and break a fever.

If nothing else, teas help counter dehydration, and the warm liquid relieves nasal congestion. Some teas may provide further benefit. Willow bark contains

Is It a Cold or the Flu?

A cold is a viral infection causing inflammation of the mucous membranes that line the nose and throat. The symptoms include a runny nose, sneezing, watery eyes, and sometimes a sore throat, aches, and coughing. Most colds will clear up within a week or so.

Influenza is a more serious illness, and usually brings with it fever, chills, muscle aches, and sometimes back pain, in addition to cold symptoms. The flu typically comes on suddenly and can lead to secondary infections, such as bronchitis and pneumonia, which require treatment with antibiotics. It can pose a serious health threat to the elderly. See a doctor if your fever lasts for more than three days or if your temperature is over 39°C (102°F). Never give aspirin to a child with a virus; this increases the risk of Reye's syndrome, a rare and life-threatening disease.

To bring down a fever, sponge the body with a lukewarm cloth. Also, drink plenty of liquids in order to prevent dehydration and loosen mucus in the respiratory tract, thereby reducing the risk of complications, such as bronchitis.

small amounts of salicin, an aspirin-like pain reliever and fever reducer. Horehound, another popular tea, is considered one of the most effective herbal expectorants. Mullein teas contain what is called mucilage, a gooey substance that soothes irritated throats and helps quell coughs.

Coltsfoot teas were drunk to relieve coughs and loosen a tight chest, and although they probably worked, coltsfoot has been shown in recent studies to be a carcinogen. A long tradition of using wild cherry bark tea for coughs accounts for the prevalence of cherry flavoring in many of today's cough syrups. The bark is indeed a mild expectorant.

There's the Rub

Chest rubs were a popular if often smelly way to ease congestion. Heated skunk oil, bear fat, goose grease, or lard was rubbed on the chest and sometimes sprinkled with nutmeg. The area was then covered with a piece of flannel. One poor soul who recalled undergoing such treatment noted, "A person can't help but wonder if a child or even a grownup, would try awfully hard to get well in order to escape that mess on their chest." Often a bit of camphor, kerosene, or turpentine was added to the mixture. Camphor penetrates the skin to reach the lungs, where it loosens phlegm. An especially aromatic variation on the chest-rub theme was a

poultice made of skunk oil and fried onions. If the remedy did not elicit a cure, at least it offered a potent distraction with its smell.

Mustard plasters made of yellow mustard powder, flour, and cold water were used almost universally. Even those people who were badly burned by falling asleep with a mustard plaster on their chests still swore by them. The plasters stimulate local blood flow and irritate the skin, thereby creating a feeling of warmth. To relieve swollen glands in the neck, some people applied crab apple poultices; others used skunk grease or some bread soaked in hot milk.

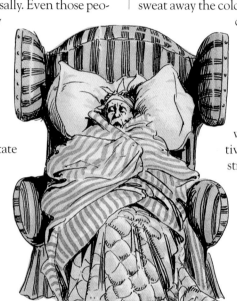

Don't Sweat It

Modern science tells us that it is impossible to "sweat" a cold out of your system, but folk medicine offered countless ways to try. Hot mustard water or ginger-water baths taken before bedtime were said to sweat away the cold overnight. (This didn't work, but the warm steam from a hot bath did help clear congestion, especially if an herb like eucalyptus, peppermint, or thyme was added.) Alternatively, one could drink a strong cup of hot ginger tea, then lie in bed under a heap of covers. Consuming

Despite the best folk treatments, influenza often demands complete surrender.

GARLIC High hopes exist for garlic's power to boost the immune system and fight viruses. Some herbalists advise eating raw cloves at the onset of cold or flu symptoms (if you cook or dry garlic, it most likely loses its antibiotic properties). Garlic capsules are becoming increasingly popular. Look for enteric coated pills, which pass through the stomach to the small intestine without being neutralized by stomach acid— and also cut down on lingering odor.

ECHINACEA In the late 19th and early 20th century this was the most widely used plant drug in North America, but only recently have scien-

tists discovered its ability to stimulate the immune system. In at least one study, echinacea was shown to relieve the severity and duration of flu symptoms. If you have a cold or the flu, take two capsules of freeze-dried extract or a dropperful of tincture in water four times a day. To prevent an illness, take half that dose for two weeks, then discontinue for two weeks. Do not take echinacea for more than eight weeks in a row, as it will lose its effectiveness.

WILLOW BARK The bark of the white willow is rich in salicin, the active ingredient in aspirin. However, it may not contain enough salicin to bring

down a fever alone, so it is best used in conjunction with aspirin or acetaminophen. To make a tea, pour 1 cup boiling water over 2 to 3 teaspoons powdered bark, sold commercially. Steep, then strain. Drink three to four times a day. Capsules are also available.

EUCALYPTUS This is a common ingredient in cough drops and vapor rubs. To relieve stuffiness and suppress coughs, put 4 drops of eucalyptus oil in a bowl of steaming water. Place a towel over your head, lean over the bowl, and inhale for a few minutes. To clear your nasal passages, breathe through your nose. This will loosen the mucus, which

ginger does in fact induce sweating, which can be useful for bringing down a fever if not for curing colds.

Perhaps nothing makes a cold-sufferer break a sweat like chili peppers, which are fiery. As any aficionado knows, they relieve stuffiness by making the nose run. Yet they also cause inflammation that, in the end, can cause more congestion.

Some families kept whiskey in the house for the sole purpose of healing the sick with hot "toddies" or "slings." One recipe called for water, sugar, whiskey, and lemon to be mixed together and brought to a boil. This was drunk before bedtime to break up the cold—and knock the patient out. An oft-repeated, if facetious, remedy for colds was to "hang a hat on the bedpost and drink whiskey until you see two hats." Despite the feeling of warmth alcohol provides, heavy consumption of alcohol actually makes the body lose heat faster by dilating the blood vessels near the surface of the skin. Alcohol also dehydrates the body and may even cause more nasal congestion.

The Warm Red Remedy

One of the most widespread cold cures was not grown in the garden or kept in the medicine chest. Rather, it was bought by the yard. The remedy? Flannel—especially red flannel, which was associated with warmth and healing. Worn next to the skin, red flannel was said to "draw out" the virus. Children were dressed in handmade flannel vests, worn under their clothing to ward off winter colds. Union suits were sewn for husbands subject to colds and the flu, and were even thought to prevent attacks of gout and rheumatism.

"Flannel" once meant wool. But in 1887 a reporter told of a "poverty-stricken article called flannelette." This "inferior" material, made of cotton, quickly gained favor because it was inexpensive and did not itch. When poultices were applied, they were covered with this friendlier form of flannel. Mothers warmed flannel squares in the oven and pinned them to the inside of their children's underclothes to treat colds. The fabric was also used to wrap premature babies. For back pain, flannel bands were worn around the waist. So-called belly bands were also made of the material: these were wrapped around a newborn's stomach and worn for five or six months to prevent a herniated navel, a disorder in which the navel swells because of a protrusion of the abdominal organs. Today flannel has lost most of its mystique, but there is still nothing that compares to the fabric for warm, cozy comfort.

---

you can then clear by blowing your nose. To clear chest congestion, breathe through your mouth. Eucalyptus oil is not only soothing but also kills some bacteria, helping to fight off secondary infections. Other substances to try as steams include menthol, camphor, rosemary, pine, and thyme.

LINDEN FLOWERS Also called lime tree flowers, linden flowers contain mucilage, which soothes the throat. They also promote sweating and may help break a fever. To make an infusion, steep 1 to 2 teaspoons dried flowers in a cup of hot water. Strain, then drink. Tea bags are available commercially.

ROSE HIPS The fruit of the rosebush, rose hips are an excellent source of vitamin C as long as you use them fresh from your garden—most of the vitamin C is lost in the drying process. For this reason, commercial rose hips tablets often contain added synthetic vitamin C. To make a tea, steep 1 to 3 teaspoons in a cup of boiling water for 15 minutes. In cases of fever, cold rose hips tea is a good thirst quencher.

HOREHOUND Horehound is an effective expectorant and is sometimes made into cough drops and hard candies. To make a tea, mix 1 to 2 teaspoons chopped leaves with 1 cup boiling water. Steep, then strain. You may safely drink several cups a day.

MYRRH A tincture of myrrh, a tree resin, makes a good gargle for sore throats. To calm the inflamed mucous membranes, gargle with 5 to 10 drops in a glass of water. Sage and acacia tinctures can be used similarly.

MULLEIN Mullein is a well-known cough remedy. The herb contains ingredients that coat and soothe sore throats. It also acts as a mild expectorant. To make a tea, pour a cup of boiling water over 3 to 4 teaspoons crushed flowers. Steep, then strain.

COLIC

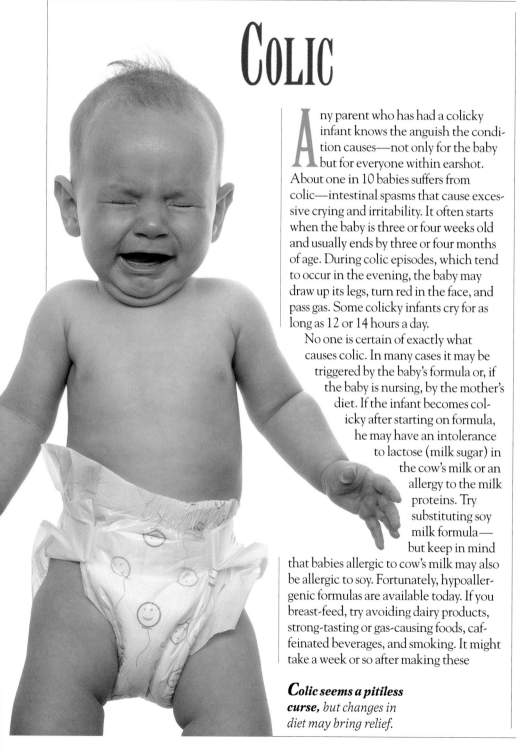

Any parent who has had a colicky infant knows the anguish the condition causes—not only for the baby but for everyone within earshot. About one in 10 babies suffers from colic—intestinal spasms that cause excessive crying and irritability. It often starts when the baby is three or four weeks old and usually ends by three or four months of age. During colic episodes, which tend to occur in the evening, the baby may draw up its legs, turn red in the face, and pass gas. Some colicky infants cry for as long as 12 or 14 hours a day.

No one is certain of exactly what causes colic. In many cases it may be triggered by the baby's formula or, if the baby is nursing, by the mother's diet. If the infant becomes colicky after starting on formula, he may have an intolerance to lactose (milk sugar) in the cow's milk or an allergy to the milk proteins. Try substituting soy milk formula— but keep in mind that babies allergic to cow's milk may also be allergic to soy. Fortunately, hypoallergenic formulas are available today. If you breast-feed, try avoiding dairy products, strong-tasting or gas-causing foods, caffeinated beverages, and smoking. It might take a week or so after making these

Colic seems a pitiless curse, but changes in diet may bring relief.

changes for the colic to disappear. If the problem continues, try cutting out wheat; some babies are allergic to it.

Some doctors believe that stressful surroundings contribute to colic. A relaxed environment, especially at feeding time, can't hurt. A gentle stomach massage can also provide relief, as can any rhythmic motion. Try giving the baby a ride in a car or swing, rocking him in a rocking chair, or holding him firmly in a car seat set atop a spinning dryer.

To make sure that the baby doesn't swallow air and add to the gas in his stomach, check that the hole in the bottle's nipple is not too large, and do not let the baby suck on an empty bottle.

Tummy Teas

Of all the folk remedies for colic, perhaps warm catnip tea, given in a bottle, was the most popular of all. Catnip helps relieve abdominal cramping and it is also a mild sleep aid. It was sometimes tied in small bags around babies' necks, probably without any beneficial effect.

Chamomile tea, another mild sedative and antispasmodic, was also popular, as was peppermint tea. Mint has been used for centuries as a digestive aid, and in America it was recommended for colic starting at the beginning of the 19th century. It is the main source of menthol, which calms the muscles of the digestive system and relaxes the opening at the base of the esophagus to let stomach gas escape. However, too much menthol can cause a choking sensation in infants. Pennyroyal, another member of the mint family, was also used, although it is not as effective. (Do not use the concentrated oils of these mints: they are toxic.)

Many swore by weak fennel seed tea (sometimes with catnip added), and for good reason. The oil in fennel seeds is a carminative, a substance that expels gas from the intestinal tract. Fennel was used to relieve flatulence as far back as Roman times. Cold infusions of crushed caraway seeds—the type found in rye bread—work the same way. Both caraway and fennel can be steeped in either water or milk. Alternatively, some modern herbalists recommend 5 to 6 drops of aniseed oil on a lump of sugar, or aniseed tea.

Cooled dill tea, called dillwater, is made from dill seeds and was yet another remedy for colic. Dill has an antifoaming action to help break up gas bubbles. Today some herbalists recommend using dill and fennel in combination. Thyme, another digestive aid, has also been long valued for colic. Besides feeding the baby these digestive teas, some herbalists recommend that mothers who are breast-feeding try drinking weak dill, anise, fennel, or catnip tea three times a day.

Other Colic Cures

Just as a glass of hot water was thought to relieve stomachaches, some found that a few tablespoons of hot water stemmed a severe attack of colic. In fact, hot water does diminish stomach spasms and relieve

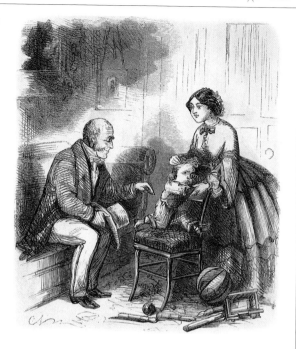

A 19th-century doctor makes a house call to calm a colicky child. His recommendation? Castor oil.

gas. (Test the water first on the back of your hand to make sure it is not hot enough to burn.) It was also believed that giving a baby two teaspoons of cold water by mouth "as soon after birth as possible" would prevent colic. Even more far-fetched (and inadvisable) was this cure: "To keep a baby from having colic, blow tobacco smoke on its stomach."

One Appalachian remedy advised tying a bag of asafetida, a foul-smelling plant resin also called devil's dung, around the baby's neck for six months. (Although asafetida is in fact a carminative, it would, of course, have to be ingested in order to work.) Another far-fetched cure was to feed the baby breast milk with a drop of kerosene. Turpentine was also considered an excellent remedy for colic, as was camphor. All three substances are

dangerous and should never be ingested. The Appalachians were right on track, however, when they prescribed massaging the baby's stomach with warm towels or warm castor oil. A hot-water bottle (or, as one old-timer suggested, a bag of hot oats) can also provide relief, as can a compress soaked in a chamomile infusion.

FENNEL The volatile oil found in fennel seeds has been shown to expel gas, thereby relieving abdominal cramps and flatulence. To make a tea, pour boiling water over 1 to 2 teaspoons crushed seeds and steep, then strain. Some herbalists recommend a combination of fennel and dill.

PEPPERMINT Long used as a digestive aid, mint leaves calm the gastrointestinal tract and stimulate bile flow, which aids digestion. To make a tea, pour 1 cup boiling water over 1 tablespoon crushed

leaves. Steep, then strain. Adults may drink several cups a day. Give the tea to infants and young children only with caution; the menthol in the peppermint may cause a choking sensation.

CHAMOMILE Traditionally used to relieve all sorts of gastrointestinal upset, chamomile flowers act as an antispasmodic, helping to calm intestinal spasms. To make a tea, pour 1 cup boiling water over 1 tablespoon crushed flowers. Steep, then strain. Those allergic to pollen may experience a reaction.

CATNIP Although scientific studies have yet to confirm the sedative qualities of catnip, it has a longstanding folk reputation as a colic remedy. To make a tea, pour 1 cup boiling water over 1 to 2 teaspoons crushed leaves or flowers. Steep for 10 minutes, then strain.

THYME Thyme contains thymol, a volatile oil that calms the gastrointestinal tract and also expels gas. To make a pleasant-tasting tea, pour 1 cup boiling water over 1 to 2 teaspoons crushed leaves. Steep, then strain.

COLTSFOOT

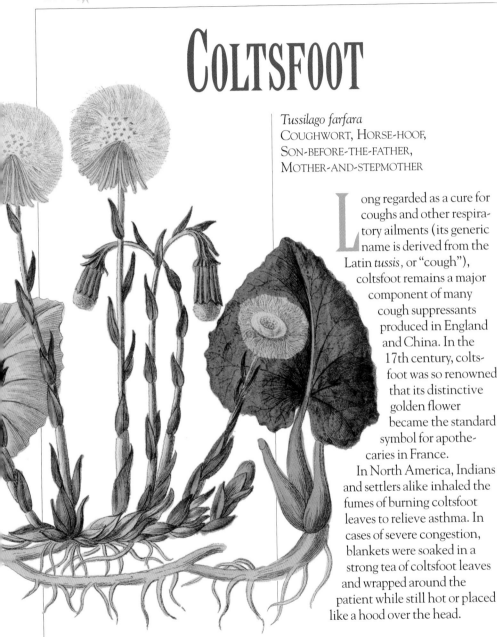

Tussilago farfara
COUGHWORT, HORSE-HOOF,
SON-BEFORE-THE-FATHER,
MOTHER-AND-STEPMOTHER

Long regarded as a cure for coughs and other respiratory ailments (its generic name is derived from the Latin *tussis*, or "cough"), coltsfoot remains a major component of many cough suppressants produced in England and China. In the 17th century, coltsfoot was so renowned that its distinctive golden flower became the standard symbol for apothecaries in France.

In North America, Indians and settlers alike inhaled the fumes of burning coltsfoot leaves to relieve asthma. In cases of severe congestion, blankets were soaked in a strong tea of coltsfoot leaves and wrapped around the patient while still hot or placed like a hood over the head.

To combat coughs, the leaves and flowers were also added to herb teas and syrups, typically sweetened with licorice and honey. Topical compresses made from infusions of bruised leaves were also used to "draw out" chest colds. Vapor steams made by boiling the leaves and flowers were prescribed for bronchitis, headaches, and fever. Headaches and nasal blockage were also frequently treated with a snuff made from the powdered root.

Very little of the plant went to waste in North America. Indian tribes in northern California valued coltsfoot so highly as a salt substitute that its possession became a cause for intertribal warfare. Settlers used extracts of the herb to flavor candy, and the silken, fuzzy seeds of the flower to stuff mattresses and pillows. Mature, woolly coltsfoot leaves wrapped in rags and soaked in saltpeter even offered a reliable form of tinder in the days before matches were readily available.

The Fall from Grace

As widely used and effective as coltsfoot was, it is now known to be dangerous in high concentrations. For this reason, it is no longer recommended as an herbal treatment. Recent studies have found the herb to contain a number of carcinogenic pyrrolizidine alkaloids (called PAs), large quantities of which can be toxic to the liver. Because of the presence of these constituents, the U.S. FDA has classified coltsfoot as an herb of "undefined safety." In Canada, coltsfoot has been limited to low-level concentrations in products approved for internal use. Great caution should be taken when considering ingestion of coltsfoot. Such external preparations as salves and ointments may be applied short-term, but for no more than six weeks a year; more extensive topical use is considered potentially hazardous.

Active plant parts Flowers, leaves
Uses Asthma, bronchitis, laryngitis
Cautions Ingestion of coltsfoot in any form, including teas, lozenges, syrups, and cigarettes, is strongly discouraged. Do not use longer than a 4- to 6-week period yearly.

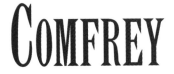

COMFREY

Symphytum officinale
KNITBONE, BLACKWORT,
BRUISEWORT, KNITBACK,
HEALING HERB

Comfrey, introduced to North America by settlers, was prized for its medicinal potency as well as for its use as a foodstuff. It was cultivated in herb gardens and was quickly naturalized in wild, marshy grasslands. Until recently, both the root and leaves were broadly used as anti-inflammatory agents for an almost universal range of maladies. Strong decoctions of the root or crushed leaves were used topically in poultices and ointments to heal bruising and reduce swelling. Comfrey was also used to treat muscle tears and sprains, as well as to set fractured bones—as evidenced by one of its common names, knitbone. Indeed, the plant's original Latin name, *conferva*, along with its botanical tag, *symphytum*, both mean "grown together."

Comfrey was prescribed internally as well—a practice that is now known to be dangerous. Plain comfrey tea was popular for easing chest congestion, healing stomach ulcers, and stabilizing the bowel. Decoctions of comfrey rootstock were gargled to relieve sore throats and were applied to bleeding gums. Gout was treated with a double dose of comfrey preparations: the powdered root was drunk as a medicine, while compresses made of a mash of fresh, chopped rootstock were applied to the affected area.

A Dangerous Drink

Comfrey contains two key compounds: a substance called allantoin, which promotes the rapid growth of new cells, and rosmarinic acid, an anti-inflammatory agent that also inhibits microvascular pulmonary injury. Along with these principal constituents, comfrey contains ample quantities of astringent tannins and binding mucilage, both of which soothe inflamed tissues.

Unfortunately, comfrey also contains pyrrolizidine alkaloids, or PAs, which can be carcinogenic and highly toxic to the liver. Since the discovery of these alkaloids—prevalent in certain varieties of the plant that are difficult to differentiate from the common variety (Russian comfrey is one)—the herb has been subject to severe restriction. Ingesting any remedy containing comfrey, including herbal tea, or applying comfrey topically to large areas of broken skin is considered to be extremely dangerous. Comfrey products intended for internal use are not permitted to be sold in Canada. Although some cosmetics and skin care products still include comfrey extracts, Health Canada does not recommend their use.

Active plant parts Leaves, roots
Uses Commercial preparations for ulcers, wounds, and fractures
Cautions Ingesting comfrey in any form, including tea, is extremely dangerous. If using topically, do not apply comfrey to large areas of broken skin. Do not harvest comfrey from the wild; it is easily confused with the similar-looking digitalis, which is lethal.

CONSTIPATION

Congested bowels—or "gripes," as constipation was once called—have forever preoccupied mankind. Our ancestors sought relief in countless ways: Epsom salts, stewed prunes, mineral oil, tea and suppositories made from senna bark, and the infamous spoonful of castor oil. Thankfully, a number of time-tested folk cures remain effective ways to put the bowels in good order; some, in fact, are key ingredients in commercial laxatives.

Until well into the 20th century, people viewed constipation as symptomatic of more serious illnesses, worrying that undigested food could remain in the intestinal tract for weeks, months, even a year. They believed that healing could be hastened and energy restored by purging the choked-up bodily systems of poisonous bile with mild laxatives, stronger cathartics, and "drastic purgatives."

Today constipation is viewed largely as a lifestyle issue. Dietary factors, lack of

Cascara sagrada candy
promised that those with
congested bowels would
soon see relief.

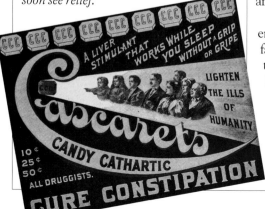

exercise, stress, and medication use are likely to interfere with bowel function, forcing the muscles of the colon to work harder at pushing a stool. Doctors say that simple adjustments, such as boosting intake of insoluble fiber and drinking more water, are good first steps before opting for a laxative, natural or otherwise. If you take their advice and are still straining, however, a laxative may be in order.

First, be cautious. Laxatives can be addictive, and they may lead to loss of important nutrients and permanent loss of bowel control. Many laxatives are, in fact, hidden in diet aids, and their abuse has been linked to colon cancer. The practice known as "purging" is now frowned upon by doctors, although colonics and other bowel evacuators remain popular in some alternative-healing circles. Chronic constipation may be a sign of an underlying health problem and should be checked out by a doctor.

Laxatives do have their place, however. All, whether over-the-counter or folk, fall into one of five categories, based on their function. One type, a stimulant laxative, irritates the cells of the colon wall, increasing muscle contractions that help move stool mass. Another type, a bulk-producing laxative, is the safest. It absorbs liquid in the intestines, swells up, and naturally triggers the urge to move the bowels;

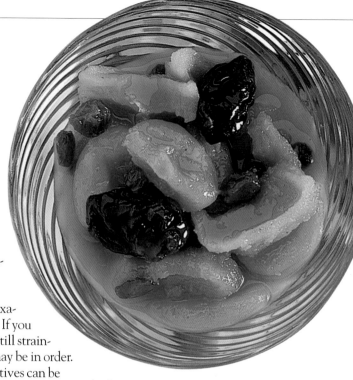

A regularity-enhancing
fruit compote *includes*
prunes, apricots, apples,
peaches, and raisins.

in this regard, it acts like high-fiber foods. A third, a hyperosmotic, is a salt- or sugar-based remedy that promotes absorption and intestinal retention of water, thereby encouraging a bowel movement. Fourth is a lubricant, which coats the contents of the stomach and eases passage of the stool. Finally, an emollient-type laxative helps liquids mix in the intestinal tract to produce a softer stool.

Helpful Herbs

Herbs have long been a regular source of laxatives; their roots, flowers, and seeds are eaten whole, pressed into oils, or made into teas and suppositories. Many have stimulant effects. At the top of the list is castor oil. As far back as the 18th century, the castor bean was known as a "powerful cathartic and gastric irritant" that could clean out the system within a few hours. Castor bean seeds, however, are poisonous, and the popularity of the oil has waned over the past decades. Other herbal stimulants include senna bark, buckthorn, and cascara sagrada. Early settlers brewed these herbs into warm teas, which have the added effect of calming the intestinal tract. All three can be found today in popular over-the-counter and prescription laxatives. A fourth stimulant, mayapple, is poisonous and no longer used.

As for bulk laxatives, one of today's most widely used is psyllium, obtained from a species of the weed plantain. Early settlers chewed the plant's mucilage-filled seeds and washed them down with water

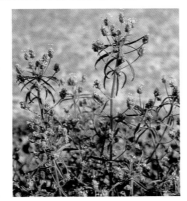

The weed called plantain is the source of psyllium, found in many over-the-counter laxatives.

or sugar or syrup to create a bulk-fiber effect.

Certain foods, particularly fruits, were also used often as bulk-fiber laxatives. Prunes, called "wild plums," were stewed and served up as "an agreeable and light article of diet for convalescence and in chronic diseases." As such, prune juice was a common ingredient in such 19th-century medicines as "Confection of Senna." Today prune juice remains a popular and gentle natural bowel regulator. Also popular were fruit-and-senna sticks and hors d'oeuvres or cocktails made with figs, raisins, dates, cloves, and cinnamon, all of which have gentle laxative effects.

First Steps

Modern folk healers and doctors alike agree that these lifestyle changes are simple and safe first choices before turning to a laxative.

◆ Drink more water and other fluids to soften hard stools.

◆ Exercise to wake up a lazy bowel and to improve intestinal tone.

◆ Boost fiber intake by eating more whole grains, fruits, legumes, vegetables, wheat germ, and brewer's yeast.

◆ Go to the bathroom when you need to; ignoring your body's signals can lead to a loss of normal bowel reflexes. A regular schedule can help.

◆ Avoid constipating medications, including loperamide, antihistamines, opiates, and scopolamine, and narcotics, such as codeine.

◆ Practice relaxation techniques: nervousness interferes with regularity.

PSYLLIUM The seeds of the plantain species *Plantago psyllium* can be an effective treatment for irritable bowel syndrome and hemorrhoids and are the laxative most recommended by modern herbalists and doctors. Add 2 teaspoons seeds to a little water and let them swell slightly. Take in the morning and at night with 1 or 2 glasses of fluid. Although rare, allergic reactions or intestinal obstruction may occur.

CASCARA SAGRADA Like other stimulant herbs, cascara contains controversial compounds that have been linked to colon cancer. But if used as directed, the herb is safe and effective. Pour ¾ cup boiling water over about ½ teaspoon powdered bark; steep for 10 to

15 minutes, then strain. Drink the fresh brew in the morning and at bedtime; use short-term only. Aged bark extracts are also available. Avoid cascara during pregnancy and lactation. Abuse can lead to permanent changes in the bowel and a potassium deficiency.

BUCKTHORN The European species of buckthorn, also known as frangula bark, is preferred over the American species in commercial preparations. A stimulant laxative, the powder is sold in bulk in some health food stores. For a tea, pour 1 cup boiling water over 1 teaspoon bark powder. Let steep for 10 minutes, then strain and drink. Overuse can lead to changes in the bowel and potassium deficiency.

SENNA Potent stimulants, the leaf, bark, and fruit of senna are found in more than 100 commercial products, including diet aids. To make a leaf infusion, pour warm or hot water over ½ to 1 teaspoon dried leaves; steep for 10 minutes, then strain. Avoid during pregnancy and lactation. Abuse can lead to permanent changes in the bowel and a potassium deficiency.

FLAXSEED Flaxseed oil, which is widely available, acts as a lubricant laxative. The usual dose is 1 tablespoon per day. The harder-to-find seeds have a bulk-fiber effect. Take 1 to 2 teaspoons crushed seeds with a glass or two of water. The seeds will swell in the intestines, providing fibrous bulk.

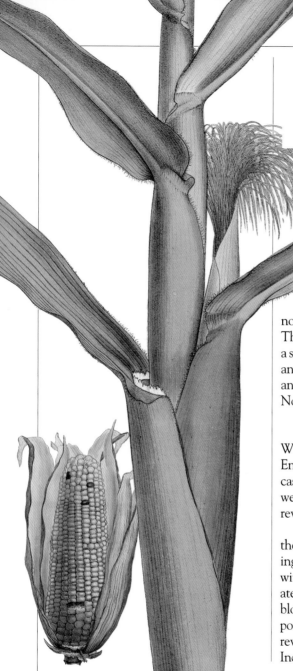

CORN

Zea mays
INDIAN CORN, MAIZE

An easy-to-grow, hardy plant that bears nutritious ears, corn is known as the Americas' greatest contribution to the world's food supply. Most researchers place its origins in what is now Mexico between 5500 and 3000 B.C. Thousands of years later, the plant played a significant role in the diet, medicine, and religious ceremonies of ancient Indian civilizations scattered throughout North and South America.

Food, Medicine, Symbol

When the Spanish explorers and the English settlers first set foot in the Americas, an estimated 200 varieties of corn were growing, and the plant was greatly revered by the Incas, Aztecs, and Maya.

The Incas made corn a diet staple, set their calendar to its planting and harvesting times, and adorned palace gardens with gold carvings of the plant. The Maya ate raw corn soaked in water to remedy blood in the urine and applied cornmeal poultices to sores and swellings. Similar reverence and uses were found among the Indians to the north. The plant's impor-

tance to the Aztecs was dramatically demonstrated by the human sacrifices performed in celebration of the corn harvest. More benignly, the Aztecs took cornmeal in water for heartburn, dysentery, and low breast milk.

When the Spanish reached the Caribbean, they called corn "maize" after the Arawak Indian word *mahiz*, meaning "giver of life" or simply "grain." In a terrible irony, Spanish conquistadors later devastated the native populations but valued the fruits of the land—especially corn. The scribe Garcilaso de la Varga reported that the Spanish were most impressed by the "remarkable curative properties of corn, which is not only the principal food in America, but is also of great benefit to the treatment of affections of the kidney and bladder."

Indian Corn

The Indians had countless uses for corn, many of which are still familiar today: tortillas, hominy grits, cornbread, popcorn, and succotash. The corn they grew, however, was quite different from the cultivars most North Americans are accustomed to today— 'Illinois Gold,' 'Silver Queen,' 'Honey and Cream' (with yellow and white kernels), or the thousands of acres of corn grown for animal feed.

Indian corn came in an array of sizes, shapes, and colors, and the kernels

---

Active plant parts Corn silk, corn oil, kernels, cob, stalks
Uses Urinary tract infections, skin inflammations; diuretic
Cautions Prolonged use of corn silk tea can cause vomiting and diarrhea. Inhaling the steam from corn silk tea can cause diarrhea, intestinal spasms, and vomiting. Dried corn silk is preferable to the fresh silk, which can quickly mold.

were harder. The Chippewa grew small ears with gold, brown, and blue-black kernels. The Yanktonai Sioux produced pale yellow corn speckled with brown and black. Apache corn was marked by bursts of red, while Pueblo corn was blue. Other corns were purple, mahogany, red, and red-orange.

Such diversity is possible because corn is easily interbred through cross-pollination. The Indians, who depended heavily on their crop yield, often planted different varieties in the same field to guard against the failure of any one strain. Many of these corn varieties are grown today.

Corn Silk Tea

When the first European settlements were founded in North America, the Indians greeted the settlers with corn—a significant event, as many of the vegetable seeds brought by the Europeans did not survive the trip. The Iroquois, for instance, greeted Jacques Cartier with corn bread on his first visit to Hochelaga in 1535. The Indians taught the settlers how to plant, cultivate, and prepare corn. One story of this early cooperation tells of an English-speaking Indian named Squanto, who showed the settlers how to grow corn in small, individual hills, fertilizing each with a fish—surprisingly, a practice he learned while visiting Europe.

A tea made from corn silk was one of the most popular medicinals among early settlers, used among rich and poor alike and by various ethnic groups, including African slaves and the Pennsylvania Dutch. The silk was taken from young ears before it turned brown, dried (the

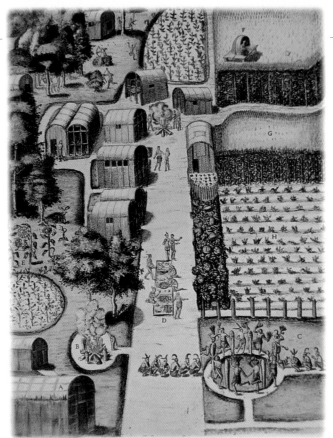

Corn raising in late-16th-century North America *was well-ordered, as depicted by traveler Theodor de Bry.*

Papago Indians of the American Southwest toasted it, using fire-heated rocks), then boiled. The boiled water was then strained and drunk for a host of ailments. The tea's diuretic action (due in part to its relatively high concentration of potassium) was used to treat conditions that affected the urinary tract, including cystitis, gout, gonorrhea, bedwetting, "congestion of the prostate," and bladder stones. It was also used as a "slimming cure" to aid weight loss, a nonirritating enema, a diabetes preventive, and a treatment for rheumatism, mumps, and respiratory problems. In earlier times, the silk was stored in glass jars through winter,

but today, when corn is out of season, 10 to 15 drops of corn silk extract in 1 cup warm water is a substitute for homemade corn silk tea.

The Whole Plant

The Indians also used many parts and by-products of the corn plant—the oil, meal, starch, stalks, popcorn, the cob and its ashes, and smut (a fungus)—for medicinal purposes. Eastern tribes used poultices of cornmeal and stalks to treat boils, burns, and inflammations. Cornmeal tea was a common Indian remedy for stomachache. The Chickasaw rubbed corn oil directly on the scalp as a dandruff remedy; to relieve itchy skin and sores, they placed the affected area in the smoke of burning cobs.

The Alabama tribe mixed cornmeal with water and poured the mixture through a sieve over the head of a patient with a stubborn fever. To remove warts, the Catawba conducted healing rituals using grains of corn. For a swollen foot, the Pueblos stood over an ear of corn on a warm hearth and rolled the cob back and forth with the affected foot; for heart ailments, they mixed blue cornmeal with some water to relieve palpitations, as well as "heart sickness" for the lovelorn.

The settlers adopted many Indian medical practices, modified others, and created their own. Corn oil was used topically and internally for eczema, granulated eyelids, and rough skin. New Englanders used a decoction of blue corn to wash out sore mouths. Other folks applied powdered corn to leg ulcers. In Appalachia, cornmeal was salted and applied to inflamed skin. Elsewhere, the meal was eaten for chills and boiled and mixed with milk to spread over burns. Cornstarch was taken as an antidote for iodine poisoning, sprinkled on wounds, and used as a body-odor powder. "Popcorn water" was drunk to settle a queasy stomach. Cob ashes were pressed against canker sores, and corn-smut tea was taken to relieve diarrhea and irregular menses.

Corn Science

Research has found that active principles in corn silk tea can induce urination, decrease blood sugar, lower blood pressure, and soothe internal irritations. As a diuretic with anti-inflammatory potential, the tea may also relieve urinary tract infections. Corn oil, which contains vitamin E and allantoin, a wound-healing substance, can aid the skin. It is also recommended to help prevent hardening of the arteries and lower cholesterol levels.

As food, corn is nutritious and high in fiber. Cornmeal and corn porridges were traditionally served to nourish invalids. Corn can also relieve constipation and reduce the risk of hemorrhoids and colon cancer. A 1981 study at Louisiana State University Medical Center found that populations with higher levels of corn consumption had lower death rates from colon, breast, and prostate cancer. And cornflakes, first made in Michigan in the late 1800s, have since become one of North America's favorite and most nutritious breakfasts.

Corn can even taste like candy. Freshly picked corn contains natural glucose, and corn syrup, converted from cornstarch, is used as a sugar substitute in processed foods and sweets. As a grain, corn was—and still is—used in North America to make beer and bourbon, as well as the fabled corn liquor of southern U.S. lore.

Hiawatha and the Mythical Origin of Corn

Many Indian tribes believed in ancient myths that glorified the origins of corn. Myths of the Woodlands Ojibwa were documented by Henry Rowe Schoolcraft in his *Algic Researches* (1839), which became the inspiration for Henry Wadsworth Longfellow's romantic epic, *The Song of Hiawatha* (1855).

Hiawatha's story unfolds in the land of Lake Gitche Gumee (Lake Superior) and Minnehaha Falls (now a park southeast of Minneapolis along the Mississippi River)—the home of the Ojibwa. At one point, Hiawatha, whom Longfellow modeled after a young Indian named Wunzh in Ojibwa lore, is sent into the forest to fast for seven days—a traditional rite of passage. He builds a forest hut and patiently awaits communication from his guardian spirit. After three days of solitude in the wild, Hiawatha is approached by a golden-haired youth named Mondamin, who is resplendent in "garments green and yellow." The visitor, sent by the "Master of Life," insists that the youths wrestle for four consecutive days, after which Mondamin will succumb.

Hiawatha is advised to bury the visitor and tend the grave as he would a garden. Although Hiawatha is weakened by hunger, he becomes stronger with each day's wrestling and kills Mondamin as the sun sets on the seventh day.

For months afterward Hiawatha tends the burial mound as instructed, "...till at length a small green feather from the earth shot slowly upward, then another and another, and before the Summer ended stood the maize in all its beauty, with its shining robes about it, and its long, soft, yellow tresses; And in rapture Hiawatha cried aloud, 'It is Mondamin!'" When the corn is harvested, Hiawatha and his people enjoy the first "... Feast of Mondamin and make known to the people this new gift of the Great Spirit." Later in the story, a glorious celebration accompanies the blessing of the cornfields and the spring planting.

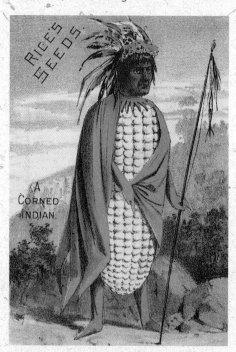

RICE'S SEEDS

A CORNED INDIAN.

The "corn Indian" on a 19th-century seed packet bespoke the perceived inseparability of the Indian and corn.

CORNS & CALLUSES

If the number of old-time remedies for corns and calluses is any indication, North Americans have been plagued with sore feet from the time of the first settlers. Folk treatments were quite innovative. Some people thought that rubbing a corn with a snail slug 19 times would remove it. Others held that the best remedy was to dissolve white fish-shell buttons in lemon juice, then rub the solution on the corns.

One folk practitioner advised touching a corn with five small pieces of flint, tying them in a rag, then discarding the rag at a fork in a road. When someone found it, the corn would disappear from the affected foot and show up on the unlucky finder—an example of the Theory of Transference, by which a disease was believed to transfer (often with the aid of incantations) to an animal, tree, or object.

Other treatments were not so odd. Nineteenth-century North Americans softened calluses with castor oil or covered them with soft soap, then wrapped the foot in a turpentine-soaked cloth. Many pioneers used white-willow bark, "burnt to ashes and steeped in vinegar."

Room for Comfort

Calluses are thickened areas of skin on the hands and bottom of the feet caused by friction. Corns are calluses on the toes (people with high foot arches are susceptible to corns because the arch increases pressure on the tips of toes when walking). More painful is a bunion, a firm, fluid-filled pad, or bursa, on the inside of the joint at the base of the big toe. It is caused by a shoe's rubbing against an abnormal outward projection of this joint; this abnormality may also be inherited.

Most foot calluses and corns can be prevented by wearing shoes that fit comfortably. If your toes rub against each other, put foam toe separators between them to prevent corns from forming. If you see a corn developing, massage it with a lotion that contains lanolin or urea to soften it. Putting a horseshoe-shaped pad or ring, available at drugstores, around the corn will ease pressure on it.

Soaking your feet will temporarily relieve pain. Medicated pads are available but should be applied only to the problem area; the pads contain salicylic acid, which is strong enough to eat through the corn and damage the healthy skin underneath. Placing a doughnut-shaped nonmedicated pad around the corn will protect the surrounding skin.

Trimming corns with scissors can cause an infection. However, shaving corns with a Credo—a German-made instrument available in most beauty-supply stores—is relatively safe. People who have diabetes or poor circulation are advised to consult a doctor instead of treating corns or calluses themselves.

Simple natural products for treating rough, hardened skin are Epsom salts and a pumice stone.

EPSOM SALTS AND PUMICE To treat calluses—not corns—soak your feet in warm water with Epsom salts for about 10 minutes, then use a pumice stone or callus file to rub the top layers off the callus. Do not use abrasives on hard corns—they will only make the area more painful.

ASPIRIN Make a paste with five or six crushed aspirin tablets and equal parts vinegar and water. Rub the paste onto the callus, then place an adhesive bandage over it to hold it in place. Wait at least 10 minutes before removing the bandage. The callused skin will easily come loose when rubbed with a pumice stone. If you are sensitive to aspirin, do not use this treatment.

WHITE WILLOW BARK A soak or wash made from white willow bark works the same way aspirin does because it contains salicin, from which aspirin was originally made. Put 1 or 2 teaspoons chopped or powdered bark into cold water, bring to a boil, and steep for 5 minutes before straining. Add to warm water as a foot soak. Use only if you are not aspirin-sensitive.

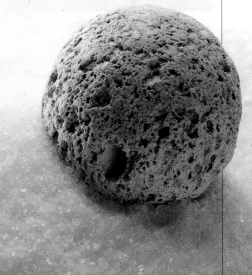

COUGHS

A cough is a social blunder. It shows lack of consideration for others. There is no excuse for it." So read an 1847 advertisement for a soon-to-be-famous Wild Cherry Cough Candy. Actually, there are many excuses for coughs, which are the body's way of ridding the respiratory tract of phlegm. They can be caused by a cold, influenza, or bronchitis, and even pneumonia, tuberculosis, or lung cancer. Dust or smoke can trigger a dry cough—as can a case of nerves. If your cough persists for more than a few days, see your doctor.

A Spate of Syrups

Today's drugstore shelves are lined with an array of elixirs designed to cure that nagging cough. Many contain ingredients that coat and soothe the throat. Some contain expectorants, which thin the mucus so that it can be brought up and expelled more easily. Lozenges serve to increase the flow of saliva, making you swallow more frequently and helping suppress the urge to cough.

Country folk had more recipes for cough syrups than you can shake a stick at. A traditional favorite was onion syrup, made with onion juice and sugar; the sugar content made the syrup popular with many children. Another syrup was made by simmering garlic cloves in apple cider vinegar, then adding honey. This was sometimes mixed with whiskey and sealed in jars. Onions and garlic are both antiseptic and irritating. Because irritants trigger the cough reflex, they help to bring up phlegm so that it can be expelled.

They also increase the watery secretions of the bronchial tubes, thereby helping to clear out the respiratory tract.

Whiskey was a popular cough syrup ingredient, although some women objected to drinking it and most children hated the taste. Sugar or even olive oil was added to make a syrup. In fact, alcohol not only acts as a solvent to help break up phlegm but also numbs a sore throat. One popular recipe called for a combination of whiskey, glycerin, lemon juice, and honey. The lemon juice, because it is acidic, helps dissolve the mucus. Vinegar works in the same way. Honey serves so well to coat and soothe the throat that a spoonful of honey was sometimes taken all by itself.

Slippery Soothers

To suppress dry coughs, Indians and early settlers boiled slippery elm bark, which produces a gel-like substance called mucilage that coats the throat. Slippery-elm throat lozenges were a staple of many medicine chests, despite their foul taste. Far more palatable was wild cherry bark, which has a mild numbing effect and was used by many Indian tribes as well as the settlers. It was often boiled and strained, then mixed with honey or stewed in molasses. It is no coincidence that many of today's cough medicines are cherry-

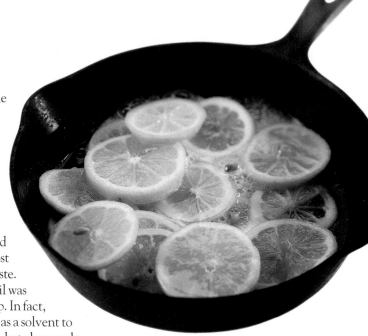

Stewed lemons, *with plenty of sugar added, make a tasty old-time cough syrup.*

flavored. But take note: wild-cherry bark can be toxic in large doses.

Other substances were boiled down to a gooey matter that would cling to the throat. Among them were pine pitch, marsh mallow root, flaxseed, and plantain leaves; the last contains astringent tannins that help allay inflammation.

Herbal Expectorants

Many different herbs were used as expectorants, often in the form of teas. Most of them not only worked well but also tasted good and were mildly antiseptic, too. European settlers brought horehound, long a traditional cough remedy, to North America, where it was popular for coughs, colds, and tuberculosis. It acts as a local irritant, just as garlic and onions do. Many Indian tribes drank sweet-tasting licorice tea for coughs, and licorice later became a standard cough remedy. Licorice is not only an expectorant, it also coats the throat and calms inflammation. Seneca root, first used by Indians, became popular among settlers for coughs and croup. In Europe it is found in some cough syrups.

Thyme was taken as a tea, often with honey. The herb acts as an expectorant and it contains substances that relax the respiratory tract. The steam from a thyme bath can calm a cough. Ginger was also popular; one recipe combined a tablespoon of whiskey, a teaspoon of honey, a dash of ginger, and a quarter cup of hot water. A simpler remedy called for chewing on a piece of gingerroot and swallowing the juice. Today ginger is still considered a good cough suppressant.

Perhaps the most basic expectorant is steam. Nineteenth-century doctors prescribed steam inhalations of eucalyptus oil for bronchitis and whooping cough. Thyme and chamomile inhalations were also effective. The Pennsylvania Dutch boiled pine tar on the stove and breathed in the steam. Others cured their coughs simply by sipping hot water. Hot liquids do indeed help dissolve phlegm. So do horseradish and hot mustard, but these have an unwanted rebound effect—they cause swelling of the nasal passages, which triggers more congestion.

The Dread Croup

In infants, croup brings on a cough like no other, one that instills terror in the hearts of parents. It is said to resemble the bark of a seal. This upper respiratory infection causes the child's windpipe to swell, which makes breathing difficult and noisy. Croup usually strikes children between the ages of three months and three years. If a child has serious trouble breathing, take him to the emergency room at once.

Aside from the adult cough remedies, there were countless methods used to cure croup. Many mothers, when their babies were "mimicking a rooster," as one said, boiled water in a pot, then held the child over it to breathe in the steam. (This is dangerous unless the child is held a safe distance away.) Steam, especially from a hot shower, is still considered the best treatment. Some parents administered a few drops of kerosene with a spoonful of sugar; this is obviously unwise. Others hung a silk ribbon around the child's neck in the belief that this cured the croup.

Sometimes a spoonful of warmed chicken fat, goose grease, butter, or skunk oil was administered as an expectorant and also to induce vomiting, which was thought to break up the congestion. Small amounts of ipecac syrup, an emetic, were occasionally mixed into expectorants; large doses of the syrup, however, can be toxic.

FOR FIFTY YEARS
I HAVE USED
AYER'S CHERRY PECTORAL
for COLDS *and* COUGHs
THREE SIZES 25¢ 50¢ $1.00 ALL

LICORICE Licorice contains the ingredient glycyrrhizin, which acts as an expectorant. Lozenges made with real licorice extract slowly release a sweet-tasting demulcent that soothes the throat and encourages the expectoration of mucus. Do not take more than a few lozenges a day, since too much real licorice can cause side effects.

SLIPPERY ELM Good for dry coughs, lozenges of slippery elm bark, available commercially, release the bark's mucilage slowly to coat the throat and keep coughing to a minimum.

THYME The essential oil contained in thyme acts not only as a soothing expectorant but also an antiseptic. To make a tea, mix 1 to 2 teaspoons crushed leaves in 1 cup boiling water, then steep and strain.

HOREHOUND Horehound, good for productive coughs, acts as a local irritant to trigger the cough reflex and help bring up phlegm. To make a tea, steep 2 teaspoons leaves or flowers in 1 cup boiling water, then strain. Lozenges are available commercially.

Cherry bark, once a cough cure, inspired cherry-flavored cough drops.

APPALACHIA & THE OZARKS

The people of the Appalachians and the Ozarks inherited a rich tradition from their forebears: at its core is a view of the world as a unified, harmonious place. When illness strikes, there is a cure somewhere—in nature, in prayer, or in a healer's magical skills.

The mountain forests of Appalachia and the Ozarks may seem a forbidding wilderness, but to the people who live there they are a cornucopia of cures. Armed with such popular medical guidebooks as *Gunn's Domestic Medicine* and their own resourcefulness, early settlers of the region quickly reaped its bounty of medicinal roots and herbs. Out of thousands of plants, they found therapeutic uses for roughly 25 percent—even higher than the remarkable 10 percent reported to have been used by Indians throughout all of North America.

Magic and Faith

Appalachian healing is based on a millenia-old tradition: the use of healing plants. The physicians of classical Greece and Rome, including the naturalist Pliny the Elder, wrote learned treatises on herbal remedies. Moreover, the Bible—an integral part of many mountain dwellers' lives—describes balms, purgatives, and other medicines made from herbs: aloe and myrrh, mint and coriander, mustard seed and rue.

The sassafras tree *is a traditional source of medicine in Appalachia.*

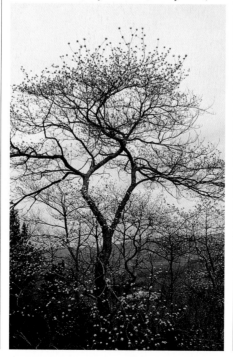

Appalachian folk medicine also adheres to the ancient theory that all living things possess four "humors"—blood, phlegm, black bile, and yellow bile. Blood is considered moist and hot; phlegm, moist and cold; black bile, dry and cold; and yellow, dry and hot. According to the theory, in a healthy body the humors are balanced; illness arises when they become unbalanced. Thus, illness can be cured by a plant that raises or lowers the level of a particular humor. A healer can boost sluggish blood circulation, for example, by prescribing a medicine from a "hot" plant.

A second ancient theory is the Doctrine of Signatures, which holds that the medicinal use of a plant is revealed by its "signature"—its color or shape. Yellow plants are deemed useful for treating jaundice. The shape and wrinkled surface of walnuts suggests that they are good for treating the brain. Some Appalachian healers believe that signatures are simply part of nature; others hold that they were established by God to direct humans to remedies. In either case, the belief in signatures reflects a more general belief in the unity of nature.

Mountain medicinals:
From the earth comes ginseng; from the tree, walnut.

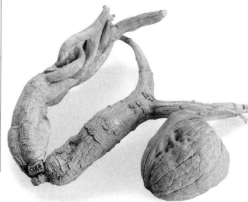

An "Old-Timer Herbalist"

From a simple shack in northeastern Alabama, A. L. "Tommie" Bass (1908–1996) dispensed herbal remedies and shared his medical wisdom. From youth, the self-described "old-timer herbalist" absorbed the backcountry ethic of self-reliance, supporting himself with a variety of skills—skinning animals, cutting timber, picking berries. At the same time, he gained knowledge of the healing traditions of the region from his parents, neighbors, and the area's Cherokee Indians.

Bass began collecting and selling herbal remedies as a youth. Through years of trial and error, he taught himself to determine a plant's medicinal value from its taste, smell, and time of harvest. Neighbors sought him out for advice, and newspaper accounts of his practice spread Bass's fame through Appalachia and beyond.

It was Bass's custom not to charge for a first dose of medicine but only when favorable results were achieved and the client returned for a follow-up dose. His theory of healing came down to an intuitive sense of the intimate connection between humans and the natural world. "Mother Nature's got her way," he once said, "and she's going to have it."

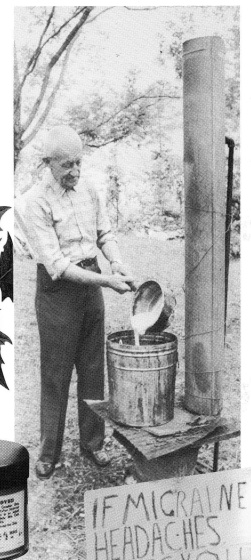

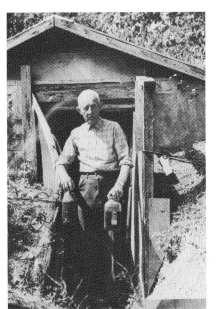

The Bass family salve, *its recipe brought from England by Bass's great-grandmother, was made from jimsonweed (above), hog lard, sulfur, and tobacco. The price was 50 cents a jar.*

Bass brewed and bottled his own elixirs *(left and top right). His answer to the common cold was a combination of boneset, mullein, rabbit tobacco, and sumac. He also knew that feverfew would ease migraines.*

A Mountain Family Tradition

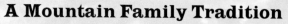

Appalachian families hand down recipes for herbal remedies from one generation to the next, passing them on orally or copying them in notebooks. While some remedies are relatively simple and can be used directly from the wild, others require more elaborate mixing and preparation. As often as not, a recipe is likely to include sassafras, continuing an age-old Appalachian tradition that survives even in the face of medical research that warns of the plant's potential dangers.

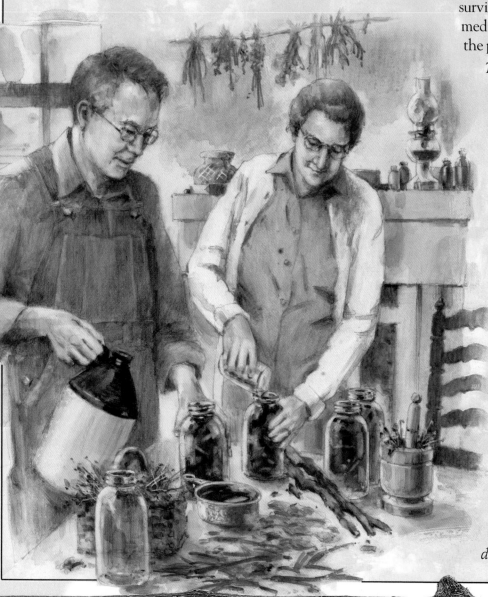

The mountain-dwelling herbalists of Appalachia and the Ozarks believe that herbs work together: some plants enhance the effectiveness of other herbs, while others lessen undesirable side effects. Here a mountain couple combine wild cherry bark with sassafras, redroot, yellow-root, and huckleberry leaves to create a tonic. The sassafras imparts a distinctive flavor and is believed to act as a blood purifier. Redroot and huckleberry are sweeteners, although honey or sugar is often also added as a preservative or for taste. Some herbal mixtures are left to steep in grain alcohol, to blend the ingredients more thoroughly.

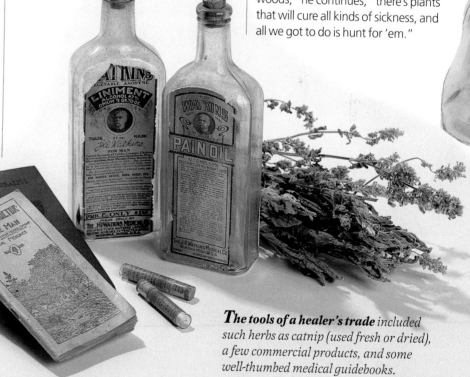

Ginseng sports tiny red fruits *before the root is harvested with a special hoe.*

Also relied upon is the Theory of Transference: the shifting of a human ailment to an object, an animal, or another person. One West Virginia practice involves plucking the feathers from a pigeon's chest and placing the bird's exposed skin against the stomach of a person suffering convulsions, which then shift to the bird. To remove warts, mountain healers rub them with a potato, place the potato in a sack, then leave it at a fork in the road. It is said that the warts will shift to the first traveler who picks up the sack.

So-called power doctors heal by "laying on hands" and uttering part of a Scripture or a religious rhyme or phrase. An example is the rhyme used to ease the pain of a bad burn: "Two little angels came from heaven/ One brought fire and the other brought frost/ Go out fire and come in frost," repeats the healer to the patient.

In the backcountry, one of the most valuable healing skills is the ability to halt severe bleeding. One approach used by "bloodstoppers" is to insert the patient's name into a verse from the Bible. This method often works, perhaps because of the power of suggestion.

Nature's Pharmacy

If magic and faith are at the core of Appalachian folk healing, plants are its tools. In addition to their reliance on ancient doctrines, inhabitants of the region added to their knowledge of herbs by observing how animals use plants. An example is their careful notation of which plants animals ate after being bitten by a poisonous snake. They also learned much from the Indians—a cultural interaction that continued into this century. Indeed, one of the best known Appalachian herbalists of recent times, Clarence Gray of West Virginia, was converted to the practice by an Indian. A series of heart attacks had left Gray near death when an Indian appeared at his house carrying pipsissewa, a local herb. The visitor instructed him to make a tea from the herb and take three spoonfuls every day for six months. To his surprise, Gray recovered.

Many mountain dwellers still incorporate herbal remedies into their daily diets, nibbling on wild violet flowers (rich in vitamin C) and sipping a tonic made from wild cherry bark—which, they believe, keeps the heart healthy. More significant, to this day the herbalists of the Appalachians and the Ozarks continue the centuries-old task of exploring nature's pharmacy to ferret out cures. With tradition on their side, they draw strength from their belief in the wholeness and unity of the world they inhabit. Blessed with an ethnobotanical Eden, Appalachian healers seek because they are certain they will find. "God Almighty never put us here without a remedy for every ailment," declares one. "Out in the woods," he continues," there's plants that will cure all kinds of sickness, and all we got to do is hunt for 'em."

The tools of a healer's trade *included such herbs as catnip (used fresh or dried), a few commercial products, and some well-thumbed medical guidebooks.*

CRANBERRY

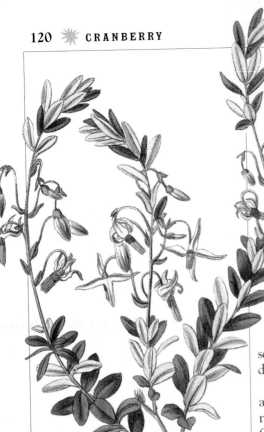

Vaccinium macrocarpon
TRAILING SWAMP CRANBERRY,
LARGE CRANBERRY

Cranberries are firmly embedded in North American folklore and history as part of the feast that the Indians and the Pilgrims enjoyed together in the autumn of 1621. At many a Thanksgiving dinner, turkey and trimmings are served, more often than not, with a delectable cranberry sauce.

The round red berries had long been an important part of the diet of the native peoples of New England, eastern Canada, and the Great Lakes region, and European colonists were not slow to follow suit. Ripening in late summer and autumn, the fruit stays on the shrub's low, trailing branches well into winter and loses nothing to the bitter cold. It is also easy to store through the winter, remaining fresh and juicy with a minimum of care, and is a valuable source of vitamin C during a season when that nutrient is hard to come by in northerly climes. Although the settlers had never heard of vitamin C,

they were undoubtably aware that sailors who ate the tart berries did not develop scurvy during their long voyages at sea.

In her 1855 *Canadian Settler's Guide*, author Catharine Parr Traill gave a recipe for cranberry sauce and praised the berries for their "great medicinal virtues." It was not until after the American Civil War, however, that the rest of the continent came to appreciate cranberries and their sauce. Surprisingly, the credit may go to American Gen. Ulysses S. Grant. Having grown partial to the nutritious berries that his New England soldiers often carried with them on the march, Grant ordered cranberry sauce to be served to his troops as part of the newly instituted American Thanksgiving Day observance in 1864. Within a few years, cranberry sauce had assumed its role as an essential component of Thanksgiving dinner.

A Changing Role

Oddly enough, apart from their obvious nutritional value and gentle diuretic properties, cranberries were not particularly honored in the folk healer's arsenal until well into the 20th century. True, some said that a tea brewed from the leaves could lower blood sugar—a doubtful prescription at best—and the acidic berries were sometimes crushed into a poultice for minor wounds and bites. One 19th-century source noted that "a split cranberry, held in position by a daub of starch paste, will quickly

Active plant parts Berries
Uses Urinary tract infections; diuretic, antiseptic
Cautions Cranberry juice is considered safe for nearly anyone who is not allergic to cranberries. Because of the calorie content of excess sweeteners in some commercial juices, pregnant or nursing women and anyone on medication for kidney or urinary tract ailments should not consume more than a glass a day. Medicinal dosages of cranberry concentrates should be taken only in consultation with a doctor.

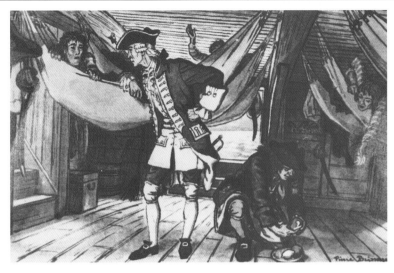

Shipboard physicians soon learned that cranberries were as effective as oranges in preventing scurvy.

relieve the pain and inflammation attending boils on the tip of the nose." Still, there was no herbal tradition avowing that drinking cranberry juice could prevent or cure infections of the urinary tract. That knowledge came not from folk tradition, as do most herbal remedies, but from laboratory tests.

As far back as the 1840s, researchers in Germany had noted that the urine of people who drank cranberry juice was high in hippuric acid; this finding was verified by American scientists in 1923. In their studies, the Americans speculated that the acid inhibited the growth of the bacterium *Escherichia coli* (*E. coli*), which caused the most common and chronic kinds of urinary tract infection, or UTI— a painful problem that mainly affects women. As a result, cranberry juice became widely used by women and appeared to be beneficial, even though further studies showed that the amount of hippuric acid generated was not sufficient to back up the claims for its efficacy. Studies in the 1990s suggest that the preventive action is much more subtle than had been believed: two constituents of cranberry juice—fructose and a polymeric compound with an extremely high molecular weight—seem to stop E. coli bacteria from adhering to infection sites in the urinary tract. In one clinical test, 125 ml to 180 ml of cranberry juice per day were enough to prevent UTIs in 19 of 28 patients; the nine other patients were found to have preexisting infections.

Even though the acidic action of cranberry juice may not be the reason for its best-known therapeutic use, it is undeniably responsible for another practical value. It has been found that the hippuric acid in the urine of those who drink cranberry juice inhibits the action of odor-creating bacteria. For this reason, cranberry juice is often incorporated into the diet of incontinent nursing home patients to control the embarrassing ammoniacal odor of urine.

Ways to Use It

Like the berries themselves, undiluted cranberry juice is too sour to be palatable for most tastes. It is usually mixed with water and an artificial sweetener, sucrose, or with other fruit juices. Commercial cranberry cocktail generally contains about one-third cranberry juice. For a homemade alternative, try simmering 2 cups of ground or mashed cranberries in a liter of water; add honey or sugar to taste. Or look for bottled cranberry concentrate at your health food store and mix it with water at a ratio of five to one.

Half a cup of cranberry juice taken twice a day is commonly regarded as a preventive of UTI; to help control or cure an existing infection, take the same amount four times a day. Capsules containing dried cranberry powder are also available at various strengths. These have more fiber and less sugar than commercial juices but should be used only with your doctor's approval.

Not to be confused with ...

Native to lowland bogs of the northeastern United States and eastern Canada, the common cranberry should not be confused with the mountain cranberry (*Vaccinium vitis-idaea*), a dwarf shrub of rocky, upland forests that is also known as lingonberry, cowberry, or foxberry. Although its small fruits are sometimes substituted for those of the common cranberry and share some of its medicinal properties, they are not known to be effective in preventing UTI. Another so-called cranberry, the highbush cranberry (*Viburnum opulus*), is not a cranberry at all: it is a member of the honeysuckle family. And although its bright red berries resemble cranberries, they contain none of cranberry's properties.

CUTS & ABRASIONS

When early settlers suffered a cut or scrape, they draped a cobweb over it to stop the bleeding or packed it with chimney soot or gunpowder. Other "mechanical" blood stanchers were chewed tobacco or sassafras leaves and a paste made from flour and vinegar. Even leather scrapings from the sole of a shoe were used. A popular herb was milkweed; its milky juice is known to constrict blood flow, allowing a clot to form. The cobweb remedy, too, was effective: though unsanitary, spider webs have been found to contain a substance that causes blood to clot.

After the bleeding had been stopped came the risk of infection, for which early pioneers had a host of treatments.

Wounds were dressed with poultices made from the bruised leaves of plantain or coltsfoot. One healer held that "the leaves of primroses make the finest salve to heal wounds ever known." Another had a recipe that called for pounded ivy leaves, rock alum, walnuts, and spring water. Probably more effective were St. Johnswort and calendula flowers, which were used by surgeons to dress bullet wounds during the American Civil War.

In World War II, extracts of garlic were used to disinfect wounds (garlic has been shown to contain allicin, a potent antibiotic). Other early practices, such as applying fresh cow manure to cuts on the feet or having dogs lick wounds, doubtlessly caused more harm than good.

Treating Wounds

Wash cuts and abrasions with mild soap and running water to get out any dirt, and pat dry with a clean cloth. Studies show that broad-spectrum antibiotic creams help wounds heal faster. Apply an antibiotic cream or hydrogen peroxide, or try an herbal remedy. If the area becomes red and swollen, or if it oozes pus, consult a doctor; it may need additional treatment.

Most cuts and scrapes are minor and stop bleeding on their own within a few minutes. If bleeding continues, remove any visible dirt or debris and apply direct pressure to the wound with a clean cloth or gauze pad; if nothing else is available, use your hand. Keep applying pressure until the bleeding stops, then tape the cloth or gauze in place. If blood soaks through the cloth, do not remove it; you may lift off clotting blood cells. Instead, add another cloth and keep pressing. Do not try to use a tourniquet; if misused, it can cut off circulation to the limb.

See a doctor if ...

When you have a cut, see a doctor in the following cases:
◆ The wound is deep, large, or has rough edges. It may need stitches to heal properly and minimize scarring.
◆ A foreign object is deeply embedded in the wound.
◆ Blood spurts from the cut or the cut continues to bleed heavily after several minutes of pressure. In this case, go to the emergency room.

A mother ministers to her child in "The Cut Finger," an 1808 engraving.

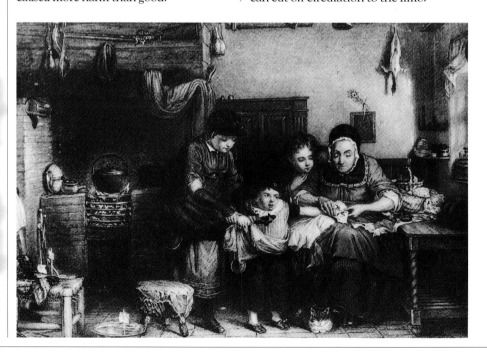

GARLIC Garlic contains allicin, which has been shown to inhibit the growth of many kinds of bacteria. To discourage infection, bruise a clove of garlic and place it on a cleaned cut.

BENZOIN Benzoin is the aromatic resin of the *Styrax* genus of trees, which grow in tropical Asia. It is an effective antiseptic and stops small cuts from bleeding. Benzoin is available as compound benzoin tincture.

ALOE VERA Aloe vera gel is a soothing emollient and has been used for centuries to hasten wound healing. If you have your own plant, cut off a lower aloe vera leaf (lower leaves are older), split it lengthwise, and squeeze the gel onto the injury. The gel forms its own bandage when dry.

CALENDULA This herb speeds the healing of wounds and reduces inflammation. Make a tea by adding 1 to 2 teaspoons minced fresh flowers to 1 cup boiling water. Let steep for 10 minutes. Or put a few drops of commercial extract in cool, boiled water. Then dip a clean cloth into it and apply it as a compress to cuts and abrasions.

ECHINACEA Preparations containing echinacea have mild antibiotic properties and stimulate the production of new tissue. Try a commercial echinacea ointment on hard-to-heal wounds.

GOLDENSEAL Medical studies show that goldenseal fights bacteria and is an effective astringent. Its major alkaloid, berberine, is a strong antibacterial agent. Sprinkle goldenseal powder on cuts to disinfect them.

TEA TREE OIL Tea tree oil, also called cajeput oil, is an effective disinfectant because of its active terpene derivatives. Stir 1½ teaspoons oil into a cup of warm water and use to rinse infected wounds. Many tea tree oil products, including soap, are also available.

If bleeding continues, lie down with your legs elevated to decrease the likelihood of fainting. If possible, lift the injured area above the heart to decrease the flow of blood to the heart and continue to apply pressure to the wound.

If a foreign object is embedded in the wound, do not try to remove it. Instead, lie down and apply direct pressure above and below the wound. When the bleeding stops, see your doctor or go to a hospital, where appropriate care can be given.

A wound may spurt blood if an artery has been cut. This is a potentially life-threatening injury that requires emergency medical assistance. Apply direct pressure to the wound, then call an ambulance or go to a hospital emergency room.

Healing Herbs

Modern research has proven many herbs to be fairly effective against infection and in the healing of wounds. Laboratory studies have supported the effectiveness of such traditional treatments as echinacea, calendula, goldenseal, and even garlic, although to varying degrees.

A study conducted in Austria in 1994 looked at 48 plants that folk tradition credits as vulneraries (substances that promote wound healing). This study found that 35 of the extracts showed antibacterial activity. Six that produced "outstanding antibacterial effects" were the leaves of sundew (drosera), witch hazel, eucalyptus, and blackberry, the bark of English oak, and the flowers of linden.

Verbal Charms

Some folk cures for bleeding were verbal "charms," or prayers, rather than herbs. "Bloodstoppers" —people believed to have a special ability to stop others from bleeding and often to help with other ills— were found in most communities and are still encountered in many parts. Sometimes this ability is believed to be inborn, as in the case of a seventh son of a seventh son.

Bloodstopping charms often incorporated Bible verses, as in Ezekiel 16:6, in which the name of the bleeding person was inserted: "I passed by you, [name], and saw you flailing about in your blood. As you lay in your blood, I said to you, 'Live!'"

These verbal charms are still used in many regions and ethnic communities. Some scientists think their apparent effectiveness is due to suggestion, which would be similar to what happens in hypnosis: healing thoughts are planted while the patient is in a deep trance. Hypnosis has, in fact, been successful in treating many conditions.

Whether using herbal or commercial products, apply a plastic bandage to cuts, both for protection and to prevent a scab from forming; scabs often make cells regenerate more slowly. Change the dressing at least once a day and try to keep the injury clean and dry. Open cuts that bleed do not require tetanus shots, but deep puncture wounds that do not bleed may. If you have not had a tetanus shot in the past five years, get a booster.

DANDELION

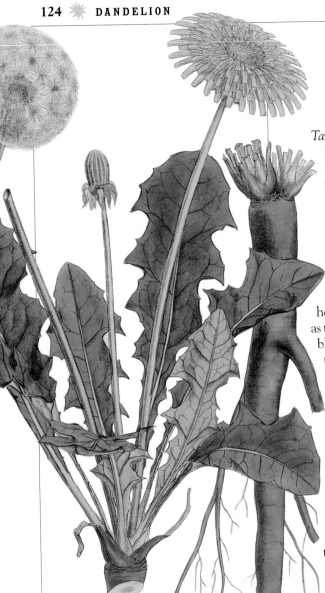

Taraxacum officinale
LION'S-TOOTH, WILD ENDIVE,
BLOWBALL, CANKERWORT,
CONSUELDA, PISS-IN-BED

To lawn caretakers, few plants are hated as much as the dandelion, considered an unwanted, stubborn intruder in any manicured patch of green. Yet few childhood memories are as pleasurable as those of plucking a dandelion, blowing hard on its fluffy white top, and gazing at the parachute seeds as they drift away. What's more, few plants have had as rich a history of medicinal use as the dandelion has.

A Persistent Traveler

Much like the plant itself, which appears in lawns time and time again, the use of dandelion has survived over hundreds of years and spanned the globe. In the 10th century the Arabs prescribed the plant as a diuretic. The Chinese drank dandelion tea for colds and applied dandelion poultices to the breasts to treat soreness, low milk production, and cancer.

In the Middle Ages, dandelions were prescribed by way of the doctrine of signatures, a longstanding folk theory that appraised a plant's usefulness by its physical characteristics. The yellow flower signaled a treatment for jaundice and liver ailments (conditions that tinted the skin yellow), and its milky juice, resembling urine, identified it as a remedy for urinary tract problems. These practices eventually found their way to North America.

English settlers introduced the plant to the New World, placing it in windowsill pots and herb gardens. Nicholas Culpeper, in his popular 17th-century herbal, called a decoction of dandelion roots and leaves in white wine a "wonderful help" when treating many conditions, including an "evil disposition." The Hudson's Bay Company, the British trading enterprise founded in 1670, exported dandelion to its Canadian outposts in the 18th and 19th centuries to balance the meaty diet of its employees.

In the spring, settlers picked dandelion's bitter leaves and added them raw to salads. As a tonic, the Pennsylvania Dutch ate them raw as a "hot salad" with a vinegar and bacon dressing. The greens were also cooked like spinach. Many settlers along the east coast harvested the roots in autumn and roasted them as a "mild" substitute for coffee. (Unknown to them, the resulting brew was mild because it was caffeine-free.) As pioneers moved westward, they spread dandelions across

Plant parts used Roots, leaves, shoots rarely
Uses Liver sluggishness, loss of appetite, constipation, yeast infection (topically)
Cautions The milky sap of the shoots may produce nausea in children; the plant should not be given to children under the age of two. Allergic reactions are rare, although handling the plant may cause contact dermatitis. Pregnant and nursing women are advised not to take diuretics, including dandelion tea. Taking the plant internally is contraindicated in bile-duct obstructions and gallstones. Anyone with disorders of the liver, kidney, gallbladder, bladder, or stomach should consult a physician before using dandelion.

the new territory to feed bees and guarantee a supply of honey. Despite the plant's many uses, by the 20th century faith in it had crumbled, and many doctors considered its medicinal value overrated. Soon alternative "bitter" preparations— especially those containing alcohol— were used to treat the internal organs.

Names Grand and Crude

The name "dandelion" comes from *dent de lion*, French for "tooth of the lion." This appellation derives from the leaf's unique shape, which resembles a row of jagged teeth. Its genus name, *Taraxacum*, has been translated in two ways: first from the Persian *tark hashgun*, or "wild endive," one of the plant's common names; the second translation is from the two Greek words *taraxos* and *akos*, "disorder" and "remedy." Coupled with *officinale*, the latter becomes the exalted "official remedy of disorders."

Conversely, during the course of its many travels the plant has been given a variety of names, some of which are decidedly unappealing: swine's snout, yellow gowan, Irish daisy, puffball, urinaria, peasant's cloak, priest's-crown, and piss-in-bed. Urinaria refers to its old name in English apothecaries, *herba urinaria*, so designated for its drug-like diuretic effect. Piss-in-bed—also piss-a-bed, piddly bed, wet-a-bed, and *pissenlit* (French)—also refers to its diuretic effect. The nickname peasant's cloak probably comes from the shedding of the seed head, similar to that of a cheap coat, while priest's-crown

The parachute seeds of dandelion will readily sprout after settling in the soil.

suggests the image of a young seminarian whose full head of hair turns white and eventually falls out as the priest ages.

A Cleansing Tea

Dandelion root tea and, to a lesser extent, the leaf tea, were favorite remedies for ailments that affected the liver, spleen, kidneys, bladder, and stomach. Both folk tradition and early medicine generally associated a bitter taste like dandelion's with the stimulation of bile and gastric secretions. First and foremost, it was thought to cleanse a "congested" liver. In fact, scientific studies have found that compounds in dandelion do mildly stimulate bile flow and may help prevent cirrhosis. The plant was commonly used to treat liver-related disorders, such as jaundice, hepatitis, bile-duct obstructions, and gallstones. But these disorders are

often only symptoms of more serious problems, and any benefit to the liver would fail to treat the underlying cause.

A tea made from the roots or leaves was also used to promote urination and dissolve kidney stones. The leaves were thought to be more potent, and extracts of the greens were so popular that one store in New York claimed to have sold 3,700 pounds (1,680 kg) of the extract in one year alone—1874. Dandelion's mild diuretic effect, for which science has yet to find a clear chemical explanation, has been found principally in the greens. Even so, use of the plant may help to prevent, minimize, and pass stones, but it will not correct the underlying causes— an unbalanced diet and metabolism.

This diuretic effect aids in the reduction of fluid retention and weight loss. However, any water or weight loss will be temporary, lasting only until the body's supply of water is replenished.

Dandelions were also taken to expedite the digestive process. For the stom-

Tagged by this Shaker label (c. 1875), the root was used to make a diuretic tea.

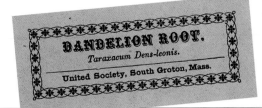

DANDELION ROOT.
Taraxacum Dens-leonis.
United Society, South Groton, Mass.

ach, they were used to relieve both loss of appetite and "fullness" as well as indigestion. Many settlers and Indians, such as the Iroquois and Pillager Ojibwa, consumed the tea (or the raw roots and greens) to facilitate the digestion of fatty meats and relieve heartburn. Teas made from the root or dried leaf were also used as laxatives. Science has found that dandelion can stimulate the appetite and produce a mild laxative effect. It may also help relieve the pain and diarrhea caused by colitis. Furthermore, its high potassium content sets it apart from other diuretics that drain the body's potassium reserves.

To prepare a tea, place 1 to 2 teaspoons fresh root or leaves, finely chopped, into 1 cup water in a small pot. Boil for 10 minutes, then strain. Beware of plants in the wild or any in your own backyard that have been sprayed with pesticides.

"Blood Builder"

Aside from its employment as a digestive and diuretic, dandelion was thought to cleanse and tone the blood. The fresh leaves, a root tea, or a wine made from dandelion flower heads were taken at the first sign of spring. One such tonic from the American Midwest was prepared by soaking pulverized dandelion and sarsaparilla roots overnight in hot water.

Dandelion was believed to lower blood pressure and remove toxins that had built up over a winter of harsh weather and salty diets. It was also taken to build endurance for springtime field work and to fortify the blood against anemia and diabetes. Remarkably, the plant's high sugar content does not aggravate diabetes. In fact, studies earlier in this century reported that the leaves showed the potential to lower blood sugar in animals.

For many, including those in Pennsylvania and the Ozarks, dandelion wine was the preferred tonic. Recipes combined dandelion blossoms, boiling water, sugar, yeast, and either lemons, oranges, grapefruits, raisins, or raspberries. The concoction was strained and left to ferment, according to different recipes, for 10 days, 30 days, or "until the hissing stops."

Past Meets Present

Many of dandelion's traditional uses have withstood scientific scrutiny. As a diuretic and mild sedative, the tea made from the roots or leaves can help calm the nerves, reduce blood pressure, and relieve menstrual cramps—uses that were well known to the Cherokee and Kiowa Indians.

Because the raw root contains calcium and vitamins A and C and has anti-inflammatory properties, eating it at the first sign of a cold is not without some merit. Nor is simply chewing the root, as the Cherokee did, to relieve toothaches and sore gums.

Several of dandelion's other, lesser-known folk uses have also received scientific attention. For example, extracts of the plant have been found to inhibit the fungus that causes yeast infections. Derivatives of the plant have also been reported to show potential antitumor activity.

As an antifungal and anti-inflammatory, the dandelion could well have soothed irritated skin, relieved bruises and arthritis, and helped remove skin papillomas, such as warts. The juice from dandelion's roots, the white latex from its stems, and its leaves themselves have all been used for a variety of skin conditions (including freckles and moles), even though contact with the plant can cause dermatitis.

Today dandelion extracts are found in diuretics, laxatives, cosmetics, antismoking products, and, in Germany, medicines for gallbladder conditions. Commercial dandelion tea bags are also sold.

Dandelion Folklore

Combine dandelion's historic medicinal reputation, the plant's abundance, and the power of the human imagination, and folk beliefs abound. Below are just a few.

◆ If you picked a dandelion today, you will wet your bed tonight. (This idea and a nickname, "piss-in-bed," come from the plant's diuretic effect.)

◆ If you are an unmarried girl and blow all the seeds from the white, fluffy seed head, the number of blows will tell how many years will pass before you marry.

◆ If you are a recently married young man or woman and blow hard once on a dandelion seed head, the remaining number of seeds indicates how many children you will have.

◆ If you blow off all of the seeds in one breath, a wish will come true.

◆ The number of seeds left after a good blow will tell you what time it is.

◆ If you whisper words to your beloved and blow the seeds in his or her direction, the seeds will relay your whispered words.

According to folk beliefs, blowing on a dandelion seed head can predict the future.

DANDRUFF

Although dandruff's white particles of skin are often spotted on the hair or the shoulders, dandruff is actually a skin condition. It has many causes: a dry or oily scalp, sunburn, an allergic reaction, a deficient diet, residue from harsh hair products—even stress. The most common cause, however, is seborrheic dermatitis, an itchy, scaly rash that can affect the scalp, face, and chest.

Mainstream treatments for the rash typically consist of steroid lotions, antiyeast creams, and antifungals, even though dandruff is neither a yeast nor a fungal infection. Controlling seborrheic dermatitis generally involves the use of antidandruff shampoos that contain zinc, selenium, sulfur compounds, tar, or tea tree oil. Alternative therapies include relaxation techniques and diet supplements—in particular lecithin and vitamins A, B complex, and E. Often, dandruff is permanent, and control of the problem requires ongoing attention. Whatever the course of treatment, avoid scouring or scratching the affected skin.

Herbs for Your Head

Goldenseal root infusion, garlic oil, and rosemary leaf oil are the most effective herbal treatments for the condition once known as "scurf." All three have been widely employed in folk medicine for a variety of skin conditions. Goldenseal and garlic were used by settlers and Indians for dandruff, ringworm, acne, and sore eyes and gums. Rosemary was traditionally used as a bath oil and hair rinse, a preventive for dandruff and baldness, and a stimulant for the blood, eyes, and hair.

Other herbal remedies have shown positive effects, but research on many is incomplete. Extracts of quillaja and yucca, both with good foaming and detergent qualities, were used to soothe an itchy scalp. Distilled tars, too, were used, and are still found in over-the-counter products. Cade oil, a tar distilled from juniper, served as a remedy for an irritated scalp and hair loss. Coal tar was used as an antiseptic and anti-itch skin ointment. Pine tar soap, which contains creosote compounds that are mildly antibacterial, was highly regarded as an antidandruff shampoo among rural Pennsylvanians.

Flaky Treatments

Many dandruff remedies were specified as prewash rinses, final rinses, shampoos, overnight conditioners, or massage oils. Prewash rinses included mint tea, witch hazel, and beet or lemon juice. Doublestrength infusions made from chives, birch leaves, catnip, celery seed, chaparral, thyme, nettle, chamomile, or wintergreen—or sometimes a combination of any of these—served as final rinses.

Aloe vera gel was applied to the scalp and left on overnight. West Virginians washed their heads with rosemary or sage leaf tea and borax three times a week.

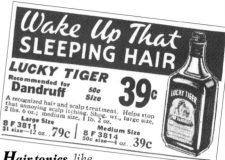

Hair tonics, like this one from the 1930s, were once thought to cure dandruff.

Kerosene and stump water were also popular, as were scalp-massage oils made from burdock root or sweet bay.

Petroleum jelly, castor oil, and the oils of peanut, corn, and olive have all served as scalp treatments. However, studies have shown that these may irritate the skin, promote rash, and worsen flaking. Other household remedies that have fallen by the wayside include a mixture of phenol, glycerin, rum, and rose water, a salve made from sesame oil and gingerroot, and a paste of salt and raw eggs.

GOLDENSEAL To make a tea, pour 1 cup boiling water over 2 teaspoons chopped root. Steep, strain, and apply as a scalp rinse three or four times a day. The constituent berberine has strong antibacterial and antifungal properties but may irritate the skin.

GARLIC Crush a raw garlic clove and apply the pulp to the affected skin. The pulp and oil both contain the antibacterial and antifungal sulfur compound allicin. Both pulp and oil may irritate the skin or cause allergic dermatitis.

ROSEMARY To make a tea, pour 1 cup boiling water over 1 teaspoon chopped leaves. Steep, strain, and apply once a day as a compress. Rosemary extracts are antiitch, antiseptic, and antifungal. Tinctures are also available. Topical use may cause allergic dermatitis.

DEPRESSION

Periodic feelings of sadness and grief are normal aspects of life. Nevertheless, feeling this way is usually referred to in everyday speech as "being depressed." It is extremely important, however, to distinguish such normal emotions from clinical depression.

An illness, clinical depression manifests itself in several forms and is not always easy to diagnose. While it is sometimes a secondary effect of another disease or a reaction to medications, it can also be caused by certain biochemical imbalances, although this is rare.

About 25 percent of Canadians experience some kind of emotional disturbance at one time or other, and 1 in 4 women (as opposed to 1 in 10 men) are likely to have a clinical depression in the course of their lives. Bipolar disorder, formerly known as manic-depressive disease, has depression as its negative pole. Many clinically depressed patients are helped today by new medications and psychotherapies.

Still, accurate professional diagnosis and treatment are of the utmost importance because of the risk of suicide.

People undergoing a moderate depression may sample traditional herbal remedies and such disciplines as yoga and meditation to complement professional treatment. These therapies may also help to combat, if not prevent, bouts of anxiety and emotional fatigue.

Treatments of Yore

"Nervines," tonics, and teas were regularly prescribed for many physical maladies now recognized as symptoms of depression: loss of appetite, sleeplessness, irritability, trembling spells, headaches, and shortness of breath. Fragrant herb pillows, along with various herbal teas, were recommended to help with insomnia.

Settlers from England brought with them myriad calmative applications for lavender. Most notably, they applied its aromatic oil directly to pressure points such as the temples to help cure headaches and induce drowsiness. In gypsy folk medicine, wines flavored with herb mixtures of valerian, clove, and rosemary were widely prepared and thought to be effective at soothing frayed nerves. Today, St. Johnswort is the herb of choice.

Prescriptions of exercise, fresh air, and abstinence from flesh-foods often accompanied traditional remedies, along with common sense orders to engage the patient in social activities. These folk treatments were not far off the mark: physical ailments notwithstanding, the damaging effects of isolation are often what perpetuate chronic episodes of depression, especially among the elderly.

See a doctor if ...

The *Diagnostic and Statistics Manual IV,* the official diagnostic manual of the psychiatric profession, outlines criteria for identifying a major depressive episode. Such episodes are signaled if five or more of the following symptoms are present for a two-week period and represent a change from the patient's previous behavior.

◆ Depressed mood for most of the day, nearly every day
◆ Diminished interest in all or most daily activities
◆ Major weight loss without dieting
◆ Increased or decreased appetite
◆ Insomnia, excess sleep, or fatigue
◆ Feelings of worthlessness or guilt nearly every day
◆ Inability to concentrate or recurrent thoughts of death or suicide

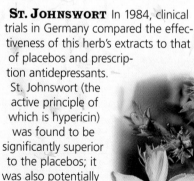

ST. JOHNSWORT In 1984, clinical trials in Germany compared the effectiveness of this herb's extracts to that of placebos and prescription antidepressants. St. Johnswort (the active principle of which is hypericin) was found to be significantly superior to the placebos; it was also potentially as effective as the

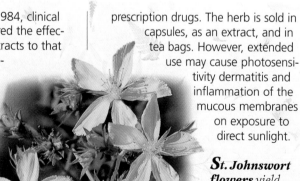

prescription drugs. The herb is sold in capsules, as an extract, and in tea bags. However, extended use may cause photosensitivity dermatitis and inflammation of the mucous membranes on exposure to direct sunlight.

St. Johnswort flowers yield valuable hypericin.

DIAPER RASH

For hundreds of years parents have found keeping a baby's bottom dry a never-ending challenge. In fact, the search for a solution has developed into a major industry, with disposable diapers of countless kinds flooding the market. Still, despite the advances in diaper design, diaper rash is as common today as it was centuries ago.

Diaper rash develops when an infant's skin is exposed to feces or urine, particularly when a diaper change is delayed. It can also result from chafing caused by rough diapers. An effective preventive is breast-feeding. Some studies have shown that when newborns are breast-fed from birth they have a lower frequency and severity of diaper rash than those given formula. The benefits are said to last even after an infant has been weaned.

Although most rashes disappear within a day, they can last longer. Avoid using commercial baby wipes and soap; the wipes contain alcohol, which irritates the skin even more, as does soap. Instead, rinse the infant's bottom with a saline solution (1 tablespoon salt to 1 liter boiled water) at room temperature. Gently dry, then apply a zinc oxide lotion to create a barrier against wetness.

Old-time diaper rash remedies included applying cornstarch or baking soda to the affected skin or placing chopped plantain leaves in the diaper. Oven-browned flour, with the same absorptive qualities as cornstarch, was also used.

Airing a baby's bottom can also help prevent diaper rash: the less time an infant's skin is covered by a diaper, the better. Wait for nap time, then place an unfastened diaper under the sleeping child. Or you can put the baby on towels placed atop a waterproof sheet.

Cloth or Plastic?

Despite the numerous varieties of diapers to choose from, today's parents still wonder whether to use cloth or plastic. If you choose cloth, follow folk practitioners' advice and add 2 tablespoons white vinegar to 4 liters water during the laundry's final rinse phase (some say that doing this helps balance the pH of the cloth diapers with that of the baby's skin). Another tip: let cloth diapers dry in the sun; ultraviolet rays act as a sterilizer, which can eliminate bacteria living on the cloth.

Babies with diaper rash are susceptible to yet another problem: the fungus candida, signaled by a fiery red rash with well-defined borders. This condition should be treated with prescription drugs.

One of the benefits of breast-feeding your baby has proved to be a lower incidence of diaper rash.

CORNSTARCH Cornstarch acts as an absorbent on wet skin. Although it can be used straight from the box, it will absorb more moisture if it is spread on a cookie sheet and dried in the oven for 10 minutes at 150°C (300°F). Let cool before using.

FENUGREEK This spice can be applied directly to the skin, like baby powder. Or you can mix it with a little water to form a paste. Apply the paste sparingly to irritated areas.

BAG BALM Originally used to soften cows' udders, bag balm has become popular among mothers as a preventive treatment for diaper rash. Today it may be found readily in farm-supply stores. After rinsing the baby's bottom with cool water, dry, then apply the bag balm directly to the skin.

DIARRHEA

The 1874 *Household Encyclopedia* offered the following advice to diarrhea sufferers: "Those who are liable to frequent returns of this disease should live temperately, avoid crude summer fruits, most kinds of vegetables, and all unwholesome food and meats of hard digestion. They ought also to beware of cold, moisture, or whatever may obstruct the perspiration, and they should invariably—winter and summer—wear flannel next to the skin."

We can only be grateful that this was not the final word on folk treatments for this common bodily disorder, characterized by frequent and abnormal liquid bowel movements. In fact, the voluminous work that folk practitioners have performed in identifying and developing cures for diarrhea could fill a large book. What they have discovered is an abundance of natural substances that are effective in treating this ubiquitous, if temporary, illness. Not so simple, however, is identifying the root cause of diarrhea, which is not so much a disorder as a symptom of underlying problems.

The fruit and roots of black-berry are shown with blueberries, scoopfuls of bilberry and witch hazel leaves, and white oak bark—all high in tannins.

Finding the Cause

The most common culprit for what in more modest days was referred to as "the summer complaint" is food poisoning. This occurs when food or water that has been contaminated with bacteria is ingested; staphylococcus and salmonella are frequently to blame. Diarrhea can begin anywhere from 2 to 48 hours later, depending on the type of bacteria. The incubation time and type of food eaten can make it easier to identify the offending bacterium: staphylococcus works fast, causing diarrhea in an hour or two, while salmonella takes about six hours.

Food poisoning, however, may not be a factor at all. Amoebic dysentery, caused by ingesting the tiny animal parasite *Entamoeba histolytica*, can cause severe diarrhea. So can such intestinal problems as colitis.

Other possible causes are chemical poisoning (after which diarrhea and vomiting begin in less than an hour), a viral infection in the digestive tract or elsewhere, and digestive problems brought on by a deficiency of certain enzymes, including lactase.

Even a simple change in eating habits—especially when adopting a diet high in roughage and fresh fruits—can cause problems until the body has had time to adjust. Moreover, diarrhea is often brought on by the food or water consumed in another country, resulting in a disruption of the balance of bacteria in the intestines. (To prevent what is often called *turista*, drink bottled carbonated beverages; avoid tap water and beverages with ice cubes.) Still another cause of diarrhea is purely psychological—the result of too much emotional stress.

Actually, most diarrhea resolves itself in a few days. It results in complications only in severe cases, with dehydration as a by-product. To replenish the fluids and minerals that have been flushed out of the system, some doctors advise drinking a liter of carbonated water in which ¼ cup sugar and ½ teaspoon each of salt and baking soda have been dissolved.

A Forestful of Cures

Over the years folk practitioners have marshaled an impressive array of treatments for diarrhea, ranging from the highly unlikely (wearing a necklace made of allspice or drinking milk that has been boiled in an iron pot) to others that were not only complicated but potentially dangerous. One such remedy called for preparing a powder out of 3 parts goldenseal and 2 parts each garlic, bayberry bark, wormwood, and chaparral (now known to be dangerous when used internally), and taking it every two hours.

Indians used a number of native plants to treat diarrhea. The Cheyenne made a decoction from the leaves and stems of ragweed, while the Oglala Sioux used the leaves of the indigo bush. Indeed, the hills and forests of North America are alive with flora, both native and naturalized, that have been brought into the service of combating this unpleasant condition. Comfrey, bayberry bark, raspberry, geranium, oregano, prickly ash, skullcap, and spearmint are but a smattering of the many plants that Indians, herbalists, and folk healers have tried.

Tea or Toast?

Whatever its cause, diarrhea occurs because irritation of the intestinal tract has stimulated stronger-than-usual bowel movements, sweeping fecal matter rapidly out of the digestive system and allowing too little time for fluids to be absorbed. To reduce intestinal irritation, folk practitioners recommend tannin-rich teas, which have an astringent effect. Even though tannic acid is found in common tea, it is present in higher concentrations in certain berries, including blackberry. Tannins are believed to reduce intestinal inflammation by binding to the surface protein layer of the inflamed mucous membrane. But take note: excessive doses of tannic acid can result in liver toxicity.

Some people believed that milk toast, the longtime breakfast favorite, would ease diarrhea if the toast were burnt — the milk would coat the intestines while the "charcoal" would act as an absorbent. Today activated charcoal capsules are indeed an effective treatment for diarrhea. Milk and other dairy products, however, are not advised: they can lead to nausea and vomiting. Instead, drink clear liquids, which will replace fluids without milk's nauseating effect.

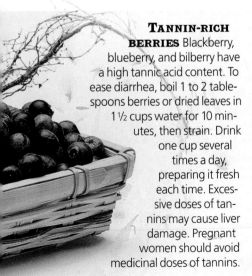

TANNIN-RICH BERRIES Blackberry, blueberry, and bilberry have a high tannic acid content. To ease diarrhea, boil 1 to 2 tablespoons berries or dried leaves in 1½ cups water for 10 minutes, then strain. Drink one cup several times a day, preparing it fresh each time. Excessive doses of tannins may cause liver damage. Pregnant women should avoid medicinal doses of tannins.

WITCH HAZEL LEAVES Although witch hazel is most often used topically, its high percentage of tannins make it an effective internal treatment for diarrhea. Combine 2 to 3 teaspoons of minced witch hazel leaves with 1 cup boiling water and let steep for 10 minutes. For mild diarrhea, drink a cup of the tea two to three times a day, but not for more than two days at this rate.

WHITE OAK BARK White oak bark contains 8 to 10 percent astringent tannins. It is commercially available as an extract and in capsules. To make your own white oak decoction, add ½ teaspoon powdered bark to 1 cup cold water. Boil for 5 minutes, then strain. Drink one cupful per day.

WILD STRAWBERRY A tea made from the leaves of wild strawberry (*Fragaria vesca*) can be drunk several times a day to treat diarrhea. Pour 1 cup boiling water over 1 teaspoon dried leaves. Steep for 10 minutes, then strain. The tea may cause an allergic reaction in people hypersensitive to strawberries.

WALNUT LEAF Place 1 to 2 teaspoons minced walnut leaves (*Juglans regia*) in 1 cup cold water and heat to boiling. Steep for five minutes; strain. Drink a cupful one to three times a day.

DIZZINESS

Dizziness generally describes a feeling of light-headedness, a loss of balance, or vertigo—a sense that one's surroundings (or oneself) are spinning. Most spells are harmless and pass quickly, causing only momentary concern; sitting or lying down for a short time is usually enough to let them pass. But feeling dizzy can also indicate more serious problems that may call for seeing a doctor. Some dizziness is accompanied by a darkening of vision or a momentary blackout. And a case of severe dizziness may cause nausea, vomiting, sweating, or fainting.

The middle ear contains much of the body's equipment for determining our sense of balance, and a number of factors can cause this machinery to malfunction. An ear infection, for example, can cause congestion that "gums up the works." Likewise, if you get a feeling of vertigo when you roll over in bed or sit up abruptly after lying down, a middle ear problem may be the cause. "Feeling faint," on the other hand, is a brief drop in blood pressure caused by insufficient blood reaching the brain, the result of either standing up suddenly or standing a long time without moving. The conventional advice to ease a dizzy spell is to sit down and put the head between the knees; doing so will help blood flow to the head return to normal. Other causes of dizziness range from simple tiredness, stress, and fever to more serious conditions requiring medical attention. These include anemia, hypoglycemia, subdural hematoma, or transient ischemic attack—a temporary blockage of the arteries to the brain due to injury or disease.

Beneficial Botanicals

Of the numerous herbs that have been traditionally used in folk medicine to treat dizziness—balm to betony, sage to shepherd's purse—a few have come to the fore. Most prominent are ginger, ginseng, and ginkgo, which are prescribed not only by folk healers but also by many physicians. Among herbalists, lavender enjoys a reputation as an effective treatment.

That shaky feeling can be eased by a few choice botanicals—ginger and ginkgo among them.

LAVENDER To lessen dizziness, suck on a sugar cube on which you've placed 1 to 4 drops lavender oil. Or make a tea by pouring 1 cup boiling water over 2 teaspoons dried lavender flowers. Steep for five minutes, then strain and drink.

GINKGO The flavonoid glycosides in ginkgo increase blood flow to the brain and have a significant effect on vertigo, especially in the elderly. Standardized extract of ginkgo leaves is available in capsules. For frequency of dosage, follow the directions on the label.

GINGER To make a tea from fresh ginger, pour 1 cup boiling water over 1 to 2 teaspoons grated gingerroot. Let steep for 10 minutes; strain, then drink. Powdered gingerroot is available as a spice at grocery stores and in capsule form at pharmacies and health food stores.

GINSENG Although ginseng is used mainly as a tonic, a ginseng compound called ginsenoside Rg_1 is known to counter loss of blood pressure associated with dizziness. To quell dizziness caused by a short-term illness, drink an infusion of ½ teaspoon dried root in 1 cup hot water, divided into two daily doses. For long-term prevention, use only ¼ teaspoon dried root daily. Ginseng extracts are also available.

DRY SKIN

Dry skin doubtless plagued our forebears, who labored in the elements and scrubbed the wash by hand with caustic lye. It is still a common problem. Occasionally, dry or itchy skin is associated with a serious disease; if the condition persists, see a doctor. More often, however, it indicates that the skin's sebaceous (oil) glands have been outmatched by nature's onslaughts—glaring sun, harsh winds, cold winter weather—as well as today's dry indoor heat. All of these exact a higher toll as we age and our sebaceous glands become less active.

To treat dry skin, early settlers slathered on such fats and oils as castor oil and lard. Also popular was lanolin, or hydrous wool fat, a yellowish fatty substance obtained from wool. All of these form a protective layer on the skin that prevents moisture from escaping. Likewise, various foods—including avocado pulp, papaya milk, and almond oil— were applied to the skin to beneficial effect. Indeed, many of these are ingredients in modern-day skin creams.

Comfrey leaves have a long history of folk use; their active ingredient, allantoin, softens dry skin and helps lock in moisture. In Germany comfrey ointment is regularly prescribed for dermatitis and eczema. In Canada, the herb has been restricted (at least for internal use) because it contains toxic pyrrolizidine alkaloids. However, it is probably safe to use comfrey leaf preparations externally on unbroken skin—although children and pregnant or lactating women should avoid the herb altogether.

Another remedy was the wildflower known to English settlers as "king's cure-all"—now called evening primrose. Today evening primrose is treasured for the oil found in its seeds, containing valuable fatty acids that, when taken internally, help maintain normal bodily functions; the oil is sold in capsule form as a dietary supplement. Some folk practitioners claim that ingestion of the supplement will also help moisturize dry skin—but in reality, the orally-taken oils' effects on dry skin have yet to be proved.

ALOE VERA The fresh gel of aloe vera contains a high level of malic acid, an alpha hydroxy acid valued for its anti-wrinkle effect. To obtain the gel, cut off a leaf at the fleshy base and split it open with a knife. Scrape out the gel with a spoon, taking care not to rupture the green rind.

COCOA BUTTER Cocoa butter is the fat extracted from roasted cocoa, or cacao, beans. The white waxy material can be applied to dry skin as needed; it melts on contact to soothe and protect. Cocoa butter is available in stick form.

AVOCADO FACIAL The oil in avocados acts as an emollient. Avocado also contains beneficial vitamin E. To treat dry facial skin, purée the pulp and pat it on the face as a mask. Leave on for 20 to 30 minutes.

Nevertheless, topical applications of evening primrose lotions and creams will help skin stay moist. (An oral, or internal, treatment that does help dry skin is vitamin E—about 800 IU per day.)

Finally, folk wisdom prescribes drinking plenty of water to hydrate the skin and bathing in tepid water scented with bath oils. But avoid too-frequent bathing, which can remove the skin's natural oils—as will harsh deodorant soaps.

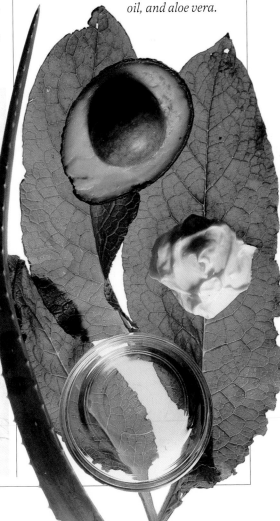

Dry skin soothers include *comfrey leaves, avocado, cocoa butter, evening primrose oil, and aloe vera.*

EARACHES

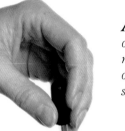

*A **drop or two** of herbal eardrops made with garlic or mullein will soothe earaches.*

Heat was the most common traditional folk remedy for earaches. Warm skunk oil or olive oil were used as eardrops, and heated cloth bags of salt served as heating pads. Indians used a poultice of licorice leaves steeped in hot water for ear pain.

Tobacco was another common remedy for earaches, although it is not recommended today. It was often mixed with the juice of roasted onion and dripped into the ear. Tobacco smoke—blown gently into the ear—was also thought to ease the pain.

Heat and liquid are still the best ways to relieve earaches. Heat increases blood flow to the affected area, which speeds healing; liquids help soften dried ear wax.

Ear Pain Relief

Earaches are most often caused by ear infections. Infection of the middle ear (otitis media) usually afflicts young children and may cause pain in the ear, hearing loss, and fever. Gargling with warm salt water when ear pain begins can help

some children: the liquid's heat increases the flow of blood to the eustachian tubes, which link the ears and throat.

Swimmer's ear (otitis externa) is an ear canal infection. If the ear feels itchy, you may prevent an infection by using over-the-counter eardrops. Herbalists advise putting a few drops of warm garlic oil or mullein oil into the ear canal. A few drops of vinegar in olive oil can also be tried.

Young children often put small objects in their ears. Do not try to remove these yourself; doing so might push them in farther. Instead, take the child to a doctor.

If an insect flies into someone's ear, shining a light in the ear in the dark may cause it to emerge. Or try removing it by tilting the person's head so that the affected ear is up, then slowly pouring in lukewarm water. If neither works, see a doctor.

See a doctor if...

Middle or inner ear infections accompanied by these symptoms require the care of a doctor.

◆ Fluid runs out of the ear
◆ Pain is severe
◆ The ear feels blocked
◆ You feel dizzy
◆ You have sudden hearing loss

HOT WATER BOTTLE A hot water bottle with a moist towel wrapped around it will soothe the pain of an earache as a temporary measure.

GARLIC Garlic has antibacterial properties due to its content of allicin, a disulfide compound. For infections of the ear canal, crush 2 cloves of garlic into ½ cup olive oil and leave it at room temperature for a few days. Strain it and keep on hand in the refrigerator. Warm it slightly before dropping it into the affected ear with an ear dropper. Lightly cover the ear opening with a cotton ball.

HYDROGEN PEROXIDE To get excess wax out of your ear, put ten drops of hydrogen peroxide in each ear and let it stay there for three minutes.

Then tilt the head so the liquid runs out—and the wax with it.

MULLEIN Despite no scientific evidence that mullein offers more than mild astringent properties, its oil has long been used to treat earaches. For eardrops, mix ½ cup crushed fresh flowers with 1 cup olive oil. Let steep overnight before straining and using.

ECHINACEA

Echinacea purpurea
CONEFLOWER, PURPLE
CONEFLOWER, BLACK SAMPSON,
COMBFLOWER, HEDGEHOG

Used for centuries by the Plains Indians for its ability to prevent and fight infections from colds to skin problems, echinacea is leading the revival of herbal medicine. At the beginning of the 20th century, the Eclectic doctor and pharmacist John Uri Lloyd studied echinacea and predicted it would be "ardently sought and widely used." By 1921 it had outsold more than 300 North American plant-based products prepared by Lloyd Brothers of Cincinnati, a premier pharmacy of the time. Indeed, Lloyd was right: today echinacea is the best-selling herbal product in the U.S. and Germany.

Species and Nicknames

Native to the plains of central North America, echinacea has three major species, all similar: *Echinacea angustifolia* (narrow-leaved purple coneflower), *E. purpurea* (purple coneflower), and *E. pallida* (pale purple coneflower). Although all three of these members of the sunflower family have been used in folk medicine, *E. purpurea* now has the widest distribution in North America and has received the most scientific attention.

The Indians used a variety of descriptive names for echinacea. Because the seed head was used to comb the hair, the Lakota called it *on'glakcapi* ("comb"). The Omaha and the Ponca names were *mika-hi* ("comb plant") and *inshtogahte-hi* ("eyewash"). The Omaha also differentiated between *nuga* (male and larger) and *miga* (female and smaller) purple coneflowers, preferring the latter—possibly the shorter *E. angustifolia*—for medicinal use. The Pawnee used two names: *ksapitahako* ("to whirl," after a children's game), and *saparidu hahts* ("mushroom medicine").

The settlers, too, had myriad names for echinacea. Snakeroot, scurvy root, and combflower all refer to specific uses. Coneflower, Indian head, black susan, black root, cock-up-hat, hedgehog (*echinos* is Greek for "hedgehog"), and sea urchin variously describe the plant's appearance—its cone-shaped flowers, its spiny, dark-colored seed head, and its dark medicinal root. Black sampson, once a popular name for the herb, was coined by slave owners after a common slave name.

Immunity Booster

Various Indian tribes found echinacea worked on a host of ailments, and often took the tea or juice from the root internally and externally at the same time. The Choctaw and the Crow used the herb for colds and coughs at the onset of symptoms. The Dakota and the Omaha treated

Active plant parts Roots, leaves, flower heads
Uses Colds and flu, cuts and abrasions, yeast infections
Cautions No toxic effects have been reported for echinacea, yet the herb is not recommended for pregnant women, nursing mothers, diabetics, or children under two. Short-term reactions may include fever, nausea, and vomiting. Allergic reactions are also possible. Echinacea should not be used by those suffering from severe illnesses, such as tuberculosis, leukemia, collagen diseases, multiple sclerosis, and all autoimmune diseases.

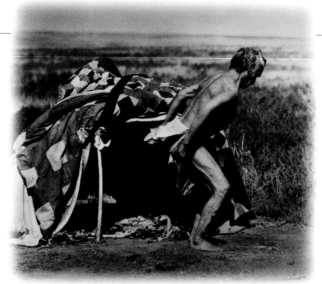

In Indian sweat lodges, echinacea was added to the steam water to help sweat out impurities in the body.

bacterial infections with echinacea, and the Sioux and the Delaware applied it to the lesions of gonorrhea and other venereal diseases. The Lakota and the Mesquakie drank the root tea to remedy stomachaches and cramps and sometimes to boost strength and alertness.

As settlers learned of echinacea's uses by the Indians, they adopted many—especially those for colds and influenza—and expanded the herb's reach to include bronchitis, whooping cough, bladder infections, allergies, and food poisoning. In fact, as its popularity grew in the late 19th century, echinacea forged a reputation as an all-around tonic that would improve the blood, clean out toxins, prevent colds, and fight any number of infections. Oklahomans even gave it to their ailing horses and cattle to stimulate the appetite. Confidence in the plant was so high that both the Indians and the settlers used the tea against rabies—a serious condition that no herb can cure.

Numerous scientific tests, most of them conducted in Germany, have confirmed echinacea's "nonspecific" boost to the immune system. It has been found that no one principle is at work, but different constituents (including echinacein and polysaccharides) work to guard the bloodstream, inhibit infection, and stimulate the production of white blood cells and new tissue. Most significant, echinacea tea and extract may help ward off colds and relieve cold symptoms.

Wider Indian Use

The Indians used echinacea in several different forms to relieve discomforts of the skin and mouth. The juice, root tea, or mashed root salve were applied to relieve skin irritations, including measles and smallpox, as well as the swelling that is symptomatic of mumps. Root applications were also used to soothe the pain of snakebite, arthritis, and sore muscles and to speed the healing of eye infections, wounds, boils, frostbite, and gangrene.

Tribes of the Great Plains, including the Cheyenne and Sioux, chewed the root or gargled the tea to numb toothaches, mouth sores, swollen tonsils, and sore throats. The Omaha and Winnebago used the salve as a local anesthetic.

In Indian rituals, the mildly numbing root juice was applied to the feet before walking on hot coals, to the mouth before holding a hot coal there, or to the hands before pulling meat from boiling water—practices that symbolized spiritual power. Believed to help purify bodily systems, the

The "Discovery" of Echinacea

Although echinacea was first mentioned in *Flora Virginica* (1762) as a remedy for saddle sores on horses, H.F.C. Meyer, a doctor and patent-medicine salesman from Pawnee City, Nebraska, is credited with its modern discovery. In 1871 he used it in his secret Blood Purifier for treatments first known to the Indians, such as those for fever and snakebite.

Fifteen years later, Meyer sent samples of the plant to both John King, author of the *American Dispensatory*, and the Lloyd Brothers pharmacy. (He even sought to show off its virtues in person—with a snake.) The Lloyds identified the plant as *Echinacea angustifolia*, and King added it to his book (although without Meyer's boasts). As a result, echinacea was said by John Uri Lloyd in 1917 to be "consumed in larger quantities" than any other North American drug "introduced in the last 30 years."

Despite no official recognition by the Canadian Medical Association, many doctors used echinacea before the rise of modern antibiotics.

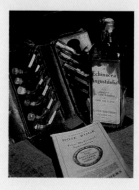

root was also added to the steam water used in sweat-lodge ceremonies.

Many of these original uses of echinacea remain valuable today. Research has found hints of anti-inflammatory, antibacterial, and wound-healing properties. The extract is also reported to be mildly insecticidal, although the plant cannot treat insect or snake bites beyond its possible anti-inflammatory activity. In Germany, it is approved for chronic respiratory and urinary tract infections and for external sores and wounds.

Researchers have also found potential new uses for echinacea. Extracts of the root may prevent and help cure yeast infections, and patients undergoing radiation treatment may experience fewer side effects when taking the herb. Other studies are looking at echinacea's effect on cancer cells and arthritis. Around the world, the herb is used topically for arthritis, burns, boils, eczema, psoriasis, and herpes and internally for colds, tonsillitis, and bladder and respiratory infections.

Buying and Using

Although more than 150 conventional medicines are made from echinacea in Germany, it is not yet recognized as bona fide by the medical community in Canada and the United States. Nevertheless, many varieties of the plant are available.

When buying the fresh herb, look for the Latin name: for years, other plants have been fraudulently sold as echinacea. In bygone days, button snakeroot (*Eryngium praealtum*) was an imposter. More recently, Missouri snakeroot (*Parthenium integrifolium*) has been substituted. Also, echinacea's old genus names—*Rudbeckia* and *Brauneria*—may still be in use.

Echinacea products are usually labeled "organically grown," "pesticide-free," or "farmed," indicating that the plant is neither from the wild nor endangered. Tinctures and extracts are the most common forms; these should produce a slight tingling sensation when applied to the tongue. Other forms are tea bags, juices, tablets, and capsules. If you are buying the raw plant material, look for either the plant's aerial parts or the powdered root.

Studies have yet to pinpoint the best form or recommended dosage, but extensive usage has determined amounts that are generally agreed upon. Tinctures are normally applied to the back of the tongue or added to drinks: 15 to 30 drops (usually a dropperful) at a time, two to five times a day. Tablets and capsules are usually taken once or twice a day.

The pressed juice of *E. purpurea* is yet another product—usually taken at 1 to 2 teaspoons a day. Teas (made from tea bags or 2 teaspoons raw root) can be taken up to three times a day but are reportedly less potent because not all of the healing components are water-soluble. For the best results, two weeks of use should be followed by two weeks of non-use. Any uninterrupted use should not exceed eight weeks. Externally, salves and ointments are also widely used, as are cotton pads soaked with the tea or extract.

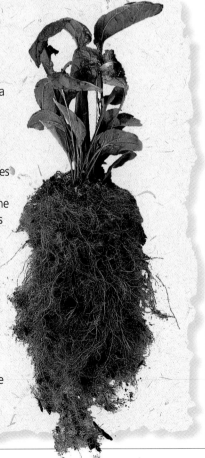

Growing Your Own

Echinacea is a hardy, drought-resistant wildflower that is popular for its colorful blooms. It generally ranges from Saskatchewan south through Nebraska, Kansas, and Oklahoma into northern Texas, but it can live in any garden that has proper soil and sun.

To grow your own, sow the seeds in January on a sandy soil surface, then tamp them down. The seeds should sprout in spring. Echinacea does not like competing with weeds or being transplanted. If you wish to harvest the roots, grow the plant for three to four years and gather the roots in autumn. To prepare the roots for medicinal use, rinse them off completely and lay them in the hot sun (or in low oven heat) to dry.

Echinacea angustifolia, which grows only 15 to 50 cm (6 to 20 in.) high, is smaller than most echinacea species. *E. purpurea* and other species grow up to 1.2 m (4 ft) high. Cultivars of *E. purpurea* are also grown, the most popular being those that produce white flowers. These include 'White Lustre' and 'White Prince,' all of which can be used medicinally.

ELDER

Sambucus nigra
EUROPEAN ELDER, BLACK ELDER,
PIPE TREE, BOURTREE

The European elder, which has been naturalized in parts of North America since the 17th century, is one of mankind's earliest and most versatile plant companions. All of its parts— root, flowers, berries, bark, leaves, and wood—have illustrious histories. In medieval Europe the plant was so widely exploited that it earned the title "nature's medicine chest." Centuries later, it even had its moment of glory in Hollywood: it was poisoned elderberry wine that two spinster aunts graciously offered their guests in the comedy classic *Arsenic and Old Lace*.

On a happier note, the elderberry found several medicinal uses on this continent. Shaker and Appalachian herbalists as well as Indians employed it for a whole battery of upper respiratory conditions. Elderberry tea made with dried elder blossoms, yarrow, and peppermint leaves was believed to cure a cold. The juice from cooked elderberries came to be prized as a purgative and a blood tonic and was considered especially good for the kidneys and liver.

A green ointment made from the young stems and leaves was a common country salve for skin irritations, chilblains, and snakebite. Elder flower infusions and elder flower vinegars were used as gargles to alleviate tonsillitis and sore throats, while coughs were often treated with sugary elderberry wine. In the kitchen, the berries made a classic pie.

Its Use Today

Today's use of elder is generally limited to remedies and digestives made with the flowers. Distilled elder flower water is widely used cosmetically, as both a skin toner and a fragrant base for lotions. Additionally, the positive diuretic, laxative, and sweat-inducing effects of the elder flowers' volatile oil have been newly confirmed in recent studies.

Although the flowers' usefulness as an expectorant is still in question, some recent studies suggest that elder's traditional use against colds may be related to an antiviral effect. This activity is currently being studied, and elder syrup and lozenges to fight colds are now marketed in Israel. Over-the-counter preparations using elder flower and elder extracts are also generally considered trustworthy.

Elderberries are still used in cooking: the deep blue-purple fruits are harvested every autumn for use in jellies, pies, pancakes, and fritters. Only the fully cooked berries should be used, however; eating raw berries is highly dangerous.

Active plant parts Flowers
Uses Astringent, diuretic, laxative
Cautions Any formulas or recipes containing root, leaf, bark, or stem parts should be avoided because of the potential toxicity of an isolated glycoside contained in elder, called sambunigrin. Children should be supervised around this plant: many who make whistles or "pop-guns" out of elder have typically suffered severe nausea after chewing on the fresh stem. Fresh or raw berries have also been reported to be toxic, causing vomiting, dizziness, and in rare cases numbness and stupor.

ELECAMPANE

Inula helenium
SCABWORT, HORSEHEAL,
ALANT, YELLOW STARWORT,
WILD SUNFLOWER

This sunflower-like plant has been in demand as a medicine since ancient times. Some say that its species name—*helenium*—comes from the legend that Helen of Troy carried the herb when she was stolen away by the Trojan prince Paris. It was also widely used in Europe and Asia to treat "thicke and clammie humours which stick in the chest and lungs"—pneumonia, tuberculosis, whooping cough, and asthma—as well as sciatica and itching. Veterinarians valued it too, using it as a treatment for skin diseases on horses and sheep—hence two of its common names: scabwort and horseheal.

The first settlers brought elecampane to the New World, where it established itself in fields and along roadsides in the eastern half of North America. A tea made from the roots was a folk remedy for lung ailments and indigestion, as well as a diuretic and menstruation promoter. Some claims were false: in Indiana, elecampane was one ingredient of what was claimed to be an "infallible treatment" for rabies, although it actually had no effect on the disease. More sensibly, in the 19th century, the herb's roots were boiled with sugar to make cough drops and throat lozenges, often in combination with licorice, bloodroot, or skunk cabbage.

Recent Findings

Modern herbalists recommend elecampane mainly for coughs, asthma, bronchitis, and emphysema. Its active principle, alantolactone, has indeed been proven an effective expectorant. Studies also show that it expels intestinal parasites, kills some types of fungi and bacteria, and has anti-inflammatory properties. Some herbalists use a wash made from the root to treat sciatica and facial neuralgia. In experimental animal studies, the herb has acted as a sedative and reduced blood pressure. If you have high blood pressure, consult your doctor before using it.

While root extracts are available and are taken mixed with water, enthusiastic gardeners may want to grow their own elecampane. Note, however, that the root is considered to have medicinal value only if harvested the second year. To make a decoction, simmer 1 to 2 teaspoons of the minced root in 3 cups of water for 30 minutes. Keep the pan covered while it cools. Take up to 2 cups a day, a tablespoon or two at a time, with honey to disguise the bitter taste.

Active plant parts Root
Uses Respiratory problems, intestinal worms; digestive aid
Cautions Nursing mothers and children under age two should avoid elecampane. Because of its traditional, yet unproven, use in bringing on menstruation, the herb should not be used by pregnant women. Laboratory studies with animals show that small amounts of elecampane lower blood sugar levels, while large amounts raise them; for this reason, diabetics should avoid it. Contact with the plant or its oil may cause a skin rash. In large doses, elecampane can induce nausea, cramps, dizziness, and paralysis.

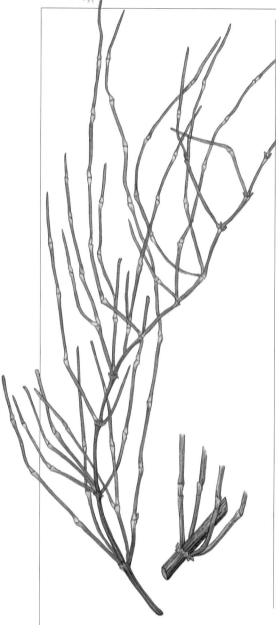

EPHEDRA

Ephedra sinica
MA HUANG

No herbal product has inspired more controversy in recent years than ephedra. Even though the species native to North America is mild enough to have been called Mormon tea, Chinese ephedra, known as ma huang, has become the focus of debate over the potential dangers of "natural" drugs.

A Chinese Import

In China, ephedra has been prized for thousands of years as a treatment (either singly or combined with other plants) for asthma, colds, and hay fever. Although it is a potent nervous system stimulant and overconsumption can cause serious side effects, it is recognized by the Chinese as safe when taken in proper dosages. The same is true in the U.S. and Canada, where authorized preparations containing ephedrine (the most active of the herb's alkaloids) have long been a favored treatment for upper respiratory problems.

In the 1920s North American drug manufacturers began importing ephedra in order to extract the ephedrine. In standard doses of 6 to 12 mg ephedrine, the herb has fewer side effects than many other over-the-counter products. Still, in excessive doses it can cause nervousness, headache, palpitations, flushed skin, and other side effects. A milder ephedra alkaloid, called pseudoephedrine, was later extracted by scientists and is a common ingredient in many commercial cold and allergy remedies today.

The story of ephedra's fall from grace began in 1993, when a clinical trial showed that ephedrine and caffeine in combination contribute to weight loss. (Ephedrine raises the rate of metabolism, thereby burning calories.) Spotting a golden opportunity, some manufacturers began marketing weight-loss products that combined ephedra with such caffeine-rich plants as kola nut. But because the general public was without the benefit of the health screening and medical supervision given the subjects of the 1993 test, dozens of cases of adverse effects were reported. Contributing to the problem was the faulty equation of "natural" with "safe," which led many women who turned to ephedra for weight loss to take higher-than-recommended doses.

As awareness of ephedra's potency as a stimulant grew, rumors spread among young people that taking two or three times the dosage cited on the label of ephedra products would produce a "legal high." Hence was born the boom in such intriguingly-named products as Herbal Ecstacy, Cloud 9, and Ultimate Xphoria, all sold by unscrupulous manufacturers as alternatives to amphetamines, or "speed."

Although in Canada these ephedra products were not approved for sale, many

---

Active plant parts Stems
Uses Asthma, allergies, colds
Cautions Consult your doctor before taking ephedra. Pregnant women and anyone with high blood pressure, heart disease, diabetes, glaucoma, or hyperthyroidism should avoid the herb. Side effects may include headache, skin irritation, insomnia, nervousness, dizziness, vomiting, heart palpitations, or psychosis. Do not use ephedra with caffeine.

were sold clandestinely in fitness centers and other establishments. Made partly or wholly from ephedra, these concoctions promised euphoria without the legal consequences of marijuana, cocaine, and speed. Ultimate Xphoria, for example, billed itself as "A 100% Herbal Alternative Supplement with Vitamin C" and urged buyers to "Experience the Magic of Ecstasy"—an obvious reference to a popular street drug.

As a result of the increased use—or more aptly, misuse—of ephedra, more than 400 reports of adverse effects were made by North American consumers, ranging from nervousness to tremors and heart attacks. Fifteen deaths in the United States were also attributed to the herb. In quick order, ephedra became a lightning rod for criticism of the medicinal herb industry.

Legislation Abused

How could such dangerous products be sold? The answer goes to the heart of the debate over herbal medicine, its regulation, benefits, and dangers.

The federal government cannot prevent Canadians from illicitly importing unauthorized herbal remedies from the United States, where such products may be available on the market. As well, many herbal products are sold as foods in Canada, making it difficult to curtail their availability.

Under the Canadian Food and Drugs Act, any product offered for sale as a therapeutic remedy—to cure, prevent, or treat disease—is defined as a drug. Many herbal products with documented health benefits are allowed to be sold in Cana-

Mormon Tea: The North American Ephedra

Several species of ephedra are native to North America, but these varieties are all but devoid of the alkaloid ephedrine. If they have some effect against asthma or any other ailment, it is unclear why, although some people swear by the herbs as a mild decongestant.

Southwestern U.S. Indian tribes used the stems to treat colds, allergies, and venereal diseases. They also introduced the species *Ephedra nevadensis* to the Mormons as a piney-smelling tonic. The new settlers found this herb an agreeable substitute for coffee and black tea, and today this species of ephedra is still called Mormon tea. Other common names for *E. nevadensis* are joint fir, squaw tea, popotillo, and teamster's tea—a reference to the wagoners who made use of the herb as they traveled through the American West.

Ironically, Mormon tea was served in brothels in the Old West because it was believed to cure syphilis and gonorrhea—hence its other (and unsavory) nickname: whorehouse tea. In truth, both North American and Chinese ephedras are powerless against these ailments.

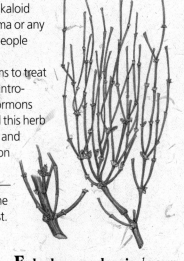

Ephedra nevadensis, *known as Mormon tea, is virtually indistinguishable from Chinese ephedra in appearance.*

da under the drug category, but they must be approved for use by Health Canada and issued a Drug Identification Number (DIN). Any authorized herbal product will sport a DIN on the front of the product label—as an eight-digit number, preceded by the letters DIN or GP (General Public).

In the controversial case of ephedra, Health Canada issued a warning in 1997, advising con-

Ephedrine-laced, *this product came cloaked in psychedelic colors.*

sumers not to purchase or consume products containing ephedrine unless the product labels carry a DIN. Only government-approved ephedrine products (including many popular over-the-counter nasal decongestants) are considered safe for use, as long as the dosage instructions and precautions are strictly followed. Many such products are only recommended for short-term use.

Interestingly, long before the controversy over ephedra began the International Olympic Committee had banned the use of ephedrine alkaloids by athletes during training or competition. Ephedra is sometimes used by bodybuilders and athletes for its purported "thermogenic" ability to burn off fat instead of muscle.

EPSOM SALTS

MAGNESIUM SULFATE, EPSOMITE

In 19th-century North America, Epsom salts were one of the few medicines readily found in medicine cabinets on farms and in small towns. Although this form of magnesium sulfate is found anywhere mineral or sea water evaporates, it takes its name from a mineral spring in Epsom, England, where one Nehemias Grew discovered it in 1694. (Canada's attempts at production came chiefly from a deposit west of Ashcroft, British Columbia, but output ceased in 1942.) Epsom salts were often taken internally as a laxative. They were also

Sea water is but one of the many sources of epsomite, another name for hydrated magnesium sulfate.

added to water to make a soaking solution used to relieve soreness and swelling. Pastes of Epsom salts and water were used to treat shingles. The salts were also rumored to cure hangovers.

Epsom salts work by osmosis. When taken internally they act as a hyperosmotic, drawing water into the bowels from surrounding tissues to soften stools. When used in a soaking solution, Epsom salts draw fluid out of the skin and shrink tissues, reducing inflammation associated with sprains, insect bites, hemorrhoids, corns, boils, poison ivy, and arthritis. The salts may also help draw out splinters.

The Spring Purge

Older North Americans may still remember when Epsom salts were given as part of the spring round of purgatives taken to rid the body of intestinal "toxins" built up over the winter months. (Castor and cod liver oils were also used for this purpose.) Although this practice has since been discounted as unnecessary and potentially harmful, small doses of Epsom salts are still occasionally used to treat constipation. Because of

their hyperosmotic activity, Epsom salts are also said to reduce blood pressure; they were once used to relieve throbbing headaches thought to result from hypertension. Because the salts dehydrate the body, they should be taken with a full glass of water, followed by a second glass. Epsom salts should be used only in the short term, since they interfere with the body's absorption of important nutrients.

Foot Soak, Face Cleanser

Tired, sore feet can be refreshed by alternately soaking them in warm water with Epsom salts, then plunging them in a basin filled with ice water. Some people recommend adding Epsom salts and five tea bags to warm water, then letting the solution cool before soaking the feet.

A teaspoon of Epsom salts can be mixed with a tablespoon of cold cream and massaged into the skin as an exfoliating cleanser. To treat blackheads, add one teaspoon Epsom salts and three drops iodine to ½ cup boiling water and let cool. Dip cotton strips into the solution and apply to the blackheads. Finally, daub the entire area with an alcohol astringent. Epsom salts and warm water can be used as a mouthwash or gargle, but do not swallow unless you want a laxative effect.

People are not the only ones to benefit from Epsom salts. Plants need magnesium sulfate, and adding a teaspoonful of Epsom salts around flowers or vegetables may stimulate their growth.

Uses Constipation, minor sprains, bruises, insect bites
Cautions See a doctor if you experience abdominal pain, nausea, vomiting, diarrhea, dizziness, or muscle weakness after taking Epsom salts internally. Consult a doctor before taking Epsom salts internally if you are allergic to laxatives, are on a low-fat or low-sugar or other special diet, are taking other medication, or have kidney disease, inflamed bowels, or abdominal pain.

EVENING PRIMROSE

Oenothera biennis
KING'S-CURE-ALL, EVENING
STAR, NIGHT WILLOW
HERB, TREE PRIMROSE

Not a true primrose, the evening primrose is a native wildflower found growing from Newfoundland to British Columbia, and south to Florida. The plant gained its name from its bright yellow flowers, which bloom for only one night. Although Indians and early settlers used it medicinally, it was not until the 20th century that attention turned to the healthful oil contained in its seeds.

A Valuable Fatty Acid

Evening primrose oil is rich in gammalinolenic acid (GLA), an essential fatty acid that is necessary to maintain normal bodily functions. Lower than normal levels may occur in diabetics, people at risk for heart attack and stroke, those with atopic eczema (an inherited dermatitis), alcoholics, and women suffering from premenstrual syndrome (PMS).

Even though our ancestors had no knowledge of GLA, some of their uses for evening primrose have been supported by modern science—an affirmation, perhaps, of the early trial-and-error approach to herbal medicine. Housewives boiled its leaves in milk and applied the infusion to skin problems. In fact, recent studies have demonstrated the oil's effectiveness in treating the itching of atopic eczema. The Cherokee treated obesity with evening primrose tea; today studies have suggested weight loss after taking the oil, particularly among those with a family history of obesity. To give strength to lacrosse players, the Iroquois chewed the root to a pulp, then rubbed it on athletes' muscles—perhaps a harbinger of its current-day (although internal) use for arthritis.

In clinical studies, GLA has also been shown to lower cholesterol and triglycerides, thereby inhibiting formation of blood clots. The oil is also claimed by some herbalists to treat the symptoms of PMS and menopause, although studies are inconclusive. More controversial are claims that the oil reverses neurological damage in diabetics and helps the damaged livers of alcoholics to regenerate.

New and Improved

Wild varieties of evening primrose contain highly variable amounts of GLA. For this reason, commercial suppliers have joined with plant breeders to develop a variety that consistently yields an oil containing 72 percent cis-linoleic acid and 9 percent GLA—making it perhaps the richest plant source of these fatty acids. Today a number of the evening primrose oil products found on the market—most often in capsule form—are derived from this new cultivar.

Active plant parts Seed oil
Uses Atopic eczema, obesity, rheumatoid arthritis, cardiovascular disease, premenstrual syndrome, alcoholism
Cautions Evening primrose can make bleeding disorders worse. Side effects may include skin rashes, nausea, and headache. People with epilepsy should avoid this herb.

EYE PROBLEMS

For early North Americans with eye problems, the family cow came in handy. At bedtime, stale bread was soaked in milk and tied over tired or sore eyes. Milk was dripped into the eyes to flush out dirt or other foreign particles. Even cow dung was used: it was mixed with honey and smeared on the eyelids to make cataracts disappear—a practice that in fact merely introduced bacteria.

The garden yielded other remedies for eye inflammations. Raw potato or cucumber slices were placed over the eyelids to soothe puffy eyes. Inflammation was treated with an infusion of eyebright (*Euphrasia officinalis*)—now more widely used in Europe than in North America.

Minor Eye Ailments

Folk remedies for eye problems are largely confined to the treatment of soreness, puffiness from lack of sleep (relieved with a cool herbal compress), pinkeye, sties, and "black eyes" (actually bruises). Cataracts are treated with surgery.

The most common problem is conjunctivitis (better known as pinkeye), which affects the conjunctiva—the mucous membrane inside the eyelid and covering the exposed surface of the eyeball. This inflammation and accompanying soreness can be caused by intense ultraviolet light, such as that reflected from snow—a good reason to wear sunglasses. It can also be caused by a viral or bacterial infection.

A sty is a red, itchy abscess at the base of an eyelash. It usually comes to a head in a few days, then ruptures and heals. It was once erroneously believed that pricking a sty with a cat's whisker or rubbing it with a gold ring would make it go away. Today's home treatments give better results: holding a warm compress to the area relieves pain and helps bring the sty to a head. A sty will also benefit—as will sore or puffy eyes—from a sterile eyewash or antibiotic ointments made for eye use.

Herbal Eyewashes

To ensure an herbal eyewash solution is sterile, simmer it for 15 minutes. Then strain it through cheesecloth to remove eye-irritating particles. Cool to lukewarm before using. Sterilize an eyecup, too, before use. Place a glass eyecup in a 160°C (325°F) oven for an hour, then rinse with boiling water. Or soak a glass or plastic eyecup for at least 30 minutes in a diluted commercial sterilizing solution.

PARSLEY To help sties heal, soak a clean cloth in an infusion made of a handful of fresh parsley that has steeped in a cup of just-boiled water for 10 minutes. Drape the cloth over closed eyes for 15 minutes twice a day until the sty is gone. If a sty does not burst or drain, consult a doctor.

GOLDENSEAL To treat a sty or itchy eyes, simmer 2 teaspoons powdered goldenseal root with 1 cup water for 15 minutes. Use a sterile eyecup to bathe the eyes with the strained, cooled liquid. A commercial goldenseal tea bag can be used as a compress when cool.

WITCH HAZEL For black eyes, pour witch hazel on a cotton pad and apply to the closed eye for half an hour. The same treatment will also soothe eye irritation caused by pollution.

TEA BAGS Soothe puffy eyes by putting wet tea bags on the eyelids for 15 or 20 minutes. Some herbalists claim that tea bags are also effective for healing black eyes.

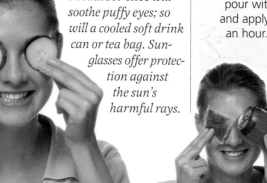

A raw potato or cucumber slice will soothe puffy eyes; so will a cooled soft drink can or tea bag. Sunglasses offer protection against the sun's harmful rays.

FAINTING

Fainting has fallen out of fashion, but it was once a hallmark of delicacy and refinement. A lady who had mastered the artful swoon could absent herself at will from an unseemly situation. The truly chaste would fall in a faint at off-color jokes or boorish behavior, although less discretionary fainting spells were often caused by constricting corsets. If necessary, a case of "the vapors" could be encouraged by wearing cold cloths in one's shoes on a hot day.

Fainting results from a sudden drop in blood pressure. The blood that normally reaches the brain is diverted to other parts of the body. Deprived of oxygen, the brain begins to shut down, cutting off hearing, vision, and, finally, consciousness. Fainting can be caused by many factors, including heat, exhaustion, hyperventilation, hypoglycemia, or an emotional trauma, such as the sight of one's own blood. People with low blood pressure are more prone to fainting, as are those taking certain drugs, including tranquilizers and high blood pressure medication. If you experience recurring episodes of fainting, consult with your doctor.

First Aid for Fainters

In the 19th century fainting was an affair for which ladies were well prepared. Fainting couches stood at the ready, elegant one-armed sofas as delicate as those whose seductive swoons they cushioned. And smelling salts were never far from reach; in fact, some women wore them in miniature glass bottles around their necks as testaments to their frailty. The bottles usually contained ammonium carbonate (a powerful nasal stimulant), to which lavender or clove oil was added. Lavender was especially popular, perhaps because its pleasant scent tempered the offensive ammonia; it also contains trace

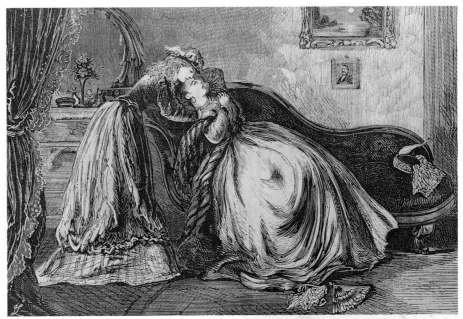

Artifice inspired many 19th-century fainting fits.

amounts of camphor, another stimulant. Black and red pepper were common stand-ins for smelling salts, but pepper—and smelling salts, too—must be used with caution: a stiff whiff can actually be toxic. Any stimulant should be held a safe distance from the person's nose.

If someone near you faints, leave him or her on the floor. Although they do it in the movies, do not splash water on the person's face—he or she may inhale the water and choke on it. If you wish, you may apply a cold damp cloth to the face. Once the person is prone and blood flows back to the brain, consciousness should return within a minute or two.

ELEVATE THE FEET If someone faints, leave the person on the ground, loosen any tight clothing, and elevate the feet. You may apply a cold cloth to the face in order to stimulate blood flow.

LIE DOWN If you feel you are going to faint, sit with your head between your knees. Better still, lie on the floor, preferably with your legs slightly elevated, and try to breathe evenly. If possible, have someone open a window for fresh air.

LAVENDER Lavender was historically mixed with ammonium carbonate as a smelling salt. If you wish, use lavender oil alone for a milder stimulant. Dip a cotton ball in the oil and wave it around under the person's nose. Rosemary oil can be used in the same way.

PRACTICES OF TRADITIONAL
PIONEER MIDWIVES

*T*he midwife was a paradox of sorts: immersed in the most natural of human events yet dabbling in the supernatural; lauded for her skill and self-sacrifice but branded by some as ignorant and impious. In reality, she was neither as benighted as critics charged nor quite so perfect as some modern advocates suggest.

On February 12, 1713, the women of Ville-Marie (in present-day Montreal) elected Catherine Guertin as their midwife—the first recorded account of a non-Indian midwife in Canada. There was never any doubt about her importance in the burgeoning New France settlement. A good midwife was indispensable to pioneer women, who on average married at age 21 and bore 12 babies over the next 18 years.

The custom of "social childbirth" lightened that formidable burden at least temporarily. Shortly before a baby was due, neighboring women took over an expectant mother's chores and continued to help for three to four weeks afterward, a "lying-in" period during which she could regain her strength and begin nursing. Social childbirth provided the new mother with invaluable

*A **typical birthing session** teamed the mother's efforts with those of midwife, husband, and neighbors.*

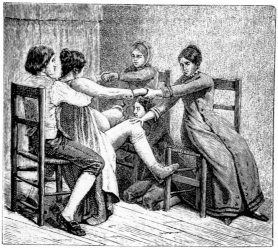

support and the other women with an equally welcome respite from their own domestic routines. When labor started, however, socializing abated: it was time for the midwife to take charge.

If a woman's labor progressed normally, the midwife actually needed to do very little, she knew that most deliveries were best left to run their own course. But if progress seemed slow, she might delve into her midwife's bag for one or more com-

*A **sign advertises** the services of midwives trained at a reputable school, one of North America's few.*

pounds—salves, lubricants, ointments, poultices, plasters, and herbal teas of goldenseal root, blue cohosh, and burdock—to ease the mother's discomfort and help nature along. Hot cloths were often applied to the mother's abdomen to relax the muscles of the uterus. Sometimes the midwife would place a quill filled with snuff powder in one of the laboring woman's nostrils, provoking a fit of sneezing that propelled the newborn into the world—a "quilled baby," as it was called. Occasionally the midwife had to reach into the birth canal to turn a baby headfirst or correct whatever else was impeding the delivery.

In theory, almost anyone could become a midwife in early North America; no formal course of study or apprenticeship was required. In reality, most were mothers past their childbearing years, with an aptitude for healing and firsthand knowledge of the

Instruments of Birthing

A traditional midwife's bag contained an assortment of herbal ingredients for use in teas, ointments, and other preparations, and this was generally the extent of her "specialized" equipment—apart from her experience and her own two hands. Natural processes usually produced healthy babies, she knew; interfering when there was no crisis tended to make matters worse, not better.

A philosophy different from that held by midwives emerged with the appearance of new tools and methods, beginning with the invention of forceps, which made it possible during difficult births to pull babies out of the birth canal without killing them. Early forceps and the skills of those using them left much to be desired, however, and countless women and infants suffered as a result. Yet physicians and man-midwives pressed on, experimenting with new devices at every opportunity, even during routine deliveries. Midwives saw firsthand the rising rate of infections, perforated organs, and other dire effects, but the tide of history would not be slowed. Science was on the march, and in medicine nothing symbolized "progress" more vividly than an array of gleaming new tools, designed by men to improve on nature.

*A **state-of-the-art** birthing chair of the late 1700s, featuring an adjustable back and a footrest, reflects the status of technology and its paraphernalia in the emerging "new midwifery."*

Ordinary household items *(above) were generally all that a midwife needed to oversee a normal delivery. She used the small brush and tapered stick to clean her hands and fingernails. The kettle was essential both for making tea for the mother as she awaited the onset of labor and for maintaining a plentiful supply of hot water (kept in the familiar washbowl) for cleansing the baby and the mother's perineal area. The cotton string was used to tie off the umbilical cord, which the midwife then cut with a pair of scissors. Soft towels (in earlier times made of cotton or linen) were kept close by for drying and wrapping the newborn, and a fresh set of linens was put on the bed in which mother and child would recuperate from the rigors of the birth.*

A New Life Safely Begun

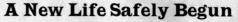

It was a scene repeated innumerable times, from pioneer days right into the 20th century. A delivery usually took place in the "borning room" —the master bedroom in a large house or a small chamber behind the central hearth, warmed by the fire and protected from drafts. "Childbed linen"— a layette—was prepared; often it was a family heirloom, handed down and stored with care until needed for the next birth in the household.

Florence Nightingale's idea that "every woman is a nurse" was realized again and again in the custom of social childbirth. This outpouring of help from an expectant mother's friends and relatives was a central part of what one historian has called the "female world of love and ritual," a network of relationships and obligations that bound most communities together. The linchpin was the midwife. Her work was more than a trade; at its best, it was an almost religious calling that set certain women apart not only for their skills but for their willingness to travel at all hours, work under difficult conditions, and attend women who could not afford to pay.

The bond between midwife and mother was stressed in the first "birth manual" published in English: "The midwife must instruct and comfort the party, not only refreshing her with good meat and drink, but also with sweet words, giving her good hope." This bond remains visible in the intimacy of three figures: the mother, her newborn, and the midwife whose hands have literally brought it into the world.

birth process. Most had also attended numerous social childbirths, observing older midwives, gradually taking a more active role, and gaining confidence in their own abilities. In addition, midwives had to master a certain body of knowledge, especially of traditional remedies made from plants they grew themselves—among them saffron, sage, and the chamomiles.

The results seemed to reflect well on North America's midwives. Fewer pioneer women died in childbirth than their English counterparts, thanks in part to better nutrition and healthier living conditions than those in many of England's teeming cities. But colonial midwives also knew

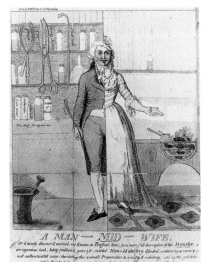

A MAN — MID — WIFE,

An early cartoon lampoons the intrusion of hardware-wielding "man-midwives" into what had been an exclusively female realm.

when to leave well enough alone, which in itself reduced the rate of infection. No known outbreak of puerperal fever among new mothers was caused by North American midwives. In fact, one historian concludes that physicians in one colony spread more infection during the 1800s than all of its "uneducated" midwives.

Men and Medicine

New techniques emerged in Europe in the 18th century that revolutionized childbirth. In particular, the increasing use of forceps by English doctors made it possible to deliver babies that would not otherwise have survived. In the 19th century, practitioners of a new midwifery by "man-midwives" equipped with forceps and other symbols of scientific progress proliferated in North Amer-

ica's cities and towns. Few traditional midwives adopted forceps; apart from being prohibitively expensive, they encouraged more intervention in the birth process than most midwives believed in—and they were no substitute for an experienced pair of hands. Forceps did help in some difficult deliveries, but they also caused injuries and infections in many women, who were left in chronic pain or unable to bear more children.

Still, the new midwifery flourished. The use of forceps in routine births defied tradition, but it saved time, enabling a man-midwife to attend more deliveries—and to collect more fees. Obstetrics soon emerged as modern medicine's first specialty, a path to status and prosperity for the entire profession. Meanwhile, traditional midwifery was vanishing from mainstream North America as more laws barred medical practice by anyone without the degree of medical doctor.

Ultimately, even as modern obstetrics achieved great technical expertise, some women began to find childbirth more stressful rather than less so because the whole process lacked an essential human dimension. As part of a "natural childbirth" movement that began in the 1960s, the midwife's traditional role was reexamined and found to offer much of value. What emerged was an attempt not to turn back the clock but to find a more balanced approach, one that made room for those basic human attributes —empathy, reassurance, voice, touch—embodied for centuries in the familiar figure of the midwife.

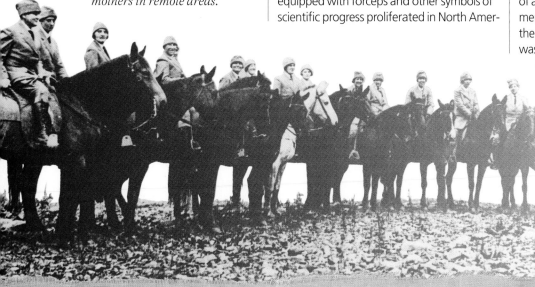

Proudly uniformed nurse-midwives of the Frontier Nursing Service, formed in Kentucky in the early 1900s, brought much needed help to mothers in remote areas.

FATIGUE

It may be the result of working too hard, sleeping too little, or living with too much stress. Or it may be the symptom of a more serious—even acute—condition. Whatever the cause, there is probably no more widespread complaint in North America today than plain old tiredness.

Before attributing fatigue solely to the complexities of modern life, it may be consoling to note that folk healers have been recommending a host of remedies, tonics, exercises, and relaxation therapies since long before two-income families became common.

"Walk barefoot in dewy grass," urged one folk practitioner as a treatment for fatigue. "Walk back and forth in several inches of cold bathwater," said another. Some folks ascribed fatigue to a "tired liver" and treated it by performing a daily exercise that involved placing the hands just above the waist and pressing in and releasing a dozen times.

Pick-me-ups

Tiredness brought on by overwork or lack of sleep is the most common kind of fatigue, and through the ages caffeine—in its many forms— has been the treatment of choice. Coffee is, in fact, the strongest natural form of caffeine. (Now that coffeehouses have become popular once again, simply taking part in the conviviality that these establishments provide may help overcome fatigue.) Still, coffee is addictive: drinking more than 3 cups a day can cause not only jangled nerves and diarrhea but may also elevate cholesterol and increase the risk of heart disease.

Other sources of caffeine include tea, colas (and sometimes other soft drinks), cocoa (a stimulant for some people), and many over-the-counter drugs. Although tea has significantly less caffeine than coffee, it contains more of a related compound called theophylline, which, in pure form, is used to treat asthma. Like caffeine, it can cause insomnia, nervousness, and increased heart rate.

Herbal Energizers

The Virginia plantation owner William Byrd wrote in the late 17th century that ginseng "frisks the spirits," but not enough to cause "those naughty effects that might make men too troublesome

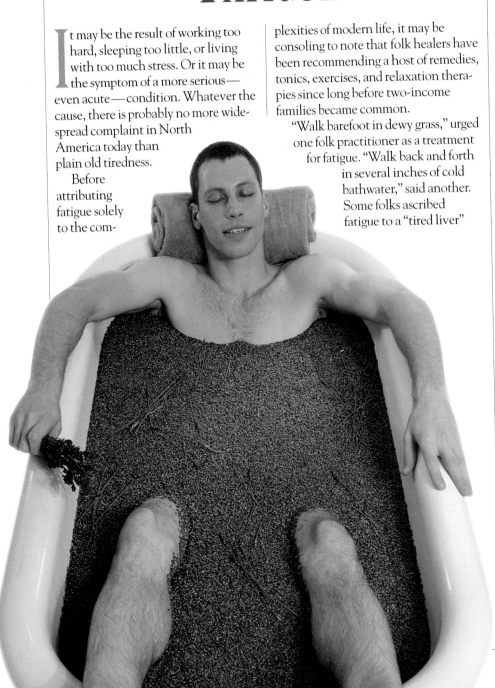

A whole tubful of lavender *really isn't necessary to ease stress-induced fatigue. A mere half-cupful in your bathwater will do.*

and impertinent to their wives." Less than a hundred years later, Canadians and Americans began using the native variety of ginseng for its purported properties as an energizer, a promoter of sexual vitality, and a cure-all for a number of age-related infirmities. Some critics have dismissed ginseng, claiming that it merely causes nervousness and diarrhea, even though these effects may be caused merely by excessive dosages. There is, in fact, considerable scientific support for ginseng's role as an adaptogen, or tonic, capable of bestowing a wide variety of benefits, including counteracting fatigue and the damage caused by stress, improving stamina, and preventing the depletion of stress-fighting hormones in the adrenal gland.

Another, more controversial, plant is the medicinal herb ma huang, or Chinese ephedra, which Asian folk healers have used for more than 5,000 years to treat asthma, colds, and allergies. A potent central nervous system stimulant, it provides an energy boost—an effect that created a following among recreational drug users. Despite Health Canada's warnings, it is still sold clandestinely in some health food stores and fitness centers as Herbal Ecstasy. Such ephedra products can be lethal when misused: through excessive dosages ma huang has caused more than 15 deaths in the U.S., as well as heart attacks, strokes, seizures, and psychosis in hundreds of others.

The Mystery of CFS

One problem our forebears did not have to contend with was the contemporary ailment labeled in 1988 as chronic fatigue syndrome. CFS sufferers, some 80 percent of whom are women and most of whom are white, are afflicted with a profound sense of fatigue, along with depression, memory problems, difficulty concentrating, and muscle and joint pains. CFS is considered a "syndrome" because it is defined by a pattern of symptoms instead of by a specific disease for which science has identified a cause. It was first thought to be linked to the Epstein-Barr virus seen in infectious mononucleosis, but blood tests have provided no evidence of a connection. Brain scans in some people show abnormalities, while the immune systems of others appear compromised; this inconsistency may exist because not all sufferers actually have CFS.

Researchers have found that some people with CFS respond to antidepressants, nonsteroidal anti-inflammatory drugs, and pain relievers. Furthermore, recent research at Johns Hopkins Hospital in Baltimore, Maryland, has linked CFS to a potentially treatable blood pressure disorder. Surprisingly, simple salt tablets, which counteract sudden drops in blood pressure, have brought significant relief, particularly to younger patients who have had CFS for only a short time.

A Good Night's Sleep

When fatigue is caused by stress, folk practitioners have prescribed herbal relaxants, including lavender, St. Johnswort, and valerian. Lavender is particularly popular as a tea; its oil (for bathing and massage) treats tension headaches, migraines, insomnia, muscle spasms, and neuralgia.

Valerian, a tall, perennial herb, has been used as a mild tranquilizer and sleep aid for more than 2,000 years. The herb has the unusual ability to act as a calmative in agitated people and as a stimulant for the weary. In Europe valerian is a leading over-the-counter tranquilizer.

BLACK TEA A cup of black tea contains about 30 mg of caffeine. Doses of roughly 60 mg—the equivalent of 2 cups—act as a stimulant to increase the activity of the central nervous system. To prepare, pour 1 cup boiling water over 1½ teaspoons black tea leaves. Let steep for 5 minutes, then strain and drink.

YERBA MATÉ This South American tea contains about the same amount of caffeine as coffee and half the amount of black tea, making it useful to those for whom coffee and tea have undesirable effects. Rarer, the canned drink is available in some markets. But take note: some yerba maté products may contain traces of cocaine substances, which will turn a urine drug test positive.

GINSENG Ginseng preparations are available as teas, tinctures, extracts, capsules, and tablets. The dried root can also be used to make a tea: add 1 teaspoon minced root to 1 cup boiling water and let steep for 5 to 10 minutes. Strain and drink one to three times a day for up to three to four weeks. Ginseng may cause nervousness and insomnia in some people.

VALERIAN Long used as a sleeping aid, valerian is useful in treating stress-induced fatigue. Use 1 cup boiling water to ½ to 1 teaspoon minced fresh roots to make a bedtime tea. Or mix a few drops of valerian extract or tincture into a glass of warm water. Use for longer than two weeks is not recommended.

LAVENDER This herb enjoys a long-standing reputation as a calmative. The dried flowers or an extract can be added to a warm bath just before retiring. Lavender oil can also be dabbed on the temples before bedtime.

FATS & OILS

The use of animal fats in early North American folk medicine was largely confined to topical skin treatments— fortunately so, considering that our ancestors had no knowledge of the dangers of high cholesterol levels and artery-hardening plaque. Occasional doses of chicken fat or even skunk oil were taken internally to cure certain ailments, but the harmful effects of fat came more from the daily diet than from self-medication.

The fat of choice was lard— obtained from rendering the fatty tissue of hogs; it is still a cooking staple in parts of the American South. Appalachian mountain dwellers mixed it with sulfur to make a chigger repellent, and with ground pokeroot to treat ringworm. An ointment for blisters was prepared from lard cooked with plantain leaves and grated carrots. For hard-to-heal sores, yellowroot or balm of Gilead was often boiled in lard to make a salve.

Lard had other uses as well. As a remedy for croup, it was spread on a cloth, sprinkled with tobacco and covered with a warm cloth, then placed on the patient's chest. (In this case, the tobacco may have had a percutaneous "nicotine patch" effect.) Kerosene, turpentine, and lard were mixed into a pungent poultice and placed on the neck for sore throats. Finely chopped horse chestnuts—which work directly on membranes— were molded with lard into suppositories for hemorrhoids. To keep the potent mustard seed in mustard plasters from burning, lard was slathered onto the skin before the plaster was applied to sprains and sore muscles.

Healthful oils come from many sources. Shown clockwise are salmon, cod, peanuts, olives, and seeds of sesame, flax, and sunflower.

Uses Base for medications, massage oils, soaps, food
Cautions Do not apply fats or oils to burns: they can trap heat and make the burn worse. Excessive consumption of animal and dairy fats raises cholesterol levels and increases the risk of arteriosclerosis, or hardening of the arteries. Excessive fat intake may also increase the risk of colon cancer. Saturated fats are more harmful than polyunsaturated fats.

Bacon and Beyond

Other animal fats, too, were used in folk remedies. In winter many children were sent to school with foul-smelling bags of camphor and goose grease around their necks to ward off influenza. This may have worked simply by keeping germ carriers—and everyone else—at a safe distance. Warmed chicken fat was fed to infants and children with croup, and beef suet was put on burns. Mutton tallow, or melted sheep fat, was mixed with white pine resin for sores or was perfumed with lemon juice and used as a hand lotion.

Raw bacon and salt pork were used to help draw out infection or poison. When wrapped around an ingrown toenail, raw bacon would soften the skin, allowing the toenail to grow out normally. Bacon or salt pork was put on warts overnight: it was said that in the morning—if you had faith—the warts would be gone. If someone stepped on a rusty nail or pitchfork, it was a common rural practice to wrap the foot with salt pork to prevent tetanus. Salt pork, sometimes sprinkled with pepper, was also wrapped around a sore throat and covered with flannel. Fatty meat of any kind was used to relieve insect bites and stings, and was said to "draw the corruption" out of boils and other pus-filled sores.

Skunk oil, also called skunk grease, was reputed to have excellent "penetrating powers." For chest congestion or pneumonia, the patient was fed 2 or 3 teaspoons of skunk oil or rendered polecat fat. (Some reported that skunk oil was odorless, although others strongly disagreed.) Wildcat oil was heated and rubbed on the skin to treat rheumatism, and bear grease was applied to the limbs when a broken bone was not healing properly.

Today animal fats are no longer recommended in salves and poultices, since they become rancid quickly and have limited value as a protective mucilaginous coating. When applied to burns, they may actually hinder the healing process. Moreover, they are too high in saturated fat to be healthy when taken internally.

Milk, cream, and butter were also ingredients in many folk treatments. An ointment for chapped hands was made from persimmon bark cooked in cream. A poultice of eggs, cream, and Epsom salts was said to remove freckles. One folk practitioner—presumably with tongue in cheek—advised milk for ridding oneself of tapeworm: the patient fasted for a few days, then inhaled deeply over a cup of warm milk, thereby attracting the tapeworm to emerge from the nose!

Butter was sometimes put on a sore so that a dog would lick it away—a result of the widespread but mistaken belief that because dogs lick their wounds, the saliva would also help human wounds to heal. For coughs, butter, pepper, resin, alum, ginger, and honey were simmered together and taken at bedtime. If a child ingested something poisonous, he was fed a few teaspoons of butter or milk to coat the stomach. Butter was also recommended before a night on the town. It was said to keep drinkers sober: perhaps a trade-off for butter's high fat content.

On the farm, *hogs—pictured in this 1932 Grant Wood painting— furnished lard for the household.*

Vegetable and Fish Oils

Vegetable oils served the same purposes as animal and dairy fats. Sunflower oil was used as an expectorant, and linseed oil was put on poison ivy, boils, and burns. A tablespoon or two of flaxseed oil was taken for constipation, and sesame oil and cocoa butter were used as laxatives.

Sweet oil (another name for olive oil) was dabbed on burns; a few drops were placed in the ear for earaches. For whooping cough, one recipe combined olive oil, brown sugar, lemon juice, and egg whites, to be taken a tablespoon at a time.

Today vegetable oils—all devoid of cholesterol—are favored over oils and fats from animal sources. Dieticians recommend a diet with no more than 30 percent of daily calories from fat, with an emphasis on the polyunsaturated and monounsaturated fats found in olive oil and the oils of corn, safflower, peanut, and canola.

Fish oils may be even more healthful. Not so long ago, cod liver oil was considered a cure-all, taken for everything from arthritis to epilepsy; it was commonly fed to undernourished children, even though the bad taste had to be masked with sugar, coffee, or brandy. Cod and other fish liver oils do contain good levels of vitamins A and D. Today people are advised to eat tuna, salmon, and other cold-water fish once or twice a week; they are good sources of omega-3 fatty acids, which help lower cholesterol.

FENNEL

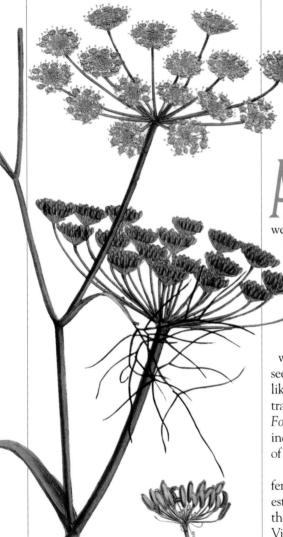

Foeniculum vulgare; F. vulgare dulce
BITTER FENNEL, WILD FENNEL,
WILD ANISE, SWEET FENNEL

A Puritan setting out for church in colonial New England often carried two things: a psalm book and a small batch of "meeting seeds." The seeds were actually the tiny dried fruit of the fennel plant, which the faithful chewed during the long religious service in order to suppress the appetite and prevent unseemly stomach rumblings. Those who decided to fortify themselves with a nip of whiskey before worship chewed the seeds in the hope that the strong licorice-like scent would mask any trace of their transgression (fennel's scientific name, *Foeniculum*, means "fragrant hay," an indication that the plant's smell was one of its dominant features).

By the time the Puritans discovered fennel, the plant already had a well-established place in the herb gardens of the New World. Both the early settlers in Virginia and the Spanish priests in the American West had brought the herb with them to North America. The plant still grows wild near some of the old mission buildings of the Spanish.

A Cure for Colic

The most important medicinal applications of fennel have remained constant for hundreds, even thousands, of years. The seed-like fruits act as carminative (from the Latin "to cleanse") agents, which expel gas from the intestinal tract. They also relieve spasms of the smooth muscle that lines the stomach and intestines. It comes as no surprise, then, that the seeds have long been used to relieve flatulence, infant colic, and indigestion. Some herbalists recommend adding fennel to purgative herbs—among them rhubarb, senna, and buckthorn—in order to counteract the tendency of such laxatives to cause cramps.

Fennel also has a reputation for loosening phlegm and calming coughs. The herb is thought to stimulate the secretions of the upper respiratory tract and may allay inflammation of the mucous membranes. In Europe fennel is found in some over-the-counter cough remedies.

To make a tea, pour 1 cup boiling water over 1 to 2 teaspoons crushed dried fennel seeds, then steep for 10 to 15 minutes and strain. Drink the tea 30 minutes before meals to prevent flatulence. To make so-called gripe water for colicky infants or children, use only ½ teaspoon of the crushed seeds, add a touch of sugar, and be sure to let the liquid cool before administering it. A few spoonfuls may be given alone or in milk or cooked cereal.

Active plant parts Seeds
Uses Gas, infant colic, indigestion, gastroenteritis, nausea, coughs, nasal congestion, obesity, water retention, and lactation and menstruation problems.
Cautions Never ingest pure fennel oil: even in small amounts it can cause vomiting, seizures, and respiratory problems. People with a history of hepatitis, alcoholism, or liver disease should not ingest medicinal amounts of fennel, nor should pregnant women; in some studies, the herb has been shown to damage the livers of laboratory animals. Do not use fennel for more than two weeks without the supervision of a doctor.

Bitter vs. Sweet

Fennel is native to the Mediterranean and Asia Minor, but gardeners now cultivate the plant worldwide. There are two main types of fennel: bitter fennel (also called common fennel) and the larger sweet fennel. These plants grow to a full height of 1.8 m (6 ft), and the fruits of both have similar medicinal value. Some people confuse sweet fennel with a shorter cousin called Florence fennel or finocchio. This subspecies has a crisp, bulbous stalk base that is eaten raw or cooked as a vegetable. Finocchio, however, is not known for any medicinal properties.

Over the centuries traditional healers have recommended infusions of fennel for gout, snakebites, insect bites, sore throat, rheumatic pains, and water retention. Teas have also been used as a mouthwash and an eyewash. Fennel was believed to be an antidote to poisonous herbs and mushrooms. Moreover, it was said to be an excellent treatment for obesity—probably because it was thought to suppress the appetite.

The fruits of the plant—*fennel seed*—*ease intestinal pain in adults and children alike.*

The 17th-century British herbalist Nicholas Culpeper recommended fennel to "break wind, to provoke urine, and ease the pains of the stone." He held that it would "take away the loathings which oftentimes happen to stomachs of sick and feverish persons" and increase a mother's milk, making it "more wholesome for the child." Fennel was also said to promote menstruation, cure hiccups, and clear the lungs and liver.

The 19th-century Eclectic physicians, relying on the plant's reputation, recommended fennel as a digestive aid and to promote menstruation and the production of breast milk, as well as to "conceal the unpleasantness of other medicines." Fennel has also been claimed to heighten the libido, facilitate childbirth, and, when applied as a poultice, relieve breast swelling in nursing mothers.

Aside from confirming fennel's ability to relieve gas and calm the digestive tract, scientists have not substantiated most of the herb's traditional uses. However, research indicates that fennel may have a mild

An Herb for the Eyes?

The Roman naturalist Pliny observed a snake rub against a fennel plant after shedding its skin, after which the snake's clouded eyes cleared. From that day, Pliny believed that fennel cured eye problems in humans. Ancient doctors prescribed extracts of the root as a remedy for cataracts and even blindness. Teas made from the crushed fruits were more recently used as an eyewash. Although there is no evidence supporting fennel's use on the eyes, its reputation prompted 19th-century American poet Henry Wadsworth Longfellow to pen the following:

Above the lower plants it towers
The Fennel with its yellow flowers,
And in an earlier age than ours
Was gifted with wondrous powers
Lost vision to restore.

estrogen-like effect, which could explain its use in promoting breast milk and menstruation. Studies notwithstanding, scientists have yet to identify the plant's estrogenic components; it is possible that, as was speculated in the 19th century, fennel may promote the production of breast milk simply because its pleasant taste encourages the baby to suckle.

Pure fennel oil is dangerous. Ingestion of even small amounts can cause nausea, vomiting, seizures, and such respiratory problems as pulmonary edema (excess accumulation of fluid in the lungs). Chewing the fruit or drinking the tea made from it, however, poses no risks aside from the rare allergic reaction.

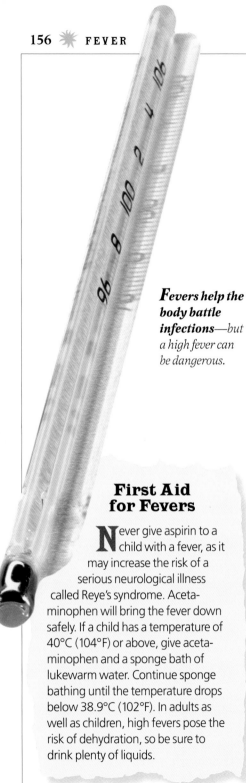

Fevers help the body battle infections—but *a high fever can be dangerous.*

First Aid for Fevers

Never give aspirin to a child with a fever, as it may increase the risk of a serious neurological illness called Reye's syndrome. Acetaminophen will bring the fever down safely. If a child has a temperature of 40°C (104°F) or above, give acetaminophen and a sponge bath of lukewarm water. Continue sponge bathing until the temperature drops below 38.9°C (102°F). In adults as well as children, high fevers pose the risk of dehydration, so be sure to drink plenty of liquids.

FEVER

A fever is defined as a body temperature over 37°C (98.6°F). It is often associated with sweating, shivering, thirst, and a rapid pulse. Bacterial or viral infections, such as tonsillitis or the flu, are usually the cause.

Fevers aren't for naught. When white blood cells flock to the body's defense, they release proteins called pyrogens. These instruct the brain to raise the body's temperature in order to kill the offending microorganisms. If a fever lasts longer than three days, rises above 39.4°C (103°F), or is accompanied by a severe headache with stiff neck, a productive cough, abdominal pain, or painful urination, see a doctor. Also consult a doctor for fever in babies under six months old or in the elderly. Note that the body's temperature varies by as much as 1.1°C (2°F) during the day, being lowest in the morning. Rectal temperature is usually about 0.6°C (1°F) higher.

The best course of action against a fever is to cover yourself with a light blanket, drink cool liquids, and use a cool (not cold) compress. If they choose, adults may take aspirin or acetaminophen.

Magic and Medicine

One folk belief held that to cure a fever, one had simply to tie a thread around one's left wrist at night, tie the thread to a tree the next morning, walk away, and never go back. Or one could place a spider inside a piece of bread and swallow it, or capture a spider and place it in a box, then hang it around one's neck. When the spider died, the fever would subside. If the patient didn't care to eat a spider, he could eat a spider web instead. It is interesting that one 19th-century study supposedly found that the webs contain a substance, termed arachnidin, which lowers fevers.

Perhaps in an effort to "rebalance the humors," various plant leaves were pressed to the heads of feverish patients. These included gourd leaves, jimsonweed, and poke leaves, often heated in vinegar for an added effect. Poultices of slippery-elm bark were applied to the belly, and onions were bound to the body.

In an attempt to draw out the fever and induce sweating, many people soaked their feet in mustard water or took mustard water baths. Cold whiskey or vinegar baths cooled the body down in a hurry when the alcohol or vinegar evaporated, but they also no doubt left the patient with a considerable chill. Today doctors advise cooling the body gradually with lukewarm sponge baths.

Good Old H$_2$O

Not surprisingly, many folk cures for fever involved cold water. One cure recommended covering the patient with a wet linen sheet, on top of which flannels and blankets were placed; this was thought to bring down the fever and correct "morbid secretions." Once the patient recovered from the chill and began to sweat, he was placed in a cold bath or "plunge" bath (perhaps in a pond, if available).

Drinking large quantities of cold water was thought to produce sweating. In some cases, this is true. The body perspires in order to cool itself down; however, if you perspire too much, the sweating stops to prevent dehydration. When liquids are ingested again, perspiration resumes. If you don't feel like drinking, suck on ice cubes. Eating fresh grapes was also thought to lower a fever; it won't, but doing so will at least provide hydration.

Hot Concoctions

Teas and toddies used to promote sweating—and thereby break a fever—abounded. One recipe called for boiling water with red pepper, honey, and orange juice. A hot mix of lemonade with whiskey or wine was also recommended. Perhaps the most popular of all was ginger tea, said to make you "sweat your eyeballs out," especially when red pepper and garlic were added. The patient was to take refuge under the covers and imbibe as much of the fiery draft as possible. Today ginger is still used to induce sweating.

Willow bark teas were also used. (Willow was thought to be so powerful that simply sitting under the tree brought a cure.) Willow contains salicin, a relative of aspirin, and may aid against fevers.

A fever marked by chills and uncontrollable shaking was referred to—with much fright—as ague, usually meaning malarial fever. The cure was boneset, also called agueweed and feverwort. Boneset, first used by the Indians, was so named because it was used against "breakbone fever," or dengue, a then-common virus that causes severe joint pain. Hot infusions of boneset were thought to cause a heavy, fever-breaking sweat. The bitter herb does promote sweating, possibly because of its nauseant properties; however, some species contain alkaloids known to cause liver impairment.

Sassafras was used by the Indians in what is now Florida to treat fevers. Settlers adopted it, and it soon became the number-two American export to Europe, second only to tobacco. Ironically, research has failed to confirm that sassafras reduces fevers. Furthermore, the root bark contains safrole oil, which increases the risk of cancer. Other herbal teas were used for fever, including thyme, saffron, and elder flower. Such teas do promote sweating, but it is unclear whether this is because of active ingredients or simply because the liquid is hot.

A folk remedy that attacks a fever's root cause is garlic, which has antibacterial and antiviral properties. Garlic teas, tinctures, and syrups were often used, although garlic is most effective when eaten raw. However, one would have to eat several cloves a day to elicit an effect.

WATER To help dissipate the body's excess heat, take lukewarm or cool sponge baths once every hour or more frequently if necessary. Alternatively, soak washcloths in cool water and apply them to the wrists, forehead, and neck. If you like, suck on ice chips flavored with a few drops of lemon juice to moisturize the lips and mouth. Finally, drink water and other liquids liberally in order to prevent dehydration.

ELDER FLOWER A hot cup of tea made from elder flowers is thought to promote sweating, which helps lower body temperature—although the effect may simply be due to the hot water. To make the tea, steep 1 to 2 teaspoons dried flowers in 1 cup boiling water, then strain. Drink one or two cups two to three times a day. Tea bags are available commercially.

LINDEN FLOWER Like elder flowers, linden flowers are believed to promote sweating and are often prescribed in cases of feverish chills. As with other herbal teas, it is unclear whether the effect is due to the flowers or to the hot liquid. To make a tea, pour 1 cup boiling water over about 1 teaspoon dried flowers. Steep, then strain. Drink one or two cups a day. Linden flower tea bags are available commercially.

Lukewarm sponge baths cool the body down slowly, while drinking liquids prevents dehydration.

FEVERFEW

Tanacetum parthenium
FEATHERFEW, FEATHERFOIL,
BACHELOR'S BUTTON, MIDSUMMER
DAISY, SANTA MARIA, WILD
CHAMOMILE, WILD QUININE

English settlers brought feverfew to the New World, planted the herb in their gardens, and used its leaves and flowers in remedies for fever, headache, and arthritis. Today it grows in the wild from southern Canada to Mexico and throughout the United States. Since its rediscovery in the late 1970s, it has become one of the most widely used and potentially effective herbal products on the market.

Migraine Muffler

Feverfew is best known today for its ability to reduce the frequency and severity of migraine headaches, a condition that modern medicine has struggled to treat successfully. Although the herb was used to ease headaches by settlers, particular mentions of its use for migraines, or "sick headaches," is scant. The ongoing resurgence of feverfew can be traced to clinical studies and word of mouth in England in the late 1970s.

Dr. E. Stewart Johnson of the City of London Migraine Clinic conducted the first surveys and clinical trials on feverfew. Using his own patients, many of whom had tried orthodox treatments without success, he reported that a large number of subjects showed significant improvement with feverfew. After his initial research, more rigorous trials were performed, including a 1988 study that confirmed reductions in both the frequency and the severity of the migraines suffered, as well as significantly less nausea and vomiting—two common migraine symptoms.

Laboratory tests have identified parthenolides as the active principles in the feverfew leaf and flower. This substance inhibits the release of serotonin, prostaglandins, and histamines into the bloodstream—all of which can inflame tissue as well as trigger and worsen migraine headaches. Furthermore, serotonin constricts blood vessels and lowers the pain threshold, while prostaglandins can cause vascular muscle spasms.

One tablet or capsule, or two or three feverfew leaves a day—at least 125 milligrams containing no less than 0.2 percent parthenolides—have been shown to prevent migraines from recurring. Unfortunately, the variable quality of the herb, even in commercial products, cannot guarantee consistent effectiveness. If the standard dose fails, larger doses may be

Active plant parts Leaves, flowers
Uses Headaches (especially migraines), arthritis, skin conditions
Cautions Taking feverfew orally may result in minor mouth ulcers and cold sores, tongue and lip irritation, temporary loss of taste, and abdominal pain. External use may result in contact dermatitis. Because of the herb's potential effect on the uterus and digestive tract, the herb is not recommended for pregnant women or children under two years of age. Feverfew withdrawal may result in the return of migraine symptoms, as well as anxiety, poor sleep, and muscle and joint stiffness.

tried. However, any ongoing use of feverfew to manage migraine headaches should be supervised by your doctor.

Once Upon a Time

Although feverfew has received much attention in the scientific community, its resurgent popularity is reportedly due to the wisdom of ordinary citizens in Great Britain. Various tales, all or none of which may be true, have been put forward as the source of feverfew's newfound fame.

One story tells of a random correspondence between a British miner and a doctor's wife. The miner, a longtime migraine sufferer who found relief from chewing feverfew leaves daily, shared his secret with another sufferer—the spouse of the chief medical officer of Britain's National Coal Board. A little over a year later, the woman's husband, upon seeing her astonishing improvement, prompted his colleagues to research the herb.

Another story tells of a Welsh miner who wrote to the editor of the local paper seeking a migraine remedy. A woman in a neighboring town supplied the answer: a daily feverfew-and-butter sandwich.

A third story involves a "Mrs. Jenkins," whose success in using feverfew for her migraines was highlighted in a 1978 article in British *Prevention* magazine and caught the interest of the Migraine Trust, a national sponsor of clinical studies.

Historical Use

The earliest recorded use of feverfew dates to first-century Greece. In A.D. 78, a physician named Dioscorides noted the plant's usefulness in reducing fever, soothing arthritis pain and skin inflammations, treating cholera, and relieving the discomfort of menstruation and childbirth. In 17th- and 18th-century England, the herb was used to ease dizziness, headache,

melancholy, and "women's complaints." Nicholas Culpeper, author of *The Complete Herbal* (1652), a medical book much used by early settlers, recommended feverfew to strengthen the womb and allay "all pains in the head." Another medical book, John Hill's *The Family Herbal* (1772), possibly referred to migraine when it noted that "in the worst headache this herb exceeds whatever else is known." Housewives commonly planted feverfew in their gardens—hence its nickname "housewife's aspirin"—and Cotton Mather, an early Puritan leader, used the herb in a heated cloth bag "bedewed with rum" for a toothache.

Nevertheless, by 1849 the *Dispensatory of the United States* reported limited use of feverfew and credited the herb only with tonic properties. When North Americans did use feverfew, they maintained faith in the herb's traditional usage and explored new possibilities. The Shakers recommended it for dizziness, colds, worms, irregular menstruation, and delayed urination. The Eclectics prescribed it for "female hysteria" and fevers. The mere

Growing Your Own

Native to the rocky soil of the Balkans, feverfew is an aromatic perennial that has long been cultivated as a medicinal and ornamental plant. Growing up to 60 cm (2 ft) tall, it is naturalized throughout the United States and southern Canada.

To grow feverfew in your garden, start with the seeds or root cuttings (which are easier and will provide more leaves in the first year). Plant in spring, 45 cm (18 in.) apart, in rich, well-drained soil. For optimal growth, choose an area in partial shade and use compost. The plant grows quickly and produces leaves early on; additional leaf growth and yellow-and-white, daisylike flowers come slowly after, from June to August. To promote bushiness and leaf development, pinch back the buds before they open.

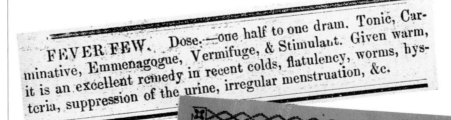

The Shakers marketed feverfew and touted it for many maladies. Headache was not one of them, as the label above attests.

presence of the plant was thought to purify the air and repel insects, and a tincture of the flowers was used to treat insect bites.

Feverfew leaves were considered especially valuable. A tea of the leaves was taken for indigestion, nervousness, and depression, and a poultice of the leaves was applied to inflamed skin and joints. The leaves themselves, fresh or dried, were the most common dosage form—usually two to three a day. Leaves were eaten to ease muscle spasms, stimulate menstruation, and discharge the placenta after birth; the herb was used as a diarrhea remedy and general tonic. The leaves even served as an emergency treatment to counter the dulling effect and convulsions of opium intoxication.

A Versatile Medicine

The renewed interest in feverfew has resulted in numerous scientific findings. The same principles that make it effective at preventing migraine headaches may also relieve a number of other ailments, including arthritis. Although rheumatoid arthritis reportedly is not helped by taking feverfew internally, the essential oil can be mildly anti-inflammatory when applied topically to the skin and joints.

A tincture of feverfew is mildly antibacterial and reportedly effective against psoriasis and skin infections. The herb is also thought to prevent blood clotting, although anyone using it for its possible anticlotting properties—especially those patients already taking anticoagulants—should consult a doctor.

Feverfew's toning effect on blood vessels may reduce blood pressure and provide a sedative effect. The herb may also have a mild soothing effect on the muscles of the uterus and digestive tract. More studies are needed to determine the

What's in a Name?

According to legend, Galen and other early Greek physicians called the plant we now know as feverfew *parthenion* after it was used to treat the injuries—indeed, save the life—of a man who had fallen from the Parthenon, the temple of Athena on the Acropolis. More likely, the name (derived from *parthenos*, Greek for "girl" or "virgin") was chosen because the plant was used to promote menstruation. Whatever its source, the word lives on in feverfew's botanical name: *Tanacetum parthenium*. In the translation of another Greek physician, Dioscorides, the plant is called *Pyrethrum parthenium*. "Pyrethrum" possibly refers to *pyretos* (Greek for "fever"), a clue that fever may have been an early medicinal use of the herb.

The plant's common name, too, has a number of possible origins. The word "feverfew" is similar to "febrifuge," the term for a fever-reducing substance (from the Latin *febrifugia,* meaning "driver out of fevers"). One view suggests that during the Middle Ages the name featherfoil replaced the name parthenion because of the feathery borders of the plant's leaves; this theory holds that featherfoil eventually became "featherfew" and, finally, "feverfew."

However the name "feverfew" originated, it took hold, and the plant was used by generations of folk practitioners and housewives to treat fevers. The sweet-smelling herb was even planted around homes to ward off fever-producing malaria. (Malaria, Italian for "foul air," was thought to be caused by bad air.) When Peruvian cinchona bark—the active principle of which is quinine—was found to remedy malaria, feverfew was briefly known as "wild quinine" on the mistaken assumption that it had a similar potency.

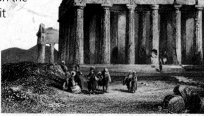

The Parthenon *may have inspired the specific name "parthenium."*

optimum form and dosage, as well as feverfew's potential as a fever reducer.

In addition to migraines and other headaches, modern herbalists recommend bitter-tasting feverfew for colds, indigestion, diarrhea, and delayed menstruation. Potential side effects include minor mouth ulcers and cold sores, tongue and lip irritation, temporary loss of taste, abdominal pain, and dermatitis. Note, too, that studies have discovered "feverfew syndrome," a withdrawal condition in numerous patients who have used feverfew for years and then stopped. It can cause migraine symptoms, anxiety, poor sleep, and muscle and joint stiffness.

FLATULENCE

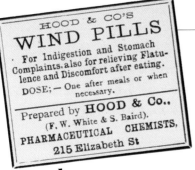

***A**ntiflatulents of yore
included this popular product.*

A normal bodily function, "passing wind" has historically been treated with delicacy and euphemism. As the ultimate faux pas, it has also been the source of much comedy. Mark Twain himself wrote of what we politely call flatulence: his essay *1601* lampooned the mores of Elizabethan England by imagining Elizabeth I, Lord Bacon, Sir Walter Raleigh, and other revered figures arguing over who in their midst had committed just such an offense.

A Bacterial By-product

The average adult produces 8 liters of abdominal gas, or flatus, per day. About fourteen times daily, small amounts are expelled rectally, totaling about 2 cups. Although excessive flatulence can cause bloating and pain, it rarely indicates a serious medical problem.

Most gas is the by-product of bacteria fermenting food in the intestines. Certain foods—especially beans, cabbage, cauliflower, broccoli, onions, apples, bananas, and cherries—have reputations as gas producers, although their effects vary from person to person. Other causes are the air from carbonated beverages, swallowing air while chewing with the mouth open, and inadequately chewed food. Less common culprits are allergies, postnasal drip, lactose intolerance, malnutrition, high-fiber foods, bulk-forming laxatives, and certain medications, including cholesterol-lowering drugs and tranquilizers. More rarely, flatulence may be a symptom of an underlying medical condition, such as irritable bowel syndrome.

Proper digestion, whereby foods are absorbed by enzymes and digestive acids or acted on by beneficial intestinal flora, can help control the problem. B-complex vitamins, vitamin C, and folic acid will aid this process. The best prevention is to determine which foods cause excess gas and to modify your eating habits accordingly. Note that it is often a combination of different—not individual—foods that makes flatulence worse.

Other aids include activated charcoal. Taken just after meals, it adsorbs gas and prevents it from binding to odor-causing substances—but it also depletes nutrients beneficial to digestion. Yogurt contains acidophilus, "good" bacteria that inhibit "bad" odor-causing bacteria.

As for the notorious beans, soaking them overnight, then cooking them with fresh water and an onion, is claimed by some to lessen their gas-producing effects.

PEPPERMINT Pour 1 cup boiling water over 1 tablespoon chopped dried leaves. Let steep for 5 to 10 minutes; strain, then drink warm three to four times a day. Tinctures and oil of peppermint may vary in their concentration.

FENNEL Fennel tea bags may be of little value unless the seeds have been crushed. Make fresh tea by pouring 1 cup boiling water over 1 to 2 teaspoons of just-crushed dried seeds. Steep 10 minutes, strain, and drink before or after meals. Alternatively, chew ¼ teaspoon seeds.

DILL Chew ½ teaspoon dill seeds. Or prepare dill water by mixing 1 teaspoon oil of dill with 4 cups warm water; take 1 cup as needed. Make a mild tea by steeping 1 teaspoon ground seeds in 1 cup boiling water for 10 to 15 minutes. Strain, then drink before or after meals.

ANISE Mix a few drops of aniseed oil into 1 cup warm water. Or make a tea by grinding 1 teaspoon seeds and covering with 1 cup boiling water; steep for 5 to 10 minutes, then strain. Drink either solution before or after meals. Some people may be allergic to anise.

CARAWAY SEED The volatile oil components of caraway seeds work as a carminative by promoting gastric secretions and stimulating appetite. To make a tea, pour 1 cup boiling water over 1 to 2 teaspoons of freshly crushed seeds. Steep for 10 to 15 minutes, then strain. Drink 1 cup two to four times a day between meals. Alternatively, chew ½ teaspoon seeds after a meal.

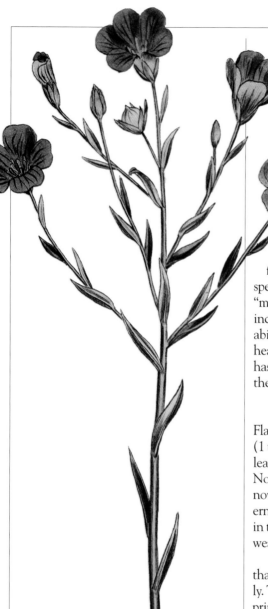

FLAXSEED

Linum usitatissimum
FLAX, LINSEED, LINT
BELLS, LINUM

Long known as the source of linen and linseed oil, flax also enjoys a reputation for its varied use in folk medicine. Its species name, *usitatissimum*, is Latin for "most useful." In recent years, the increased attention to grains and their ability to lower cholesterol, help the heart, and potentially reduce cancer risks has also put the seeds of this plant under the microscope—with interesting results.

Functional Fiber

Flax, an annual that grows 30 to 90 cm (1 to 3 ft) high with pale green alternate leaves and blue flowers, was introduced to North America by European settlers and now grows prominently in the northwestern United States and Canada. The fibers in the plant's stem have been coveted by weavers for more than 10,000 years.

However, it is the seed's dietary fiber that was—and still is—useful medicinally. The oil, meal, or seeds themselves were primarily used as a laxative for both humans and animals. Because flaxseed is a "bulk forming" laxative, prompting quicker, more frequent bowel movements, it was used to treat constipation, remedy the diarrhea associated with dysentery, and help relieve hemorrhoids. The oil was also used as an enema for these ailments, even though the fiber's effect was lost. The nutritious grain is now commonly included in fiber-rich multigrain breads and muffins.

In the 19th century the Eclectics recommended flaxseed for intestinal pinworms in children. The complicated remedy called for a teaspoon of oil mixed with sugar or molasses to be given "morning, night, and morning; that is, three times, then miss three, then give it again, and so repeat it until the child has taken it nine times." Today laxatives and anthelmintic drugs are commonly prescribed together to kill worms and promote bowel movements so that surviving worms cannot cling to the intestinal walls.

Soothing Mucilage

Flaxseed is mildly anti-inflammatory, and doses were taken as a demulcent to relieve ulcers and gastritis. The seeds' mucilaginous components expand in water and potentially coat and protect an inflamed stomach lining from painful contact with acid and bile. One recipe advised those with gastrointestinal problems to add a teaspoon of flaxseed to water, cover the pot, let stand, and stir before drinking—seeds and all—"every night before going to bed for two or three months." Other users witnessed results much sooner.

The mucilage (from the boiled seeds), mixed with honey, lemon juice, and

Active plant parts Seeds
Uses Constipation, diarrhea; source of dietary fiber
Cautions Only flaxseed oil or edible linseed oil should be taken internally. Do not ingest or apply commercial linseed oil to the skin. In any form, flaxseed taken internally may cause gas, and it is contraindicated in cases of intestinal obstruction.

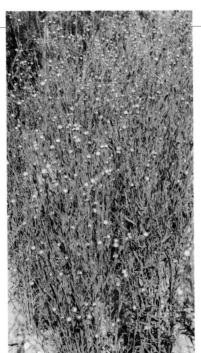

Linum species are graced with yellow, blue, red, or white flowers before they yield flaxseed.

alcohol, also made a popular sore throat syrup, taken 1 tablespoon at a time.

Flaxseed's effects on stomach acid and the stomach lining also helped relieve heartburn—the inflammation of the esophagus and upper stomach caused by a reflux of stomach acid. However, stale seeds or rancid oil taken internally can actually cause indigestion and irritate the stomach. The oil spoils quickly and should be kept refrigerated. Also, as with most high-fiber foods taken without water, consuming large portions of flaxseed can cause gas.

For Many Ills

Flaxseed's medicinal value was enhanced by the many forms in which it could be used. A tea made from boiled seeds and sweetened with honey or sugar and lemon was taken for colic, colds and coughs, sore throats, urinary tract infections, and respiratory conditions. It was also mixed with lime-water and applied to burns.

A single flaxseed was used to remove foreign objects, like specks of dirt, from the eye. The moistened seed was inserted underneath the eyelid; the object would adhere to the seed and would come out as the seed was removed. Although this remedy may work, it is not recommended: the seed may cause further irritation.

Flaxseed poultices were made by grinding, then boiling the seeds to activate the mucilage in the seed coat. The powdered seed and the seed cake (which results when the oil has been pressed out) were also used. The seed material, often mixed with cornmeal, was heated and placed between two clean cloths (to retain its heat and protect the skin) before it was applied.

The poultice's emollient action brought boils to a head and mildly relieved sore skin, although flaxseed is not antiseptic. Flaxseed poultices were also applied to the chest to relieve a cold and to the throat for hoarseness or painful swallowing. The effect on the skin is harmless, although the Eclectics reported that the skin became "blanched, sodden, and wrinkled."

Conflicting Views

Renewed interest in fiber-rich grains, flaxseed included, has produced promising, albeit incomplete, findings. Many reports cite that both the seed and the oil of flax contain high levels of omega-3 fatty acids. These acids, found mostly in fish oil, are believed to lower LDL ("bad") cholesterol levels without affecting HDL ("good") cholesterol and thus lower the risk of heart disease, rheumatoid arthritis, viral infections, and cancer.

Disputing these findings, the *University of California-Berkeley Wellness Letter* reported in October 1995 that flaxseed "is no better for you than oatmeal, and the oil is no better for you than most other oils." It also stated that flaxseed does not contain the prized omega-3 fatty acids but a similar substance called linolenic acid, which is difficult for the body to convert into a helpful amount of omega-3s.

Such findings do not entirely undercut flaxseed's benefits. As a source of polyunsaturated oil, the grain does lower cholesterol. It is also rich in compounds called lignans (found in the seed, not the oil), which are being studied for their potential to reduce and prevent cancers of the breast, colon, and prostate.

Linseed Oil

In some parts of North America, "flaxseed oil" and "edible linseed oil" are interchangeable. The latter is the vegetable oil used in cooking and folk medicine and should not be confused with commercially treated linseed oil, which is best known as a furniture polish or leather softener—especially for baseball gloves. This treated linseed oil is also found in paints and varnishes and is not safe to ingest or to apply to the skin.

Flaxseed oil can be mildly anti-inflammatory and was used in folk medicine, internally for constipation and stomach pains and topically for burns, styes, and hemorrhoids. Today the nutty-tasting oil is used in cooking and on salads. It is highly unsaturated and can help lower cholesterol and the long-term risk of heart disease. However, its nutritional benefits can be compromised by spoiling or excessive heat.

FLUID RETENTION

Well over a hundred folk remedies for fluid accumulation in the tissues (edema) have been tried. They range from the poetic—queen-of-the-meadow and bittersweet—to the surprising. In an 1873 herb catalog, Shakers recommended poison ivy for "paralysis of the bladder," and the Parke Davis pharmaceutical company marketed preparations of poison oak in the 1890s.

Peter Smith's 1812 *The Indian Doctor's Dispensatory* suggested this cure for edema, then known as dropsy: "In a very weak case, a jelly of calf's feet is to be eaten cold, with vinegar." Smith's specific reference to a "weak case" of dropsy

The diuretic effect of corn silk tea may be due to its high potassium content.

underscores what is now generally accepted about herbal diuretics: they are, at best, safe, but usually produce only a modest effect. When treating fluid retention related to serious conditions, such as hypertension, a doctor's supervision is the best medicine. A doctor may prescribe synthetic diuretics that are stronger and more effective than herbal versions.

Natural Diuretics

Nevertheless, for minor forms of fluid retention—including premenstrual bloating—some folk remedies are still useful. Such herbal diuretics as corn silk, uva ursi, dandelion, and buchu are among

CORN SILK Put 1 teaspoon of corn silk in cold water, boil for two to three minutes, and strain. Drink 1 cup several times a day. Corn silk extracts are also available commercially and should be taken as directed.

DANDELION Boil 1 to 2 teaspoons of dried dandelion herb (all parts of the plant before flowering) or root for about 15 minutes in 1 cup water. Strain. Drink 1 cup morning and evening. Alternatively, take 10 to 15 drops of tincture three times a day. Use dandelion with caution if gallstones or obstructions of the bile duct or bowel are present.

See a doctor if...

◆ Swelling in your extremities or abdomen lasts for more than a week. Fluid retention can be the sign of a serious heart or kidney problem.
◆ In pregnant women, fluid retention can be a symptom of so-called "toxemia"—high blood pressure, protein in the urine, and kidney dysfunctions.

those that can help relieve the discomfort of temporary water retention.

Caffeine also acts as a diuretic; in fact, it is an active ingredient in most diuretics bought over the counter. For those who find the caffeine in coffee too harsh, black tea will work. Another natural way to prevent fluid retention is to cut back considerably on your daily intake of salt.

BLACK TEA Black tea can contain up to 4 percent caffeine and related compounds; these increase the production of urine. Prepare a tea with 1 teaspoon dried black tea leaves per cupful of boiling water. Let steep for five minutes, and drink warm three to four times a day. Black tea, like coffee, may cause nervousness or insomnia.

UVA URSI Uva ursi, traditionally known as bearberry, contains hydroquinone derivatives (mainly arbutin), along with tannins, triterpenes, and pheno-carbosylic acid. The diuretic effect is minimal: the tea is better known for its effect on inflammation of the lower urinary tract. Pour 1 to 2 cups boiling water over 1 teaspoon coarsely powdered leaf or add to cold water and boil for 15 minutes. Drink 1 cup three to four times a day.

FOOD POISONING

A diner's worst nightmare, food poisoning is often the result of eating food contaminated by such bacteria as staphylococcus, which can develop on the potato salad left in the sun at a picnic, or salmonella, sometimes found in older eggs or in poultry. Bacteria can also be transferred to food prepared by someone with unclean hands. Less commonly, food poisoning results from eating poisonous mushrooms or certain foods, such as puffer fish, that are toxic—even lethal—if improperly prepared. Symptoms include stomach cramps, nausea, vomiting, and diarrhea. If the person experiences persistent vomiting, dehydration, bloody diarrhea, dizziness, or a high fever, take him to the hospital. Do so also if he has trouble speaking, swallowing, or breathing: these are signs of botulism, a life-threatening illness.

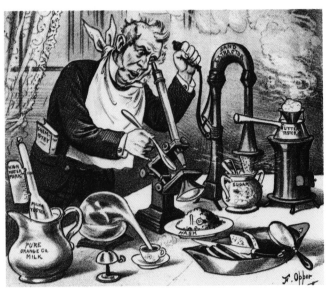

Fearful of food contamination, a 19th-century diner looks before he eats.

In their agony, some people attempt to induce vomiting, but this may be futile; if the food has already left the stomach, it cannot be brought up. Most bouts of food poisoning pass in a matter of hours without medical treatment, although you may choose to take an over-the-counter anti-diarrheal. To counter dehydration, drink a

How to Avoid Food Poisoning

◆ Wash hands before handling food.
◆ Wash cutting boards and kitchen implements used for raw meat or poultry before reusing.
◆ Thaw frozen meats and poultry in the refrigerator, not on the counter; thaw completely before cooking.
◆ Cook food thoroughly and avoid raw meat, fish, and eggs.
◆ Avoid mussels that do not open completely, dented tin cans, and any food that smells or looks spoiled.
◆ Promptly refrigerate leftover food.
◆ Store eggs in the back of the refrigerator, not in the door.

little water as soon as you are able. Then switch to clear fruit juices or broth.

Easing the Anguish

In the 19th century there were no remedies for food poisoning per se; the term did not even exist until 1887. But there were many attempts to treat the symptoms. To induce vomiting, the Indians relied on lobelia, also called pukeweed and vomitwort. Settlers took pulverized lobelia seeds and a pinch of red pepper in warm water. (Although it works, lobelia is now known to be poisonous.) Mustard seeds, once called pukes, are safer. Table mustard in water will also induce vomiting.

To check nausea, some people soaked chunks of charcoal in water, then drank the resulting liquid. Today only activated charcoal is used for treating chemical poisoning, although it may not be effective against food poisoning. Ginger and chamomile were also used, to some effect, to soothe the stomach and ease cramps.

CHAMOMILE Chamomile settles the stomach and calms cramps. In test tubes, German chamomile kills certain bacteria, including *Staphylococcus aureus,* a common cause of food poisoning. To make a tea, pour 1 cup boiling water over 2 to 3 teaspoons dried chopped flowers. Steep, then strain.

GINGER Ginger is known to quell nausea, a common symptom of food poisoning. Capsules of ground ginger-root are available commercially. Take 2 grams with a glass of water once a day. Or make a tea by pouring 1 cup boiling water over ½ teaspoon coarsely ground root. Steep, then strain.

FOOT ODOR

In earlier times, when the health benefits of regular bathing went unrecognized, body odors were considered a normal part of life. Especially ripe smells might be masked with perfumes, but little attempt was made to eliminate the cause. Today we think otherwise, and foot odor in particular is considered an embarrassment.

Foot odor originates in a warm, airless environment—namely, shoes—that encourages bacterial and fungal growth. This begins with secretions from the eccrine (sweat) glands, which open directly onto the skin surface on the soles of the feet. Anything from overexertion to hot, humid weather or fever can trigger sweating, which serves to cool the body. Anxiety and fear can also induce a sweat, especially on the soles of the feet.

Sweat itself is odorless. Odor is caused by bacterial or fungal action on odorous compounds in skin, such as butyric acid. Feet are most susceptible because they are enclosed for long periods.

The best way to discourage foot odor is to wash your feet regularly in warm soapy water; deodorant or antibacterial soaps

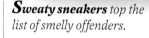

Sweaty sneakers *top the list of smelly offenders.*

work best. Frequent airing of the feet will encourage evaporation of sweat. Airing shoes will discourage mold growth, as will changing your shoes to allow moisture buildup to dry fully.

Sprinkles and Soaks

A number of materials can be sprinkled into shoes to absorb sweat and discourage bacterial activity—among them cornstarch, a fine, odorless powder derived from corn seeds. It has the ability to absorb about 24 percent of its weight in water without losing its dry appearance. Other absorbents, such as bran and oatmeal, will also keep feet dry.

Activated charcoal, used primarily as an antidote to chemical poisons, can also be used. Its large surface area allows it to adsorb a variety of both liquid and gas

compounds. Charcoal encourages the decomposition of organic substances, thus adsorbing sweat and the gases given off by bacterial action. It is an ingredient in many commercial foot-odor products, but can discolor shoes, socks, and hosiery.

Aside from absorbents and charcoal, try a footbath. Epsom salts not only help kill odor but have a soothing effect. Or use regular tea (2 tea bags to half a liter of water); the tannins act as an astringent and exhibit some antibacterial properties. Soak the feet for about half an hour.

Foot odor may be caused by pitted keratolysis, a condition in which the soles of the feet appear whitish, with tiny pits; because it may be due to the same organism responsible for acne, try applying an acne medication containing 10 percent benzoyl peroxide to clear up the skin.

ACTIVATED CHARCOAL This product can be sprinkled in shoes to adsorb odor particles and reduce shoe odor. It is usually sold in capsule form.

BAKING SODA Sprinkle baking soda liberally into your shoes; the surface area of the soda neutralizes odors. Also, pat the powder on feet before putting

on your socks. This can help neutralize skin acids that promote the growth of bacteria and hence foot odor.

EPSOM SALTS Pour 2 cups of Epsom salts into 4 to 8 liters of warm water. Place the solution in a bucket or footbath. Soak feet for 15 minutes twice daily. This magnesium sulfate solution is

astringent and possibly antibacterial, promoting a healthy environment for the skin of the foot.

CORNSTARCH Cornstarch absorbs sweat. Once or twice daily, sprinkle it liberally onto feet before putting on your socks. Do not use if your feet have sores or open wounds.

FOXGLOVE

Digitalis purpurea
DEADMEN'S BELLS, WITCH'S BELLS

The foxglove is one of nature's most valuable gifts to modern medicine. It is also one of the most deadly. Digitalis drugs derived from the leaves of this showy biennial have long been employed as a treatment for congestive heart failure. The cardiac glycosides that are naturally present in foxglove are put to use in medications that save millions of lives every year. Foxglove is that rare medicinal plant that yields the complete pharmacological compound needed to restore a weakened vital function—in this case, strengthening contractions of the heart. The substance itself can be toxic, however, if too much is administered. Moreover, foxglove is often superseded by new vasodilator drugs today.

Foxglove was naturalized in North America in colonial times and was likely prescribed as a sedative and diuretic by both Indians in the Rocky Mountain region and immigrant folk healers. However, early use of the plant in the preparation of home remedies was generally discouraged because of the dangers associated with overdosing. The plant caused severe nausea, visual disturbances, seizures, and ultimately fatal cardiac arrhythmia—all side effects of its then unknown benefits for heart disease.

Today, although foxglove is still cultivated for ornamental purposes, the plant's medicinal principles remain far too powerful for inclusion in any herbal remedies. It is important to avoid foxglove altogether in all medications that are not prescribed by a doctor, and keep children away from the plant at all times.

From Dropsy to Digitalis

Foxglove's emergent use in the treatment of heart ailments started with a case of dropsy, a condition of severe and sometimes deadly fluid retention. In the late 1700s, an English doctor named William Withering detected foxglove in an herbal folk remedy that cured a case of dropsy he had formerly diagnosed as fatal. After 12 years of careful study and experimentation, Withering discovered that therapeutic doses of foxglove must be administered at nearly poisonous levels, then be adjusted continually over the period of the ailment. Withering's use of foxglove in cases of dropsy helped reveal the links between kidney function and heart disease, confirming that the plant's previously recognized diuretic effect was tied to its action on the heart. His findings on foxglove's ability to stabilize blood pressure in a weakened heart, as well as lower it in hypertensive ailments, laid the groundwork for the field of digitalis therapy as it exists today.

Although foxglove was widely used throughout the 19th century as a cardiotonic, the continuing dangers of working with it eventually caused most herbalists to downplay its relevance outside of mainstream medicine. Its folk use has now been consigned to the annals of history.

Active plant parts Leaves
Uses Prescription drugs for heart disease
Cautions Foxglove is extremely dangerous: even if only one leaf is chewed, it may cause paralysis and sudden heart failure. Gardeners with small children are advised not to grow foxglove as an ornamental plant because of its extreme toxicity.

FROSTBITE

Prolonged exposure to freezing temperatures can lead to frostbite—tissue damage (particularly in the extremities) brought on by frozen skin and severely reduced circulation. Persistent pain or numbness, blisters, and skin discoloration signify a serious condition and should be seen by a doctor.

Only minor frostbite and chilblains (itchy, red swellings due to the cold) can be treated with home remedies, the most effective of which is extract of ginkgo biloba. Long used in China (either before or after exposure), ginkgo improves circulation to the skin and extremities.

Prepare for the Cold

Prevention of frostbite includes wearing proper clothing, keeping the extremities covered, and avoiding alcohol. Once you are out in the cold, drinking water and moving around also helps.

Unfortunately, even the best preparations can fail. The first symptom of frostbite is the familiar "pins and needles" effect, followed by complete numbness. The skin appears white and hard, then turns red and swells. Once frostbitten skin thaws, blisters commonly form. Badly damaged skin can turn black, indicating dead tissue that requires amputation.

Orthodox first aid calls for immediate shelter. If the victim is also suffering from hypothermia, this must be treated first. Once the victim is no longer exposed to the cold, remove clothing from the affected area and place warm hands or lukewarm water—no hotter than 43.3°C (110°F)—on the skin. Hands can be warmed in the victim's own armpits.

Folk Cures and Myths

To provide warmth and stimulate local circulation, many early settlers turned to herbal poultices. Red pepper and mustard powder, two irritating rubefacients, were often included in poultices for frostbite, but neither should be used on tender skin. (However, simply sprinkling a little of either into socks or gloves can provide toasty warmth.) Poultices of beech or oak leaves make use of astringent tannins that can soothe and help thaw the skin.

Lukewarm footbaths, prepared with teas made from alum root or balm of Gilead buds can provide relief. Old remedies that obviously should no longer be considered include pouring whiskey into your boots, putting your hands in a kettle of boiled pine needles, and rubbing kerosene on frostbitten ears.

Several popular frostbite treatments are dangerous. Rubbing the affected area with snow does not raise the skin's temperature, and any rubbing or massaging of the skin can worsen the damage. Also, because frostbitten skin is often numb, direct heat from a heating pad, campfire, or hot water can easily burn the skin.

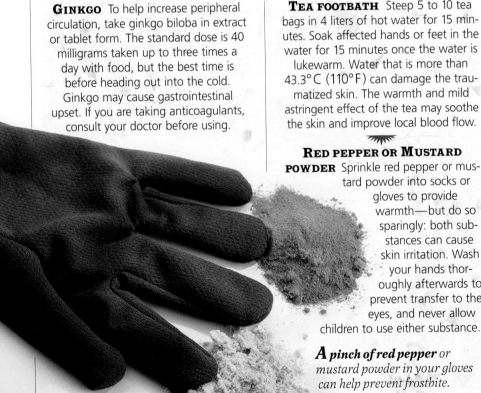

GINKGO To help increase peripheral circulation, take ginkgo biloba in extract or tablet form. The standard dose is 40 milligrams taken up to three times a day with food, but the best time is before heading out into the cold. Ginkgo may cause gastrointestinal upset. If you are taking anticoagulants, consult your doctor before using.

TEA FOOTBATH Steep 5 to 10 tea bags in 4 liters of hot water for 15 minutes. Soak affected hands or feet in the water for 15 minutes once the water is lukewarm. Water that is more than 43.3°C (110°F) can damage the traumatized skin. The warmth and mild astringent effect of the tea may soothe the skin and improve local blood flow.

RED PEPPER OR MUSTARD POWDER Sprinkle red pepper or mustard powder into socks or gloves to provide warmth—but do so sparingly: both substances can cause skin irritation. Wash your hands thoroughly afterwards to prevent transfer to the eyes, and never allow children to use either substance.

A pinch of red pepper or mustard powder in your gloves can help prevent frostbite.

GARLIC

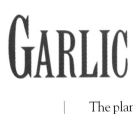

Allium sativum
THE STINKING ROSE, POOR MAN'S TREA-
CLE, RUSTIC TREACLE, NECTAR OF THE
GODS, CAMPHOR OF THE POOR

Never has so humble a plant enjoyed a more exalted history than that of the "stinking rose." This famously foul-smelling bulb has been treasured since the beginning of recorded time, both as a food and a medicine. A garlic prescription written in cuneiform was discovered on a Sumerian clay tablet dating back to 3000 BC. Garlic might even be the secret behind the great pyramids: the Egyptians rationed it to the pyramid builders to boost their strength (and prevent dysentery).

An ancient papyrus recommended garlic for everything from headaches to tumors to snakebite, worms, and heart trouble. The Egyptians consumed so much of the herb that they were dubbed "the stinking ones." When they took a solemn oath, it was garlic on which they swore. King Tutankhamen himself was buried not only with a superfluity of gilded finery but also with six cloves of garlic.

The plant has alternately been viewed with reverence and scorn. The Greeks and Romans ate garlic before going into battle, and Greek athletes fortified themselves with garlic before races. The Greek physician Hippocrates valued it for use against constipation and even cancer. But upper-class Greeks and Romans turned their noses up at garlic, or more specifically, at garlic breath, which they took as sign of low birth. In medieval Europe the rich shunned garlic, which became known as the poor man's treacle, or cure-all.

Worldly Healer

If garlic's odor was legendary, so eventually were its healing powers. Many Europeans ate garlic daily to protect themselves against the plague. They also tied braids of freshly harvested bulbs to their doorposts in order to ward off evil spirits. In India, lepers became known as "peelgarlics" because they ate so much garlic. (Modern research supports garlic's use against leprosy, and it is actually administered for that purpose today.)

During World War I, garlic juice was used by the British, French, and Russian armies to treat wounds and prevent gangrene. During World War II, garlic earned the nickname "Russian penicillin" because it was used by the Russian army when the supply of antibiotics ran low. In China, it is still used to treat diarrhea, dysentery, and tuberculosis. Beyond its renown for healing, garlic had a long-standing reputation as an aphrodisiac; it was therefore eliminated from the diets of many yogis, monks, and nuns.

Active plant parts Bulb
Uses High blood pressure, high cholesterol, arteriosclerosis, colds, respiratory infections, intestinal worms, gastrointestinal ailments
Cautions Large amounts (five or more cloves a day) can result in heartburn, flatulence, and intestinal distress. Those taking aspirin or anticoagulant drugs should consult a doctor before taking large amounts of garlic. People with clotting disorders should not take medicinal amounts of garlic. In rare cases, garlic may cause an allergic reaction.

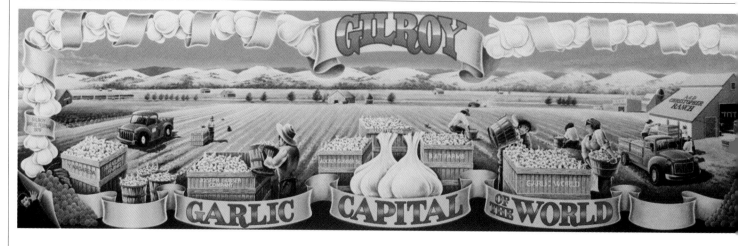

Garlic in North America

The Indians used a native species of wild garlic to treat snakebite, intestinal worms, and more. Cultivated garlic varieties from Europe arrived with the settlers, along with the practice of strapping peeled garlic cloves to the feet of smallpox victims and those with fevers in order to draw out the infection. The 19th-century Kings Eclectics prescribed poultices of garlic to treat pneumonia. Garlic tea was recommended for intestinal disorders and stomach ulcers.

Garlic juice was poured into the ear, often mixed with warm olive oil, to cure the "deafness" caused by ear blockage. Cloves were wrapped in gauze and placed in the ear to cure earaches. For pinworms, chopped garlic or enemas of garlic juice were employed. Dogs were commonly fed garlic cloves to rid them of worms.

To heal wounds, people made a crude antibiotic ointment of mashed garlic mixed with honey or milk. Garlic was also called upon to cure aches, pains, and fevers. Peeled cloves were placed on aching teeth and cut cloves were rubbed on arthritic joints. An early headache remedy called for a teaspoon of honey mixed with ½ teaspoon of garlic juice.

Above all, garlic was a treasured cough and cold remedy. Many people wore it around their necks, not so much to ward off vampires as to ward off illness. Those who could bear it ate it raw. Poor souls who suffered from whooping cough also suffered from this cure: a mixture of garlic and lard rubbed on the chest. Finally there were the innumerable cough syrups. One recipe called for simmering ten garlic cloves in a half-liter of milk and adding honey to taste. Another required soaking four peeled cloves in a half-liter of brandy for two weeks; the resulting elixir was said to aid coughs and asthma. Also recommended for asthma was a syrup made with garlic, apple cider vinegar, and honey.

An Edible Antibiotic

Even more amazing than the number of ailments people treated with garlic is the number of uses that have since been justified by science. Louis Pasteur confirmed garlic's antiseptic activity in 1858. More recently, scientists have identified garlic's main active components, one of which is a substance called alliin. When a clove is crushed, bruised, or chewed, the alliin is converted into allicin, a potent antibiotic—and also the source of garlic's

In Gilroy, California, a world-renowned garlic festival held in late July celebrates the local bumper crop.

characteristic odor. Allicin is highly unstable; it cannot survive the heat of cooking or the acid in your stomach. But when fresh garlic is chewed, the allicin is quickly absorbed in the mouth.

Garlic exhibits antibacterial, antimicrobial, and antifungal activity, which supports its external use on wounds, worms, and athlete's foot. In one Chinese study, garlic was used effectively to treat patients with cryptococcal meningitis, one of the most serious fungal infections. It also works against the bacteria that cause typhus, dysentery, and enteritis. In fact, garlic can inhibit the growth of some bacteria that have become immune to standard antibiotics. Research indicates that it may also protect the stomach lining from ulcers.

When garlic is eaten, its essential oil is excreted principally through the lungs, making it especially useful against respiratory ailments. Also, garlic extracts have been found to have significant anti-inflammatory activity, perhaps supporting garlic's traditional use against arthritis.

Cancer Safeguard?

Garlic's potential for preventing certain types of cancer is promising. In mice, garlic extracts have been shown to inhibit the growth of cancer cells. What's more, a Chinese study found that residents of one region who regularly ate large amounts of garlic were far less likely to have stomach cancer than residents of another region where garlic is rarely consumed.

Garlic is an antioxidant, an agent that helps eliminate compounds known as free radicals, products of the oxidation process that contribute to aging, arthritis, and cancer. Researchers have also discovered that garlic helps eliminate toxic levels of lead and mercury from the body. It has also been used to help treat diabetes.

Heart Help

Currently enjoying top billing among garlic's seemingly endless powers is its apparent ability to help prevent heart disease and strokes. Garlic has been shown to lower serum cholesterol and triglyceride levels while raising the level of high density lipoproteins, or "good" lipids, thereby lowering the risk of cardiovascular disease. Garlic is thought responsible for the low incidence of arteriosclerosis (hardening of the arteries) in parts of Italy and Spain, where large amounts of garlic are eaten. One study found that eating as little as one clove a day of fresh garlic can help lower serum cholesterol levels.

Moreover, the substance in garlic called ajoene, a by-product of allicin, is at least as effective as aspirin in thinning the blood and preventing blood clots, which can lead to heart attacks and stroke. Garlic may also lower blood pressure.

Unfortunately, allicin (the compound that gives garlic much of its medicinal value) also gives it its smell. Garlic tablets or capsules impart less odor than fresh garlic. In order to be effective, however, they must be enteric coated so that they pass through the stomach and release their contents in the small intestine, where the alliin is converted to allicin; otherwise, the alliin is destroyed by the stomach acid before it can be converted. Garlic pills vary widely in alliin content. The daily dose should be at least 10 milligrams of alliin, which equals about one clove of fresh garlic, but just how much of it each pill contains will tend to fluctuate from one product to another. Still, to get the most benefits from garlic, eat it raw.

To solve the problem of garlic's lingering odor, try chewing fennel seeds or fenugreek seeds, or using a mouthwash made of baking soda and hydrogen peroxide. A folk remedy suggests taking a long, hot bath to draw out the garlic oils, which emanate from the skin. Even if this fails, the smell of garlic may be a small price to pay for the health benefits it brings. An old Welsh rhyme advised, "Eat leeks in March and wild garlic in May, and all the year after physicians may play."

Garlic: Cooked or Raw?

There is no doubt that garlic offers the greatest medicinal value when eaten raw. But what benefits does the cooked herb provide? Scientists aren't sure, since most of the studies performed on garlic have involved garlic pills or extracts. We do know that the compound called allicin, which is thought to be responsible for many of garlic's healing properties, is destroyed by heat. Nevertheless, it appears that garlic contains other compounds that may also be beneficial, considering that people who consume a lot of cooked garlic have a lower incidence of stomach cancer. The degree of cooking may be a factor: garlic baked until mild and sweet is probably devoid of active compounds, whereas garlic that is lightly stir-fried may retain some pharmacologic activity.

Garlic is strong medicine, with an odor to match. Enteric coated pills will help eliminate its offensiveness.

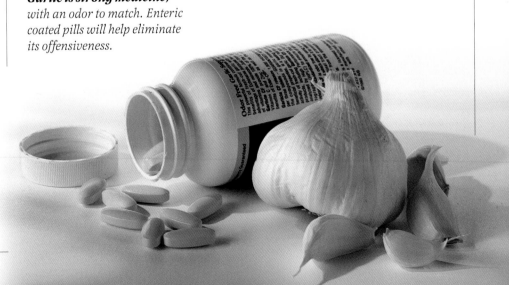

GINGER

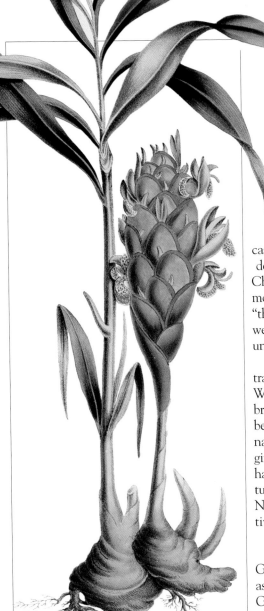

Zingiber officinale

This exotic spice, prized for its culinary and medicinal qualities, actually lent a hand in the discovery of the Americas. In the 15th century, Europe grew desperate for easier access to the riches of China and India, including ginger, cinnamon, pepper, and silk. Speculation that "the Indies" could be reached by sailing west rather than east led Columbus unknowingly to the New World in 1492.

North America itself soon became a trading hub and ginger a standard import. When English settlers arrived, they brought with them a fondness for ginger beer, a forerunner of ginger ale. Medicinally, the same uses that were part of ginger's mystique in the spice trade (and have been valued in China for 25 centuries) quickly took hold in colonial North America: those of food preservative, digestive aid, and nausea reducer.

Stomach Soother

Ginger's primary medicinal use has been as a remedy for indigestion and nausea. Ginger beer, made in Jamaica and England, provided the early settlers with relief from diarrhea, nausea, and vomiting. In 19th-century North America the Eclectics endorsed the root tea for diarrhea, indigestion, nausea, dysentery, and other ailments. The Eclectic medical reference, *King's American Dispensatory*, gave recipes for ginger beer and wine, and noted that "cakes of ginger and molasses and flour" (what we now call gingerbread) helped the stomach "when eaten in moderation." The root tea, crystallized ginger candy, and ginger cookies were all used to relieve gas and hangover, stimulate the appetite, and aid the digestion of fatty meats, beans, and yams.

The ginger ale that your mother gave you to quell nausea when you were a child may have provided more than tender loving care. In the early 1980s American scientists reported that ginger prevented motion sickness better than Dramamine, a popular commercial product. Subsequent research in the United States, Sweden, Germany, and Britain has reported that ginger acts on the gastrointestinal tract, as well as on the inner ear and the central nervous system—which monitor balance—to reduce dizziness, anesthesia-related nausea, and the vomiting and cold sweats associated with seasickness. A recent study found that low doses of ginger may also relieve morning sickness; because of its potential effect on the uterus, however, its use during pregnancy should be supervised by a doctor.

The same principles that provide ginger's aroma—compounds called gingerols and shogaols—soothe the muscles of the gastrointestinal tract. To relieve nausea,

Active plant parts Rhizome
Uses Nausea, indigestion, arthritis, coughs
Cautions Ingestion of ginger may cause sweating. Although the herb is allowed for sale in therapeutic products in Canada, the safety of large doses and continuous use has not been adequately determined. Overdoses may depress the central nervous system and cause cardiac arrhythmia. Because of its potential effect on the uterus, ginger's use during pregnancy should be supervised by a doctor.

the standard dose is 1 to 2 grams of the powdered root every four hours while symptoms persist. In Germany the recommended daily dose for indigestion and motion sickness is 2 to 4 grams.

Teas can also be made with ½ to 2 teaspoons grated root. Weaker teas are recommended for colicky children under two. A glass of ginger ale with natural flavoring reportedly provides relief of motion sickness. (Note: many ginger ales are made with artificial flavoring.) However, since dehydration is often associated with nausea, the benefit of ginger ale may stem more from the liquid than from the ginger. In culinary quantities, the spice lacks any medicinal effect.

Beyond ginger's use for gastrointestinal problems, early settlers enjoyed a warm bath or footbath that contained juice pressed from the grated root to invigorate the body and soothe bruises and tired muscles. When mixed in sesame seed oil, the juice was also used as a massage rub. Chewing the root soothed a sore throat, and grated ginger in olive oil treated dandruff. Warm ginger compresses were used to treat sinus congestion, menstrual cramps, and general achiness and fatigue.

Wonder Spice?

Research on ginger's other folk uses has produced some positive results. Taken as a tea, tincture, or capsule, ginger can produce sweating and help reduce fever. It also helps to relieve chills and stimulate circulation. By interfering with the release of histamines and prostaglandins into the bloodstream, ginger may reduce arthritis inflammation and the severity of allergic reactions and migraines.

Ginger may help to fight intestinal infections, prevent ulcers, and provide a cleansing, antioxidant effect on the kidneys, liver, and gallbladder, while its effect on uterine muscles may stimulate menstruation and soothe cramps. Ginger may also help lower cholesterol, blood pressure, and the risk of blood clots. The root tea is said to be a mild cough suppressant and expectorant. Still, additional research is needed to validate these effects—as well as ginger's potential to tone blood vessels, help prevent heart disease, boost immunity, and fight tumors.

Although the effectiveness of many of ginger's external, or topical, applications remain unsupported, a recent study has confirmed the use of its fresh juice or volatile oil to relieve minor burns and skin infections. Ginger folk remedies for snakebite and baldness are not likely to work, but applying the juice or oil to sore muscles and joints, earache, or toothache may provide a mild degree of relief.

A North American "Ginger"

The ginger plant, *Zingiber officinale*—the aromatic herb that grows in hot, moist climates—has a North American counterpart. Called wild ginger or Indian ginger, *Asarum canadense* emits a rotten odor and grows from Quebec to Ontario, south to Florida, and west to Minnesota and Illinois.

The North American plant was used in many of the same ways as its tropical namesake. Indians and pioneers used the root for indigestion, loss of appetite, fevers, coughs, sore throats, colds, and menstrual problems. A strong root tea was drunk as a heart medication. In a culinary, if not medical, appreciation of wild ginger, George Washington Carver—famous for his exhaustive studies of the peanut—made use of the root to spice his tea and the leaves to flavor salads. Today the plant is being studied for its potential to fight bacteria and tumors.

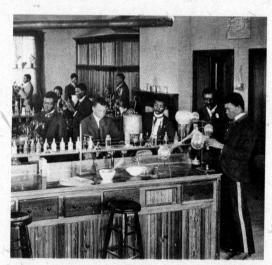

George Washington Carver, *shown second from right in his laboratory at Tuskegee Institute in Alabama, was fond of wild ginger.*

Although similar in taste, cultivated ginger and wild ginger are totally distinct plants, each with its own colorful names. Cultivated ginger's distribution is reflected in its nomenclature: Jamaican, African, or Cochin ginger; in China it is called *chiang*. Wild ginger is also called heartleaf, Canada snakeroot, false coltsfoot, and colicroot.

GINSENG

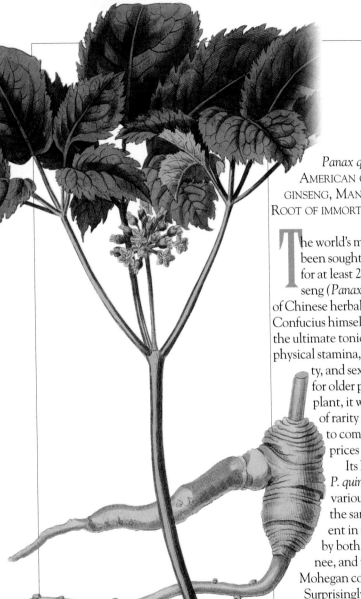

Panax quinquefolius
AMERICAN GINSENG, WESTERN
GINSENG, MANROOT, LIFE ROOT,
ROOT OF IMMORTALITY, HEAL-ALL

The world's most costly plant root has been sought for medicinal purposes for at least 2,000 years. Asian ginseng (*Panax ginseng*), a cornerstone of Chinese herbal medicine praised by Confucius himself, was long regarded as the ultimate tonic—an enhancer of physical stamina, mental acuity, longevity, and sexual prowess—especially for older people. A slow-growing plant, it was harvested into a state of rarity centuries ago and came to command astronomical prices in its native land.

Its North American cousin, *P. quinquefolius*, was used by various Indian tribes in much the same way: it was an ingredient in a love potion concocted by both the Meskwaki and Pawnee, and the Delaware and the Mohegan considered it a cure-all. Surprisingly, European settlers learned about ginseng not from the Indians but by way of China. In 1714 a French Jesuit missionary in China published a report on the plant's uses and its exorbitant cost. Noting that the conditions in which ginseng grew—on northerly, forest-shaded slopes in soils enriched with leaf mold—were highly similar to those of the forests of eastern Canada, he predicted that if the plant was to be found anywhere else in the world, it would be there. The following year, a Jesuit priest in Canada read his words and set out in search of the wondrous medicinal plant. He discovered American ginseng, later found to contain active principles closely related to those of its Asian counterpart. He sent samples to China, and thus set in motion a highly profitable export business that continues to this day.

The majority of ginseng products found on the North American market today contain Asian ginseng grown in China or Korea, while most American ginseng is channeled to Asian markets. The reason for this ironic twist? In traditional Chinese medicine, American ginseng is preferred for

The root's resemblance *to the human form led to its Chinese name: jen-shen, or "manroot."*

Active plant parts Root
Uses Stimulant; general tonic; stress resistance; appetite and digestion enhancement; immune system booster
Cautions Because of its stimulant properties, anyone suffering from high blood pressure or heart disease should consult a physician before using ginseng. Similarly, its effects on the glandular and hormonal balance could make its use dangerous to persons with pituitary, adrenal, or thyroid problems. It is also said to reduce blood sugar levels: diabetics should consume ginseng only under a doctor's supervision.

what is said to be its *yin* (or "cooling") effect on weak, convalescing patients and the elderly, as well as its ability to replenish *ch'i*, or vital energy. Asian ginseng is the *yang* (or "warming") herb, valued as a tonic for blood and circulatory problems.

Made in North America

Panax quinquefolius is a low-growing herb that inhabits rich woodlands from Quebec to parts of the American Southeast and from eastern Oklahoma to southern Manitoba. Like its Asian relative, it is harvested for its multi-branched root, which often resembles the human body and accounts for at least part of its reputation in folklore. The more humanoid its

Not to be confused with...

American ginseng is native to shady woodlands in eastern and midwestern North America. Asian ginseng grows in similar habitats in China and Korea. Neither should be confused with Siberian ginseng *(Eleutherococcus senticosus),* an unrelated shrub native to northeast Asia; its root is often sold as a substitute for the rarer and more expensive roots of the true ginsengs. Nor should either be confused with dwarf ginseng *(Panax trifolius),* a smaller North American cousin whose globular root is of far lesser medicinal value.

Given ginseng's high price, many imposters have masqueraded as ginseng. For example, desert dock *(Rumex hymenosepalus),* native to the western U.S., was sold for a time as "wild red desert ginseng."

shape, the more valuable it is. Such roots may be 10 years old or more: it takes at least six years for them to reach marketable size.

The allure of these treasures led to intensive hunting, which made American ginseng relatively rare in the wild. (The Ojibwa always planted a seed for each herb taken, but others disregarded this practice.) Today the herb is regulated under an international treaty that governs trade in endangered flora and fauna.

Today most American ginseng found in ginseng products is grown commercially rather than harvested in the wild. In Canada, growers are concentrated in British Columbia and Ontario. Canada's production accounts for about 45 percent of the world's supply of American ginseng, with estimates that it may reach 75 percent by the end of the 1990s.

A deceptive practice by some ginseng suppliers is mixing *P. quinquefolius* grown in North America with that grown in China, which has been shown to have lower levels of active principles. Chinese-grown American ginseng is known in the trade as "China white."

Helpful Ginsenosides

Studies have isolated several active constituents, called ginsenosides, in both American and Asian ginseng and analyzed their properties. The constituents vary depending on the species, the age of the plant, when it was harvested, and how it was processed. Moreover, they may have different effects on different people.

Oddly enough, many ginsenosides seem to have opposing effects: some raise blood pressure while others lower it; some stimulate the central nervous system, but others depress it. Taken together, ginsenosides are believed to act as an adaptogen, or tonic, that helps the body adjust to

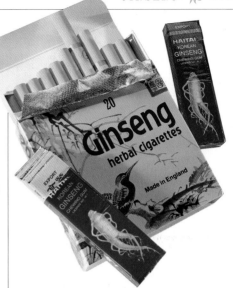

Questionable ginseng products *that may have little or no effect range from cigarettes to chewing gum.*

stresses of all sorts, combating fatigue and increasing general resistance.

European clinical studies have shown that Asian ginseng extracts containing up to 7 percent ginsenosides can lead to more efficient visual and auditory performance, increased respiratory efficiency, heightened alertness and concentration, and increased motor coordination—even though researchers agree that more clinical studies are necessary. American ginseng is not as extensively researched: of more than 2,900 scientific studies on ginseng, the vast majority have centered on Asian ginseng. Still, American ginseng has been found to contain higher levels of the ginsenoside Rb_1, which is believed to have an anti-stress effect.

Ginseng root can be chewed raw or dried, or it may be powdered and brewed into a tea. It is also available in a number of suspect forms, including cigarettes, candy, and chewing gums, the effectiveness of which cannot be gauged.

Spiritual Elements in
African-Based Folk Medicine

From the rural South to urban centers across North America, many African descendants keep alive a holistic perception of health that stems from age-old concepts of being and spirituality found in their ancestral homelands. Illness is seen as a disequilibrium caused by outside forces of either natural or supernatural origin.

The perception on the part of many African descendants that illness is the result of either natural or unnatural causes is inextricably tied to religion: wellness versus sickness is equated with good versus evil. Natural illnesses are those that stem from cold, heat, or dampness and the condition of the body—the balance of its working parts and the nature of the blood. Given the belief that events occur in the world as God made it, natural illness can also be seen as divine punishment. Unnatural illnesses, on the other hand, arise from the occult, the result of sorcery by "root doctors," conjurers, or individuals who have the awful power to hex, "witch," or "root" someone.

Said to "build" the blood are red foods like pork, red wine, and beets. White or clear substances thought to "lower" the blood include lemon juice, vinegar, and tonics made from aloe vera gel.

An African-based holistic view holds that one stays well by avoiding extremes of temperature, eating properly, keeping clean (both inside and out), and exercising. Proper behavior is also essential to health. There is little sympathy for someone who breaks the rules; if a person gets sick, it is said, he brought it upon himself. Among many folk of African ancestry, the diagnosis of illness has as much to do with determining the ways in which the patient has not taken care of himself as with the symptoms.

Ebb and Flow

The state of the blood reflects health as a whole. Spoken of as being high or low, thick or thin, fast or slow, hot or cold, good or bad, blood is said to always be in flux and to vary depending on its quality and quanti-

The Healer from the Piedmont

In the hamlet of Moncure in the North Carolina Piedmont, John Lee and his family have been a vital resource in community health care for more than a century. Lee learned the old-time healing arts from his father, a respected herbalist and "bloodstopper"(a person believed to staunch bleeding by magical means) and from his mother, who drew on an ancestry that combined African, Cherokee, and Lumbee healing traditions with those of the Irish and English. Even as a boy Lee enjoyed respect because he had been born with a caul—the "veil" over his face that was a sign he had been gifted with special insight. His mother took him along on visits to her patients, sending him out to gather the appropriate herbs. Today his diagnoses are based on years of practical experience and intuition as well as dreams and spiritual divination. Lee is also adept at interpreting vague symptoms and has brought relief to many people who were not helped by conventional doctors.

The satisfactions of Lee's calling are deep, and he views his ability as a gift to be shared with the community. "It's good to have knowledge," he says, "and if you don't use what you have, you might as well bury it."

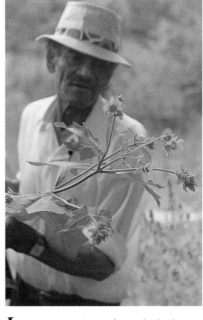

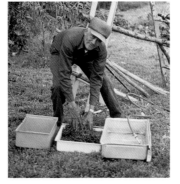

Lee gathers plants from the lush foothills and riversides of the Piedmont. At left, he washes the roots of yellow sarsaparilla (Menispermum canadense), *later to be paired with black cohosh in an all-purpose tonic.*

Familiar with some 100 herbs, Lee uses a basic pharmacopeia of about 60, which he usually selects and harvests himself. The strong, acrid taste of a plant like poke (below right) warns Lee that it should be used in small doses, while the milder taste of mint-family plants (below) signals the relative safety of larger doses.

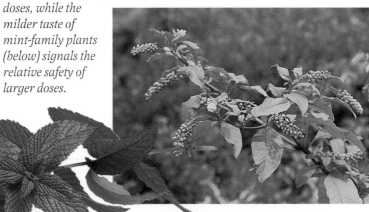

The speed of the patient's response is another indicator used by Lee to categorize botanicals. The potency of gripgrass, or Sisyrinchium (above left), is revealed because the patient can immediately "feel it working." Catnip (above right), on the other hand, produces only a mild response.

ers use magic and various substances to put a "fix" on people. Both faith healers and root doctors are also thought to have the power to "deroot" someone who is being controlled: the faith healer renders the rooting harmless, while the root doctor has the power to harm or even kill the individual responsible for the rooting.

Aside from its use against illness, magic is common where the cultural environment is seen as hostile and where people have little control over what happens in their lives. "Magic vendors" and candle shops, found in many North American cities, sell oils, incense, religious artifacts, powders, charms, and amulets that are variously used to win love, bring luck, keep a spouse from straying, or avenge a slight from a neighbor.

A Modern Blend

In keeping with the resurgence of interest in medicinal herbs, many people of African ancestry are using folk medicine to treat such common ailments as colds and flu as well as, in some instances, more serious illnesses. Young people in particular are returning to their spiritual and cultural roots and to what they see as a more natural approach to health care, looking anew at the "things the old people used." This phenomenon results in part from distrust of conventional medicine. Furthermore, many believe that folk practitioners provide a sense of nurturing that is sometimes missing under a physician's routine care.

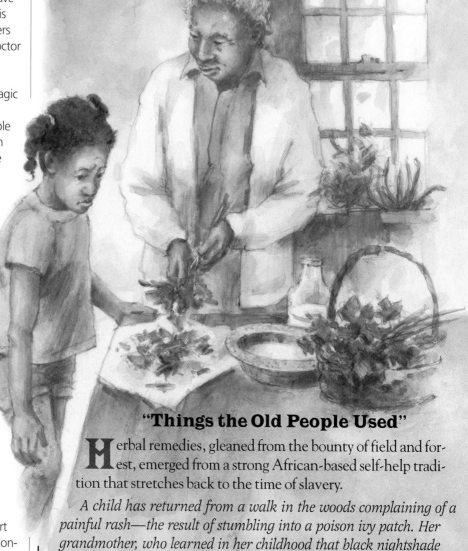

"Things the Old People Used"

Herbal remedies, gleaned from the bounty of field and forest, emerged from a strong African-based self-help tradition that stretches back to the time of slavery.

A child has returned from a walk in the woods complaining of a painful rash—the result of stumbling into a poison ivy patch. Her grandmother, who learned in her childhood that black nightshade heals such rashes, has ventured into the woods and returned with a basketful of the plants. After bruising the leaves and berries, she wraps them in cloth, dips them into a bowl of milk, and gently swabs the girl's legs. Two days later, the girl tells her grandmother that she can "hardly tell" she has poison ivy.

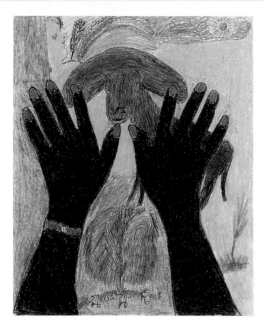

Healing and peace are personified by hands in African-based folk art, as in this work by Georgia artist Nellie Mae Rowe (1900–82).

ty, the season, one's age, and one's life circumstances.

"High blood," the symptoms of which are headache, dizziness, blurred vision, and "falling out" (sudden collapse), refers to too much blood, a shift of blood to the head, or high blood pressure. Emotional pressures or foods that are "too rich" or red in color are said to be the cause. "Low blood," evidenced by muscle weakness, lethargy, and fatigue, is blood that is either insufficient in quantity or circulating too far down in the body; it includes anemia and is often semantically confused with low blood pressure. Clear or colorless foods, too little red meat in the diet, and, in women, menstruation are believed to be at fault.

Normal blood should automatically thicken in winter to protect against problems associated with cold. These include colds, flu, bronchitis, pneumonia, and a disorder known as "quick TB," greatly feared by many women in the American South, black and white alike. As spring approaches, the blood should "thin down," readying the body for hot weather. Treatments, based on folk medicine practices formed three centuries ago among slaves, Indians, and Europeans, include herbal teas that "bring down" the blood or rid it of impurities caused by cold.

Some of these remedies, such as ginger and lemon juice, serve to open the pores so that impurities are "sweated out." Others, among them dandelion root and Epsom salts, eliminate impurities by opening the bowels.

While cold is linked to upper respiratory disorders, heat is associated with fevers, inflammations, and skin eruptions—the last, from measles to skin cancers, signaling "something in the body trying to come out."

"Unnatural" Threats

Almost any health problem may be seen as unnatural if it fails to respond to ordinary treatment. Some descendants of Africa believe that those who wish you ill can "do something to you" by magic. Problems of love and envy are the reasons given for most "rooting," or hexing. Abnormal control of a person causes physical or behavioral changes or both. Personifying impersonal forces—the stress caused by being laid off work or by family or money problems— allows the victim to identify the source of the problem and to

take action. Because they exist outside nature, such illnesses are very frightening, and ordinary people—especially physicians— are unable to deal with them.

Methods of Healing

As they were in earlier times, family members are the first to be called on for medical needs. If their ministrations fail to work, herbalists or religious leaders may be brought in. Herbalists (usually part-time practitioners well versed in botanical remedies, which they prepare themselves) treat illnesses seen as "natural." At times, they may also perform rituals.

If an illness is deemed "unnatural," only a healer with "the power"—a faith healer or, in some cases, a root doctor or conjurer—can treat it. Faith healers, from either mainstream or storefront churches, call upon supernatural forces by using prayer and the "laying-on of hands." Conversely, root doctors and conjur-

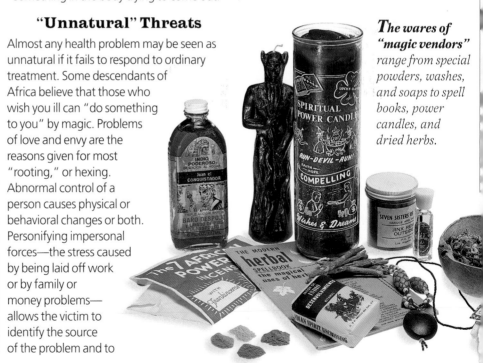

The wares of "magic vendors" range from special powders, washes, and soaps to spell books, power candles, and dried herbs.

GOLDENSEAL

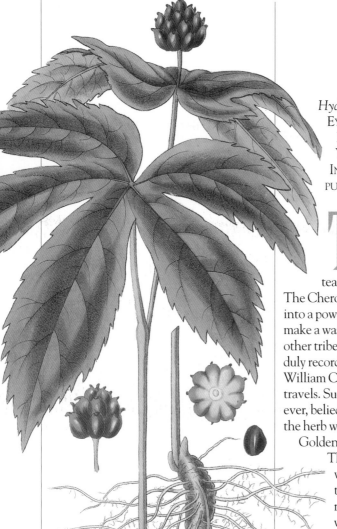

Hydrastis canadensis
EYEROOT, GROUND RASPBERRY,
INDIAN DYE, ORANGEROOT,
YELLOW INDIAN PAINT,
INDIAN TURMERIC, YELLOW
PUCCOON, YELLOWROOT

The earliest uses of the North American plant known as goldenseal—as a dye, face paint, medicinal wash, and tea—originated with the Indians. The Cherokee dried the root, ground it into a powder, and mixed it with water to make a wash for eye infections. Its use by other tribes as an eye and ear wash was duly recorded by Meriwether Lewis and William Clark on their fabled frontier travels. Such limited applications, however, belied the immense popularity that the herb would later enjoy.

Goldenseal was first used topically. The powdered root and wash were applied to skin inflammations, swellings, acne, and ringworm. The powdered root was also mixed with bear fat to make an insect repellent. Later, tea made from the root was drunk to treat nasal congestion,

fatigue, and loss of appetite. The Iroquois used a root decoction for "sour stomach," diarrhea, jaundice, whooping cough, fever, pneumonia, and heart problems.

Early settlers gargled with tinctures of goldenseal to soothe a sore throat. They also drank the tea as a general tonic and to relieve indigestion; as an astringent and antiseptic wash, they used it to treat bleeding wounds, dandruff, vaginal infections, and hemorrhoids.

Many women drank goldenseal tea to reduce excessive menstrual bleeding and to prevent hemorrhaging after childbirth. Large doses of the tea were also consumed in an attempt to induce abortions. Today, however, pregnant women are urged not to use goldenseal; it may stimulate the uterine muscles and cause a miscarriage.

Golden Age

In the mid-1800s, the Thomsonians—followers of New Englander Samuel Thomson (1769–1843), a prominent medical botanist—gave goldenseal its name and popularity. The name was chosen because the plant's scarred golden rhizome resembled the marks made in a wax stamp once commonly used to seal letters. Prior to that, the plant was known by a variety of names, including eyeroot, Indian dye, and yellowroot (not to be confused with *Xanthorhiza simplicissima*, another medicinal yellowroot).

As the Thomsonians continued to promote the usefulness of goldenseal, the herb caught the attention of John King and the Eclectic physicians. King included the herb in the first edition of his *King's*

Active plant parts Rhizome, roots
Uses Diarrhea, indigestion, irritations of the eye, lips, mouth, and throat
Cautions Because of goldenseal's potential effects on blood pressure, blood sugar, and the uterus, pregnant women and people at risk for heart disease, diabetes, glaucoma, or stroke should not use it. Large doses and long-term use can irritate the mouth and throat and cause exaggerated reflexes, hypertension, nausea, vomiting, diarrhea, and difficulty breathing. Any kind of homemade eyewash must be properly sterilized.

American Dispensatory in 1852, and the herb quickly became a favorite among the Eclectics. Solidly grounded in folk medicine and embraced by the leading medical botanists in the land, goldenseal experienced a golden age. In fact, because of its many uses, it was gathered nearly to extinction. After the American Civil War the price of goldenseal root soared, placing it among the most expensive of medicinal herbs. By 1900 it was a well-advertised ingredient in many "miracle cure" patent medicines, including Dr. Pierce's Golden Medical Discovery.

Goldenseal's folk uses grew to include cracked lips and nipples. The root was chewed to relieve canker sores, the leaves were macerated in vinegar and applied to snakebites, and the fresh leaf juice was ingested to calm "fits." Inhabitants of the Missouri Ozarks added the powdered root to mineral oil to treat stomach ulcers. They also stirred freshly chopped root into maple syrup and rubbed the mixture on the gums to treat infant thrush.

In the 20th century, famed Appalachian folk practitioner Tommie Bass called goldenseal "the king and queen of the herbs that the good Lord put in the ground." But he, too, noticed that "it's become hard to find in this part of the country and it don't grow around me."

The goldenseal in this product made it known as "golden medical discovery."

Today, the root is sold in capsules, tablets, tinctures, extracts, and tea bags, alone or in combination (often with echinacea).

Goldenseal's Secret

Like those for most cure-alls, the wilder claims for goldenseal are little more than a charlatan's bombast—it has even been said to mask drugs. However, there is good scientific evidence to explain why folk healers found the herb so effective against the core ailments they used it to treat. Goldenseal contains berberine and hydrastine, two antiseptics that effectively treat mucous membranes, such as those of the eyes, mouth, throat, and intestines.

In the late 1960s, research in Canada indicated that hydrastine stimulates the autonomic nervous system and constricts blood vessels. Berberine has been shown to be effective against the bacteria and protozoa that cause diarrhea. In addition, ingesting it stimulates bile secretion, which soothes stomach upset by aiding the digestion of fats. Sterile washes containing antiseptic and astringent berberine can also reduce eye inflammation.

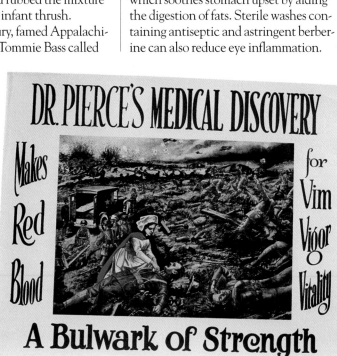

DR. PIERCE'S MEDICAL DISCOVERY

Makes Red Blood

for Vim Vigor Vitality

A Bulwark of Strength

The Drug-Test Myth

Beginning in the late 1970s, goldenseal root found a huge—if nefarious—market among drug users, who believed it would mask traces of morphine, cocaine, and marijuana in urine samples. Similar claims existed in folk medicine. The herb—thought to prevent drug and alcohol addiction by cleansing the liver, kidney, and blood of these toxins—was used to treat alcoholism.

Furthering goldenseal's reputation as a concealer of illicit drugs was the novel *Stringtown on the Pike,* a murder mystery published in 1900. In the story, the forensic chemist who examined the alleged victim believed the death to have been caused by strychnine poisoning. In fact, the dead man had merely partaken of a medicinal "bitters" of morphine and hydrastine (the latter being a major chemical component of goldenseal), which leaves the same chemical signature as strychnine. Moreover, the hydrastine had masked the morphine, leaving it undetected.

Because the novel was authored by none other than John Uri Lloyd, the renowned Eclectic plant pharmacist, the public took notice. Soon afterwards goldenseal was given to race horses to mask the morphine used to enhance performance.

Clinical studies have proven that goldenseal root cannot mask opiates and, in the process, deceive modern drug-test procedures. Furthermore, studies suggest that it can increase the potential of a false-positive result.

GOUT

Once known as "rich man's disease," gout is a hereditary metabolic disorder that causes uric acid—which is naturally secreted by the kidneys—to be deposited in and near the joints. The result is swelling, redness, and severe pain. Factors that increase the risk of gout include drinking alcohol, eating rich meaty foods, and being overweight—common circumstances of privileged men, particularly in times past.

Benjamin Franklin, Charles Darwin, Sir Isaac Newton, and Theodore Roosevelt were all noted sufferers of gout. The condition also afflicted Sitting Bull and the members of many Indian tribes. Today, postpubescent men—and to a much lesser extent, postmenopausal women—are most susceptible to gout.

A gout attack typically lasts only a few days and affects only one joint (usually, the big toe) and less commonly the hands, elbows, hips, or knees. Swelling and localized warmth are common, and the pain

Males are more prone to gout, the ailment affecting this troubled soul.

can be so excruciatingly intense that the joint cannot tolerate the weight of a sheet. Preventive measures include changes in diet and drinking habits (including a high water intake and less alcohol) and prescription drugs.

Anything That Soothes

In use for more than 500 years and still prominent today, meadow saffron (also known as autumn crocus) is the most fabled gout remedy. It is the source of colchicine, a specially extracted alkaloid that is valued for its ability to lessen the buildup of uric acid in the body. However, the alkaloid is highly toxic and can cause severe diarrhea. For this reason, colchicine is available only by prescription.

Many topical liniments and diuretic teas were used to soothe the swelling and cleanse the kidneys. Drinking nettle tea (and applying its juice topically) was common. Nettle is a diuretic, but its effect on gout has not been verified; it may also irritate the digestive tract. In a practice that dates back to ancient Rome, nettle was also used to "sting" the afflicted joint; although this is no longer recommended, it may numb the swelling by confusing pain feedback and irritating the skin. Other remedies were liniments made with evening primrose, garlic, and mullein,

and poultices of elderberries, burdock, flax, and rotten apples.

The long list of teas with diuretic, analgesic, or anti-inflammatory properties is headed by bilberry, burdock, echinacea, and willow bark. A remedy used by Henry VIII and brought to the New World was drinking the distilled water of "broome flowers." Gout remedies that are now known to be potentially toxic include teas made from sassafras, blue cohosh, calamus, horsetail, and woody nightshade.

"40 Cherries of Any Kind"

Both orthodox and folk medicine advocate simple dietary changes to prevent gout. Gout sufferers should consume more fruits, vegetables, and grains, and less shellfish, anchovies, asparagus, spinach, mushrooms, and high-protein foods, such as meat (especially kidney and liver) and beans. Hawaiian folk wisdom enlists watercress soup and a vegetarian diet. The Pennsylvania Dutch and countless other folk recommend eating cherries, anywhere from 10 to 40 a day, regardless of the variety. Strawberries, pineapples, raw carrots, and fish oil are also taken, but such measures lack scientific support.

BURDOCK Although this traditional tea has not been proven to relieve gout, it may be mildly diuretic and soothing. To prepare, pour boiling water over 2 to 3 teaspoons dried root, steep, then strain. Drink three times a day. Do not take during pregnancy or lactation.

WILLOW Glycosides give this tea anti-inflammatory, antirheumatic, and analgesic potential. To prepare, pour boiling water over 1 to 2 teaspoons bark, steep, then strain. Drink three times a day.

HANGOVER

As a surefire remedy for hangover, sauerkraut juice has long been drunk by the Pennsylvania Dutch in the belief that it restores lost oxygen and vitamin B. Centuries earlier, Europeans drank cabbage broth the morning after as a "laxative and diuretick" and even sniffed it up their nostrils, swearing "the cabbage purgeth the head ... [and] withstandeth drunkenness."

Cabbage notwithstanding, early physicians were convinced that a "headache of dissipation" meant a loss of bodily energy, and they were not far from the truth. Drinking too much alcohol overwhelms the capacity of the enzyme known as alcohol dehydrogenase (ADH), which metabolizes alcohol through the liver. Meanwhile, the head pounds as dilated blood vessels stretch like rubber bands and contract to their original shape, the stomach rebels, and the now-dehydrated body gives in to enormous fatigue. At this point, there is little one can do to counter a bout of overindulgence other than to drink copious amounts of water and eat crackers or other bland foods. While rates of alcohol metabolism vary somewhat from beverage to beverage, choosing beer or wine over bourbon or brandy is less important than eating food, which will delay absorption of alcohol and result in lower levels in the blood.

Nevertheless, folk remedies for hangover abound. In addition to sauerkraut

juice (which probably helps replenish lost liquids), a cup of bouillon replaces salt and potassium (as do sports drinks), and a homemade antacid (baking soda and a touch of lemon juice in a glass of water) can help calm an upset stomach. Eating fatty foods before and during drinking can help slow alcohol absorption. A capsule of activated charcoal may help as well.

The vaunted vanilla milk shake and ice cream soda probably have more value as comfort foods than as safe coatings for the stomach, and inhaling pure oxygen or taking vitamins will not work, say doctors. Moreover, drinking more alcohol (the ever-popular "hair of the dog") will provide only a temporary sedating effect—and a prolonged hangover. Clearly, temperance in drinking or abstinence is the best method of prevention.

FRUIT JUICE Rich in the simple sugar called fructose, fruit juices help give the body a much needed boost of energy in the form of converted glucose. Drinking a glass of fruit juice also helps to rehydrate the body.

KUDZU A traditional Chinese treatment for alcohol poisoning, kudzu is available as an extract. Mix 30 to 40 drops in 1½ cups water. Take once before rising and every 3 to 4 hours—up to four times daily if symptoms persist.

GOLDENSEAL The root of this herb contains berberine, shown to stimulate the secretion of bile in humans, which may ease the liver's job. Mix 5 to 10 drops extract or tincture with 1 cup of water.

COFFEE Caffeine, a central nervous system stimulant and vasoconstrictor, may temporarily ease a headache and perk you up. Still, a cup of coffee should never encourage a newly-alert yet still hungover person to drive: only time will eliminate alcohol from the bloodstream.

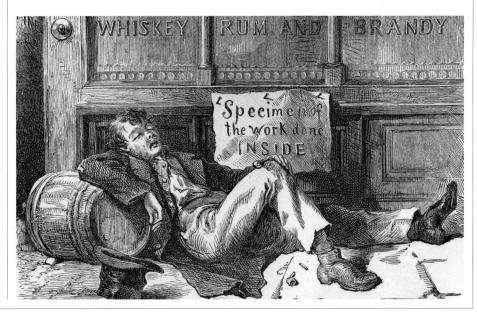

An overimbiber serves as proof of alcohol's pitfalls in this 19th-century poster.

HAWTHORN

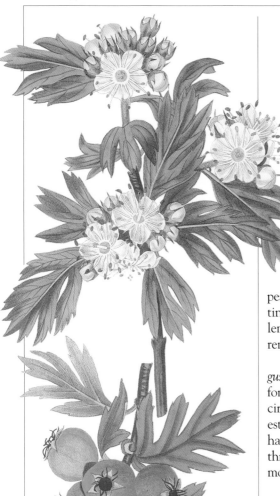

Crataegus laevigata
ENGLISH HAWTHORN, HAW, MAY,
MAYBUSH, WHITETHORN

English settlers brought hawthorn bushes to North America and used them as hedgerows between their fields. In fact, the Pilgrims' ship *Mayflower* was named for this plant's blossoms. Like other Europeans, the settlers took hawthorn teas and tinctures for stomach and bladder problems and used the tea externally to help remove thorns and splinters.

Indians used native species of *Crataegus* for similar ailments. The Cherokee, for example, used *C. spathulata* to improve circulation and fight fatigue. Today, it is estimated that hundreds of species of hawthorn grow in North America; throughout the world, *C. laevigata* is the most widely used medicinally.

An Old World folk belief held that bringing hawthorn branches into one's house would cause a death in the family. The plant was also linked with the plague because of the foul odor of some European species. Despite these associations, hawthorn enjoyed a long medicinal history in both Europe and Asia. However, its most popular use—as a heart remedy—was not discovered until the late 1800s. At that time, a doctor in Ireland began prescribing a "secret medication" for heart ailments. After he died in 1894, his daughter revealed his "secret" to be a tincture of hawthorn berries. It became a popular treatment in North America and Europe.

Help for the Heart

Recent research suggests that hawthorn may indeed be a helpful heart medication. Extracts from the leaves, berries, and flowers have been shown to expand blood vessels, thereby lowering blood pressure, reducing cholesterol buildup, and allowing blood to flow more freely, especially in the heart itself. Hawthorn may also help tone the heart muscles, reduce the frequency of recurring angina attacks, and normalize irregular patterns of heartbeat (arrhythmia). Although the most active compounds in hawthorn—flavonoids and procyanidines—have been found to tone the heart, its overall effect results from many constituents working together.

Even though hawthorn is available as a tea, extract, and capsule, it should not be used in any form to treat a heart condition. Generally, the herb must be taken for months to be effective; it will not provide relief from such acute problems as an angina attack. In standard, supervised dosages, no toxic buildup has been noted, but Health Canada has not approved over-the-counter hawthorn products intended for therapeutic internal use to treat heart problems. It is ill-advised to attempt self-medication for heart disease.

Active plant parts Berries, flowers, leaves
Uses Preventive for heart conditions, high blood pressure
Cautions Heart disease is a life-threatening condition. It is ill-advised and dangerous to attempt self-medication of a heart problem with hawthorn or any other medicine. Consult a physician immediately if you believe that you have a heart problem. In large doses, hawthorn is a sedative and may lead to a sudden drop in blood pressure.

excrete proteins that cause allergic reactions. To keep the mite population to a minimum, dustproof your home—especially the bedroom. Cover bedding in allergen-proof coverings, which have a vinyl or polyurethane skin on one side. To kill the mites, wash bedding weekly in water that is at least 48.9°C (120°F).

Wet-dust furniture once a week. On carpets, use a powerful vacuum cleaner and use it often; models are now designed for people with allergies. If you have a cat or a dog, reduce animal dander (invisible shreds of protein sloughed off the hide) by washing the pet on a regular basis.

The Low-Pollen Yard

Planting relatively pollen-free trees, shrubs, grass, and flowers in your landscape can go a long way toward lessening the threat of hay fever. Avoid plants that are wind-pollinated, such as walnut and oak, and all ornamental grasses; these are usually more allergenic than insect-pollinated plants, which include most ornamentals and bulbs. (In general, wind-pollinated plants are drab and have inconspicuous flowers, while insect-pollinated plants are more colorful and showy.) If you are fond of conifers, choose pines over cedar and juniper; even though pines produce an abundance of pollen, the pollen grains are resinous, making it difficult for the grains to be absorbed into the nasal membrane.

Low-pollen trees and shrubs include dogwood, ash, birch, elm, and cypress. Flowering plants that will remain relatively pollen-free include azalea, begonia, peony, viburnum, tulips, and other bulbs in general.

Avoid gardening in the early morning; pollen counts are usually at their highest before 10 A.M. Early afternoon is the best time to be out in the garden, since pollen counts tend to rise as the sun sets.

CHAMOMILE In those allergic to ragweed (a relative of chamomile), chamomile can actually aggravate hay fever. Despite this, European doctors prescribe chamomile preparations for respiratory tract inflammations in non-allergic people because of the herb's azulene content, which may have antiallergenic properties. For a tea, pour 1 cup boiling water over 2 to 3 teaspoons minced German chamomile flower heads. Steep for 10 minutes; strain. Drink three to four times daily.

KHELLA This Middle Eastern fruit (*Ammi visnaga*) is rarely sold in North America. The herb possesses the same properties available from the synthesized prescription drug cromolyn, used to treat asthma and other bronchial disorders. Studies have shown the herb to be an effective preventive against hay fever. To make a tea, pour boiling water over ¼ teaspoon powdered fruit. Steep for 10 to 15 minutes, then strain. Drink one cup daily. Do not exceed suggested dosage: prolonged use may cause nausea, sleeplessness, and headaches. Photosensitivity may occur in some people.

PEPPERMINT Indians, as well as 19th-century Eclectic physicians, used peppermint to treat respiratory problems. The herb's volatile oils may act as an antispasmodic, which can help relieve congested nasal and other breathing passages. Place 4 to 10 drops peppermint oil in a basin of just-boiled water. Make a steam tent by draping a towel over your head and inhale the vapors for 15 to 30 minutes, adding fresh water as needed. Do not place your face too close to the hot steam.

SALT-WATER NOSE SPRAY

Many leading herbalists recommend this treatment as an effective therapy. Prepare a soothing 0.9% isosmotic solution by dissolving 2 teaspoons salt in 1 liter warm water. Cool and store at room temperature. (Discard unused solution after two days, as it may become contaminated.) Spray or instill several drops into each nostril as needed throughout the day.

The 0.9% solution is the same concentration normally found in the body and is the mildest way to flush the nasal passages.

NETTLE Folk healers used this popular herb for a wide variety of ills—although hay fever was not one of them. Today, however, leading herbalists claim that nettle is a safe and effective alternative to prescription drugs and over-the-counter antihistamines, even though scientists have not identified the active principles responsible. The preferred form of administration is the freeze-dried leaf extract, available in capsules. Take one or two capsules every two to four hours to control hay fever symptoms.

Freeze-dried nettle leaves, easily found in capsules, are newly popular among hay fever sufferers.

HEADACHE

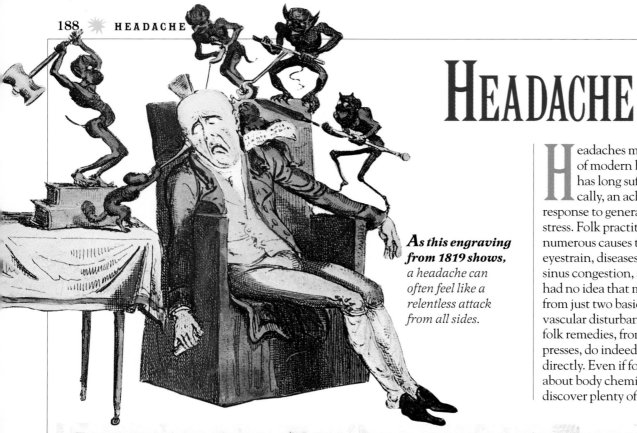

As this engraving from 1819 shows, *a headache can often feel like a relentless attack from all sides.*

Headaches may seem like products of modern life, but in fact mankind has long suffered their evils. Typically, an aching head is the body's response to general physical or emotional stress. Folk practitioners attributed numerous causes to headaches, including eyestrain, diseases of the womb, poor diet, sinus congestion, and constipation. They had no idea that most headaches arise from just two basic causes—tension and vascular disturbances. Nonetheless, many folk remedies, from herb teas to hot compresses, do indeed treat these causes directly. Even if folk healers knew little about body chemistry, they managed to discover plenty of remedies that worked.

TIE A BAND TIGHTLY AROUND YOUR HEAD This remedy, which has been used in many folk traditions, can actually help. The tight band reduces the flow of blood through the scalp, which may alleviate the throbbing of a vascular headache.

HOT FOOTBATHS Soak your feet in hot water in order to draw blood to your feet. This will reduce the pressure in the blood vessels in your head, which may soothe a throbbing vascular headache. Folk wisdom holds that adding mustard powder to the footbath produces a stronger effect.

HOT COMPRESS Place a hot compress on your forehead or the back of your neck to relax the tight muscles that are often the cause of a tension headache.

COLD COMPRESS Apply a cold compress to your forehead or the back of your neck. This will constrict the blood vessels and reduce blood flow, which may relieve a vascular headache.

FEVERFEW Chewing two or three leaves of feverfew daily may prevent the onset of migraines by controlling the body's release of serotonin, a chemical that causes the blood vessels to constrict. Continued use over several months may be necessary to achieve results. Some people develop mouth ulcers from chewing feverfew leaves. Capsules are available; however, the quality of feverfew they contain varies widely.

WILLOW BARK The bark of the white willow contains salicin, a compound chemically related to aspirin.

It was traditionally used against headaches, although scientists believe the bark may not contain enough salicin to stop the pain. To make a decoction, mix 2 teaspoons minced or powdered bark in 1 cup cold water. Heat to boiling, boil for five minutes, then steep and strain. Drink one cup three to four times a day. Willow bark is also available in capsules.

VALERIAN For tension headaches, try a cup of valerian tea, a mild sedative. To make the tea, add 1 teaspoon minced dried root to 1 cup boiling water and steep. Valerian, which has a strong, disagreeable odor, can also be taken as a tincture or in capsule form. Stop using the herb and consult a physician if you experience nausea, blurred vision, or other side effects.

Tension headaches are caused by muscle contractions in the head and neck and often feel like bands of dull, constant pressure. They tend to be the result of stress, lack of sleep, or holding one's neck and head in a stationary or rigid position for long periods of time, such as while reading or working at a computer. Chewing gum and grinding one's teeth can also trigger tension headaches.

Vascular headaches, including the migraine and cluster varieties, are thought to result from the constriction and later expansion of blood vessels in a particular area of the head. These are experienced as sharp, throbbing pains.

An occasional trigger of headaches is sinus congestion, which puts pressure on the nerves and blood vessels in the front of the face or just above the eyes, causing pain in those areas. Sinus headaches typically worsen when you bend over. Tooth, jaw, or ear problems also may

contribute to headaches. Very high blood pressure can cause frequent headaches, usually upon waking. These headaches most often occur in the back of the head.

Despite the discomfort, a headache is not usually cause for worry. It is not a pain in the brain—which contains no sensory nerves—but in the scalp or the meninges, the membranes that surround the brain. However, frequent or sudden severe headaches may occasionally signal a serious medical condition and should be discussed with a doctor.

Aspirin's Ancestors

Before the advent of aspirin, folks had many ways to rid themselves of this most common of ailments. Not all of them were advisable. For instance, the practice of bleeding to alleviate headaches was still in vogue at the dawn of the 19th century. Some remedies were intended for specific types of headaches, which included "sick

See a doctor if ...

If your headache is accompanied by any of the following, see a doctor immediately. You may have a serious medical problem, such as glaucoma, an aneurysm, a brain tumor, or meningitis.
◆ Sudden awakenings from sleep
◆ Blurry vision
◆ Confusion or slurred speech, especially after a blow to the head
◆ Difficulty moving any one part of your body
◆ Fever and a stiff neck
◆ Nausea
◆ Pain in or around your eyes
◆ Pain that is sudden and severe
◆ Frequent or chronic recurrence, especially if you are over 35 and the problem is new

CATNIP Like valerian, catnip is a mild natural sedative that may bring relief from stress-related headaches. To make a tea, mix 1 or 2 teaspoons dried leaves in 1 cup boiling water. Let steep, then strain and drink.

ESSENTIAL OILS To relieve the tension behind a tension headache, dab a small amount of lavender or peppermint oil on each temple and on your forehead. Rub gently into the skin, then remain quiet for several minutes.

GINGER Ginger was traditionally believed to cure headache pain. Today it is postulated that ginger may work against migraines by inhibiting prostaglandin synthesis, although more research is needed. If nothing else, ginger helps quell the nausea that

often accompanies migraines. Take up to 2 grams (between ½ and ¾ teaspoon) of ground gingerroot in a glass of water. Or, to make a decoction, pour 1 cup boiling water over ½ teaspoon ground root. Let steep, then strain. People with gallstones should not take ginger.

Feverfew leaves, taken fresh or in capsule form, can help prevent migraines.

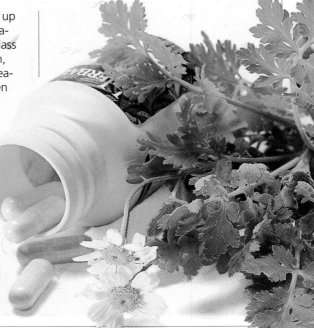

Migraine Medicine

A migraine is a vascular headache triggered by abnormal dilation of the blood vessels in the head or neck. It often occurs on only one side of the head and may be accompanied by nausea or vomiting, visual disturbances, and sensitivity to light. The underlying causes are not fully understood. In some people, such foods as cheese, chocolate, and red wine trigger migraines. Migraines are more common in women than men; they seem to occur more frequently before menstruation and less often during pregnancy and menopause.

For so-called sick headaches, boiled cabbage leaves, onion poultices, or, in the case of the Indians, tobacco leaves were placed on the forehead and back of the neck to "draw out" the pain. According to *King's American Dispensatory,* "Ginger in powder, formed into a plaster with warm water, and applied on paper or cloth to the forehead, has relieved violent headache." In Alabama, ginger (right) was administered as a hot tea or in whiskey. Ongoing research has yet to confirm—or deny—ginger's traditional use against migraines, but ginger has been proven effective against nausea, which often accompanies migraines.

Recently, scientists have discovered that feverfew, which was long used to fight fever, may prevent the onset of the headaches altogether. During a migraine attack, the brain releases a hormone called serotonin, which constricts the blood vessels. Feverfew leaves contain a substance called parthenolide, which limits the release of serotonin. Studies show that with long-term use feverfew reduces the frequency of migraines; however, the herb has little effect on the pain once it has set in.

Alternatively, a number of new prescription drugs are now available for migraine headaches. For more information, consult your physician.

headaches" (migraines), "nervous headaches" (tension headaches), and "bilious headaches," associated with stomach upset.

Two folk treatments were precursors of the wonder drug called aspirin. One of them, willow bark, was among the most popular headache remedies. The Indians used the roots of red willow or mashed the bark and bound it to the forehead. Inhabi-

tants of the Appalachians made tea from small willow branches. Another mountain "cure" involved chewing willow twigs "until your ears ring." Willow bark contains salicin, a close chemical relative of aspirin. In truth, most willow bark contains so little salicin that, taken in safe doses, it probably cannot cure a headache. Because the amount of salicin in the bark varies, consuming larger amounts of bark

may result in a overdose, which would cause ringing in the ears.

Wintergreen tea was another common headache remedy. Wintergreen contains methyl salicylate, also a relative of aspirin. However, today the herb is considered unsafe for internal use; several deaths have resulted from the ingestion of wintergreen oil. In the late 1880s, synthetic versions of salicin and salicylate, most notably aspirin, became popular, antiquating most folk remedies for headaches.

Calming Cures

Unlike aspirin, which works directly on headache pain, myriad sedatives soothed the tension behind tension headaches. These included several members of the mint family: catnip, sage, pennyroyal, and, of course, peppermint. Indians and settlers alike drank catnip tea to assuage the "nervous headaches of females," and catnip does indeed have modest sedative powers. Sage was also thought to soothe the nerves. According to one proponent, it made you sleep like a baby, but scientists have failed to confirm the existence of any sedative properties. The Indians favored pennyroyal and introduced it to the settlers for headache; however, one cup of the tea won't stop the pain, and in large doses the herb is toxic.

In the early 1900s peppermint water was the therapy of choice for "nervous headache." Handkerchiefs were perfumed with peppermint, and peppermint oil was rubbed on the temples—probably to some effect. A German study found that rubbing peppermint oil on the forehead and temples was more effective than a placebo in relieving headache symptoms. (Like peppermint, lavender oil was used as a "cooling lotion" for so-called nervous headache. The pleasantly scented oil acts as a mild sedative.)

Aside from members of the mint family, other popular "nerve tonics" included passion flower tea. Passion flower has both sedative and mild painkilling properties. The Indians also made teas from valerian, another sedative. One physician prominent in the late 1880s, William Gowers, prescribed a combination of bromide (a sedative) and marijuana. For acute attacks he gave his patients injections of morphine. (These treatments are no longer recommended, of course.) Today another opiate narcotic, Demerol, is often given by emergency physicians to people with severe migraines that do not respond to other treatments.

To ease headaches and induce sleep, many country folk thought of stuffing pillows with various aromatic herbs, including sage and pine needles. The Indians stuffed their pillows with hops, which may indeed have sedative effects. Using an early form of inhalation therapy, the Navajo made infusions of herbs including sage, juniper, and prickly pear cactus and poured them over hot stones to form steam, which they then inhaled.

Compresses

There were also many attempts to attack the pain from outside the head. To draw out headache pain, the Indians sliced wild potatoes and bound them to the forehead or applied bruised poppy flower heads. The Pawnee dusted powdered root of Indian turnip on top of the head and temples, while the Choctaw applied mullein leaves and the Ojibwa relied on crushed white pine needles.

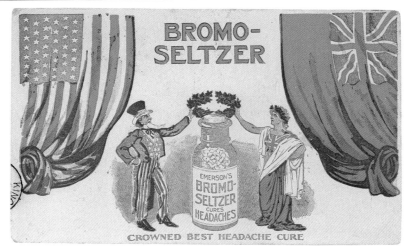

BROMO-SELTZER

EMERSON'S BROMO-SELTZER CURES HEADACHES

CROWNED BEST HEADACHE CURE

Popular for headaches and hangovers, Bromo-Seltzer mixed sodium bicarbonate and acetaminophen.

The settlers used compresses of boiled sage leaves or soaked handkerchiefs or brown paper bags in vinegar, then pressed them to the forehead. Some people will recall verse two of a certain Mother Goose nursery rhyme, after Jack falls down and breaks his crown:

Up Jack got, and home did trot,
As fast as he could caper,
To old Dame Dob,
Who patched his knob
With vinegar and brown paper.

Vinegar compresses are still recommended by folk healers, probably because of the cooling effect that takes place when the vinegar evaporates from the skin.

Since headaches were regarded by some as a fever of the stomach, compresses were also routinely applied to the abdomen. Mustard seeds were ground and moistened, then spread on a cloth and applied in order to draw out the "fever."

Some compresses were beneficial simply because they provided heat or cold. The raw potatoes favored by the Indians and settlers acted as cool compresses, as did sliced apples, which were also tried. Applying anything cold may confuse the nerves that carry the pain signals and temporarily limit their ability to transmit pain. Fried onions and cooked potatoes provided heat, which may have eased the muscle tension that contributes to tension headaches. Today a cloth soaked in hot or cold water and applied to the forehead and the back of the neck is considered effective.

The Caffeine Paradox

At the close of the 19th century, the seeds of the guarana plant, native to Venezuela and Brazil, were crushed, dried, and used to make a stimulating tonic. Because the drink had a high caffeine content—about three times as much as coffee—it was used as a remedy for certain forms of headache, particularly "nervous headaches," menstrual headaches, and migraines.

By relaxing the smooth muscles, including those of the blood vessels in the head, caffeine helps alleviate certain types of headaches for those who do not normally consume caffeine. It also increases the effectiveness of pain relievers such as aspirin and acetaminophen, and it is in fact an ingredient in some over-the-counter headache remedies. However, caffeine is only a short-term cure; in the long run, it can actually cause the muscle tension that sometimes triggers headaches in the first place. What's more, throbbing vascular headaches can be the result of caffeine withdrawal.

HEAT EXHAUSTION

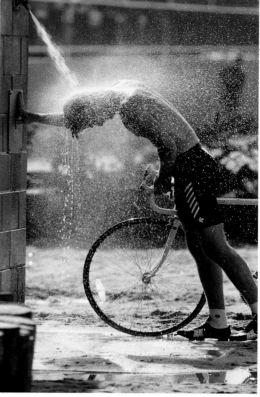

Heat exhaustion is caused by dehydration and is preceded by increasing fatigue, anxiety, and heavy sweating—warnings that the victim should quickly get out of the sun and drink plenty of liquids. The skin often becomes pale and clammy. If fainting occurs, it is usually because the sufferer has stood too long in the heat, allowing the blood to pool in the legs.

When heat exhaustion strikes, lay the patient down in a cool place and elevate the feet about 30 cm (12 in.). Offer sips of water, juice, or a sports drink containing electrolytes. Remove or loosen any tight clothing. You may also want to apply cool compresses. If the person is unconscious, lay him or her down in a cool place, elevate the feet, and wait until consciousness returns, usually in a few minutes.

Heat stroke, a more serious condition, is caused by the body's inability to cool itself under extremely hot conditions. The victim feels weak, has a severe headache, then suddenly loses consciousness. The skin is red, dry, and hot to the

*A **spray on the skin** helps cool the body down, although it is no substitute for drinking liquids.*

touch, with little perspiration. The victim requires emergency cooling and immediate hospitalization, or he or she may suffer permanent brain damage or even death.

Folk medicine offers little in the way of cures for heat exhaustion. Eating mayapple fruits was said to combat the condition, and they do provide beneficial sugar and electrolytes. However, so do many other fruits and vegetables, which also provide water and are more readily available today. (What's more, mayapple fruits are known to cause gastrointestinal upset and purging.)

Running cold water on one's wrists was long thought to cool down the entire body, but it merely cools down the wrists. Salt tablets, too, were thought to prevent heat exhaustion; today they are no longer recommended because they cause fluid retention, which leaves less fluid available for sweat production. Also, the tablets can cause vomiting, which leads to further dehydration.

Prevention: The Best Cure

Preventing heat exhaustion is fairly simple. If possible, minimize your activity during hot, humid weather, and stay out of the sun. When vacationing in hot climates, give your body time to adjust to the heat gradually. If you must exert yourself, drink plenty of liquids—even if you don't feel thirsty. Avoid caffeine and alcohol, which cause dehydration. Eat light meals and wear lightweight, light-colored clothing. (Note: loosely woven fabrics breathe better than tight weaves.) If possible, break for a cool shower or a swim. Alternatively, soak a towel in cold water and apply it as a compress. Finally, wear a hat to shield yourself from the sun.

FRUIT JUICE OR SPORTS DRINKS To combat heat exhaustion, it is essential to drink liquids in order to counter dehydration. The best choices are fruit juices or sports drinks, which replenish the sugar, potassium, and sodium lost during sweating. Although the drinks should be cool, they should not contain ice.

COOL COMPRESS Soak a rag or washcloth in cool water and apply it to the person's face and torso. This will help cool down the body, although it will not counter dehydration.

COOL BATH OR SHOWER If it happens to be convenient, a cool shower or bath, or even a spritz with a garden hose or sprinkler, will help cool and refresh the person, although, again, it is no substitute for drinking liquids. Never immerse a person who is unconscious.

HEAT RASH

When sweat remains unevaporated and the skin's pores become blocked, heat rash is likely to develop. The irritating rash, also known as prickly heat and medically as miliaria, is characterized by tiny, itchy red splotches, inflamed skin, and miniature blisters. While folk remedies aim to soothe the skin, absorb moisture, and inhibit infection, the best treatment may simply be cool showers and plenty of air.

Heat rash is usually associated with excessive sweating, but it can also be caused by the body's slow acclimation to hot weather. It typically occurs where we sweat: the neck, armpits, groin, waist, upper chest, and back. Mild cases clear up quickly without treatment. For standard cases, at-home measures can help. Keep the skin clean and avoid infection with cool showers, baths, or spongings (without soap) and regular applications of calamine lotion and dusting powder. Try not to scratch the itchy skin, and air the affected area as much as possible. Orthodox treatments also include over-the-counter cortisone creams and lotions and antihistamines for severe itching. Do not apply moisturizing creams or oils.

The best way to prevent heat rash is to reduce sweating. Limit activity during uncomfortably hot and humid weather, avoid strenuous exercise, and wear loose-fitting clothing made of cotton. New parents should be especially careful: infants are vulnerable because of their underdeveloped sweat glands, many layers of clothing, and wet diapers. Diaper rash can be caused by heat rash.

Red millet seed—"miliaria" in Latin—was the inspiration for heat rash's medical name.

Powders and Cool Washes

Many folk remedies are powders that are dusted on the affected skin, where they form a protective layer. Both cornstarch and baking soda effectively absorb some of the irritating dampness on the skin and make it more difficult for bacterial infections to occur. The powdered root of bull nettle and "dry, pulverized sulfur" were once used for the same purpose. Another powder was a half cup of flour, browned in the oven and sprinkled on the rash.

Cool, soothing remedies were also popular. The Indians and the early settlers applied washes made from yellow dock, which contains astringent tannins, to inflamed skin. A poultice of grated potatoes was also tried. Cold compresses were made by soaking a clean cloth in water, milk, apple cider vinegar, or infusions of chaparral, burdock, chickweed, blue flag, prickly ash bark, sweet fern, or red clover flowers. Similar 20th-century remedies include baths made with oatmeal, baking soda, vinegar, or thyme and fresh aloe vera gel—a soothing emollient that has long been used to relieve itching, prevent infection, and promote healing.

Offbeat folk treatments for skin rashes included rubbing the skin with the inside of a watermelon rind and taking "more exercise in the great outdoors"—unwise in hot weather, but a good way to air out the skin. There was also this three-pronged remedy: wash with witch hazel, "keep the bowels open," and drink plenty of lemonade. In fact, witch hazel can be good for the skin, and a cool lemonade drink can help the body endure a hot day.

CORNSTARCH OR BAKING SODA Dust the affected area liberally. Both powders, available at supermarkets, will absorb moisture. Do not get in the eyes, ears, or mouth. Rinse the skin every few hours and reapply.

YELLOW DOCK To make a cleansing and itch-relieving wash, boil 125 grams minced fresh root in 2 cups water for 10 minutes. Strain, let cool, and apply several times a day. The wash may irritate tender skin; discontinue use if irritation persists.

ALOE VERA Carefully slice open the inner portion of the fleshy leaf and scrape out the mucilaginous gel. Apply the gel to the affected skin two to three times a day. Wash the skin before reapplying.

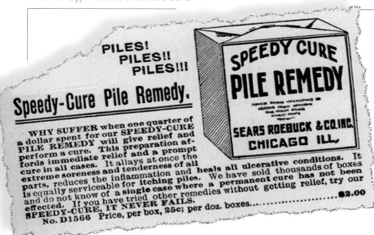

PILES!
PILES!!
PILES!!!

Speedy-Cure Pile Remedy.

WHY SUFFER when one quarter of a dollar spent for our SPEEDY-CURE PILE REMEDY will give relief and perform a cure. This preparation affords immediate relief and a prompt cure in all cases. It allays at once the extreme soreness and tenderness of all parts, reduces the inflammation and heals all ulcerative conditions. It is equally serviceable for itching piles. We have sold thousands of boxes and do not know of a single case where a permanent cure has not been effected. If you have tried other remedies without getting relief, try our SPEEDY-CURE, IT NEVER FAILS........$2.00
No. D1566 Price, per box, 25c; per doz. boxes.

SPEEDY-CURE
PILE REMEDY

SEARS ROEBUCK & CO.INC.
CHICAGO ILL.

HEMORRHOIDS

An 1897 Sears Roebuck catalog *offered this "speedy" hemorrhoid treatment among its wealth of goods.*

Our forebears had dozens of folk cures for "piles"—among them garlic and cocoa butter suppositories, witch hazel wipes, cod liver oil or horse chestnut salves, and pine resin steam baths. Many of these remedies were based on commonsense use of herbs and soothing heat, and some remain popular today. Others, such as carrying a stoneroot in one's pocket, still require a leap of faith.

Hemorrhoids—varicose veins in or around the anus caused by increased pressure—have a variety of causes. Constipation (common during pregnancy) and dry stools rank high on the list. Also to blame are prolonged sitting or standing. Exchanging bad habits for good ones can eliminate straining during elimination and help prevent piles: lose weight, increase water and fiber intake, and eat fresh fruits and dried figs, prunes, and dates, which have laxative properties.

Sitz Baths and Herbs

Heat, in the form of a sitz bath (sitting in a tub of warm water), a compress, or prescription and over-the-counter topical creams and suppositories all help soothe and heal both internal and external hemorrhoids. See a physician, however, for an accurate diagnosis. Severe pain can be a sign of a thrombosed hemorrhoid; if such hemorrhoids are treated within 24 hours, the blood clot can be removed with a local anesthetic. Bleeding hemorrhoids can be a sign of more serious problems.

An earlier version of the sitz bath involved sitting wrapped in a blanket on a bucket of steaming hot mullein leaves or pine resin. But as soothing as these substances might have been, steam had its risks. (One old-timer remembers his father's reaction after trying this remedy: "A jump that would put a kangaroo to shame.") Today, a safer alternative is a sitz bath of Epsom salts, which helps reduce inflammation. Some herbalists also suggest bathing in witch hazel, which is anti-inflammatory.

Salves and suppositories were often made with lard and astringent, antiseptic substances such as gum benzoin—a key ingredient in compound tincture of benzoin—and pine resins, including turpentine. (Pine resins have since been replaced by more effective and less irritating corticosteroid and zinc products.)

White oak bark continues to be used for reducing external inflammations. Extracts of butcher's broom (*Ruscus aculeatus*) and horse chestnut seed (also known as buckeye) are also widely prescribed today by European doctors to strengthen weak veins, although some experts debate their efficacy.

EPSOM SALTS Sit in a tub of warm water in which Epsom salts have been dissolved. The warm water eases pain and the salts constrict the hemorrhoid. Do not try if hemorrhoids are bleeding.

PSYLLIUM Also known as plantain, psyllium is a highly effective bulk-fiber laxative and will ease the passage of stools. Mix 1 tablespoon commercial psyllium with 1 cup water or fruit juice and drink once or twice a day. People with serious digestive ailments should consult with their doctor before using psyllium or any other laxative.

WITCH HAZEL Undistilled witch hazel extract or ointment is rich in tannins that help shrink hemorrhoids. Apply to the hemorrhoid two or three times a day. Distilled witch hazel contains alcohol, which can be irritating.

COD LIVER OIL OINTMENT Widely used in the early 20th century, this fish oil contains the wound-healing vitamins A and D. The same nutrients are found in shark oil, a key ingredient in leading commercial hemorrhoid products. Mix either oil with petroleum jelly and apply to external hemorrhoids only.

HICCUPS

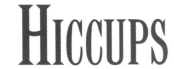

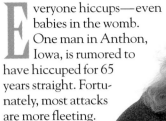

Everyone hiccups—even babies in the womb. One man in Anthon, Iowa, is rumored to have hiccuped for 65 years straight. Fortunately, most attacks are more fleeting.

A hiccup is simply an involuntary contraction of the diaphragm. This causes a sudden intake of breath, which is checked by the abrupt closing of the glottis (the space between the vocal cords). The result is the characteristic hiccup sound.

Hiccups are usually harmless. However, in rare cases they can last for days, making it difficult to eat or sleep. If this occurs, see a doctor: a serious condition may be the cause.

Paper Bags and More

Most people have heard of breathing into a paper bag, swallowing a spoonful of sugar, or having someone startle you in order to stop the hiccups. Other cures that have been put forth include drinking vinegar, pressing a cold knife or coin to the back of the neck, or pulling on

Holding your breath is one of many time-tested "cures" for hiccups.

the tongue. Sniffing black pepper to make yourself sneeze was also said to help, as was eating a spoonful of peanut butter or a lump of sulfur.

Some people drank pineapple juice to end the hiccups. Others advised swallowing three gulps of water without taking a breath or taking nine sips of water, three at a time. Even today some still swear by bending over and drinking a glass of water from the "wrong" side of the glass.

One curious remedy called on the imagination as cure: if you could recall the last place you saw a frog that had been run over by a car, your hiccups would stop.

More logical was the use of certain teas, including peppermint and dill, for their antispasmodic activity. Many Indians relied on juniper tea (no longer considered safe) or valerian root tea, a sedative.

Many homespun hiccup "cures" may have some merit. Holding one's breath or breathing into a paper bag prompts the diaphragm to contract more deeply in order to bring in more oxygen, which may interrupt the spasms. So may taking a sudden deep breath as if startled.

Other folk remedies may work by irritating the phrenic nerves, which extend from the neck to the chest. These nerves are responsible for the normal contractions of the diaphragm; when one of them is irritated, it causes spasms of the diaphragm, which in turn cause hiccups. Further irritation, such as eating sugar or mustard or drinking vinegar or pineapple juice, may jolt the nerve back into its normal state. Moreover, the act of swallowing opens the glottis and may help stop the hiccups. Eating dry bread or crackers is one way to ensure a lot of swallowing. Some modern-day doctors recommend tickling the roof of the mouth with a cotton swab, which also opens the glottis. So does a simpler, if childish, remedy: sticking out the tongue.

SUGAR One of the most persevering hiccup remedies is to swallow a teaspoonful of sugar. Follow it with a glass of water. The grainy sugar may slightly irritate the esophagus, causing the phrenic nerves to "reset" themselves, although there is no proof of this.

BROWN PAPER BAG Breathe slowly and deeply into a small paper bag. (Stop if you feel light-headed.) This increases the carbon dioxide level in the blood, making the diaphragm contract more deeply to bring in more oxygen, which may stop the spasms.

DILL OR PEPPERMINT Pour 1 cup boiling water over 2 teaspoons minced dill or peppermint leaves. Steep for 10 minutes, then drink slowly. Both herbs act as antispasmodics, and the simple act of swallowing the tea may also help stop the hiccups.

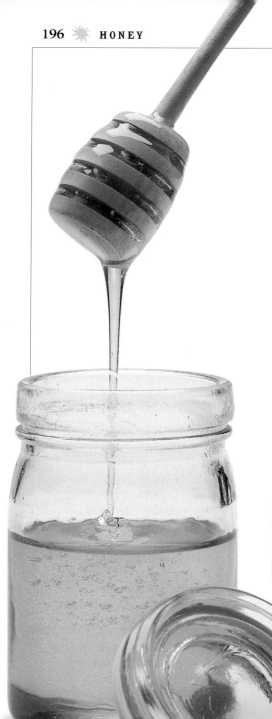

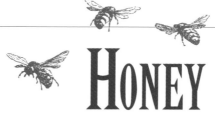

HONEY

Before the development of refined sugar in the mid-1800s, honey was the world's major sweetener, and one of its primary medical uses was to make ill-tasting remedies more palatable. Folks blended it with tinctures to concoct syrups and stirred it into poultices and liniments to make them thicker and easier to apply. Honey was also used to dress wounds, skin rashes, and boils.

Honey's success as a skin ointment lies in its high sugar content. The sugar absorbs water, denying infection-causing bacteria the moisture they need to survive. Honey is also slightly acidic, which may point to antibacterial properties that go beyond the activity of its sugars.

A Sweet Antiseptic

Renewed medical interest in honey was spurred on in the United States by two doctors who leaned on folk wisdom. Rooted in the self-care practices of his home state, Vermont, D. C. Jarvis, an ear, nose, and throat specialist, praised the medicinal merits of honey in his 1958 book, *Folk Medicine*. Although many of his claims need further investigation, he surmised that honey's "moisture-pulling" power made it useful for everything from bedwetting to muscle cramps.

The other doctor was Richard Knutson, an orthopedic surgeon in Mississippi. In 1975 he began looking for a new treatment to combat stubborn infected wounds that did not respond to common antibacterial drugs. On the advice of a retired nurse who had worked in the American South before the age of antibiotics, he investigated "sugar-coating wounds." He treated thousands of cases ranging from burns to bullet wounds with a salve of sugar mixed with mildly antibacterial iodine. A growing number of physicians, especially in Europe, are now using sugar compounds to treat wounds and to disinfect incisions after surgery. Honey, which is almost 80 percent sugar, may also provide the same benefits.

Sore Throat Relief

Today honey's most common medicinal use is as a sore throat and cough remedy. Honey provides a soothing coating over inflamed areas and promotes healing. It is applied directly inside the throat or mixed

Uses Sore throat, minor skin wounds, and inflammations
Cautions Honey or honey-sweetened milk should not be given to children under one year of age. It can carry bacterial botulism spores, which germinate in a baby's immature intestines and make a deadly toxin. (Children over the age of one year and adults have more developed digestive systems.) Honey and other bee products contain pollens that can trigger allergic reactions; they should not be taken for hay fever and other allergies without a doctor's supervision. Beware of honey harvested from the wild; if it was made from the pollen of certain toxic plants, it could be poisonous. Honey may promote tooth decay.

in a glass of hot water or lemonade and employed as either a drink or a gargle.

Honey was once used in remedies for ulcers, diarrhea, and bladder conditions and in topical applications for baldness and eye problems (even cataracts), treatments that lack scientific support. Also, the long-standing folk claim of honey's nutritional value is incorrect; honey is high in calories (64 per tablespoon), high in sugar, and low in nutrients.

Following the lead of Dr. Jarvis, some practitioners now endorse a folk tradition recommending honey to treat hay fever and seasonal respiratory congestion. The theory is that if you ingest small amounts of pollen found in locally produced honey for a few months, you will be less sensitive to the pollens in your region when allergy season arrives. Although many doctors hotly dispute this treatment, allergy shots work in a similar manner.

Researchers in Germany are experimenting with a pollen drink that, working on the same principle, may provide similar desensitization over time. Critics claim that the tiny amounts of pollen in honey do not survive digestion in a form that can effectively desensitize. A final answer awaits further medical research.

"Bee Products"

In addition to honey, other "bee products," such as bee pollen, honeycomb, royal jelly, and propolis (bee glue) were all used medicinally. Bee pollen and honeycomb are now believed to be without medicinal value, and bee pollen may even provoke allergic reactions. Royal jelly, once thought to prevent wrinkles, also lacks benefits and may trigger severe asthma attacks. Propolis, used to treat dermatitis and as a tonic, is being studied for its anti-inflammatory, antitumor, and antioxidant potential.

Colonies of Bees Come to North America

Honeybees were introduced to North America in the 1620s by English colonists, who brought these precious pollinators to the New World from their gardens back home. As in Europe, honey was a staple of cooking and health care in New England and New France. By 1640, the town of Newbury, Massachusetts, had established a municipally run apiary, where the price of a colony of bees was equivalent to 15 days of skilled labor. Straw skeps (homemade beehives) were common sights in gardens. By 1863, large apiaries were operating in Ontario and Quebec.

As pioneers moved west, they took their honeybees with them. Indians referred to the bees as "white man's flies" because wherever they saw a swarm, they knew that a white settlement was likely to be close by. Frontiersmen hunted swarms that had reverted to the wild. Using honey or sweets as bait, the hunter waited until the bees headed for home. Following them, he hoped to be led to a large store of honey, often 45 kilograms (100 lb) or more. After cutting down the tree or removing the branch that contained the nest, the hunter used smoke to scatter the agitated bees, which either fled or reentered the hive. After sealing the hive's entrance, the hunter would take the remaining bees home to add to his own collection.

It is reported that bees did not cross the Mississippi River until 1797, and their westward migration was literally "stopped cold" by the high elevation, chilly nights, and barren terrain of the Rocky Mountains. In 1853, during the California gold rush, a honeybee colony was brought by boat from the East Coast to San Francisco. The bees thrived in the mild climate, and their conquest of the continent was complete.

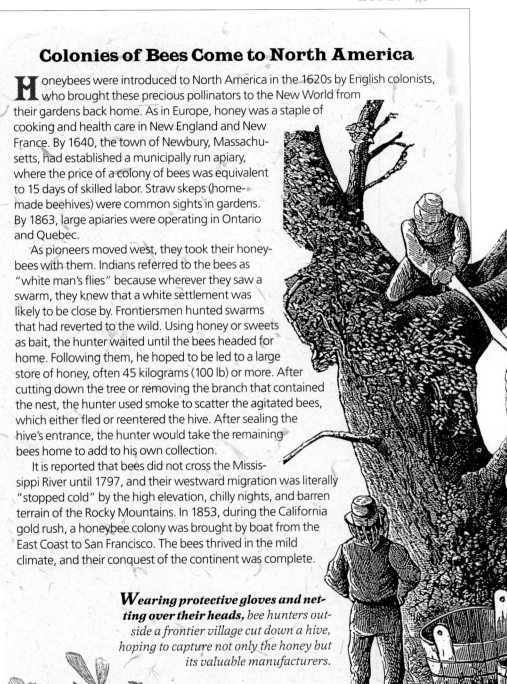

Wearing protective gloves and netting over their heads, bee hunters outside a frontier village cut down a hive, hoping to capture not only the honey but its valuable manufacturers.

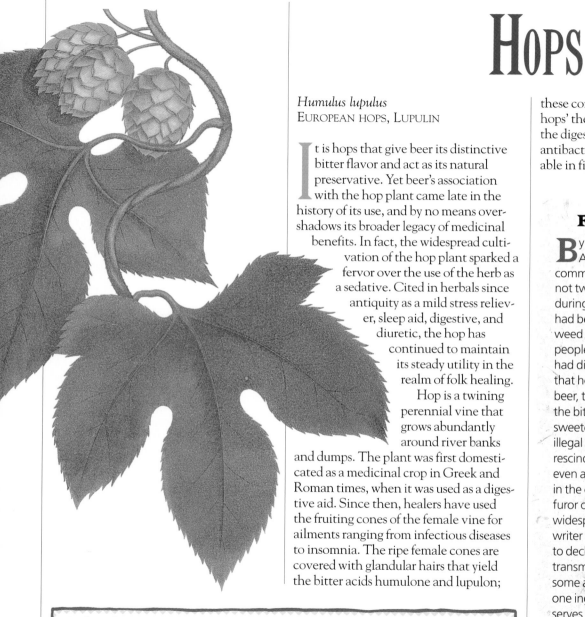

HOPS

Humulus lupulus
EUROPEAN HOPS, LUPULIN

It is hops that give beer its distinctive bitter flavor and act as its natural preservative. Yet beer's association with the hop plant came late in the history of its use, and by no means overshadows its broader legacy of medicinal benefits. In fact, the widespread cultivation of the hop plant sparked a fervor over the use of the herb as a sedative. Cited in herbals since antiquity as a mild stress reliever, sleep aid, digestive, and diuretic, the hop has continued to maintain its steady utility in the realm of folk healing.

Hop is a twining perennial vine that grows abundantly around river banks and dumps. The plant was first domesticated as a medicinal crop in Greek and Roman times, when it was used as a digestive aid. Since then, healers have used the fruiting cones of the female vine for ailments ranging from infectious diseases to insomnia. The ripe female cones are covered with glandular hairs that yield the bitter acids humulone and lupulon; these components are responsible for hops' therapeutic and anodyne effect on the digestive tract. Hops bitters also have antibacterial agents, making them valuable in fighting infection.

From Ale to Beer

By the 17th century, both North American and English beers were commonly brewed with hops. Yet not two centuries before in England, during the reign of Henry VIII, hops had been outlawed as a "wicked weed that would endanger the people." Although German brewers had discovered in the ninth century that hops had a preservative effect in beer, the English were up in arms at the bitter taste hops imparted to their sweeter national ale. Hops remained illegal in England until the ban was rescinded in 1552. A century later, even as bitter beers had taken hold in the colonies, the English furor over hops was still widespread. One writer went so far as to declare, "Hop transmuted our wholesome ale into beer. This one ingredient preserves the drink indeed, but repays the pleasure in tormenting diseases and a shorter life."

> **Active plant parts** Fruiting cones of the female vine
> **Uses** Indigestion, anxiety
> **Cautions** Hops are considered safe when taken intermittently as a tea for digestive or sedative purposes; larger medicinal amounts should be used only in consultation with a doctor. Hops may cause diarrhea, stomachache, or contact dermatitis in some people.

Traditions of Use

Indigenous to North America as well as Europe, hops were used by Indians well before settlers brought their knowledge of the plant to this country. Accounts by explorers traveling west reveal that, among some tribes, hops were being cultivated agriculturally.

Unaware of the Indians' domestication of the vine, settlers brought their own staple hop seeds from abroad. They also discovered and harvested this valuable commodity in the wild; native hop plants were documented as far north as New Brunswick and as far west as Montana and New Mexico. Folk healers cataloged many uses for hops: earaches and tooth-aches were treated with small, warm bags of hops, wet with alcohol and tied with a kerchief to the afflicted area. Digestive teas were prepared with fresh hops. Tinctures were employed in cases of anxiety, stomach cramps, and cystitis.

Well into the 19th century, hops bitters were promoted as veritable elixirs in many patent digestive medicines, with such slogans as "Take Hop Bitters three times a day, and you will have no doctor bills to pay." Settlers and Indians alike harvested the new buds and asparagus-like shoots in the spring as foodstuffs, and they used frothy infusions of fermented hops to raise large batches of bread. Also, hops were indispensable to the brewing of that most potent of "tonics," beer.

Hop-Picker Fatigue

By the late 18th century, beer brewing had transformed hops from a localized medicinal herb into a cash crop. Hops' previously modest reputation as a sedative grew with commercial cultivation of the vine as growers began to notice a condition among field workers that they called "hop-picker fatigue." Numerous cases of unexplained fatigue were documented in people who picked hops; moreover, many women working in hop fields began to report menstruating early. As a result, folk use of the plant became more and more widespread. Hop's notoriety escalated, its medicinal use as a sedative and menstruation promoter now widely touted.

The swift upswing in the plant's popularity provoked the mainstream medical community, which dismissed much of the folklore surrounding hop's sedative properties as being more magical than medicinal. Laboratory tests to isolate functional sedative principles in the plant's volatile oils uncovered no definitive proof to support its use. Consequently, by the end of the 19th century, sedatives made with hops remained relegated largely to the practice of herbal medicine.

The Original Sleeping Pillow

Abraham Lincoln counted on them, and many other North Americans today are returning to them as a natural way to get to sleep: small pillows filled with hops are making a comeback as an herbal alternative to many prescription sedatives. Choose very dry, whole cones and moisten them slightly with glycerine and water before stuffing them into a pillow (the moisture helps cut down on the noisy rustling and chafing of the hops inside). For those who do not like hops' distinctively acrid smell, try adding a few handfuls of lavender to the stuffing. Lavender provides its own sedative effect, and its sweet fragrance will mask the odor of the hops within.

Today new research shows that dried hops release a volatile depressant alcohol, methylnonyl carbinol, as they oxidize over time. Present only in trace amounts in fresh hops, this substance may account for at least part of dried hops' reputed sedative effect. Because it can be absorbed through inhalation and skin contact as well as ingestion, the compound helps explain both the sedation brought on by hops pillows and the fatigue experienced by hop pickers. In the case of early menstruation, however, there remains no conclusive evidence of any substance in hops that might influence estrogenic or other hormonal activity. Hops are now being studied for potential antidiabetic use: recent tests have found that its principal components, humulone and lupulone, lower blood sugar dramatically.

Horehound

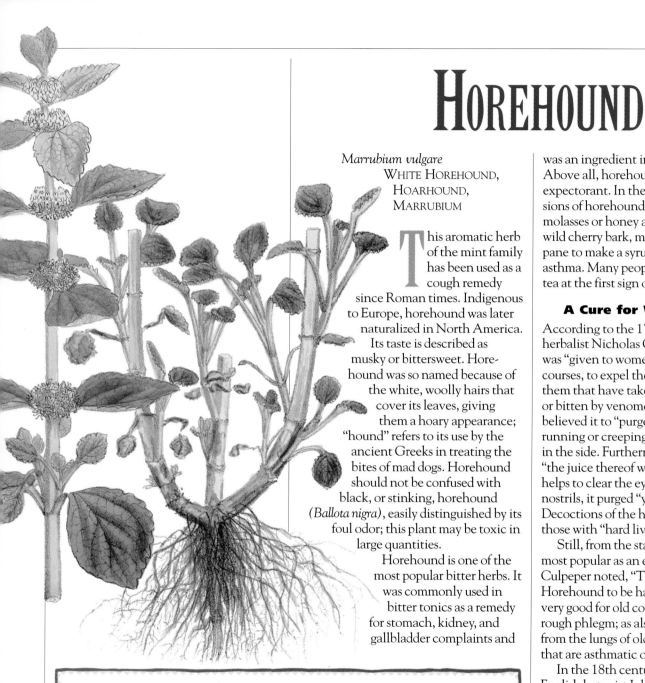

Marrubium vulgare
WHITE HOREHOUND,
HOARHOUND,
MARRUBIUM

This aromatic herb of the mint family has been used as a cough remedy since Roman times. Indigenous to Europe, horehound was later naturalized in North America. Its taste is described as musky or bittersweet. Horehound was so named because of the white, woolly hairs that cover its leaves, giving them a hoary appearance; "hound" refers to its use by the ancient Greeks in treating the bites of mad dogs. Horehound should not be confused with black, or stinking, horehound (*Ballota nigra*), easily distinguished by its foul odor; this plant may be toxic in large quantities.

Horehound is one of the most popular bitter herbs. It was commonly used in bitter tonics as a remedy for stomach, kidney, and gallbladder complaints and was an ingredient in liver and bile teas. Above all, horehound was a trusted expectorant. In the 19th century infusions of horehound were thickened with molasses or honey and often mixed with wild cherry bark, mullein, and elecampane to make a syrup for coughs and asthma. Many people brewed horehound tea at the first sign of a cold.

A Cure for What Ails You

According to the 17th-century British herbalist Nicholas Culpeper, horehound was "given to women to bring down their courses, to expel the after-birth, and to them that have taken poison, or are stung or bitten by venomous serpents." He also believed it to "purge foul ulcers and stay running or creeping sores" and ease pains in the side. Furthermore, he wrote that "the juice thereof with wine and honey, helps to clear the eyesight"; sniffed up the nostrils, it purged "yellow jaundice." Decoctions of the herb were said to aid those with "hard livers."

Still, from the start, horehound was most popular as an expectorant. As Culpeper noted, "There is a syrup made of Horehound to be had at the apothecaries, very good for old coughs, to get rid [of] the rough phlegm; as also to void cold rheums from the lungs of old folks, and for those that are asthmatic or short-winded."

In the 18th century the prominent English botanist John Hill wrote that horehound was "famous for the relief it gives in moist asthmas, and in all diseases of the breasts and lungs, in which a thick and viscous matter is the cause." It was

---

Active plant parts Leaves, flower tops
Uses Coughs, congestion, indigestion, loss of appetite
Cautions In large doses horehound disturbs heart rhythm. People with heart disease should avoid this herb. The plant juice may cause dermatitis.

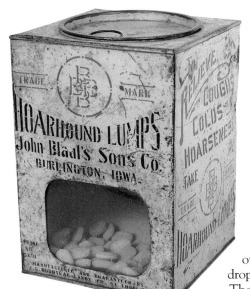

These hore-hound "lumps," circa 1900, were said to relieve *"coughs, colds, and hoarseness."*

later noted that horehound was useful in treating yellow jaundice resulting from a "viscidity of the bile" and that it promoted all manner of fluid secretions. (Marrubic acid, derived from a constituent of the herb, has been shown to stimulate the flow of bile in rats.) In large doses the herb was believed to exert a diuretic effect and to expel worms. Perhaps because of its bitter taste, horehound was also valued as a general stimulant and tonic.

Bearing in mind horehound's reputation, 19th-century Eclectic physicians prescribed the herb as a laxative and a remedy for asthma, tuberculosis, jaundice, leukemia, malaria, intestinal worms, and hysteria, as well as for "female complaints." However, they were quick to determine that, in fact, the plant was powerless against these ailments. Its use was largely discontinued, except against coughs and colds, for which it has remained popular in the 20th century. Today horehound is also used as a flavoring in alcoholic bitters and liqueurs.

Cough Syrup Controversy

To treat coughs, horehound was usually taken in the form of syrups or teas. It was also popular in steam inhalations. Many people made their own horehound candy, which they used as cough drops or even so-called asthma lozenges. (Some modern cookbooks still include recipes for horehound candy.) Horehound was also found in a variety of over-the-counter cough drops and cold formulas.

The German Commission E, the government-run regulatory committee that provides data on herbs for medicinal use in Germany, found horehound to be an effective expectorant as well as a decongestant and an appetite stimulant. The herb contains a bitter principle known as marrubiin, which provokes bronchial secretions, thereby thinning bronchial mucus. Like all bitter herbs, horehound is commonly thought to whet the appetite by promoting the production of stomach acid. And, because it is believed to stimulate the secretion of bile, it is also thought to provide relief from indigestion caused by insufficient bile production. Research indicates that bitter herbs may also help prevent the formation of gallstones.

Many herbalists in Canada continue to recommend horehound for colds; it is interesting, however, that in 1989 the U.S. FDA declared the herb ineffective as an expectorant because of a lack of scientific evidence (although it conceded the herb's safety). Horehound is still available, as are cough drops that contain the herb, so consumers may decide for themselves whether or not it actually works.

Horehound may prove to have other uses. Recent studies show that in small doses horehound helps normalize heart rhythm. However, in large doses it can actually cause cardiac arrhythmia. Research indicates that the herb may also lower blood sugar levels. Be aware that large doses may have a laxative effect.

A Dandy Candy

Horehound candies and cough syrups, bought in the store or made on the stovetop, were standard weapons against colds. The home-made varieties began with infusions, made by steeping 2 tablespoons of leaves in a half-liter of hot water, then straining. To make a cough syrup, twice as much honey as liquid was added. This goo was then bottled and stored. Lozenges were made by adding sugar to the infusion, and boiling the mixture until it thickened. It was then poured into a shallow pan. When the mixture was cool, it was cut into squares to form lozenges, which were taken at the first tickle in the throat.

Menthol and horehound helped these *1930s cough drops "stop that tickling cough."*

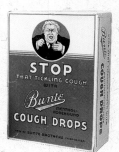

HORSE CHESTNUT

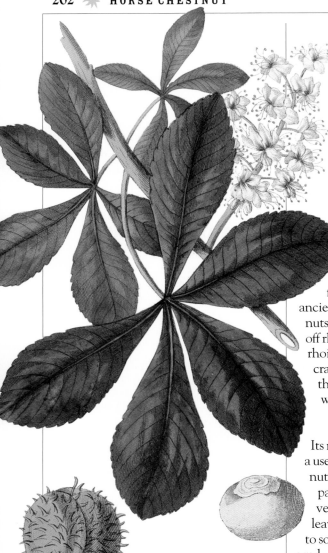

Aesculus hippocastanum
BUCKEYE

The first horse chestnut tree introduced into North America is believed to have been planted in Pennsylvania in 1763. Since then, the tree and its knuckle-size chestnuts have made a unique contribution to North American folk medicine. Continuing an ancient practice, men carried the chestnuts in their front pants pockets to ward off rheumatism, arthritis, and hemorrhoids. When the chestnuts dried or cracked, their healing powers were thought to pass into the body; they would be replaced with fresh ones.

For Healthy Veins

Its nuts, bark, and leaves made the tree a useful medicinal source. Horse chestnut was most effective at treating painful swellings, including varicose veins and hemorrhoids. Both the leaves and the nuts were used in pastes to soothe inflamed skin and tone damaged underlying veins. Extracts of the nut—namely, aescin and aesculus—have been found to have anti-inflammatory and vein-strengthening properties and are used today to treat joint and muscle inflammations, varicose veins, contusions, and swollen wounds. Another constituent, saponin, is still used in cough remedies; the leaf tea mixed with brown sugar was once a popular cough syrup.

Although parts of the plant were taken internally as foods and medicines, the nuts, leaves, flowers, and young sprouts of the Aesculus species—including Ohio and California buckeye (*A. glabra* and *A. californica*)—are toxic and no longer recommended for use in home remedies.

Not to be confused with ...

The horse chestnut tree, *Aesculus hippocastanum*, grows up to 23 m (75 ft) tall and sports prickly seed sacs and clusters of red, yellow, and white flowers. It should not be confused with the *Castanea* genus of chestnut trees—the source of edible chestnuts. This genus includes American chestnut (*Castanea dentata*) and sweet chestnut (*C. sativa*).

The mighty American chestnut of lore once grew throughout the northeastern United States—and on the northern shore of Lake Erie in Canada—until a fungus virtually wiped out the tree in the late 1800s. Most sweet, edible chestnuts are now imported from Italy.

Active plant parts Nuts, bark, leaves
Uses Varicose veins, hemorrhoids
Cautions The nut is poisonous and should not be ingested in any form. The leaves, flowers, and young sprouts are also toxic. Symptoms of poisoning include nervous muscle twitching, weakness, dilated pupils, vomiting, diarrhea, depression, paralysis, and stupor. Homemade remedies of the nuts should be avoided. Horse chestnut pollen is allergenic.

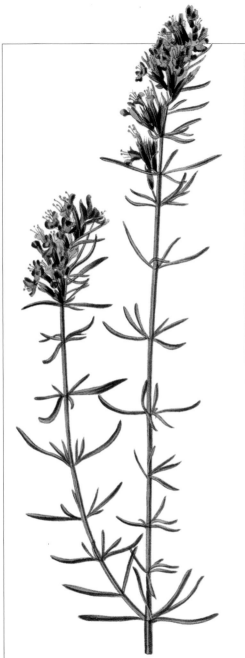

HYSSOP

Hyssopus officinalis

A low-growing perennial with pretty blue or pink flowers, hyssop is often grown in gardens for ornamental purposes. Its name means "holy herb," and Jewish priests in Jerusalem used the plant some 2,500 years ago to cleanse temples and other sacred sites. Even so, experts speculate that *Hyssopus officinalis* is probably not the plant referred to in the Bible by David: "Purge me with hyssop and I shall be clean…."

Hyssop is a member of the mint family and has a strong camphorous odor. During the Middle Ages it was used to mask the taste of spoiling meat. In Europe the herb was strewn about the house to disguise foul odors. The plant's volatile oil is found in such liqueurs as Benedictine and Chartreuse. Hyssop should not be confused with giant hyssop, hedge hyssop, or water hyssop, which are entirely different species and should not be ingested.

Minty Cough Medicine

In North America hyssop was used mainly for coughs, sore throats, and respiratory problems, a tradition that dates back to the ancient Greeks, who made a syrup from the herb, water, and honey to relieve tightness of the chest. The Cherokee of southern Appalachia used a hyssop syrup for colds, coughs, and asthma and other "lung and breast diseases," as a tea for fevers, and to bring on menses.

The 1898 *King's American Dispensatory* noted that the herb possessed stimulant and tonic properties and was "principally used in quinsy [tonsillitis] and other sore throats, as a gargle, combined with sage and alum, in infusion sweetened with honey. Also recommended in asthma, coughs, and other affections of the chest, as an expectorant."

Hyssop was renowned as a wound healer as well. According to the same reference, "The leaves, applied to bruises, speedily relieve the pain, and disperse every spot or mark from the parts affected." The plant was thought to cleanse wounds caused by rusty nails because the penicillin mold grows on its leaves. (This fact is irrelevant: the mold grows in many places, in insignificant quantities.)

Despite these early claims, hyssop was used little after the 18th century, except against sore throats and congestion, although modern folk literature suggests that it kills lice and eases rheumatism. Some recommend a steaming facial made with hyssop, recalling the British practice of mixing the herb's juice in ale and drinking it for the complexion.

Hyssop acts as a demulcent and a mild expectorant, perhaps justifying its use against respiratory problems. Despite its medicinal smell, there is no evidence that the herb has antibacterial properties; however, recent research suggests that it may have antiviral action against the herpes simplex and HIV viruses.

Active plant parts Leaves, flowers
Uses Sore throat, coughs
Cautions Do not take hyssop in large doses: it causes convulsions in laboratory rats.

IMPOTENCE

A man's inability to achieve or maintain an erection and engage in sexual intercourse, impotence is estimated to affect every man at least once in his life. Most occurrences are temporary; usually caused by fatigue or stress, they last only a day or two. However, for more than 22.5 million North American men, impotence is a chronic condition that can interrupt the sex life, threaten the passion of a marriage, and damage a man's self-image.

Although countless "potency-enhancing" herbs and mythical aphrodisiacs have been touted throughout history—from ginseng to oysters to "Love Potion #9," a hit song by the Searchers in 1965—few are known to produce any direct stimulation at all. Nevertheless, simply believing in aphrodisiacs may provide a rousing placebo effect. Two of the oldest known love enhancers are apples, shared by Adam and Eve, and honey. (In ancient Greece, newlyweds ate honey during the moon's first waxing and waning of their marriage—from which came the term "honeymoon.") Chocolate, once rare, was also thought to pique desire. Now common, it has lost this saucy reputation.

"Lost manhood" was once a euphemism for impotence.

Sometimes the physical shape of a plant added to its mystique. The roots of ginseng (also called "manroot") and mandrake, which resemble the human body, were thought to invigorate sexual energy. Rhinoceros horn, the unicorn plant, snakeroot, and oysters were used for similar reasons. The sexual organs from libidinous animals, such as goats and rabbits, were also used to help humans.

Potent Plants

Although a variety of love potions have been concocted over the years—ingredients have included garlic, celery, mint, cayenne, peaches, and licorice—only a few plant remedies can safely treat impotence. Saw palmetto has been used over the past century for prostate pain and discomfort and reportedly vitalizes the reproductive system. Because nearly 90

Rescue FOR Weak Men

Prof. Jules Laborde's Wonderful French Preparation of "CALTHOS" that Restores Lost Manhood.

FIVE DAYS' TRIAL TREATMENT
Absolutely Free by Sealed Mail.

NO C.O.D. OR DEPOSIT SCHEME.

The marvelous French remedy, "CALTHOS," recently introduced in this country by the Von Mohl Co., of Cincinnati, Ohio, one of the largest, richest and most responsible business firms in the United States, has attracted the attention of the entire medical profession because of the wonderful cures it has effected. If you suffer from Lost Manhood, Varicocele, Weakness of any nature in the Sexual Organs or Nerves, (no matter how caused), or if the parts are undeveloped or have shrunken or wasted away "CALTHOS" will restore you.

"CALTHOS" is a French discovery by Prof. Jules Laborde, famed in Paris as France's foremost specialist.

"CALTHOS" is the only remedy recognized by the medical profession as a specific cure for weak men.

It has the endorsement of the German and French governments, and is largely used in the standing armies of those countries.

"CALTHOS" is put before you on its merits alone. Try it and put it to the test. **Try it FREE**. There is no security required—no C.O.D. scheme.

Send us your name and address, and we will send you enough "CALTHOS" to last five days. **It will be sent in a sealed package by mail.** In the quiet of your home you **can** try it and see what it does.

All correspondence relating to the "CALTHOS" department of our business is strictly confidential. We neither publish nor furnish testimonials.

Address applications for trial treatment to

THE VON MOHL COMPANY, 761 B, Cincinnati, O. | Largest Importers of Standard Preparations in the United States

percent of impotence cases have physical causes, saw palmetto can restore sexual health by helping the prostate. Similarly, burdock, once thought to "stir up lust," may tone the blood and urogenital tract. Ginkgo biloba, relatively new to North America, can increase circulation to the body's extremities, including the penis.

One of the most potent plants used for impotence was the bark of the African yohimbé tree, which causes blood engorgement in the pelvic region. Today yohimbé is considered too dangerous to use as an herbal remedy. Spanish fly, obtained by pulverizing insects of the *Cantharides* genus, is also potentially dangerous; it causes blood to rush to the penis by irritating the urogenital tract.

Onion, jasmine, damiana, snails, bran, and other plants and foods have been eaten to stoke love's fire; from a scientific perspective, though, they are not thought to work. Many Chinese herbs, such as ginseng and dong quai, have also found favor in North America today.

SAW PALMETTO To tone the reproductive system, take the standardized extract in capsule form, one 160-milligram capsule, twice a day.

ST. JOHNSWORT To counter depression and relax muscles, pour boiling water over 1 to 2 teaspoons dried flower tops, steep, then strain. Drink up to 4 cups a day for a few weeks. St. Johnswort tea bags are also available.

ABSTINENCE To overcome distractions, anxiety, or sexual boredom and trigger a return of focus and energy, abstain from sex for a few days.

INDIGESTION

Indigestion is a term used to describe any discomfort related to eating, whether it is heartburn, abdominal pain, nausea, or flatulence. Its causes are many: stress, eating too quickly (or eating rich or gas-producing foods), or drinking wine or carbonated drinks. Smokers, pregnant women, and the obese are especially susceptible. Persistent indigestion can indicate an ulcer, a gallstone, or inflammation of the esophagus.

Heartburn, a burning sensation in the chest and sometimes the throat or mouth, is caused by acid rising from the stomach into the esophagus. To avoid heartburn, drink sparingly during meals and eat a low-fat, high-fiber diet. Do not eat just before going to bed. Also, pass up fried and spicy foods, citrus fruits, tomatoes, alcohol, caffeine, and tobacco—all of which are acid producing. Avoid chocolate and mints, which relax the opening at the base of the esophagus, letting acid in. Finally, do not take aspirin.

Antacids soothe heartburn as well as acid indigestion; the oldest of these is baking soda. Commercial antacids often contain calcium carbonate (which may neutralize as much as twice the acid as baking soda), aluminum hydroxide (which tends to cause constipation), and magnesium salts (which tend to have a laxative effect). Combined, magnesium salts and aluminum hydroxide are more potent, and their side effects may negate each other. Besides antacids, which neutralize stomach acid, acid reducers are now available.

Age-old Stomach Settlers

Early pioneers concocted countless ways to settle their churning tummies, from drinking chamomile tea to eating sand. Bitter-tasting "stomach teas" were standard; they contained a combination of such ingredients as strawberry leaves, powdered rhubarb, gentian, wormwood, and dandelion root. (Bitters are still believed by many to aid digestion by stimulating the production of gastric enzymes.) Some chose instead to eat dried orange or grapefruit peel after meals or to take a nip of whiskey and sugar in water. Colic cures, including fennel and caraway seeds, anise, dill, catnip, and peppermint, were also called on for use against bilious afflictions because they help expel gas.

Gingerroot was prized, and for good reason: it is known to quell nausea and aid digestion. Powdered cinnamon in water was thought to soothe indigestion, and it probably does. There is also scientific support behind the practice of adding cayenne pepper to food to stimulate digestion. Eating papaya after meals is beneficial, too, because of a potent enzyme called papain. Even garlic and wild onions were once used as after-dinner digestives.

An older word for indigestion was "dyspepsia."

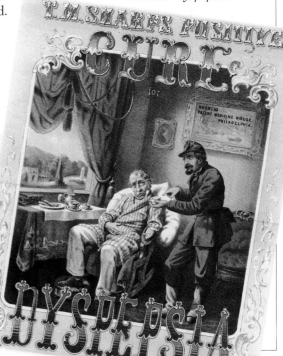

CHAMOMILE This herb calms gastric spasms and soothes the digestive tract. To make a tea, pour 1 cup boiling water over 2 to 3 teaspoons (or one tea bag) of finely chopped flowers. Let steep, then strain before drinking.

FENNEL Fennel is well known as a carminative, an agent that helps dispel gas from the intestines. To make a tea, steep 1 teaspoon crushed dried seeds in 1 cup boiling water, then strain. Or chew ¼ teaspoon seeds after a meal.

ANISE Anise works similarly to fennel. To make a tea, grind 1 teaspoon seeds and cover them with 1 cup boiling water. Steep, then strain. Or drink a few drops of aniseed oil in warm water.

PEPPERMINT The volatile oil in peppermint dispels gas and calms cramps. Pour 1 cup boiling water over 1 tablespoon chopped dried leaves. Steep, then strain and drink.

THE HEALING TRADITIONS OF
THE LOUISIANA CAJUNS

In the steamy, Spanish moss draped bayous of Louisiana, the Cajuns preserve a rich variety of folk healing traditions— techniques that range from natural remedies to magical practices. Virtually every community has a traiteur, *or "faith healer," who is well versed in the medicinal powers of the plants of the region.*

For more than two centuries, southern Louisiana has been home to the Cajuns, descendants of the exiled French Acadians who arrived there around the time of the American Revolutionary War. In both Canada and Louisiana they learned from the healing traditions of their neighbors—Indians and people of British, Spanish, African, and West Indian descent. Later they absorbed many of the traditions of so-called backdoor Cajuns—the German, Lebanese, and Irish immigrants who married into the culture. Today the Cajuns' religion, language, foodways, music, and healing practices are unique in all of North America.

A Link to the Divine

The ancient practice of faith healing, or *traitement,* remains vital to this culture. Called *traiteurs* if they are male and *traiteuses* if they are female, Cajun faith healers share many similarities with Appalachian "power doctors." Traiteurs are believed to possess special powers imparted by God, and they heal through the laying on

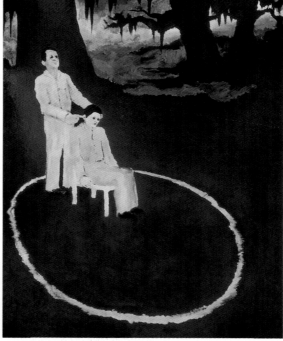

Cajun painter George Rodrigue's *"Doc Moses, Cajun Traiteur" depicts a healer curing an earache. The circle of powder is a barrier against evil spirits.*

of hands while uttering prayers or religious phrases, which they must keep secret.

Certain customs must be respected if the treatment is to be effective. Traiteurs cannot charge for their services, nor can they offer them—the patient must seek their help. When treatment is finished, the patient cannot thank the traiteur or leave a payment, although tips or gifts of food are acceptable. More important, the patient must have faith in the healer. "You have to believe in the treatment," says one older traiteur. "Both people have to believe: the one who's giving it and the one who's receiving it, or it won't work." As one anthropologist has written, "The traiteur represents a link with the divine."

Traitement is generally quite simple, without elaborate ceremonies. Some traiteurs use water or Roman Catholic religious artifacts, such as a crucifix or candles, whereas others do not. Some use knives to symbolically "cut" pain; others schedule treatments according to the phases of the moon.

The power of the traiteur's utterance is the key element in *traitement.* Traditionally this power was thought to be blocked by water, yet in this age of modern conveniences, the belief has largely been discarded. Many traiteurs minister over the telephone to patients who live far away, and the intervening bodies of water are no longer thought to hinder their capabilities.

Accoutrements of Healing

The Cajuns share a belief in the power of magic with other traditional North American cultures. Many magical cures do not require specialists and so are generally practiced in the community. One such cure is that based on transference—the shifting of an ailment to another person, an animal, or an inanimate object. For example, it is said that a copper penny or white bean passed over an infected area will carry the patient's malady away with it when it is tossed into a bayou as the tide goes out.

In the old days, many people wore amulets of various kinds to heal or deflect ailments. Parents draped necklaces of alligator teeth or rattlesnake rings on infants to hasten teething. Some people believed that wearing a gold earring would remedy eye trouble.

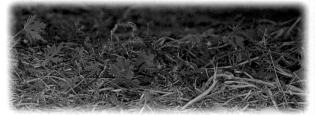

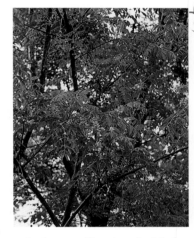

La mauve grass (Modiola caroliniana) *is used to make a poultice for infections and a healthful tonic, while the leaves of the chinaball tree (right) are used to cure sunstroke. Another tree, the willow, is invested with mystical powers. To cure childhood asthma, the child's height is marked on a willow trunk. A hole is cut at the mark, stuffed with a lock of the child's hair, then plugged back up. It is believed that when the child grows higher than the mark, he will be cured.*

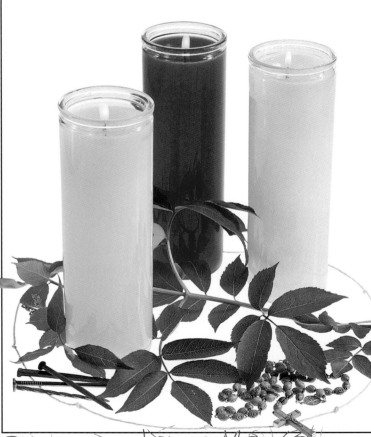

Among the traiteur's tools are candles (one for each patient), kept lit and prayed over for the duration of the treatment. Traiteurs also find a use for nails: getting rid of a bad tooth. It is said that if the traiteur touches the tooth with a nail while uttering his prayers, it will soon fall out. Aside from consulting traiteurs, Cajuns make use of plants and such religious objects as rosary beads. Elderberry leaves are tucked into clothing to draw out illness, and a string, usually knotted nine times, is worn around the finger to remove warts; to cure shingles, it is worn around the waist. The string is left on until it falls off, by which time the patient is cured.

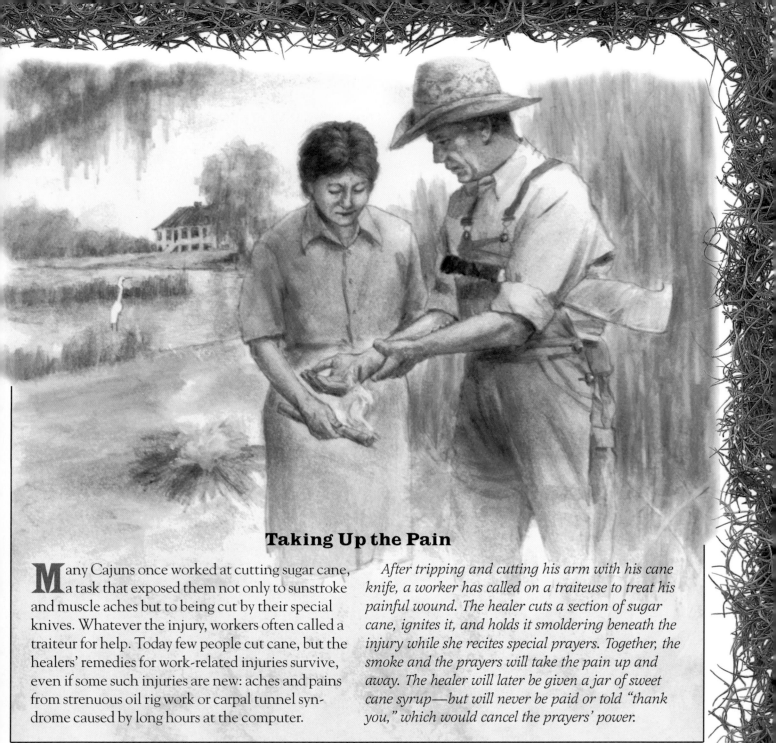

Taking Up the Pain

Many Cajuns once worked at cutting sugar cane, a task that exposed them not only to sunstroke and muscle aches but to being cut by their special knives. Whatever the injury, workers often called a traiteur for help. Today few people cut cane, but the healers' remedies for work-related injuries survive, even if some such injuries are new: aches and pains from strenuous oil rig work or carpal tunnel syndrome caused by long hours at the computer.

After tripping and cutting his arm with his cane knife, a worker has called on a traiteuse to treat his painful wound. The healer cuts a section of sugar cane, ignites it, and holds it smoldering beneath the injury while she recites special prayers. Together, the smoke and the prayers will take the pain up and away. The healer will later be given a jar of sweet cane syrup—but will never be paid or told "thank you," which would cancel the prayers' power.

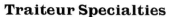

Traiteur Specialties

Traiteurs often have a specialty, treating particular ailments ranging from snakebites to blood poisoning. Some even treat hyperactivity in children. Because of the strict taboo against offering their services, traiteurs cannot announce their specialties. The community knows what each traiteur can do; when a sufferer needs special treatment, word of mouth directs him to the appropriate healer.

When treating a patient, the traiteur utters a prayer, repeating it for as long as he feels is necessary. So deeply is the practice of traitement ingrained in Cajun life that orthodox physicians, by and large, respect it. In fact, many doctors refer patients to traiteurs when their medicines fail to work for stress-related illnesses—shingles, for example. One doctor wrote, "There are plenty of things I can't understand. One is the power of these people. I've seen them bring about what looked like cures in cases I thought doomed."

If their treatments do not work immediately, traiteurs advise seeing a doctor. Indeed, they insist that acute cases be treated by professionals. They view themselves as the partners of orthodox practitioners, but are set apart in one remarkable respect: As they lay their hands on a sufferer, some actually feel the patient's pain—for a brief moment a stab of pain passes through the healer as it departs from the patient. Traiteurs say that this is God's way of letting them know that the treatment is working. It is a sign of their power, and the price they pay for their gift.

Natural Remedies

Cajuns have long made use of herbs and other natural remedies. Records note that they learned much from the Indians, who were skilled at concocting poultices for wounds and sores. Not surprisingly, the hot climate of Louisiana also led the Cajuns to devise many treatments for the potentially fatal fever caused by sunstroke. Even today the leaves of the chinaball tree *(Melia azadarach)* are made into a crown to draw out the heat. Another cure involves draping a red cloth over the head of the patient, then placing a jar of water on top. The water is said to draw the heat from the head, and some traiteurs insist that the water may boil.

Other remedies include teas made from horsetail (locally called *prele*) to tone the kidneys. A plant called *mamou (Erithrena herbacea)* yields a syrup that relieves throat ailments and even pneumonia. Citronelle, or lemongrass *(Cymbopogon citratus)*, is drunk as a tea to reduce nausea, especially in pregnant women. Cajun healers also use the plant lizard's tail *(Saururus cernuus)*, which they know as *herbe à malot,* to brew a tea for treating colds, fevers, and such ordinary childhood ailments as teething and colic.

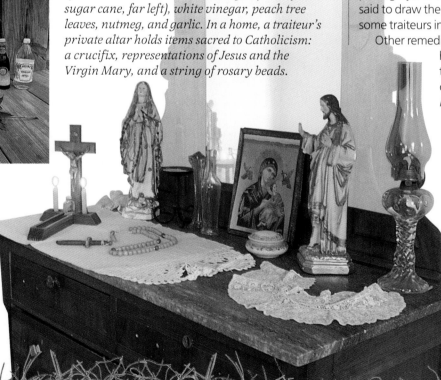

Dressed in early Cajun garb, a woman from southern Louisiana displays an assortment of often-used medicinals: cane vinegar (made from sugar cane, far left), white vinegar, peach tree leaves, nutmeg, and garlic. In a home, a traiteur's private altar holds items sacred to Catholicism: a crucifix, representations of Jesus and the Virgin Mary, and a string of rosary beads.

INGROWN TOENAIL

The Indians of the West Indies may have provided the first North American remedy for ingrown toenail. Early Spanish explorers reported that the natives put pineapple poultices on inflammations, including those affecting the toes. The remedy worked because pineapple juice contains bromelain, an anti-inflammatory enzyme that is sometimes found in commercial ointments. Among early settlers, fat—which softened the skin and allowed the nail to grow out—was a popular remedy, although it is no longer advised today. Raw bacon was wrapped around the affected toe, or a fat-or-oil-based salve was applied. A typical recipe started with

Soothing bromelain is extracted from the pineapple.

beef tallow or lard, to which such substances as turpentine, camphor oil, salt, or brown sugar were added.

Another common treatment was to cut a V in the center of the nail; doing so was thought to make the sides grow toward the middle. (This practice has been discredited; today we know that a nail actually grows from back to front.) Fat, too, has fallen out of favor. Animal fats grow rancid quickly and do little to provide the protective mucilaginous coating that helps inflammations to heal. Nowadays, soaking the toes in warm water is the preferred treatment.

A Pain in the Toe

The condition known as ingrown toenail results when one edge or both edges of the nail—most often, that of the big toe—press into the adjacent skin, causing inflammation, redness, and possibly infection. The painful affliction is usually caused by nails that are unnaturally curved or cut incorrectly. Tight-fitting shoes can also be at fault, while poor personal hygiene can increase the risk of infection.

To decrease the chances of getting an ingrown nail, cut it straight across instead of into a half-moon. You will avoid cutting tender skin, which can become infected if a splinter of nail from the cut edge grows into it. For the same reason, do not cut nails too short.

Toenails grow more slowly than fingernails, but their edges grow faster than the center. You should check toenails every week to see if it is time for a trim. Thicker than fingernails, toenails are easiest to trim just after a bath or shower, when they are softer.

Also make sure that your shoes fit properly. Women who regularly wear high heels with pointed toes are particularly susceptible to ingrown toenails. Wear open-toed shoes when possible, and avoid tight socks.

If a toenail is only slightly ingrown, soak the toe in warm water to soften the nail, then trim the excess and put a tiny piece of sterile cotton under the edge to lift it. Change the cotton daily until the nail grows out.

If the toe is swollen or there is a discharge of pus, see your doctor, who may prescribe an antibiotic and remove the part of the nail causing the problem. And take note: People with diabetes or circulatory problems should not treat an ingrown toenail themselves; see a podiatrist or your doctor.

BROMELAIN Apply a commercial ointment containing bromelain to the affected area to reduce inflammation. In some people, skin sensitization may occur after using bromelain.

YARROW Crush yarrow flowers or leaves and put them on the skin around the toenail to prevent or reduce infection. Ointments containing yarrow are also available. Yarrow can cause dermatitis in some people.

EPSOM SALTS Soak the affected toe in warm water and Epsom salts. A 10-minute soak twice a day will relieve the pain and reduce the inflammation of an ingrown toenail.

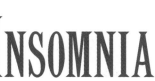

INSOMNIA

Mark Twain offered the following cure for insomnia: "Lie near the edge of the bed and you'll drop off." Some people prefer counting sheep, although many others turn to prescription sleeping pills in an attempt to summon the elusive sandman.

On any given night, about a third of all North Americans have trouble catching all forty winks. Why can we not, as Longfellow described, "drift gently down the tides of sleep"? According to folk wisdom, dirty dishes left in the sink are one reason. Indeed, anxiety over unfinished business or other worries can keep sleep at bay. So can physical discomfort, whether from asthma, arthritis, angina, migraines, ulcers, or some other ailment. Medications are sometimes responsible for lost sleep, including barbiturates, cortisone, some decongestants, theophylline and other respiratory drugs, and certain thyroid drugs, antidepressants, and heart medicines. Add to the list caffeine, nicotine, and alcohol, which may induce sleep at first but then make for fitful rest.

Depression can disrupt sleep, too, often causing early-morning awakenings. Anxiety, on the other hand, makes it harder to fall asleep. Any physical or psychological stress can cause transient insomnia, which generally ends when the stress does. However, insomnia can become chronic, especially if one develops anxiety over falling asleep.

Finally, some people are genetically predisposed to be light sleepers. During the night these people not only awaken more often but have faster heartbeats and higher body temperatures. Women are more prone to sleeplessness than men and become more likely to experience insomnia after the age of 40, possibly because of hormonal changes. With increasing age, both men and women experience lighter, more fragmented, and shorter sleep, although this is no cause for concern.

Fighting Insomnia

To help combat insomnia, keep a regular sleep schedule. Get up at the same time every day and avoid taking naps, no matter how sleepy you are. At night, do not go to bed unless you are tired. And make certain to get regular exercise—but not too close to bedtime. Studies show that people in good physical condition fall asleep faster and sleep more deeply.

Sleeping pills should be used only on a short-term basis, if at all. Such drugs as benzodiazepines (which work by reducing the activity of the brain) and sedative hypnotics lose their effectiveness over time. Moreover, withdrawal from these drugs often causes rebound insomnia that is worse than the original. Antihistamines depress the central nervous system, and are therefore the active ingredients in many over-the-counter sleeping aids.

The hormone melatonin is currently popular in the United States for treating

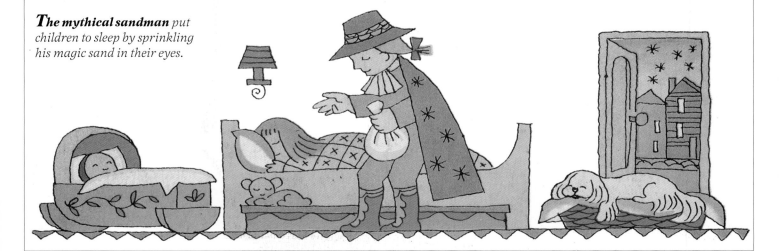

The mythical sandman put children to sleep by sprinkling his magic sand in their eyes.

Getting a Better Night's Sleep

The cure for insomnia depends on the cause. Your doctor may help you diagnose the problem. If you think your insomnia could be caused by depression, consult a psychiatrist. The following are general tips for falling and staying asleep.

Avoid caffeine, alcoholic beverages, and tobacco.

Do not eat heavy meals close to your bedtime.

Avoid foods that contain tyrosine, which can cause heart palpitations. These include chocolate, Cheddar cheese, and Chianti wine.

Exercise regularly, but not within two to four hours of bedtime.

Make sure your bedroom is comfortable: not too hot, too cold, too noisy, or too bright.

Develop and maintain a relaxing bedtime routine.

Get up at the same time each day, even on weekends.

Avoid reading, eating, or watching television in bed so that you associate the bed only with sleep.

Learn a relaxation technique, such as meditation or breathing exercises, to use before bedtime.

If you don't fall asleep within 20 minutes, get out of bed and read or perform some other relaxing activity until you can no longer keep your eyes open. If you still can't sleep, repeat the process. The next day, get up at your regular time and do not nap. In two to three weeks, you should notice an improvement.

insomnia. Preliminary studies show that low doses of melatonin may indeed be effective in treating some sleep disorders and especially in helping to counter the effects of jet lag; however, more information is needed on the safety of long-term use. Since no manufacturer of melatonin has yet submitted supporting scientific evidence of the safety and effectiveness of the hormone to Health Canada, melatonin is not approved for sale as a drug in Canada.

Herbal Nightcaps

Before the advent of barbiturates in the early 20th century, the wide-awake turned to herbal teas to help them sleep. Foremost among the herbs used was valerian. Recent studies have confirmed that valerian helps people fall asleep faster and sleep better, without the morning-after "hangover" effect of sleeping pills; it is as effective as small doses of barbiturates or benzodiazepines and is not habit-forming. However, if you try valerian, do not expect it to be aromatic: simply put, the herb stinks. Some herbalists recommend combining it with other herbs, such as lemon balm or passion flower, to mask the unpleasant odor.

Catnip, which stimulates cats (as does valerian), seems to have the opposite effect on humans. It has had a long tradition of use as a sedative, although it has not been proven to have sedative properties. Passion flower, another widely used herbal sedative, was appreciated by the

Milk, turkey, and pumpkin seeds all contain tryptophan, which may help induce sleep.

Indians and the settlers. The herb is popular in Britain and has been approved in Germany to treat "nervous unrest." Likewise, lemon balm, which has demonstrated sedative properties in laboratory studies, is used in sedatives sold in Europe. (Note that lemon balm can interfere with a thyroid-stimulating hormone. For this reason, those with thyroid problems should consult a physician before using it.)

Many of the sedative teas used by the settlers involved a mixture of herbs. One recipe combined skullcap with passion flower and lemon balm. Another called for skullcap, valerian, gentian, and hops. In fact, skullcap, which was used by Indians for "nervous irritation," has been found to have no sedative properties.

Other herbs used as sedatives included black cohosh, which probably had some effect; lady's slipper, called American valerian because it acts like valerian; and squaw vine, or partridgeberry, used by the Menominee Indians for insomnia and later adopted by the settlers. Wild lettuce also had a reputation for inducing sleep. The stalks contain a milky white sap, called lettuce opium because it was thought to look and act like that of the opium poppy. However, studies have failed to confirm any sedative effect.

Hops-Scented Slumber

Indians and settlers alike used hops to put themselves to sleep. A pinch of hops was added to boiling water to make a soothing tea. Alternatively, one could sleep on a hops pillow. Folk wisdom advised sprinkling the hops with alcohol before stuffing the pillowcase in order to "bring out the active principles." When dried hops are stored, they eventually release a volatile depressant alcohol, which is absorbed through inhalation as well as through surface contact and ingestion. This may explain the supposed sleep-inducing powers of these pillows.

Milk and Honey

For generations mothers have administered warm milk to induce sleep. Scientists have since studied milk's potential sedative effects and found mixed results. Milk contains tryptophan, an amino acid that increases the amount of serotonin in the brain, and serotonin acts as a sedative. In addition, the milk's warmth in itself may be relaxing. However, in one study, instead of putting people to sleep, milk actually had the opposite effect. Even though high doses of tryptophan do help induce sleep, because of a chemical quirk, drinking milk was found not to increase the level of tryptophan in the brain but to decrease it. What's more, drinking milk raises the levels of dopamine and norepinephrine in the brain, which increase the brain's activity.

Nevertheless, milk may be useful. Because carbohydrates facilitate the entry of tryptophan into the brain, drinking milk along with a carbohydrate—such as a spoonful of honey—may in fact summon the sandman. A sprinkling of cinnamon, which itself has mild sedative properties, may enhance the effect. And whole milk, which contains fat, tends to slow down the brain's functions.

Over the years, some people also ate pumpkin to help them sleep. This may have worked—if they consumed the seeds, which are high in tryptophan. In truth, one might have to eat several kilograms of pumpkin seeds to notice any effect. Other foods, notably turkey, also contain high levels of tryptophan. It is less clear why anyone would eat onions to make them drop off, but many did. Folk wisdom advised a cup of onion tea before bedtime, and many cultures believed in eating raw onion before retiring. Some people kept a jar of chopped onions next to their bed and took a whiff whenever sleep eluded them (the worth of doing this has yet to be proved).

Sheepish Dreams

Finally, some people employed mental tricks, such as counting sheep, to lull themselves to sleep. Believe it or not, this age-old ritual is not mere folly. Picturing the woolly mammals engages the right side of the brain, while counting them uses the left, effectively preventing one from concentrating on anything else: work problems, worries, or the fear of not falling asleep. Some swore by other tricks, including breathing deeply six times, counting to 100, then breathing deeply six more times. In fact, any such strategy may work, especially if one has faith in it.

VALERIAN Valerian is an effective sedative, although its aroma is off-putting. It is not habit-forming. To make a bedtime tea, pour 1 cup boiling water over ½ to 1 teaspoon chopped root. Drink 1 cup before retiring. The tea may also be taken two to three times during the day. Valerian root capsules and tinctures are available.

PASSION FLOWER This herb's mild sedative effects have been documented. To make a tea, pour 1 cup boiling water over 1 teaspoon chopped dried flower-tops. Steep and strain. Drink 1 cup 2 to 4 times a day.

CHAMOMILE Chamomile tea has traditionally been drunk as a bedtime beverage, but its sedative effects have not been adequately proven. To make a tea, pour 1 cup boiling water over 2 to 3 teaspoons minced flowers. Steep, then strain. Tea bags are available.

ST. JOHNSWORT This herb is a treatment not only for depression but also for nervous unrest. It may work by inhibiting an enzyme known as MAO. It is most effective when taken for four to six weeks. To make a tea, steep 1 to 2 teaspoons dried flowering tops in 1 cup boiling water, then strain.

JUNIPER

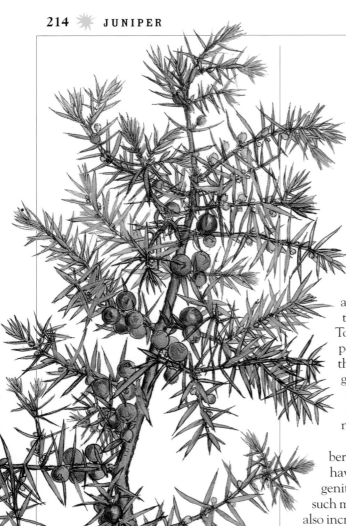

Juniperus communis

In the 1600s a Dutch medical professor named Franciscus Sylvius developed an alcoholic extract of juniper berries as an inexpensive diuretic. The British, for reasons entirely nonmedical, took a liking to the new drink and called it gin (from *jenever*, the Dutch word for "juniper"). Today gin is by far juniper's most popular incarnation. Yet over the course of history, the evergreen's berries and needles were first and foremost a medical cure—one whose safety has now come into question.

For centuries ripe juniper berries (actually mature cones) have been used as a diuretic and a genitourinary antiseptic to benefit such minor infections as cystitis; they also increase the production of urine, which helps prevent kidney stones. Perhaps because of their diuretic properties, the berries have also been eaten to ease the pain of rheumatism, which was thought to result from "poor elimination"

and "imperfect drainage of the system" due to a rich diet. (Today, it is known that diuretics may in fact be of some use in treating arthritis pain.) Similarly, juniper was used to treat gout, a condition involving painful inflammation of the joints caused by high uric-acid content in the blood. Acidic fruits, such as juniper berries, are reputed to break down and promote the excretion of uric acid. In Germany, juniper is prescribed today for both arthritis and gout.

An Indian Favorite

Indians flavored their buffalo stews with juniper and ate the shrubby plant's inner bark to fight starvation in winter. They also used the herb for medical purposes. Many western Indian tribes treated rheumatic pains by warming the twigs and berries over hot coals and applying them to the ache. The Comanche believed that the leaves had a purifying effect, and they were not alone. In some other tribes, people nursing patients with serious illnesses were advised to chew juniper berries to ward off diseases that might enter through the nose or the mouth. (Among Europeans, this same practice existed since the Middle Ages, when juniper was used to protect against leprosy and the plague.)

Teas made from small juniper twigs were used externally as an astringent for hemorrhages and internally to treat colds and stomachaches. The berries were used as a diuretic and blood tonic, and they were distilled in oil for clearing uterine obstructions. Berry teas were even used

---

Active plant parts Ripe berries, dried needles
Uses Indigestion
Cautions Do not take more than 20–100 mg of the volatile oil (or 2–10 g of berries) per day. Do not take juniper for more than six weeks in a row. The oil may cause kidney damage, gastric irritation, and possibly diarrhea. Anyone with a kidney disorder should not take juniper. Some people with hay fever develop allergy symptoms from juniper. Pregnant women should avoid taking juniper, as it may stimulate uterine contractions.

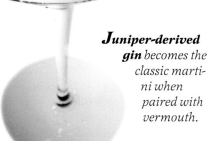

A juniper elixir promised relief from kidney deposits, rheumatism, and bladder irritation.

for birth control. And as far back as the 16th century, Zuni Indians in what is now New Mexico used juniper to speed the healing of the uterus after delivery.

From England to North America

The 17th-century British herbalist Nicholas Culpeper, on whose wisdom early North Americans relied, extolled the virtues of juniper. He called the berries a "great resister of the pestilence" and "excellent good against the bitings of venomous beasts." He also noted the diuretic quality of the berries, professing that they "provoke urine exceedingly." In his opinion, juniper was "so powerful a remedy against the dropsy [the old name for edema, or fluid retention in the body] that the very lye made of the ashes of the herb being drank, cures the disease." Today diuretics are still used in treating edema, although their effect is modest.

Culpeper also prescribed juniper for sciatica and gout, and advised that rubbing the gums with it would cure scurvy. Like the Indians, Culpeper believed that the herb stimulated the muscles of the uterus, noting that it would "give safe and speedy delivery to women with child."

Despite the distinguished doctor's advice, the 19th-century Eclectic physicians rejected the use of juniper to aid childbirth but did recommend it internally for edema and bladder or kidney infections, and externally for eczema and psoriasis. The berries were noted in the U.S. Pharmacopeia for bringing on menstruation and were also used to cure colic, flatulence, and intestinal worms.

Safety Concerns

For all the claims made for juniper, North American doctors gradually realized that the herb works by way of irritating the kidneys; therefore, its long-term use was discontinued. Although juniper is indeed one of the most potent diuretic herbs, it should not be used by itself. It is, however, found as one of several ingredients in some over-the-counter diuretics. The herb should be avoided entirely by any-

Juniper-derived gin becomes the classic martini when paired with vermouth.

Evil Spirits, Away!

In many cultures, from the Chinese to the Pueblo Indians, juniper was used not only to treat specific ills but to guard against "bad magic." The Tewa Indians were known to carry juniper leaves in pouches as a safeguard against evil. The ancient Greeks burned juniper berries and branches to appease the gods of the underworld. In the Victorian Language of Flowers, in which common flowers were imbued with symbolic meaning, the berries represented protection from one's enemies.

Juniper was once burned during childbirth because the smoke was thought to keep fairies from substituting a changeling for the newborn baby. The shrubs were also planted near the front door of people's homes in order to keep witches out of the house, but such magic was not foolproof—any witches who could guess the number of needles on the tree's branches were free to enter.

one with a kidney disorder. It is not effective against bladder or kidney infections, as was previously believed.

The oil distilled from juniper berries is known to have a calming effect on the smooth muscle of the gastrointestinal tract, possibly justifying its traditional use against colic. It is recommended for treating indigestion (which requires only short-term use) by the German Commission E. Note that the volatile oil is much more plentiful in the fresh ripe berries than in the dried berries.

KIDNEY PROBLEMS

Among the veritable slew of old-time folk remedies for kidney ailments were these juniper-based drafts: a shot of "good gin" mixed with crushed pumpkin seeds and a cup of juniper berry tea. Quite simply, both did more harm than good. Juniper was once thought to work because it is a diuretic, but it actually irritates the kidneys. For this reason, it should never be used by anyone with a kidney disorder.

In truth, plain old water does a better job of preventing kidney infections, kidney stones, and nephritis than most folk remedies do. Because it dilutes urine, drink at least two liters of water each day—more after exercise or in hot weather. Some herbal diuretics also may act as preventives by helping to flush out fluids and salts, including the minerals that accumulate to form kidney stones. However, take note: diuretics should be used in cases of serious kidney problems only under the supervision of a doctor.

The Body's Regulator

The kidneys' main functions are to regulate salt and water balance and to eliminate waste products. The organs also help to regulate the body's pH, or acidity versus alkalinity. Another regulatory function is to excrete excess water when it accumulates in the body and, conversely, to retain reserves when excessive water is lost, most often through diarrhea or sweating.

Among the most common kidney-related ailments are kidney stones and hypertension (high blood pressure). Less often, kidney problems may be congenital, autoimmune-related, or caused by diabetes, injury, or drug interactions.

Types of Stones

Kidney stones form when minerals, which are normally flushed away in the urine, crystallize to form clumps that range in size from a grain of sand to coarse gravel. The most common cause is excessive calcium or vitamin D intake, followed by gout or other metabolic disorders. When kidney stones block any part of the urinary tract, especially the ureter ducts or the bladder, intense colicky pain results. Many stones pass through the urinary tract, but others must be removed surgically or by sound-wave treatment, called lithotripsy.

Most kidney stones are formed from one of two kinds of calcium: calcium phosphate or calcium oxalate. Less commonly, stones may form from uric acid crystals, especially in people with gout. Symptoms of kidney stones include severe flank pain and blood in the urine. If you suspect you have a kidney stone, collect your urine in a clean container and strain it through a nylon stocking to obtain any stone, which can then be analyzed by your doctor. Knowing whether the stone is made of calcium phosphate, calcium oxalate, or uric acid will help you alter your diet accordingly.

Although most stones contain calcium, do not cut down on calcium unless your doctor advises you to do so. If the body fails to get enough, it will rob the bones to get the mineral, increasing the risk of osteoporosis. Do, however, increase your intake of fluids to keep the urine from becoming too concentrated.

Vitamin A-rich, kidney-friendly foods include winter squash, carrots, apricots, and cantaloupe, all low in protein.

Calcium phosphate stones are caused in part by the consumption of phosphorus-rich foods. But take note: the balance of phosphorus and calcium in the diet is delicate, and restricting the intake of one may interfere with the absorption of the other. You should consult your doctor before adjusting your intake of either of these two essential minerals.

Likewise, stones formed of calcium oxalate may result from eating certain oxalate-rich foods. These include berries, grapes, and citrus fruits. Among vegetables to cut down on are those of the turnip family, beets, rhubarb, green peppers, and dark greens, such as spinach. (Eliminating all of the problem vegetables, however, would deplete your body of essential vitamins and minerals.) Also go easy on chocolate, beer, and cola. Your doctor can provide a list of the foods that can be eaten in moderation with little risk of causing calcium oxalate stones.

Uric acid stones, often associated with gout, result from a diet rich in high-protein foods containing purines, which promote the overproduction of uric acid; the excess uric acid crystallizes to form stones. Among foods high in purines are sardines and anchovies (perhaps the worst offenders), organ meats, processed meats, meat broths and extracts, lentils and other legumes, chocolate, beer, and red wine.

Watch that Protein

As a first step in preventing kidney problems, watch your protein intake. While protein is essential in the diet (the recommended daily allowance for adults is at least 60 grams per day, the amount in a 250-gram sirloin), excess protein increases the kidneys' workload and can accelerate kidney failure.

Also add to your diet foods that are high in vitamin A—especially those low in protein, including winter squash, carrots, apricots, and cantaloupe. Vitamin A and beta-carotene are excellent antioxidants and help reduce oxidative damage to cells. What's more, they are known anticarcinogens.

Also kidney-friendly is the cranberry, which has an antiseptic effect because of its acidity. Drinking a half cup of cranberry juice daily will help prevent urinary tract infections from spreading from the bladder to the kidneys.

STAY HYDRATED To keep urine from becoming so concentrated that it crystallizes and forms a kidney stone, drink at least 2 liters of water per day—more in hot weather or when exercising strenuously.

FRUIT JUICES The ascorbic and citric acids in fruit juices acidify the urine and have an antiseptic effect on the kidneys. But don't overdo it: limit fruit juice intake to 250 to 375 ml per day.

DANDELION This common weed is often used to treat fluid retention resulting from kidney disorders. Boil 1 to 2 teaspoons of dried dandelion (all parts of the plant) or root for about 15 minutes. Strain.

Drink 1 cup morning and evening. Use dandelion with caution if gallstones or obstructions of the bowel are present.

GOLDENROD European goldenrod (*Solidago virgaurea*) is considered by experts to be one of the most effective and safest herbal diuretics. Although scientists disagree on its active principles, goldenrod is widely prescribed by German physicians to treat urinary tract inflammation and kidney stones.

PARSLEY A parsley tea may facilitate the passage of small kidney stones. Add 1 teaspoon minced leaves to 1 cup boiling water; steep for 5 minutes. Avoid the seeds and oil, which can be toxic. People with kidney disease should consult a doctor before using parsley, and pregnant women should avoid it.

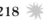

LAVENDER

Lavandula officinalis
ENGLISH LAVENDER, FRENCH
LAVENDER, LAVANDIN

Lavender's name derives from the Latin *lavare*, meaning "to wash"— evidence of the plant's uses ever since antiquity. Lavender water and soap have long been used to refresh the skin, and lavender vinegar made with arnica flowers was once popular for treating inflammations. In hospitals, lavender oil was a staple in dressings for serious wounds and burns.

In the 20th century, this strongly scented herb is best known for its use in soaps, oils, and perfumery. More important, it is enjoying a revival as a mild tranquilizer, even though scientists have yet to pinpoint the particular constituents responsible for its purported sedative action.

A Calmative Herb

Lavender's reputation as a calmative made remedies containing lavender all the rage in Victorian days: lavender water or oil was prescribed for hysteria and cramps, and nearly every refined lady kept a lavender-scented handkerchief on hand for fainting spells. Direct application of lavender essence to the temples was said to cure a headache and put a baby to sleep. Many herbalists also prescribed ingesting lavender for its sedative and antispasmodic effects. The flowers or oil were added to mint or chamomile teas in cases of nausea and were considered useful for treating insomnia and nervousness.

It is important to distinguish lavender extract, which is mixed with water and taken internally, from the essential oil. The oil is highly volatile and may be poisonous; only external use is advised. For a calmative or sleep aid, dab the oil onto the temples and forehead. Then go to bed or sit quietly for a few minutes.

Not to be confused with ...

The essences of various lavender species have different fragrance characteristics and degrees of purity. English lavender (*Lavandula angustifolia*) is particularly prized for the complexity and delicacy of its scent. It is also called "true" lavender. French lavender (*L. dentata*) is the woodsier variety recognized by the ancient world. Do not confuse these lavenders with those that are grown largely for the perfume trade: spike lavender (*L. latifolia*), Spanish lavender (*L. stoechas*), and the hybrid lavandin (*L. x intermedia*).

Active plant parts Flower spikes
Uses Anxiety, insomnia, stomachache; diuretic
Cautions Lavender oil should never be taken orally without supervision; in large doses it is a soporific poison. Pregnant women, in particular, should never ingest lavender oil.

LEMON

Citrus limon

Maud Grieve's popular 1931 herbal asserted "it is probable that the lemon is the most valuable of all fruit for preserving health." So many folk practitioners agreed that one might today be tempted to substitute lemon for apple in the old adage: "An apple a day keeps the doctor away."

Aware of lemon's use in the 17th century to prevent scurvy among seafarers (hence "limey"), folk healers relied on lemon for almost every common ailment. For head colds, coughs, and sore throats, lemon juice or the oil from the peel was widely prescribed. All manner of herbal syrups and hot toddies included lemon as an essential.

Appalachian healers prescribed the juice for gall and kidney stones: treatment for the former required drinking a cup of olive oil, followed directly by a half cup of lemon juice; for the latter, the patient had to take the juice of 12 lemons straight. Descendants of slaves from parts of Africa and the Caribbean popularized a cleansing citrus tonic for the intestines and the liver, made with the pulp and juice of half a lemon, a dash of cayenne pepper, a pinch of turmeric, and a cup of boiling water. Today, preventing and treating constipation with a simple infusion of lemon juice and hot water, drunk within the first few hours of the day, remains a common practice in many parts of North America.

Lemon benefited the skin as well. The fresh juice was applied (either straight or mixed with olive oil) to soothe sunburn, fade freckles and age spots, and smooth wrinkles. A lemon squeezed over an open cut served both to stop any bleeding and to disinfect the wound. Lemon rinds were often placed against insect bites and stings to draw out poisons and were applied directly to the temples to cure headaches.

Rubbing the foot briskly with lemon juice was said to ease cramps and aches. Some folk healers even prescribed rubbing a quarter lemon under each armpit to ease the discomfort of a hangover.

Vitamin C Plus

Modern studies confirm lemon's historic link to wellness. The fruit contains valuable quantities of calcium, potassium, and magnesium, and has a vitamin C content higher than that of any other citrus fruit. Its natural citric acid works safely as a gastric stimulant, digestive bitter, mild antiseptic, and topical exfoliant. Aromatic extracts from the peel and leaves are widely used to enhance many over-the-counter remedies such as lozenges and flu teas. What's more, limonene, the most important volatile oil derived from the outer peel, may possess an anti-tumor action that is now being investigated for use in certain cancer therapies.

Active plant parts Fruit juice, rind
Uses Astringent, disinfectant, antiscorbutic
Cautions Excessive consumption of lemon juice can cause stomach or esophageal irritation, leading to heartburn. It may also cause tooth enamel to erode.

LEMON BALM

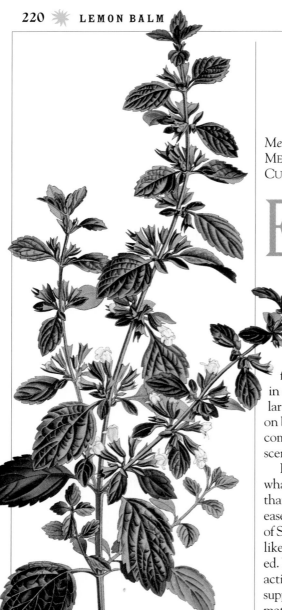

Melissa officinalis
MELISSA, BEE BALM, SWEET BALM,
CUREALL, HONEY PLANT

Even though lemon balm has long been highly regarded and extensively used throughout Western Europe, it started off in the New World as a culinary herb. It is still considered an attractive garden staple today, but its potential therapeutic capabilities have only recently been recognized in North America.

The plant's genus, *Melissa*, comes from the Greek word for "bee." In fact, in ancient times, lemon balm was popular with beekeepers, who rubbed the herb on beehives to attract the insects. Its common name comes from the citrus-like scent given off by the crushed leaves.

Because lemon balm's leaves are somewhat heart-shaped, it was once thought that the herb could help fight heart disease. This notion grew from the Doctrine of Signatures (based on "like things for like things"), but has since been discounted. Nevertheless, lemon balm's sedative action, which has received scientific support, may in fact help calm psychosomatic cardiac problems or heart palpitations brought on by anxiety.

Herpes Fighter

Among the more than 70 components of lemon balm's volatile oil are monoterpenes and sesquiterpenes, which have been shown to inhibit not only the herpes simplex type 1 virus, which causes cold sores, but herpes simplex type 2, or genital herpes. Applying a lemon balm infusion or a commercial cream containing the herb has been found to shorten the time it takes herpes lesions to heal and to lengthen the time span between recurrences.

Modern herbalists recommend drinking a tea made from fresh or dried lemon balm leaves to calm the nerves and aid sleep. You can also stuff the fragrant leaves into a small pillow and then slip it inside your bed pillow. Or add the crushed leaves to warm bathwater for a quick way to unwind before going to bed.

The active principles responsible for lemon balm's sedative effect have not been fully identified, but some investigators believe them to be certain psychoneuro-immunological principles that act through the brain to release peptides, which have a calming effect. Still, lemon balm's sedative ability is controversial: the herb is advised as a sedative in Europe, but it has not been officially recognized as an effective sleep aid by many countries.

More certain are the antibacterial effects of lemon balm oil, which can help heal wounds and soothe insect bites. Lemon balm is also often recommended as a carminative to soothe a nervous stomach and relieve flatulence. Both the leaves and the volatile oils distilled from the plant can be used for this purpose.

Active plant parts Leaves, flowers
Uses Anxiety, insomnia, wounds, insect bites, flatulence, stomach upset
Cautions People suffering from thyroid-related problems, such as Graves' disease, should consult a doctor before using lemon balm.

LICE

Lice are tiny wingless insects that infest the hair of the human body. Of its most common forms—head, body, and pubic lice (also known as "crabs")—the latter are the easiest to see. Usually, lice are apparent only when they cause a severe itch and reddened skin. Tiny white egg sacs, called nits, may also be seen in the hair or, in the case of body lice, in the folds of clothing or bedding. The condition can make one feel disgusting and unclean—in a word, lousy.

Folk remedies for lice were hit-and-miss. Removing the egg sacs by hand was time-consuming, frustrating, and useless; it may have given rise to the term "nit-picking," a synonym for trifling and unjust criticism. Most remedies, the majority of which were herbal rinses and washes—including vinegar and parsley oil—may have cleaned and soothed the itchy skin, but they were unlikely to clear up the lice infestation. Other methods, like applying kerosene or shaving the head, were too drastic (even if they worked), as they irritated the skin or removed clumps of hair.

Cooties Be Gone

The best lice treatments were also commonly used as insecticides. The pyrethrum plant, of the chrysanthemum family, is one of the most effective natural insecticides ever known. It contains pyrethrins, which speedily paralyze and kill insects. Because the plant can irritate the eyes, skin, and lungs, only commercial extracts of pyrethrum should be used.

A synthetic pyrethrum extract, permethrin, at a 1 percent concentration in a liquid cream rinse, is approved by Health Canada for treating head lice among adults and children over the age of two. Other natural insecticides and folk cures for lice that may still be effective include hair rinses made from alder leaves and bark, tobacco leaves, and indigo seeds.

Various topical anti-lice remedies have been tried. Some, including turpentine, sulfur, eucalyptus oil, and infusions or salves of pokeroot, are potentially toxic. The Indians used the fresh leaf juice of black Indian hemp, infusions of the inner bark of white ash, and the powdered seeds of pawpaw (*Asimina triloba*), which contain mild insecticidal constituents. An infusion of the leaves and flowers of larkspur was popular among American soldiers during the Revolutionary War.

Interestingly, even as modern lice treatments improve, infestations are increasing. Standard treatment consists of special pesticide lotions and shampoos containing malathion or carbaryl. At-home measures can also help. The nits can be removed with a fine-toothed lice comb. The chance of spreading lice, particularly among family members, can be reduced by washing hairbrushes, combs, bedding, and hats in hot, soapy water. An infested child should be kept home from school: outbreaks are most common in classes of schoolchildren, where lice are often called "cooties."

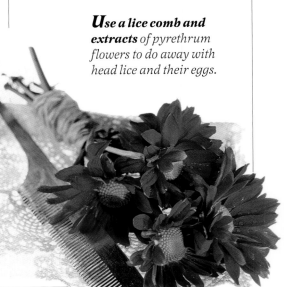

Use a lice comb and extracts of pyrethrum flowers to do away with head lice and their eggs.

LICE COMB To help remove lice nits (dead or alive), comb the hair with a fine-toothed metal lice comb, available at most pharmacies.

PERMETHRIN CREAM To kill lice and their eggs, use a 1 percent liquid cream rinse, available commercially. Apply to the itchy scalp or skin for 10 minutes. Rinse. One application is usually sufficient. Permethrin is the synthetic form of pyrethrin, a natural insecticide found in the pyrethrum plant. Tingling and irritation may occur.

ALDER Boil the inner bark of *Alnus glutinosa* in vinegar for 10 minutes. Use 1 teaspoon bark for each cup of vinegar. Strain and apply to the scalp up to four times a day. Beware: Alder may color the skin and should not be ingested.

TEA TREE OIL Add 5 to 10 drops of this germicidal oil to your shampoo or hair rinse. Repeat daily. Adding a few drops of tea tree oil to a fine comb and combing the hair may also help. Irritation may occur in sensitive individuals.

LICORICE

Glycyrrhiza glabra

For licorice lovers, a little-known fact: the shiny black jelly bean you struggled to fish out of the package as a child probably wasn't the real thing. Most "licorice" candy manufactured in the United States and Canada is actually flavored with similar-tasting anise oil. This ongoing deception has its positive side, however: although true licorice root is considered safe by Health Canada when consumed as food, excessive intake can bring about serious side effects, including high blood pressure and edema. Medical literature is full of references to cases of poisoning produced by overconsumption of licorice candy or licorice-containing tobacco.

Sweeter Than Sugar

Licorice is best known as a sweetener in candy and a flavoring for tobacco and medicines. The genus name, *Glycyrrhiza* (the Greek word from which "licorice" is derived), means "sweet root"—an apt description, considering that licorice's most important active principle, glycyrrhizin, is 50 times sweeter than sugar.

Although licorice was long treasured by the Chinese as "the great unifier" (it was believed to enhance the effectiveness of other herbs it was combined with and to detoxify poisonous drugs), its use in the Western world was largely confined to that of a laxative, expectorant, or cough suppressant; it was frequently used to treat symptoms associated with the common cold. Early North Americans were advised by Nicholas Culpeper, the Englishman whose *Complete Herbal* was highly regarded, that "liquorice boiled in fair water, with some Maiden-hair [a fern] and figs, makes a good drink for those that have a dry cough or hoarseness, wheezing or shortness of breath, and for all the griefs of the breast and lungs."

As the result of trials conducted by a Dutch physician during World War II, licorice found a medical application in Europe and North America as a treatment for duodenal ulcers. Dr. F. E. Revers took an interest in a purported "ulcer-curing" licorice paste prepared by a pharmacist in Heerenveen, a small city in the northern part of the Netherlands. Curious to learn whether the paste (which contained 40 percent licorice extract) was as beneficial as claimed, he prescribed it to a number of peptic-ulcer patients, all of whom improved markedly. However, Revers also noted a serious side effect: about 20 percent of his patients developed edema, usually of the face and extremities. These effects disappeared promptly, however, when the licorice-paste treatment was discontinued.

Today, the effectiveness of glycyrrhizin in counteracting inflammation and

---

Active plant parts Root
Uses Upper respiratory tract problems, stomach and duodenal ulcers
Cautions People with high blood pressure, cardiovascular disease, liver or kidney problems, or potassium deficiency should take licorice only under the supervision of a doctor. Do not use licorice for more than four to six weeks: prolonged use can cause edema, potassium loss, and high blood pressure. Do not consume large quantities at any time.

Not to be confused with ...

Although wild licorice (*Glycyrrhiza lepidota*) is similar to true licorice, it has undergone little investigation. Inhabiting much of North America from Mexico to Canada, this perennial was used by Indians. The leaves were soaked in water to make a poultice for earaches. The fresh root was chewed to treat toothaches, and a root tea was drunk to reduce fevers in children. Because wild licorice contains glycyrrhizin, take the same precautions that apply to true licorice (*G. glabra*)—mainly, avoid overconsumption. Also avoid if pregnant or suffering from hypertension.

diminishing the abdominal spasms caused by gastritis and stomach ulcers has been proved both experimentally and clinically, even though its activity is not fully understood. The German Commission E has approved the use of licorice in ulcer therapy (at a dosage level of 200 to 600 milligrams of glycyrrhizin daily) but cautions that the treatment should not be continued longer than four to six weeks.

When eating licorice candy, don't overindulge. In one controlled experiment, consumption of 100 to 220 grams of licorice twists (which contain .07 to 1.4 grams glycyrrhizin), eaten daily for one to

four weeks, produced high blood pressure, potassium loss, and other serious side effects in a group of volunteers.

Potential Uses

In addition to licorice's antiulcer and upper respiratory activities, other potential uses have been studied in small animals and, in some cases, in humans. These studies suggest that the herb may lower cholesterol and triglyceride levels, reduce plaque and tooth decay, and reduce liver toxicity. Licorice is also thought to have antimicrobial, antiviral, and antianemia properties. There has even been conjecture that licorice may help the hydrocortisone in topical skin-rash preparations to work more effectively. However, adequate evidence has not come forth to support the herb's efficacy for any of these uses.

When using licorice medicinally, take care to compensate for the potassium loss that glycyrrhizin causes. Eat plenty of bananas, dried apricots, and other potassium-rich foods. High doses of glycyrrhizin for long periods can cause headache, lethargy, edema, and hypertension. Eventually, even heart failure may result.

Tobacco-Chewers Beware

Licorice is responsible for much of the sweetness and flavor in many commercial tobacco blends. In fact, some 90 percent of imported true licorice ends up in tobacco products. But beware: people who

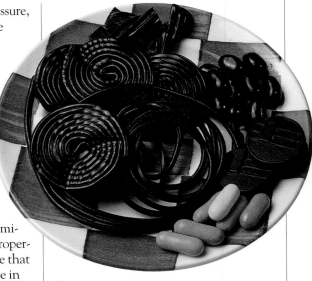

Is it real? *When buying licorice candy, check the ingredients on the label. "Artificial flavor" usually means anise instead of licorice. Of the "licorice" candies above, only the pinwheels are the real article.*

chew tobacco or use snuff are especially vulnerable to the hazards of excessive licorice intake for licorice is absorbed by the body through the mucous membranes and swallowed saliva. (It can also be absorbed through cigarette and pipe smoke, although less so.) Researchers at a Rhode Island hospital analyzed three common brands of chewing tobacco and found that they contained 1.5 to 4.1 milligrams of licorice per gram of tobacco. Absorbed in these amounts over a long period of time, licorice can raise blood pressure and cause muscle weakness.

On a less serious note, licorice has other applications, albeit nonmedicinal. The secret ingredient that brings beer to an extra-frothy head, licorice is added to the brew as a foaming agent. It is also used as a foaming agent in fire extinguishers.

Once popular as a laxative, *licorice is now used more for its expectorant and ulcer-healing properties.*

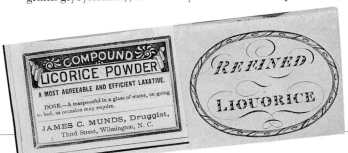

COMPOUND
LICORICE POWDER
A MOST AGREEABLE AND EFFICIENT LAXATIVE.
DOSE.—A teaspoonful in a glass of water, on going to bed, as occasion may require.
JAMES C. MUNDS, Druggist,
Third Street, Wilmington, N. C.

REFINED LIQUORICE

LIVER PROBLEMS

The words "liverish" and "bilious" have long described a sour kind of temper, often accompanied by a yellow cast to the skin and eyes, caused by jaundice. (This association may have originated in the "humors" theory of Greek medicine, which emphasized bile and its effect on the personality.) Indeed, the words bespeak the fact that people recognized the signs of a system poisoned by a sick liver long before modern medicine understood the various ways that the organ produces such symptoms.

A Complex Filter

The body's largest internal organ, the liver is a complex recycling center and filtering device. It absorbs and breaks down used substances in the blood, reconstitutes them, and sends them on their way back into the bloodstream or out through the digestive tract. The liver also manufactures many blood-coagulating enzymes and vitamin K.

The oxygen-carrying pigment called hemoglobin is taken from aging red blood cells and recycled by the liver into a substance called bilirubin. This is channeled, along with cholesterol and waste substances, into the gallbladder in the form of bile. There it waits until you eat a meal, after which the bile flows through the bile duct into the duodenum, where it performs its dual function of digesting fats and counteracting the destructive effects of stomach acid. If, however, the liver cannot recycle the bilirubin as fast as it should, the substance accumulates in the bloodstream. The result is jaundice.

An invigorated liver *was avidly sought by health-conscious North Americans in the 1800s.*

Other substances—ranging from hormones and fatty acids to drugs and toxins—may also build up in the bloodstream or liver tissues, throwing some of the body's systems out of balance and further damaging the liver itself. The resulting progressive degeneration of liver tissue is called cirrhosis; its most common cause is alcohol abuse. A strong, healthy liver can process and dispose of moderate amounts of alcohol without much problem, but if it is overloaded regularly, its cells become poisoned and it is eventually destroyed. Other causes of cirrhosis may include abscesses and tumors, as well as hepatitis.

Hepatitis (inflammation of the liver) is caused by one of two viruses. Hepatitis type A (infectious hepatitis) and type B (serum hepatitis) are called hepatotropic viruses, meaning that the liver is their primary target. The first is present in the feces of infected people, who may transmit the virus through the handling of food. Hepatitis type B is present in the blood and other body fluids of infected

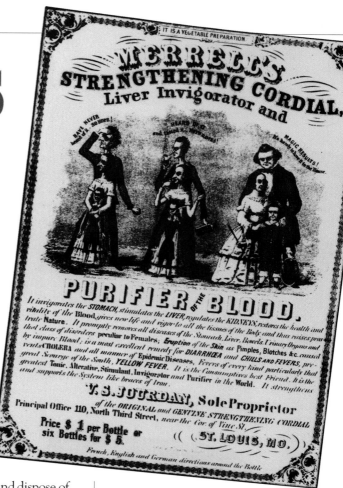

people and can be spread through sexual contact and intravenous needles used for drug abuse. Vaccines for hepatitis A and B are available. Other less common forms of viral hepatitis—C, D, and E—have recently been diagnosed.

Helpful Herbs

On the basis of the ancient Doctrine of Signatures, a tea or other concoction made from the liver-shaped leaves of the liverwort plant (*Hepatica* spp.) was regularly prescribed to ease the symptoms of a failing liver. In truth, they had no effect. Among other plants that were tried, with varying degrees of success, were burdock, boldo, gentian, rosemary, barberry, and dandelion root. Decoctions were made from the bark of such trees as white oak, hickory, Indian arrowwood, and wild cherry. Meadow saffron was found to yield colchicine, a gout remedy that has shown promise in medical trials conducted on patients in the final stages of cirrhosis.

Even though many herbal remedies are said to ease the symptoms of a "sluggish liver" (weariness and slight jaundice), only a few—including milk thistle, turmeric, yarrow, and schisandra—seem to act as more than a "feel-good" tonic. Moreover, some old-time plant remedies —such as chenopodium oil and deer-tongue leaves—have been found to damage the liver rather than heal it.

Herbs can indeed help a sound liver stay healthy and may ease many symptoms of liver damage, but they have no effect on the root causes of cirrhosis— alcohol abuse, hepatitis, or tumors. Nor can herbs do more than slow down the process of degeneration once it has begun. Treating a diseased liver involves either eliminating alcohol, augmenting the immune system, excising diseased tissue, or undergoing a transplant.

The Doctrine of Signatures

One of the "laws" of folk medicine since the Middle Ages, the Doctrine of Signatures is based on the principle *similia similibus,* or "like things for like things." In the case of phytomedicines (medicines derived from botanicals), plants whose characteristics matched those of the body's organs or mimicked the effects of an illness were believed to have a curative effect. It therefore was believed that a plant with heart-shaped leaves—motherwort, for example— had the power to cure heart trouble. Likewise, an herb with yellow blossoms, such as celandine, was thought to cure jaundice, the liver ailment that causes the skin to become yellow. A plant with blood-red sap—including St. Johnswort, which releases red sap from the glands on its leaves—was applied to bleeding wounds. The fuzziness of the burrs of the burdock plant, according to the doctrine, showed that this common weed would prevent baldness.

Although the doctrine is deeply rooted in folk-healing belief, it is also related to certain ideas in Greek and Hellenistic philosophy. Its foundation is the belief in an inherent affinity, or sympathy, between living things and the forces of the universe; for this reason, it is sometimes referred to as "sympathetic magic." In the modern era, a connection between a plant's physical appearance and its healing powers has been disproved. Nevertheless, the tenets of the doctrine remain in force among many old-time folk practitioners.

The liver-shaped leaves of liverwort inspired the belief that the plant had the power to cure liver disorders.

SCHISANDRA Studies have shown that this Chinese herb's lignan compounds, called schizandrins, may protect the liver from the effects of liver toxins. Although extracts are available, few are standardized. Look for a product that contains 19 percent schizandrins. Side effects, which are rare, include upset stomach and depressed appetite.

MILK THISTLE Milk thistle contains silymarin, a substance that alters the structure of the outer cell membrane of liver cells to prevent the penetration of liver toxins. Silymarin also aids cell regeneration. Milk thistle extracts and capsules should contain 200 to 400 milligrams of silymarin. The only side effect that has been reported is a possible mild laxative effect.

TURMERIC The curcuminoids and essential oils in turmeric have antihepatotoxic properties. Because tea made with turmeric has a bitter taste, standardized preparations of the powdered drug are preferable. Take ¼ teaspoon several times a day between meals, sprinkling it on a cracker. People with gallstones should not use turmeric.

YARROW The chamazulene and flavonoids in yarrow's essential oil have been shown to stimulate the flow of bile from the gallbladder. To make a tea, pour 1 cup boiling water over 1 to 2 teaspoons minced dried flowers. Cover, let steep for 10 minutes, then strain. Drink 1 cup three to four times a day between meals. Except for a possible allergic reaction to the flower's pollen, side effects are rare.

LOBELIA

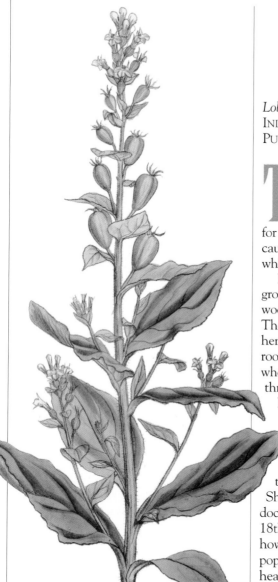

Lobelia inflata
INDIAN TOBACCO, ASTHMA WEED,
PUKE WEED, GAGROOT

Today lobelia is known to be poisonous, yet for centuries many North Americans believed that smoking or chewing the plant's leaves was good for their health. This was because lobelia caused one to vomit and sweat profusely, which was thought to cleanse the body.

Lobelia, native to North America, grows along roadsides and in fields and woodlands throughout the continent. The Indians used the herb as an emetic, hence the names "puke weed" and "gagroot." They also used it to treat asthma, whooping cough, bronchitis, and sore throat. Some tribes even believed that lobelia had magical powers: the Creek used it to scare off ghosts.

The colonists and early settlers followed the Indians' example and used the herb as an emetic and a treatment for breathing disorders. The Shakers grew it for sale overseas, and doctors began to prescribe it by the late 18th century. It was not until the 1820s, however, that lobelia became wildly popular—the favorite of New England healer Samuel Thomson, who claimed amazing powers for the herb. He advised it as a muscle relaxant during childbirth and for the treatment of ailments from epilepsy to tetanus. Thomson attracted a huge following and trained countless folk practitioners, whom jealous physicians scornfully dismissed as "lobelia doctors." But even then, the plant was notorious. After one of his patients died from an overdose of lobelia, Thomson was jailed and tried for murder. The outcome? The trial judge ruled that killing a patient while attempting to cure him was not a crime, and Thomson was set free.

Today lobelia is an ingredient in some products marketed to help people stop smoking. The herb is chemically similar to nicotine and supposedly reduces one's craving without being addictive. However, there is no evidence that it works. It is also claimed that smoking lobelia helps you lose weight; if it does, that is only because it induces vomiting. In short, any use of lobelia poses substantial risks.

Toxic Chemistry

Lobelia's principal ingredient is lobeline, a nicotine-like alkaloid that first stimulates, then severely depresses, the central nervous system. In correct dosages, it opens the bronchial tubes, which explains its use as a folk treatment for respiratory disorders. However, there are no standardized preparations, and an overdose can slow respiration, cause rapid heartbeat and a drastic drop in blood pressure, and lead to convulsions, coma, and even death. Dangerous side effects have resulted from as little as 50 milligrams of dried lobelia or one milligram of tincture.

Active plant parts Leaves and tops
Uses Historically used for respiratory problems
Cautions Because a safe dosage has not been determined and lobelia is toxic in large doses, it should never be taken internally.

MARSH MALLOW

Althaea officinalis
SWEETWEED, MORTIFICATION ROOT

Used by ancient Greeks, esteemed by Charlemagne and Henry VIII, and grown by Puritan leader Cotton Mather in his own garden, the marsh mallow has been valued as a medicinal and ornamental plant for more than 2,000 years. Its roots, which yield a beneficial mucilage, were peeled, boiled, and made into soft white candied sticks—precursors of marshmallows, the spongy sweets that are roasted at campfires.

Protective Goo

Nicholas Culpeper, the 17th-century British herbalist, endorsed marsh mallow roots and leaves for many ailments, including "head-colds" and "a raging disease called bloody flux [dysentery]" along with splinters and rough skin. He and many users of the plant took advantage of the root's juice, which forms a gel when mixed with water.

Syrups made with the boiled root, honey, and orange juice alleviated a sore throat and cough. The sweet-tasting root was also taken, either raw or in a tea, to relieve gastrointestinal inflammations. The mucilage has, in fact, shown the potential to soothe the body's mucous membranes in the digestive, respiratory, and urogenital tracts. It may also help relieve an upset stomach.

Externally, the roots and leaves were used for their demulcent and emollient mucilage, which soothed wounds and skin irritations. Freshly bruised leaves were applied to insect bites. The chopped root was used in poultices on bruises, sprains, and burns. Today, extracts are included in ointments for chilblains and chapped, scraped, or sunburned skin.

S'more Uses

The plant's botanical name, *Althaea officinalis*, means "official cure," and use of the herb carried high expectations. One of its nicknames, mortification root, arose from the belief that it could "kill" infectious diseases; accordingly, the tea was drunk or used as a douche, enema, and wash for the eyes and mouth. Although marsh mallow is not antibacterial, extracts of the plant may boost overall immunity. Its derivatives have also shown hypoglycemic activity and may therefore be useful in managing diabetes.

The use of marsh mallow as a food goes back to ancient times. The French were first to candy the root and use the sugary mucilage in pastries and candies. Today the fluffy sweets used in marshmallow fudge and "s'mores" (made with graham crackers and chocolate) may be inspired by the plant, but they no longer contain any plant parts.

Active plant parts Root; to a lesser extent, leaves and bark
Uses Sore throat, cough, stomach and urinary tract irritations, cuts, sunburn
Cautions Marsh mallow has no known toxicity, although excessive use may cause diarrhea. Marsh mallow may cause a delay in the absorption of other drugs.

MAYAPPLE

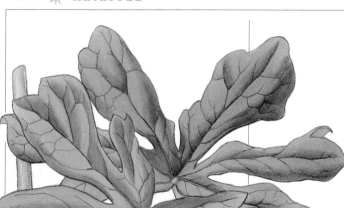

Podophyllum peltatum
AMERICAN MANDRAKE,
DEVIL'S-APPLE, INDIAN
APPLE, GROUND
LEMON, DUCK'S-FOOT,
RACCOONBERRY,
VEGETABLE MERCURY

Described once as a prized plant, the humble mayapple is now known to be highly toxic and is no longer recommended in any way for at-home use. However, the tiny, attractive plant—which grows in southern Ontario, western Quebec, and south to Florida—was a favorite of the Indians and the Eclectics, and modern medicine uses its derivatives to treat cancer.

Although the potent rhizome and root were used medicinally, the low-growing mayapple got its name from its white, May-blooming flowers and its almost flavorless fruits, which turn from green to yellow during the growing season and resemble small apples. Both its genus, *Podophyllum*, meaning "foot leaf," and species, *peltatum*, or "shield-shaped," reflect the large-lobed leaves. Many of mayapple's common names, such as duck's-foot, umbrella plant, and ground lemon, also describe the leaves or fruit.

An Indian Medicinal

In his two-volume botanical reference *American Medicinal Plants* (1892), Charles Millspaugh noted that mayapple was "one of the principal remedies used by the American aborigines." Mayapple root was known to Indians all over North America, most commonly as a powerful laxative. The Cherokee gathered the root in late fall and dried it in the shade. They believed that only the joints between the roots were poisonous and used the underground parts to treat chronic constipation and expel worms. To treat rheumatism, they drank a tincture made by soaking the root in whiskey. They applied the powdered root to skin ulcers. The Cherokee also dropped fresh juice squeezed from the root into the ear to improve hearing. Before planting corn, they soaked the seed in the root resin in order to protect the sprouts from crows and insects.

The Indians understood mayapple's severe toxicity, using the root to induce vomiting, cleanse "liver congestion," and, in larger doses, to terminate pregnancies and commit suicide. But such potency did not discourage various tribes from using other toxic parts of the plant. The Algonquin, for example, used the unripe fruits to make a spring tonic, while New England tribes used them to remove warts. Nevertheless, regardless of its overwhelm-

Active plant parts Rhizome, root
Uses Prescription drugs for cancer and skin conditions
Cautions Podophyllin, a toxic resin, is found in the entire plant, except for the ripe fruit. Ingesting any part of the plant, including the seeds, can cause toxic poisoning, the symptoms of which may be nausea and vomiting, fever, hypotension, anxiety, muscle paralysis, respiratory and renal failure, seizures, and death. Pregnant women should avoid the plant: ingestion has been known to cause birth defects and fetal death. Handling the plant can irritate the eyes and skin and cause an allergic reaction. Resins and ointments containing the resin (podophyllin) can cause painful ulceration if left on the skin longer than six hours.

ing effect on the body, mayapple was unable, as an old Indian belief held, to cause young women who pull up its roots to become pregnant.

Early Official Recognition

The first immigrants to the New World also made use of mayapple's strong laxative effect; over time, only limited doses were recommended for a "gentle" purge. The settlers also took the powdered root to induce menstruation, relieve fever, edema, and rheumatism, and to cleanse the liver and bowels in order to remedy jaundice, hepatitis, cholera, dysentery, and "dry belly-ache." Ironically, the toxic resin, extracted from both the rhizome and the roots, was even used as an antidote to snake venom. Beginning in the 18th century, the resin was used externally against venereal warts and other sexually transmitted diseases. Mayapple was also used (by both the Indians and the settlers) as a substitute for mercury, thus earning it the nickname "vegetable mercury."

Mayapple was used all over the map. In Indiana, the fruits were eaten to replenish salts lost through heat exhaustion. In the American South, mayapple juice, mixed with wine and sugar, was an alternative to lemonade, and mayapples were often substituted for lemons in marmalades and jellies. The dried rhizome and roots were included in the first *Pharmacopeia of the Massachusetts Medical Society* in 1808. Those two plant parts also made the "primary list" of the first United States Pharmacopeia in 1820, and the plant's resin was added in 1863. All three are still listed today, although only for their pharmaceutical use in prescription drugs.

The Eclectic physicians studied mayapple closely and claimed that one of their own, John King, introduced the resin to the medical establishment in 1844. *King's American Dispensatory* (1898), an Eclectic reference, boasted that mayapple was "one of the earliest favorites of our school of practice" and prescribed the resin for a number of ailments, including syphilis, scrofula (a form of tuberculosis), and menstrual pain.

Mayapple was also a popular ingredient in patent medicines, such as Ayer's Sarsaparilla and Carter's Little Liver Pills.

Cancer Stopper?

The toxin found in mayapple (called podophyllotoxin) and compounds called peltatins have shown antitumor potential and are used today in some countries to treat testicular tumors, lymphomas, small-cell lung cancer, and certain types of leukemia. These compounds have been found to stunt cell mitosis, which in turn helps stop the spread of cancer. Some countries allow similar derivatives to be used in commercial tinctures, just as the powdered root and resin were used in folk medicine: for the treatment of plantar and genital warts and other papillomas. Derivatives of the resin are also a part of medications for psoriasis and rheumatism.

Health Canada has not approved products containing mayapple for internal use. Handling mayapple and the toxic resin, found in every part of the mayapple plant except the ripe fruit, can inflame the skin and eyes. Taken internally, the root, rhizome, and resin irritate the gastrointestinal tract. Large amounts of the resin (called podophyllin), when taken internally or spread on the skin, can cause poisoning, the symptoms of which occur within 12 hours. The symptoms include nausea, hypotension, fever, hallucinations, muscle paralysis, and even death by respiratory or renal failure. Mayapple and its derivatives are especially dangerous for children and pregnant women.

Not to be confused with …

Although mayapple is also known as American mandrake, the plant should not be mistaken for "true," or European, mandrake (*Mandragora officinarum*). Mandrake was once used as a sedative, pain reliever, and anesthetic, but, like mayapple, it is now considered unsafe for use in home remedies. Today, its derivatives are used to treat arthritis.

Part of mayapple's intrigue—the plant is known to some as devil's-apple—is directly attributable to its association with mandrake, whose roots were thought to have magical properties. Since ancient times, the plant has been allied with Aphrodite, the Greek goddess of love, and the rhizome's mild narcotic effect has been used to stir the desires of impotent men.

A number of folk beliefs exist about harvesting mandrake's stubborn roots. Witches reportedly believed that, to avoid a curse, the root could be pulled up only by a dog at midnight. Folklore held that if the root was dug up, it would emit a shriek that would cause insanity. Furthermore, if a man screamed while pulling up a mandrake root, all who heard him would die.

MEADOW SAFFRON

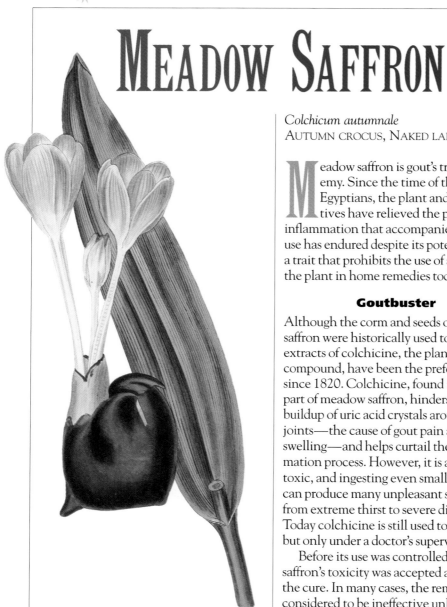

Colchicum autumnale
AUTUMN CROCUS, NAKED LADIES

Meadow saffron is gout's true archenemy. Since the time of the ancient Egyptians, the plant and its derivatives have relieved the painful inflammation that accompanies gout. Its use has endured despite its potent toxicity, a trait that prohibits the use of any part of the plant in home remedies today.

Goutbuster

Although the corm and seeds of meadow saffron were historically used to treat gout, extracts of colchicine, the plant's active compound, have been the preferred form since 1820. Colchicine, found in every part of meadow saffron, hinders the buildup of uric acid crystals around the joints—the cause of gout pain and swelling—and helps curtail the inflammation process. However, it is also very toxic, and ingesting even small amounts can produce many unpleasant side effects, from extreme thirst to severe diarrhea. Today colchicine is still used to treat gout, but only under a doctor's supervision.

Before its use was controlled, meadow saffron's toxicity was accepted as part of the cure. In many cases, the remedy was considered to be ineffective unless some

Active plant parts Corm, seeds
Uses Prescription drugs to treat gout
Cautions All parts of the plant are toxic, including the seeds. Symptoms of poisoning are nausea, extreme thirst, abdominal pain, vomiting, severe diarrhea, and coldness and pain in the extremities. Poisoning can damage the kidneys and blood vessels and cause death.

Not to be confused with ...

Meadow saffron, a crocus-like lily, is often mistaken for saffron (*Crocus sativus*), a lily-like crocus, and safflower (*Carthamus tinctorius*), a native plant also known as false or American saffron. Both saffron and safflower were once used as dyes, and medicinally, as a treatment for measles and menstrual problems. Safflower is still a source of cooking oil.

Saffron, indigenous to southern Europe and brought to North America by exploring Spaniards, was used by the Indians and the settlers as a scent and spice. The Pennsylvania Dutch flavored and colored breads, puddings, and chicken with it. An expensive "gourmet" item today, saffron is also being studied for its potential in treating cancer and atherosclerosis.

nausea, vomiting, or diarrhea—all symptoms of mild poisoning—occurred. In *King's American Dispensatory* (1898), meadow saffron was valued as "a sedative, cathartic, diuretic, and emetic," but it was also known to be a "powerful poison."

The focus on colchicine's potential to treat cirrhosis and cancer may enhance the herb's image, but its flowers are perhaps easier to appreciate. A perennial that grows no higher than 30 cm (1 ft), with striking pink or lavender flowers, meadow saffron is widely cultivated in the United States and Canada.

Although meadow saffron is a lily and not a crocus, it is known as autumn crocus; autumn is when the flowers bloom. Another tag is "naked ladies," for the flowers shoot up without any leaves for cover.

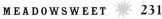

MEADOWSWEET

Filipendula ulmaria
QUEEN-OF-THE-MEADOW, BRIDEWORT

Meadowsweet has been called "herbal aspirin," and with good reason. Long before the discovery of modern painkillers, its fragrant white flowers were plucked from the damp meadows where it grows and used as an antidote to fever, headaches, and the sore muscles and painful joints caused by influenza, arthritis, and rheumatism.

It was not until the early 19th century, however, that the plant was found to contain low levels of salicin, a chemical that had earlier been isolated from the bark of the white willow and was known to have powerful pain-relieving properties. When acetylsalicylic acid was later synthesized from meadowsweet extracts, the name "aspirin" was applied to one of the world's first patent medicines in tribute to *Spirea*, the genus name later replaced by *Filipendula*.

Nature's Painkiller

Salicin by itself can cause unwanted side effects, such as gastric bleeding, nausea, diarrhea, and an upset stomach. Meadowsweet, however, contains tannins and mucilage, which buffer the undesirable actions of the salicin. Scientific studies have shown that the herb actually protects against aspirin-induced stomach ulcers.

These findings lend scientific support to the belief long held by folk practitioners that meadowsweet is easy on the stomach and thus a remedy for nausea, heartburn, indigestion, and other digestive problems. Further credibility for the herb's use as a gentle cure for diarrhea in children has come from a European study that has proven the herb's effectiveness against one of the types of bacteria that cause the condition.

Herbalists have also prescribed meadowsweet for a variety of other ills, including hyperactivity, edema, and urogenital irritation, although there is no scientific support for these claims. There is evidence, however, that the plant's active principles help promote excretion of uric acid, preventing the formation of crystals in the joints of gout sufferers.

A tall perennial with small yellow-white flowers, meadowsweet can be brewed as a tea by pouring boiling water over 2 tablespoons fresh flowers or leaves. A stronger decoction can be made by soaking 2 tablespoons dried, crushed meadowsweet root in a cup of water for six hours before boiling and straining.

There are other uses, too, for the aromatic flowers, which smell of honey and almonds. Brides have long carried meadowsweet bouquets (hence one of the plant's names: bridewort), and Queen Elizabeth I, in a time when people bathed less often, used to scatter the flowers over the floors of her private apartment.

Active plant parts Flowers, leaves, roots
Uses Headache, influenza, colds, fever, children's diarrhea, upset stomach, heartburn
Cautions Pregnant or nursing women and people allergic to aspirin should avoid taking meadowsweet in any form. Children should take the herb only with a doctor's supervision.

MEASLES

When it came to catching measles, the children of early settlers were in for double trouble. Not only did they suffer the itchy rash, chills, fever, aches, and sore eyes that characterize this once-common childhood affliction, but they also had to endure some of the most ill-advised folk remedies ever devised.

Because of the widely held misconception that the measles rash would break out on the inside of a child (and perhaps cause a deadly illness) if it did not quickly show up on the skin, early pioneers plied their sick children with all manner of teas and hot baths that they believed would speed up the arrival of the rash. Many a child in the early stages of the illness was forced to drink a foul concoction known as "nanny tea," which was made from boiling goat dung. If this unsanitary practice did not work—and there is no evidence that it did—another treatment option was sassafras tea, a brew that is known today to be dangerous to consume.

A Thing of the Past?

Measles, or rubeola, is a highly contagious viral disease spread by physical contact or airborne germs. It affects mainly children, and usually runs its course in 10 to 14 days. Some complications, such as ear infections, are common. In rare adult cases, measles may lead to more serious illnesses, such as pneumonia and encephalitis.

At one time, immunity from measles was acquired only after catching the disease, but the development of a vaccine given in early childhood has resulted in a dramatic reduction in the incidence of measles in developed countries. However, outbreaks in the 1980s among children who were immunized before 1985 have led doctors to recommend a two-dose measles vaccination schedule.

Today there is little scientific evidence to support the notion that hot teas and warm baths will "bring out" the measles. The best that can be done for measles sufferers is to keep them warm and in a darkened room (the eyes tend to become light-sensitive during the illness), and to provide relief from the infernal itch that accompanies measles. To this end, baking soda and herbal washes or lotions made with sage or myrrh are ideal.

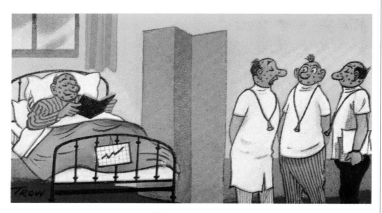

"Well, we now know one thing," says the doctor in this 1920s cartoon. "It's catching!"

BAKING SODA Soaking in a baking soda bath once the measles rash has emerged is a simple way to temporarily relieve the itching that accompanies the rash. Sprinkle ½ cup baking soda in warm bathwater and soak in it.

GOLDENSEAL Although goldenseal is one of the most popular folk remedies, many of the claims for its healing properties have been poorly researched. Numerous Indian tribes used the plant's roots as a wash for localized inflammations, fever, and sore eyes. To make a strong tea to apply to measles lesions, add 2 teaspoons dried root to 1 cup boiling water. Let the root steep for five to 10 minutes, then strain.

SAGE Sage has mild anti-inflammatory and antiseptic properties. To make a tea for topical use, pour boiling water over 2 to 3 teaspoons dried chopped leaves. Steep for 10 minutes, then strain and apply two or three times a day. Do not drink the tea: the thujones in sage are dangerous when ingested.

MYRRH Myrrh is astringent and mildly antiseptic. To soothe lesions, mix 5 to 10 drops commercial tincture with 1 cup water and dab onto the affected area two to three times a day. Test the mixture on healthy skin first to make sure that irritation does not occur. Do not use myrrh on open sores.

MENOPAUSE

Generations ago, menopause was referred to, in hushed tones, as the "change of life." Not only did it signal the end of a woman's childbearing years, it marked the beginning of old age. As recently as the start of the 20th century, menopause occurred on average at age 46; life expectancy was 51.

Menopause is the cessation of ovulation and menstruation due to a decline in estrogen production. Other effects may include hot flashes, night sweats, heart palpitations, and vaginal dryness. The thinning of the urethra and bladder tissue may cause stress incontinence, triggered by sneezing, coughing, or lifting.

Today most women reach menopause between the ages of 48 and 55. Doctors often prescribe hormone replacement therapy, which may lessen the symptoms and prevent osteoporosis. Limiting one's intake of caffeine, alcohol, sugar, and spicy foods may discourage hot flashes. Some women claim that taking vitamin E supplements relieves hot flashes, but this has not been proven.

Help for "The Change"

Doctors once believed that inflammation and obstruction of the womb posed the greatest threat. Decoctions of motherwort were given to "cleanse the womb." Some herbalists still consider motherwort a gynecological tonic, along with lemon balm, sage, goldenseal, and St. Johnswort.

Remedies for "flooding" were said to lessen the heavy bleeding that sometimes signals the onset of menopause. These included sage, cinnamon bark, raspberry leaves, alum root, and witch hazel bark, taken as douches or teas. The settlers introduced the Indians to yarrow, or squaw-weed, which became known as a "female regulator." Yarrow does check bleeding, but probably not the menstrual sort. In large doses it is toxic.

Widely popular with both Indians and settlers was black cohosh, found in Lydia E. Pinkham's Vegetable Compound. The herb may work because it contains phytohormones, plant substances that mimic hormones. However, long-term use poses serious risks. Other "female tonics" containing phytohormones include false unicorn root, red clover, marigold, sage, wild yam, aniseed, and licorice root. (Licorice should not be taken in large amounts or for extended periods.) Wild yam contains a hormonal compound called diosgenin, synthetic versions of which are used in contraceptive pills and menopause drugs. Dong quai, popular in Chinese medicine, alleviates hot flashes but contains furocoumarins, which may cause cancer.

Soy—one form of which is tofu—may help ease hot flashes.

SOY Soybeans are an excellent source of plant estrogens and therefore may ease hot flashes and other symptoms of menopause. Soy can be included in the diet in the form of tofu or miso. It is also available as a powder, which can be mixed with a liquid or added to cereal.

BLACK COHOSH Studies show that black cohosh relieves hot flashes, depression, and vaginal atrophy. Take ½ teaspoon liquid extract or ½ to 1 teaspoon tincture two to three times daily for at least six weeks. Overdoses can cause nausea, vomiting, and other, more serious, side effects. Do not take the herb for longer than six months.

CHASTE TREE Used by women for some 2,000 years, the berries of chaste tree (*Vitex agnus-castus*) restore progesterone levels, which greatly decrease during menopause. Take ¼ teaspoon crushed dried fruit or 1 to 2 teaspoons standardized extract. The herb may cause a rash.

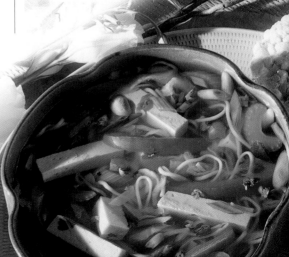

MENSTRUAL PROBLEMS

In the days before modern medicine, menstruation was cloaked in a haze of misunderstanding and myth. Swimming and bathing during "that time" were said to be dangerous, since these were believed to suppress the menstrual flow. Catching a chill, it was thought, could either stop the flow or, as was commonly believed in the American South, cause tuberculosis. Even "cold" foods, such as fruit, were to be avoided, except when used to treat excessive bleeding. Lemon juice, because of its astringency, was believed to stanch the flow. On the other hand, "hot" herbs—including oregano, basil, and garlic—were thought to "bring down the courses." It was also considered bad luck by some if one's menstrual periods began before age 14.

Hormonal Havoc

Menstrual discomforts were, until recently, considered psychosomatic disorders by many doctors. Today cramps are known to be caused by a high level of hormone-like substances called prostaglandins, the production of which is triggered during ovulation. Prostaglandins cause contractions of the uterine muscles, and cramps are the result. Whereas warm gin was once used to provide relief, today aspirin and ibuprofen, which suppress prostaglandin synthesis, have taken its place. Oral contraceptives, which prevent ovulation, also help alleviate cramps.

Premenstrual syndrome, or PMS, may strike a week or two before the onset of menstruation, bringing with it depression, irritability, water retention, breast tenderness, and cravings for sweets. According to one theory, PMS is caused by an increase in the ratio of estrogen to progesterone. In proper doses, licorice may help offset the symptoms; it contains two acids that bind with estrogen receptors and suppress the breakdown of progesterone. However, licorice is not safe for long-term use or use by cardiac patients or people with kidney problems or hypertension.

Many herbalists recommend evening primrose oil for PMS. The oil, derived from the seeds of the evening primrose plant, is a rich source of essential fatty acids, particularly gamma-linolenic acid (GLA), also found in black currant and borage seeds. Women who suffer from premenstrual syndrome have been shown to have below-normal levels of GLA. Clinical studies of evening primrose oil, however, have yielded conflicting results.

Another menstrual problem is an absence of menstruation, which may be caused by stress, a hormone imbalance, anorexia nervosa, or of course, pregnancy. At the other extreme is excessive bleeding, which may be the result of fibroids, polyps, an intrauterine device, or cancer. In either event, see your doctor.

Herbal Cramp Relief

Of all the folk remedies used to combat cramps, ginger was perhaps foremost. A scant teaspoon of powdered ginger in hot water or milk was thought to warm the stomach and relieve cramps. It was also said to increase scanty blood flow. (Ironically, ginger was used to stanch excessive bleeding as well.) Ginger may in fact ease cramps because it contains a compound that inhibits prostaglandin synthesis.

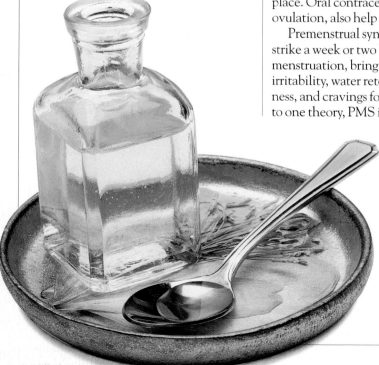

Evening primrose oil is often prescribed by modern herbalists for the relief of PMS, but studies have yielded conflicting results.

Squaw-weed, or yarrow—popular as as an astringent and wound healer—was also used for painful periods and to check "flooding" (excessive bleeding). It has been shown to have antispasmodic activity in laboratory studies. Another astringent, raspberry leaf tea, was also popular; research supporting its use is meager, but animal studies suggest that the herb may both stimulate and calm the smooth muscles of the uterus, depending on its state. Black haw tea, used by Indians and settlers alike, may have been good for cramps, since the bark contains uterine relaxants.

Two other cramp remedies were peppermint and chamomile, both of which contain substances that calm uterine spasms. Another herb, motherwort, was used in cases of heavy or painful periods and also to stimulate menstruation—and rightly so: motherwort contains a chemi-

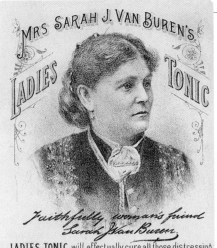

MRS SARAH J. VAN BUREN'S
LADIES TONIC
Faithfully woman's friend
Sarah J. Van Buren

LADIES TONIC will effectually cure all those distressing weaknesses so common to womankind. One bottle will do wonders for a broken-down wife or mother. It will cure cases of years standing and has never failed to give relief FOR SALE BY ALL DRUGGISTS, Price $1.00

An 1885 bill *touted a cure for "all those distressing weaknesses" of womankind.*

cal that encourages uterine contractions. American slaves used the root bark of the cotton plant to treat painful and "obstructed" menses. Cotton was also considered a "female medicine" by the Indians, who used it to ease childbirth. Relevant research on cotton root bark is spare.

Hot water was the simplest cramp remedy of all. Hot water bottles, hot baths, and even drinking hot water were said to relax cramps—and probably did.

Menstrual "Regulators"

Many astringent teas were drunk to remedy flooding, but to little effect; astringents may check the bleeding of small wounds, but they have no styptic effect when ingested. Still, cinnamon tea was espe-

cially popular, as were raspberry leaf, bayberry, and witch hazel brews.

The Aztecs and some settlers believed that if a woman did not bleed regularly, toxins would accumulate. Therefore, teas were drunk to induce bleeding, including those made with sumac root, basil, ginger, and, above all, tansy leaf. (Tansy is potentially toxic, with no evidence to support its use.) Pennyroyal was said to remedy "suppressed menses" and may have worked by irritating the uterine lining; however, pure pennyroyal oil is toxic. The Manchester Drug Company of Canada once touted French Tansy and Pennyroyal Cotton Root Pills as "Reliable Female Regulating Pills."

Smartweed (*Polygonum hydropiper* and *P. punctatum*) was used both to promote menses and to stanch blood flow; it may have contraceptive effects. At the turn of the 19th century, nutmeg was used to induce menstruation. It did not work, but the spice, a hallucinogen in large doses, caused many cases of intoxication.

The Algonquins used black cohosh to treat irregular menstruation. The herb is still prescribed by some herbalists for delayed menstruation. However, it is dangerous in large doses and should not be taken for longer than six months.

CHAMOMILE A popular remedy for stomach upset, chamomile has antispasmodic properties to calm cramps, and it may have mild sedative effects. To make a tea, pour 1 cup boiling water over 2 to 4 heaping teaspoons crushed flowers. Steep, then strain.

GINGER Ginger inhibits the production of prostaglandins, easing menstrual cramps associated with increased prostaglandin synthesis. To make a tea,

pour 1 cup boiling water over 2 grams (between ½ and ¾ teaspoon) chopped rhizome. Steep, then strain. Drink just before menstruation and then as needed. Take no more than 2 grams daily.

CHASTE TREE Also known as vitex, this tree (*Vitex agnus-castus*) yields berries that have been used for menstrual disorders since ancient times. Chaste tree has been found to alleviate premenstrual discomfort and to correct irregu-

larities of the menstrual cycle. It is thought to act on the pituitary gland. The daily dose is 30 to 40 milligrams of standardized extract.

PEPPERMINT Peppermint's antispasmodic activity helps soothe cramps. To make a tea, pour 1 cup boiling water over 1 tablespoon chopped leaves; let steep, then strain. Peppermint oil is available, but use caution and take only as directed: very high doses may be fatal.

THE HEALING TRADITIONS OF
MEXICAN AMERICANS

*T*he essential ingredient in curanderismo, *the folk medicine of Mexican Americans, is not an herb or a tonic but a belief: in God and in the healers who carry out His will.* En el nombre de Dios te voy a curar— *"In the name of God, I will heal you"—chant many of the practitioners, who rely foremost on faith to help their patients.*

As constant and vital as the Rio Grande, folk medicine is a current that wends through the Mexican American community, flowing in an unbroken stream from the 1700s, when Mexican settlers began colonizing the American Southwest, to the present day.

The tradition of *curanderismo* sprang in part from the healing practices of the Aztecs, but it was also shaped by the 16th-century Spanish conquistadores, who brought to the New World the doctrine of the Catholic Church and a medical science descended from the medieval Moorish occupation. It was tempered by the typical way of life—farming and ranching in isolated rural villages— and by the wealth of native flora, many with medicinal properties. Over the centuries these diverse branches merged into an integrated health-care system—with its own theories, healers, ailments, and remedies—developed specifically to meet the needs of Mexican Americans.

A Hierarchy of Healers

Mexican Americans maintain that illness stems from either natural causes, such as sleeping in a draft or offending God, or supernatural ones, namely witchcraft. The choice of a cure and healer is determined by the cause, and patients can turn to three groups of practitioners for help.

At the most basic level are female elders: grandmothers, mothers, and aunts who are experienced with household remedies, or *remedios caseros*. Relying on knowledge passed through the generations, these women handle such complaints as cuts, colds, and headaches. Their arsenal comprises herbal remedies, from homegrown to store-bought plants.

The sick and poor call on San Martin de Porres (left) for help. Amulets (right and above) symbolize ailing body parts to be healed.

Those suffering from more complicated problems seek out *barrio*, or neighborhood, healers, both men and women who offer specialized expertise. The *sobador(a)*, a folk chiropractor, uses massage and other means to treat sprains, bruises, or broken bones. The *yerbero(a)* is an herbalist with advanced skills in transforming medicinal plants—such as *manzanilla* (chamomile), *alhucema* (lavender), and *zabila* (aloe vera)—into healing teas, tinctures, salves, and poultices. And the *partera*, or midwife, assists at babies' births and with prenatal and postnatal care.

While household members and lay specialists can treat simple maladies, the most serious ailments can be cured only by the healers known as *curanderos(as)*.

*U*sing only holy *water* and prayer, *Don Pedrito Jaramillo treated his patients.*

The Chosen Ones

A combination of physician, psychiatrist, and pharmacist, *curanderos* are endowed by God with a *don*, or gift, of healing power. They are renowned and respected not only in their local areas, but

An Ounce of Prevention

When it comes to preventing disease, *curanderismo* leaves nothing to chance. Not only do healers encourage sensible daily habits, such as proper nutrition and good morals, but a range of measures—both secular and sacred—can be taken to ensure continued good health and ward off sickness or misfortune. There are specific rituals, for example, including the symbolic cleansing called *barrida*, which involves "sweeping" the body with an egg, a lemon, herbs, or other objects to draw off any negative vibrations while saying prayers. There are also formulas to prevent being hexed by a witch—such as tying red ribbons and a lime to an aloe plant—and numerous charms, or *amuletos*, that keep illnesses at bay.

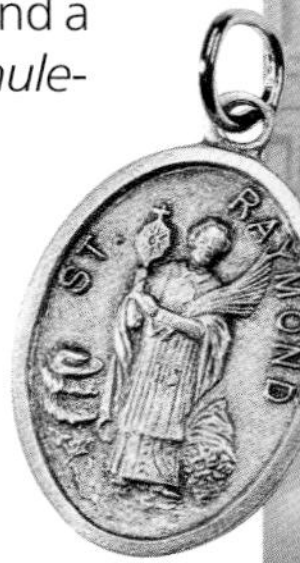

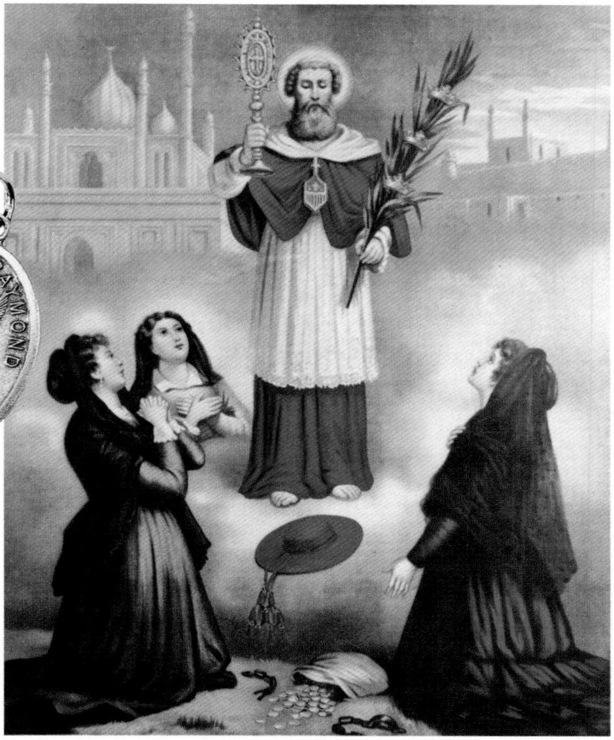

Religion plays as important a role in preventing disease as it does in curing it. Special holy water, or agua preparada, *for instance, may be rubbed on the patient's forehead for protection. Or a person seeking protection from the Virgin Mary or a saint can light a candle and pray to that entity. One saint whose grace is frequently sought is San Ramón (right), a 13th-century Dominican preacher from Spain. Pregnant women are advised to burn pink incense while looking at a portrait of the saint, which is said to protect both mother and unborn child. Those who want to prevent others from speaking evil about them can place a coin in the mouth of a statue of the saint. Medals depicting San Ramón (above) and other holy figures are also worn or carried for protection.*

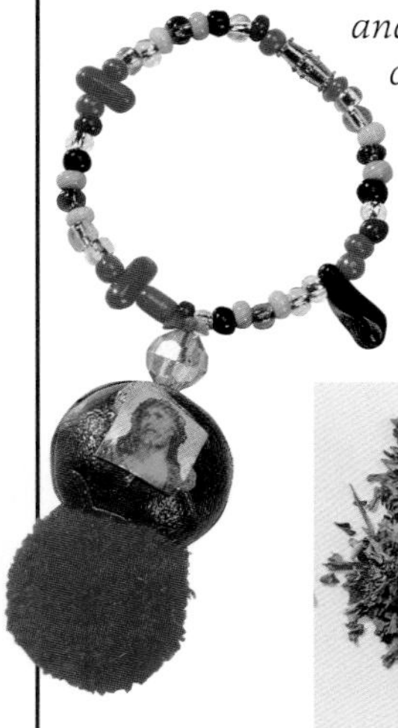

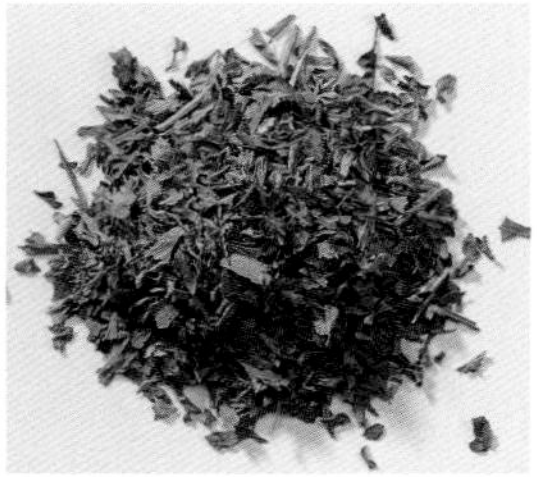

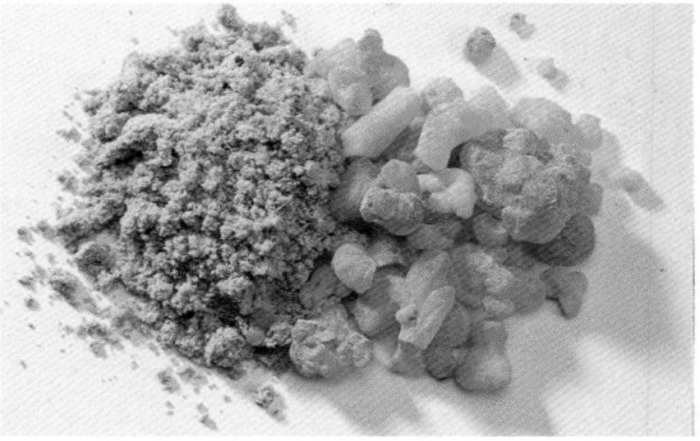

Secular measures are also effective in preserving health and welfare. To guard against evil spirits or mal de ojo, *Mexican Americans may carry the so-called deer's eye, or* ojo de venado *(far left), which is a brown seed that is shown here attached to a bead bracelet and adorned with a picture of Christ. Oshá, or wild parsley (left), is effective in preventing rattlesnake bites and colds and helps wounds from becoming more serious; it is often worn in a sack around the neck. Frankincense (above) is burned as incense to court good luck; it is said that benevolent spirits find the fragrance pleasing.*

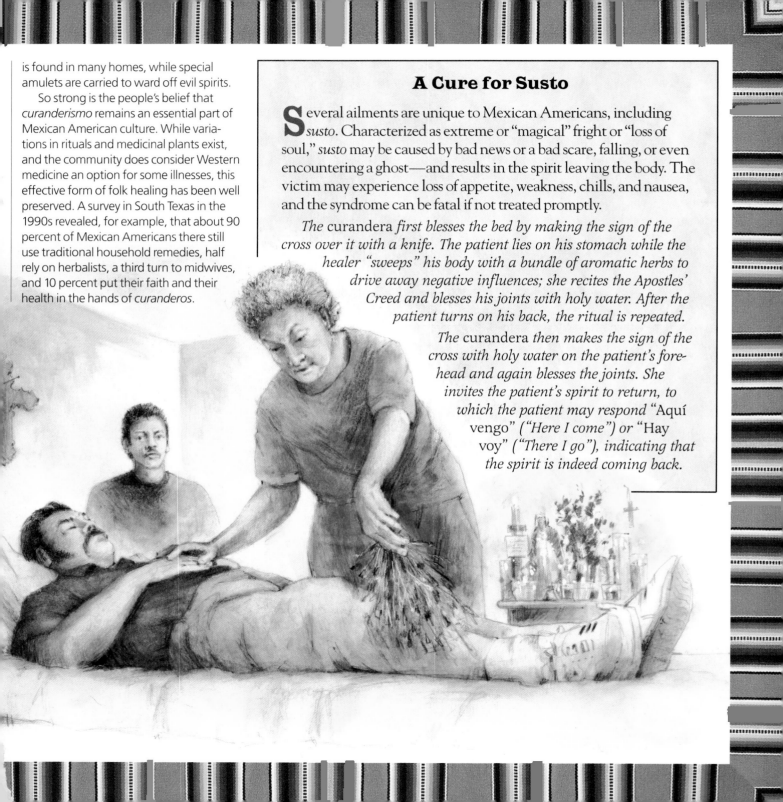

is found in many homes, while special amulets are carried to ward off evil spirits.

So strong is the people's belief that *curanderismo* remains an essential part of Mexican American culture. While variations in rituals and medicinal plants exist, and the community does consider Western medicine an option for some illnesses, this effective form of folk healing has been well preserved. A survey in South Texas in the 1990s revealed, for example, that about 90 percent of Mexican Americans there still use traditional household remedies, half rely on herbalists, a third turn to midwives, and 10 percent put their faith and their health in the hands of *curanderos*.

A Cure for Susto

Several ailments are unique to Mexican Americans, including *susto*. Characterized as extreme or "magical" fright or "loss of soul," *susto* may be caused by bad news or a bad scare, falling, or even encountering a ghost—and results in the spirit leaving the body. The victim may experience loss of appetite, weakness, chills, and nausea, and the syndrome can be fatal if not treated promptly.

The curandera *first blesses the bed by making the sign of the cross over it with a knife. The patient lies on his stomach while the healer "sweeps" his body with a bundle of aromatic herbs to drive away negative influences; she recites the Apostles' Creed and blesses his joints with holy water. After the patient turns on his back, the ritual is repeated.*

The curandera *then makes the sign of the cross with holy water on the patient's forehead and again blesses the joints. She invites the patient's spirit to return, to which the patient may respond "Aquí vengo" ("Here I come") or "Hay voy" ("There I go"), indicating that the spirit is indeed coming back.*

often throughout the Mexican American community. Indeed, some attract followers from far away and have been elevated to the status of folk saint. Don Pedrito Jaramillo, for one, a *curandero* who died in 1907, still draws pilgrims to the South Texas shrine erected in his honor.

These trusted practitioners treat life-threatening and chronic illnesses and are the only recourse against miseries—from insanity to bankruptcy—unleashed by *brujos*, or sorcerers, who are agents of Satan. *Curanderos* are also sought to combat certain maladies peculiar to Mexican Americans. *Empacho*, for instance, is an intestinal blockage that is cured by pulling the skin along the spine or abdomen, then letting it "snap" into place. The most common folk illness is *mal de ojo*, which occurs when a person, usually a child, is admired too much. One ritual cure involves making the sign of the cross over the patient's body several times with an egg, which draws out negative influences and pain, while reciting a prayer.

The Role of Faith

Curanderos have many methods of treatment at their disposal, as they have mastered all the knowledge held by household and neighborhood healers; in recent times, they may even refer patients to "Anglo" physicians. But their work is guided primarily by faith, with the Bible, holy water, rosary, and other spiritual aids playing as important a role as herbs and rituals. It is the healers' piety that allows them to channel God's will, helps them endure hours-long treatment sessions, and inspires confidence and calm in their patients. Their belief also sustains them through inevitable "failures." Suffering is part of life, and sin may be punished by illness or death, so they believe. If a patient recovers, it is by divine grace; if not, then that, too, is part of God's plan.

Likewise, their patients must have unshakable faith. "I have no healing power," Don Pedrito would modestly tell his patients. "It is the power of God released through your faith which heals you." Mexican Americans solicit God's aid through prayers, priests, and devotions to patron saints; they also employ an array of symbolic objects to protect against sickness. A small altar with votive candles, a crucifix, and pictures of the Blessed Virgin

Healers employ a range of objects *(right) in* curanderismo, *such as herbs, garlic, religious articles, oils, and candles portraying various saints. The* milagros *of a heart with a dagger (above) represents a "broken" or ailing heart.*

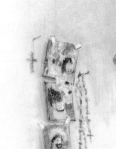

MORNING SICKNESS

Herbs taken for morning sickness by 19th-century mothers-to-be were most frequently steeped to make tea or mixed with "good old spirits." Before ginger beer appeared on the market, tea made from freshly cut rhizomes of ginger was often pre-scribed as a digestive aid. (Researchers now know that ginger contains anti-nausea compounds.) The spice, often combined with stomach-soothing chamomile or peppermint, was added to another well-known (and alcoholic) digestive aid—a bitter. Such aromatic herbs, along with cinnamon and lemon, have another distinction noted by herbalists: their scent helps to dis-tract the brain from sensations of nau-sea. For this reason, stewed mint or a lavender-laudanum compound was sometimes rubbed on pregnant bellies.

Other remedies included raspberry leaf, still touted as a pregnancy herb. However, any pregnancy-related prin-ciples remain unidentified, and research is inconclusive. Today herbalists and doctors agree that the less medicine a mother-to-be takes, the safer both she and the fetus are. Toxicity studies have been insufficient, and quality control remains a problem for many products.

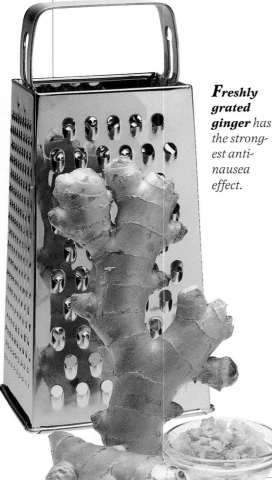

Freshly grated ginger has the strongest anti-nausea effect.

Easing the Quease

Nausea and vomiting occur during pregnancy because of changing hor-mone levels, which activate the brain's signals to the emetic, or vomiting, center. Roughly half of all pregnant women experience morning sickness at some point during their pregnancies. Symptoms occur by six weeks and last until about the 12th week. They usual-ly affect women in the morning, but they can occur at any time of the day. Everyday odors—a spouse's favorite cologne or food, for example—can suddenly trigger a run to the bathroom. Travel and stress also play a role.

A bland diet and small, light meals throughout the day are the standard recommendations. Eating soda crack-ers, sipping ginger ale, or sniffing a cut lemon before getting out of bed in the morning may also calm a queasy stom-ach. If vomiting is severe and pro-longed, prescription drugs and hospitalization may be required to prevent harm to the fetus and mother. Some over-the-counter products can be used as well, but—as with medicinal herbs—no drug should be taken during pregnancy unless approved by a doctor.

GINGER Studies show that ginger is often more effective for nausea than motion sickness medications and lacks their unpleasant side effects. It evident-ly affects the stomach, not the central nervous system, as do some commercial products. To ease morning sickness, make a tea by pouring 1 cup boiling water over ½ teaspoon freshly grated gingerroot. Steep for 5 minutes, then strain. Pregnant women should avoid ginger in capsules, which, doctors advise, are unsafe during pregnancy.

CHAMOMILE Its antispasmodic properties have made chamomile a favorite traditional remedy for indiges-tion. Pour 1 cup boiling water over 2 to 3 teaspoons minced German chamomile flowers. Steep for 5 to 10 minutes, then strain. Drink two or three times a day. Avoid chamomile oil.

LEMON Sniffing a slice of this aromatic citrus fruit is said to combat indigestion and mask the discomfort of an upset stomach.

MOTHERWORT

Leonurus cardiaca
LION'S-TAIL, LION'S-EAR

The various names for motherwort, a member of the mint family, say much about the herb. Its genus name, *Leonurus*, and the common names "lion's-ear" and "lion's-tail" come from its shaggy-looking leaves. The name "motherwort" reflects its use to regulate menstruation and to aid the expelling of the afterbirth from as far back as the days of ancient China.

Herb for the Heart?

Motherwort's species, *cardiaca* (from the Latin for "heart"), provides a clue to the ancient Greeks' use of the herb for heart palpitations—for which many modern herbalists still recommend it, even though its cardiac activity is largely confined to problems caused by anxiety and stress. Despite this, many leading herbalists sang the praises of this perennial herb and its benefits to the heart. Nicholas Culpeper proclaimed in his 17th-century herbal, "There is no herb better to drive melancholy vapours from the heart, to strengthen it, and to make [a] merry, cheerful, blithe soul..."

Today motherwort flourishes in fields, roadsides, and vacant lots across the continent. English settlers brought the herb here as a medicine for menstrual cramps. Later, the 19th-century Eclectics recommended it for everything from constipation to "nervous complaints" and "pains peculiar to females."

Today, some herbalists still recommend motherwort as a sedative and to promote menstruation, the latter due to leonurine, a chemical that acts as a uterine stimulant. German doctors often prescribe motherwort for psychosomatic cardiac disorders and as an adjunctive treatment for hyperthyroidism.

Mixed Findings

Modern research supports some of motherwort's traditional uses as a uterine tonic and heart medicine. Nevertheless, the herb is absent from many leading medicinal plant references. Clinical studies have reported antispasmodic, blood-thinning, antiviral, tumor-inhibiting, and cancer-fighting properties, but these studies have included species of *Leonurus* other than *L. cardiaca*—wholly different plants that share the common name "motherwort." Because of this, scientists are not only unsure of the presence of the active compounds in *L. cardiaca* and their effects, but also question the therapeutic value.

Furthermore, no data have been published on motherwort's toxicity. Given these uncertainties, many leading herbalists no longer recommend motherwort. Most agree that other sedative herbs, such as valerian or kava, are more effective.

Active plant parts Flower
Uses Menstrual inducer and regulator, sedative, cardiac tonic
Cautions Some people may experience allergic reactions to motherwort. Pregnant and nursing women should avoid the herb because of a lack of data on toxicity, its reputed effect on the menstrual cycle, and its documented effects on the uterus. Excessive use of motherwort may interfere with medications for heart problems. If a heart ailment is suspected, consult a doctor for diagnosis and medication.

MOTION SICKNESS

Among early North American settlers, motion sickness was a common ailment. Few could have escaped this torment during the voyage across the roiling Atlantic—especially those who traveled in the ship's steerage section, usually located near the rudder.

Motion sickness, caused by constant movement, begins in the organ of balance within the inner ear, which sends signals to the vomiting center in the brain stem. It can also be triggered by signals originating in the digestive tract. Drugs that suppress vomiting, called antiemetics, usually function by blocking these signals. Antihistamines, such as cyclizine, Dimenhydrinate, and Meclizine, block the signals and may also reduce the sensitivity of the vomiting center. Anticholinergics (drugs that suppress the parasympathetic nervous system), such as atropine, are also effective. However, many of these medications cause side effects, including drowsiness, dry mouth, sweating, and blurred vision. They should not be used during pregnancy.

To prevent motion sickness, sit near a window if possible, and focus on a point on the horizon. Sit in the middle of airplanes, not the rear. At sea, stay amidships and above deck. Above all, keep yourself

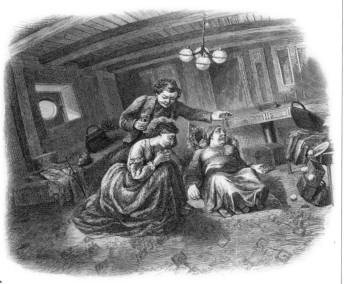

For those without sea legs, *ship travel can be a torment, as this 1863 engraving depicts.*

mentally busy. Studies have shown that those who keep their minds off their stomachs tend to get sick less often. Finally, avoid traveling on an empty stomach.

Cures for the Qualmish

Motion sickness has been the mother of many unusual cures. One remedy was to pinch the skin of one's inner wrist, about 2.5 cm (1 in.) from the palm. (Today some people wear bracelets that apply pressure to this point.) More dubious remedies involved taping a copper penny to the navel and wearing a cut-open paper bag around the chest under one's clothes.

Herbal cures included peppermint tea, which helps expels excess gas from the

intestines and also has a mild anaesthetizing effect on the stomach lining. Children were often given spearmint, which is less potent. Fennel and chamomile, which also expel gas and calm the gastrointestinal tract, were used as well.

Many put faith in bitter or acidic remedies—ingesting green tea or wormwood tinctures, chewing green olives, or sucking on lemons. Some drank the white of an egg and the juice of one lemon, beaten together and slightly sweetened. Others advised taking as much red pepper as possible in a bowl of hot soup to dispel all "sickness, nausea, and squeamishness." Except for small sips of green tea, which may help settle the stomach, there is no scientific explanation why any of these remedies would work.

The most effective motion sickness cure—ginger—was given minor billing by our forebears, although the Eclectic physicians used it in the late 1800s as a carminative and an appetite stimulant. In China, ginger has been valued for thousands of years for treating nausea and stomachache. A 1990 study found ginger to be superior to commercial products in relieving postoperative nausea. Ginger is thought to calm the gastrointestinal tract rather than the central nervous system. For best results, use fresh ginger, and take it up to four hours before traveling.

GINGER Ginger is the most effective herbal remedy for motion sickness. Take 1 gram in capsule form at least 30 minutes before travel and ½ to 1 gram more every 4 hours as symptoms occur. Do not exceed 2 to 4 grams in one day. Ginger is also available in the form of ginger candy. Large doses may cause stomach upset. Ginger is not recommended for those with gallstones.

MULLEIN

Verbascum thapsus
GREAT MULLEIN, CANDLEWICK PLANT, BLANKET LEAF, VELVET PLANT, HAG'S TAPER, FELTWORT, FLUFFWEED

Fuzzy as newborn kittens, the thickly furred leaves of great mullein have given this Eurasian native a host of names, including beggar's flannel and velvet dock. But its hidden properties are what sparked the interest of healers through the centuries, making mullein one of the most used plants in folk medicine. Respiratory ailments, including tuberculosis, asthma, colds, and coughs, topped the list. A tea made from a teaspoon of dried leaves in a cup of boiling water was not only a long-standing remedy for cold symptoms but for diarrhea as well. Of more questionable value was the widespread practice of smoking the leaves to relieve lung complaints.

Mullein was listed in the U.S. *National Formulary* in the late 19th and early 20th centuries, but was deleted in 1936 as ineffective. Still, the tea has remained popular as a home remedy. However, caution is required: The same hairs that make the plant so soft can be irritating when consumed and must be filtered out.

Great mullein is one of a half-dozen mullein species found in North America, all of them brought by European settlers. The herb quickly spread across the continent and now thrives on roadsides, in fields, and in other dry, sunny locations. A striking plant, great mullein raises a central stalk of yellow flowers that may reach 1.8 m (6 ft) in height. The closely related moth mullein is shorter and smooth-leaved, bearing large white or pale yellow flowers. Although abundant in the wild (and a favorite among wildflower gardeners), it is rarely used as a medicinal herb.

Promise Unfulfilled

Although mullein was one of the most respected of wild medicinal plants, scientists have found that it has surprisingly few active compounds. The leaves and flowers do contain relatively small amounts of gelatinous mucilage, which can soothe irritated tissues, giving credence to mullein's use in sore throat remedies. It also contains saponins, which help loosen phlegm. The crushed leaves are a mild astringent; combined with the plant's limited anti-inflammatory properties, this may explain mullein's frequent use in compresses for hemorrhoids.

Its pharmacological value may be minimal, but mullein has an undisputed attribute, one that was appreciated by generations of country women unwilling (often because of religious beliefs) to use makeup. Rubbed gently on the face, the thick, velvety leaves give a flush of healthy pink to the cheeks—and yet another name, Quaker rouge, to this multifaceted plant.

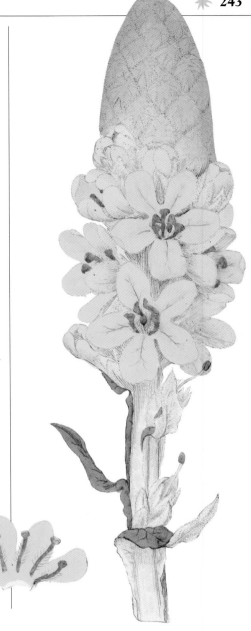

Active plant parts Flowers, leaves
Uses Coughs and other respiratory disorders, sore throat, irritated skin
Cautions When preparing mullein tea, strain the liquid through a fine mesh cloth to filter out the irritating hairs before drinking. The plant's seeds are toxic.

MUMPS

The mumps vaccine, usually given to children in their second year, has dramatically reduced the incidence of the disease. Before the vaccine, however, almost every child got mumps, and it is still common in unimmunized children and adults. A flu-like virus, mumps cannot be cured, but home remedies can be used to relieve some of its unpleasant symptoms.

Grimace and Bear It

Mumps (the word derives from "mump," an old word for "grimace") is characterized by the swelling of the salivary glands between the ear and the angle of the jaw on one or both sides of the face; this often causes a sore throat and makes swallowing difficult. Sufferers are bound to grimace while symptoms persist, usually about 10 days. Symptoms include fatigue, fever, headache, diarrhea, and, in teenagers and adults, swollen testicles (in men) or sore breasts and abdominal pain (in women).

The best treatments for mumps have helped relieve discomfort in the face and throat. Goldenseal root tea, with its proven anti-inflammatory effect on the mucous membranes (in the nose, mouth, throat, and sinuses), was drunk and gargled to treat sore gums. Sage, myrrh, and rhatany were also used to treat soreness in the mouth and throat; Indians of the American Southwest used rhatany for "spongy gums." Other favorites were yarrow, boneset, and echinacea; the latter was thought to reduce the swelling of the salivary glands. A spoonful of honey was taken to make swallowing easier.

Adults who have not previously had mumps and have never been immunized are still vulnerable. The usual treatment for mumps includes liquids (avoid citrus juices which stimulate the salivary glands), analgesics, and rest.

Although serious complications, including meningitis, pancreatitis, and sterility, are rare, see a doctor if you experience sore testicles or breasts, a fever higher than 39.4°C (103°F), vomiting, severe headaches, fatigue, or ringing in the ears.

"Tied 'Round the Head"

A most common treatment was a rope or scarf wrapped around the head and tied on top. Flannel and silk wrappings were said to keep mumps from "descending" (affecting the breasts or testicles). Commonly bound to the swelling were the grease from a hog's jaw, cudweed leaves, fish oils, camphor, and bread and milk.

The North American settlers also drank teas made from chamomile, catnip, and poke; some drew crosses with charcoal on their cheeks. Indian remedies included prickly pear "leaves" (roasted without the spines), boiled cedar sprigs, and highbush cranberry tea.

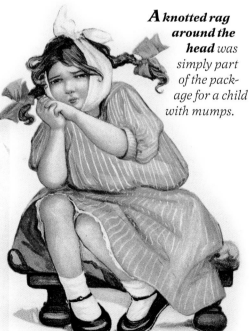

A knotted rag around the head *was simply part of the package for a child with mumps.*

PEPPERMINT Peppermint has reported activity against the mumps virus. To make a tea, pour boiling water over 1 tablespoon finely chopped leaves, steep, then strain. Drink 3 to 4 cups a day. Or take 1 to 2 capsules of the oil (available commercially) up to four times a day. Large doses of the oil are toxic.

HONEY Honey can soothe a sore throat. Take 1 teaspoon straight up or mix 1 to 3 teaspoons into a favorite tea and drink up to four times a day. Do not give to infants. Cough drops are also available.

LEMON BALM To make a sedative tea, pour boiling water over 2 to 4 teaspoons finely chopped leaves, steep, then strain. Drink 3 to 4 cups a day. This herb's antiviral effect, which has shown the potential to work against the mumps virus, may be due to polyphenolic compounds.

MYRRH Add 5 to 10 drops of anti-inflammatory tincture (available commercially) to a glass of water. Gargle up to three times a day. Ingesting myrrh may affect the menstrual cycle and interfere with diabetes treatments.

MUSCLE CRAMPS

Nobody knows why muscle cramps are called "charley horses"—the term arose among baseball players around 1890—but anyone who has had a cramp knows it can be a real pain. Happily, several folk remedies are still viable today, including stretching, applying herbal oils, and taking a walk.

Rub It Up ...

Most common in the legs and abdomen, a cramp is the overcontraction of a muscle. It is a spasm, not a strain, that may result from dehydration, fatigue, aging, or simply pointing the toes. Another cause of cramping, especially among the elderly, is a lack of blood flow to the affected tissue. In such a case, massaging the muscle can bring safe and effective relief; "rubbing out" a cramp stimulates local circulation.

Liniments—made from mustard seed, turpentine, peppermint, camphor, and cayenne pepper—have long been used to relieve tight muscles. Generally, these rubs only mask pain by causing a sensation on the skin. More effective, perhaps, are oils made from wintergreen and sweet birch, which contain painkillers like those in aspirin. All of these remedies, however, can irritate the skin and are toxic if ingested; they should not be used on small children.

Taking ginkgo biloba can improve circulation and prevent cramps. Quinine has long been taken to ward off leg cramps at night, and it is still used in Canada. To prevent nighttime leg cramps, take vitamin E at bedtime and sleep on your back, with your feet slightly elevated. Also, untuck your covers to keep your toes from pointing.

... And Work It Out

To quickly relieve a cramp, slowly stretch the muscle and massage it. For a thigh cramp, straighten your leg. For a cramped calf, pull your toes gently toward your knee. (Similarly, John Wesley, in his 1747 *Primitive Physick*, endorsed "jutting out

Hawaiian folk healers roll warm, round stones over cramped muscles. The warm massage brings relief.

the heel." He also ate apple jelly on toast for a stitch in the side.) A brisk walk and a hot bath can also help. If a cramp occurs during exercise, take a water break.

Prevention of chronic muscle cramping entails eating foods high in potassium, calcium, or magnesium, and drinking lots of water. Regular stretching and mild exercise also help. Consult a physician if muscle cramps occur frequently or for a long period of time; they may indicate a neurological or circulatory problem.

WINTERGREEN OR BIRCH OIL Rub a cramp with a mixture of 1 part wintergreen or sweet birch oil to 4 parts vegetable oil. Both contain analgesic methyl salicylate and stimulate blood flow. Use up to four times a day. Do not ingest or apply after exercise, in hot, humid weather, while using a heating pad, or on sensitive or broken skin.

ARNICA Potentially toxic, arnica should only be used in commercial ointments that contain no more than 15 percent arnica oil. Apply to sore muscles up to three times a day, every one to two hours. Do not ingest or use on broken skin.

KNEE BANDS Tie a cord snugly just under your knee to prevent calf cramps brought on by exercise. Modern athletes still use this old folk remedy, but exactly why it works is not understood. Do not cut off circulation with too tight a band.

COLD FLOORS To relieve a leg cramp, stand barefoot on a cold floor. The coolness underfoot decreases blood flow and may help relax the tightened muscle.

MUSTARD

Brassica nigra (BLACK MUSTARD)
B. juncea (BROWN MUSTARD)
Sinapis alba (WHITE MUSTARD)

Used since the Middle Ages as a condiment, mustard also has a respectable medicinal history. The three varieties of mustard—black, brown, and white—were used similarly in folk medicine and share common chemical properties. To the Indians and the pioneers, mustard was a versatile medicine. The seeds were chewed to soothe a toothache and eaten to relieve fever and bronchial conditions. Ground seeds made a snuff for headaches and head colds. Less than a teaspoon of the powdered seed in a glass of water served as a laxative.

A Traditional Plaster

Mustard seed's most common use was as a plaster, applied with a clean cloth to relieve arthritis pain and cold symptoms.

Swallow ¼ teaspoon mustard powder mixed with 2 tablespoons honey to loosen chest congestion.

Made by mixing the powdered seed with flour and just enough warm (not hot) water to form a paste, the plaster can relieve muscle and joint pain by stimulating heat and local circulation. Applied to the chest, the plaster's heat and pungent aroma can relieve congestion and cough.

A mustard plaster produces heat without being hot to the touch. Mixing water with the powdered seed forms a volatile oil, called allylisothiocyanate, that irritates (and can burn) the skin, increasing blood flow. Although mustard oil can be harmful, Health Canada allows its use in commercial liniments in low concentrations (0.5 to 5 percent).

When using a mustard plaster, do not let the skin become too red. To soothe any burning, wash the area with cold water. Protect the skin beforehand by applying petroleum jelly to the area. To make a milder plaster, use less mustard powder or replace the water with milk or an egg.

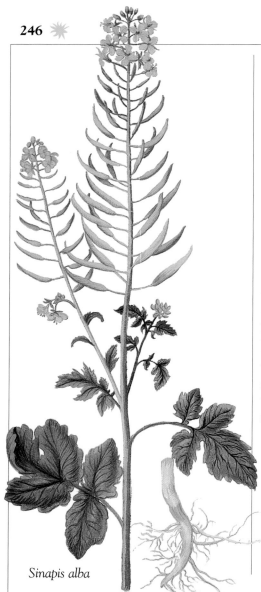

Sinapis alba

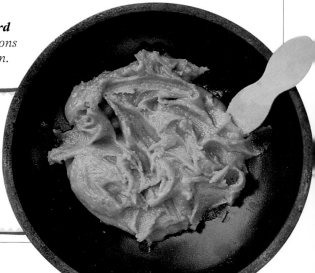

Active plant parts Seeds
Uses Sinus and chest congestion, foot problems, indigestion, joint and muscle pain
Cautions Mustard plasters can burn and blister sensitive skin after only 15 minutes. Prolonged external use can result in skin and nerve damage and should not exceed two weeks. The undiluted volatile oil should not be ingested, inhaled, or applied to the skin. Mustard fumes may irritate the eyes, nose, and lungs (in fact, mustard derivatives are used as chemical weapons). Ingesting more than 1 teaspoon of mustard powder can cause blotchy skin, vomiting, and gastrointestinal problems. Children under the age of six and people with kidney problems should not ingest the seed or oil.

NAUSEA & VOMITING

Considering the lengths to which people have gone to check vomiting, it is almost surprising that some of the measures, such as eating the lining of a chicken's gizzard, did not have the opposite effect. Of course, as the settlers knew, brief vomiting does serve a purpose, and is often followed by relief of nausea and stomach pain. Repeated vomiting, however, is pointless, and may cause dehydration. (In this case, drink clear liquids as soon as you are able.)

Many things can trigger vomiting, which is controlled by its own center in the brain stem. Food poisoning, alcohol, motion sickness, migraines, and pregnancy are common culprits. Other causes include some medications, head injuries, and disorders of the stomach or intestine.

To prevent vomiting, some people tied a dishcloth around the throat; others applied cold water. More standard were peppermint water (or candy) and ginger or chamomile tea—all good choices. Ginger has been proven to allay nausea and prevent motion sickness. Peppermint, which has a mild anesthetizing effect on the lining of the stomach, is also recommended. Chamomile calms the stomach and may have a sedative effect.

Feverfew was commonly used as a stomach tonic and also to quell nausea.

Today the herb has been found to be most useful against migraine headaches—and the nausea and vomiting that often accompany them.

Popular among the Indians and the settlers alike was tea made from the bark of the peach tree, which contains a compound that inhibits spasms of the gastrointestinal tract. Some people placed chunks of charcoal in water, let them stand, and drained off the water, which they drank every 5 to 10 minutes. Today, activated charcoal tablets are the preferred form of administration. Charcoal briquettes like those used in barbecues won't do: they contain substances that should not be ingested.

Finally, the Eclectics prescribed extracts of the kola nut (which first made its way to the continent after the American Civil War) for seasickness and morning sickness. Later, coke syrup became a popular elixir. Its anti-emetic properties are likely due to the ginger and cassia it is flavored with. Today many moms still offer sips of flat cola to their ailing children.

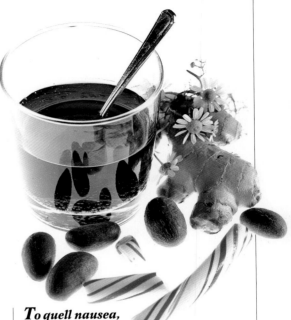

To quell nausea, *try cola (from the kola nut), ginger, chamomile, or peppermint.*

See a doctor if...

◆ You have severe abdominal pain that is not relieved by vomiting.
◆ You have diarrhea or a temperature of 37.8°C (100°F) or above.
◆ You have vomited red blood or black or dark brown matter.
◆ You have a headache accompanied by pain when you bend your head forward.
◆ Your vision is blurred and you have severe pain in or around one eye.

GINGER Ginger is excellent at relieving nausea, and also quells motion sickness. To make a tea, steep ¼ to ½ teaspoon minced root in 1 cup boiling water, then strain. Capsules and candies are also available.

COKE SYRUP Coke syrup eases nausea, probably because of its ginger and cassia content. Ask for some at the soda counter of a local restaurant, and sip ½ to 1 teaspoon at a time. Or stir a glass of cola until the bubbles disappear, then take small sips.

PEPPERMINT Peppermint calms the stomach and expels gas from the intestines, which may help allay nausea. To make a tea, pour 1 cup boiling water over 1 tablespoon chopped leaves. Steep, then strain. Peppermint capsules are also available.

NETTLE

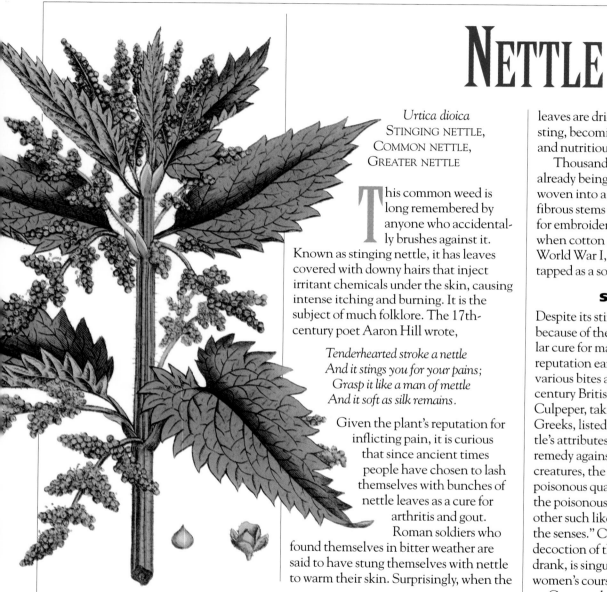

Urtica dioica
STINGING NETTLE,
COMMON NETTLE,
GREATER NETTLE

This common weed is long remembered by anyone who accidentally brushes against it. Known as stinging nettle, it has leaves covered with downy hairs that inject irritant chemicals under the skin, causing intense itching and burning. It is the subject of much folklore. The 17th-century poet Aaron Hill wrote,

Tenderhearted stroke a nettle
And it stings you for your pains;
Grasp it like a man of mettle
And it soft as silk remains.

Given the plant's reputation for inflicting pain, it is curious that since ancient times people have chosen to lash themselves with bunches of nettle leaves as a cure for arthritis and gout. Roman soldiers who found themselves in bitter weather are said to have stung themselves with nettle to warm their skin. Surprisingly, when the leaves are dried or cooked, they lose their sting, becoming a source of a pleasant tea and nutritious cooked greens.

Thousands of years ago nettle was already being harvested for its fiber and woven into a linen-like material. Its long, fibrous stems were used by many Indians for embroidery and fishing nets. Later, when cotton supplies dwindled during World War I, nettle was once again tapped as a source of fabric.

Stinging Cure

Despite its stinging hairs—or more likely because of them—nettle became a popular cure for many ills. The herb gained a reputation early on as an antidote to various bites and poisons. The 17th-century British herbalist Nicholas Culpeper, taking his cue from the ancient Greeks, listed the following among nettle's attributes: "The seed being drank, is a remedy against the stinging of venomous creatures, the biting of mad dogs, the poisonous qualities of hemlock, henbane, the poisonous nightshade, mandrake, or other such like herbs that stupify or dull the senses." Culpeper also advised, "The decoction of the leaves in wine, being drank, is singularly good to provoke women's courses."

Conversely, nettle was also used to treat hemorrhages of the uterus, infant diarrhea, and hemorrhoids, probably because of its astringent properties. *King's American Dispensatory* called nettle "an excellent styptic." The dried, crushed leaf was sniffed to cure nosebleeds. Indian women drank nettle tea to stop bleeding

---

Active plant parts Leaves, roots, and seeds
Uses Rheumatic complaints, gout, urinary and kidney problems
Cautions Do not give nettle to children under two years of age. Give the herb to older children and people over 65 with caution. Nettle stimulates uterine contractions in rabbits; therefore, pregnant women should not use nettle internally. The herb should not be used for water retention as a result of impaired cardiac or renal function.

after childbirth. The settlers followed suit and also drank the tea to increase the mother's production of milk. Scientists have since confirmed that nettle does in fact check bleeding.

In both Europe and North America, nettle tea was drunk as an expectorant to treat coughs and tuberculosis, and dried nettle leaves were smoked to ease asthma attacks—a practice considered ill-advised today. Perhaps inspired by the hairy appearance of the plant's leaves, some people rubbed nettle juice, pressed from the leaves and stems, into the scalp to stimulate hair growth; the juice was found in many hair-growth nostrums well into the 19th century. Today nettle is sometimes added to shampoo or used as a conditioner to add luster to hair.

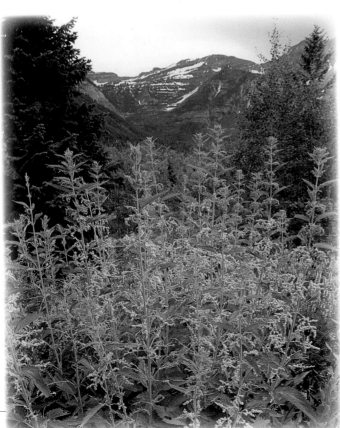

A Nutritious Tonic

Nettle was perhaps best known as a diuretic and spring tonic, and both uses were noted by Culpeper: "Nettle Tops eaten in the Spring consume the phlegmatic superfluities in the body of man, that the coldness and moistness of Winter hath left behind." Nettle was also thought to reverse anemia and boost poor circulation. The herb is indeed rich in iron, which makes it useful in treating anemia's symptoms but not the underlying cause.

Moreover, young nettle stalks are good sources of protein and vitamins A and C. The herb's vitamin C content may explain why herbalists once prescribed nettle to treat scurvy. Indian women may have known about nettle's nutritional merits because they drank nettle tea during pregnancy to strengthen the fetus. Also, eating the young leaves was said to improve the complexion.

North America's 19th-century Eclectic physicians used nettle as a diuretic to treat urinary, bladder, and kidney problems. Today, because of its diuretic action, nettle is considered useful in treating urinary difficulties associated with benign prostate conditions. The root has been found to be mildly effective in treating an enlarged prostate.

Although it is wind-pollinated, *nettle may provide welcome relief from hay fever.*

An Edible Herb

In many parts of the world, nettle is used as a pot herb. Fortunately, boiling or drying the plant eliminates its fearsome sting. Look for nettle in weedy places, usually near water. Harvest the leaves in late spring or summer wearing gloves, long pants, and a long-sleeved shirt. The leaves can be steamed like spinach or simmered in soups. Tender shoots do not sting and may be used raw in salads.

Even if you don't care for nettle as food, your houseplants may: a strong infusion is said to help them grow.

Hay Fever Medicine

Nettle may have several other modern uses. There is some evidence that the herb is effective against arthritis, possibly because of its diuretic action. Since the days of ancient Rome, gout sufferers have stung themselves with nettle leaves to relieve the pain. Although this practice may have succeeded in numbing the affected joint, it is not recommended today. Some herbalists believe that painless, long-term topical applications of the juice may provide relief, although there is no proof of this. It has also been postulated that the consumption of nettle may work against gout inflammation by lowering the amount of uric acid in the blood, but further studies are needed.

Finally, some herbalists propose nettle as an alternative to antihistamines for use against hay fever, although no one is sure why it works. The recommended dosage is one or two capsules of freeze-dried extract every two to four hours. At least one study has shown that these capsules provide significant relief among some people.

NETTLE BURN

When you brush up against or handle the nettle plant, its stinging hairs inject amines (similar to the body's histamines) into the skin and cause a burning rash. This condition is called nettle burn or nettle rash, terms that have come to cover all rashes and wheals that result from contact with the resins and "mechanical" parts of plants—namely, thorns, bristles, and hairs.

Folk healers used an arsenal of plants directly on the skin in a healing capacity. Before folk remedies are applied, however, the affected skin should first be cleaned using rubbing alcohol or soap and water.

Guilty Bystanders

The nettle family (Urticaceae), which contains an estimated 500 plants, is only one group of plants that can cause a rash. Species of *Toxicodendron*, such as poison ivy, contain irritating urushiol. Other known irritants are sinigrin, of the mustard family; anemonin, of the buttercup family; and bromelain, from pineapple husks. Daffodil and hyacinth bulbs can cause wheals on the fingers—a condition known as "bulb fingers." Roses, artichokes, and cacti can also do harm.

Good Neighbors

After gently cleaning away any bristles, dirt, or resin (which, if left on the skin, can spread the rash), several plants can be used to soothe the effects of their more caustic brethren. Plantain, which often grows near nettle, was used to heal nettle burn; however, plantain can also cause dermatitis. Jewelweed, deemed by *King's American Dispensatory* (1898) to relieve "the effects of stinging nettle," has been used on many rashes, such as poison ivy. Calendula ointment, nondistilled witch hazel, and arnica ex-tract have also proven their healing value.

ARNICA Arnica's counterirritant effect helps relieve the inflammation of a rash. Use a commercial ointment that contains no more than 15 percent arnica oil. Apply up to three times a day, every one to two hours. Arnica is potentially toxic; do not ingest or use on broken skin.

GINKGO Take standardized ginkgo biloba extract in tablet form (40 milligrams) three times a day with meals. Ginkgo reduces a rash's initial flare-up.

PLANTAIN To make a soothing wash, add one part commercial plantain leaf extract to one part alcohol (25 percent) solution. Apply three times a day. Long-term use of plantain can cause dermatitis.

GOLDENSEAL To make an anti-inflammatory wash, add 1 teaspoon goldenseal tincture to ½ cup water. Alternatively, moisten the crushed dried rhizome with water and apply as a paste. Apply either one to the affected skin three times a day.

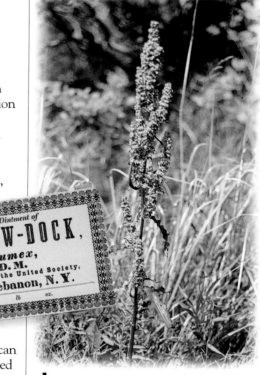

Astringent ointments *made from the root of the yellow dock plant were sold by 19th-century Shaker communities.*

Another old-fashioned soother is the oatmeal bath. Oat extracts have been used as emollients for more than a century, and studies have shown that the gluten content of oatmeal can effectively treat dry, itchy skin. Rubbing the skin with the leaves of rosemary, sage, and mint has also been tried, although in these cases mild relief may come only from the rubbing itself. The root of yellow dock (the subject of an old rhyme: "Nettle in, dock out/Dock rub the nettle out!") can be made into a soothing, astringent wash. Washes of goldenseal or chamomile can also help, as can applications of evening primrose oil and fresh aloe vera gel.

NIGHTSHADE

Solanum nigrum (BLACK NIGHTSHADE)
S. dulcamara (WOODY NIGHTSHADE)
Atropa belladonna (DEADLY NIGHTSHADE)

The nightshades, of which black, woody, and deadly are the most common, are one tough bunch. Although they have been widely used in folk medicine, the plants are extremely toxic—the black sheep in a large plant family (Solanaceae) that includes such familiar relatives as tomato, potato, pepper, eggplant, and tobacco.

"Sleeping Even Unto Death"

The genus of both black and woody nightshade, *Solanum*, derives from *solamen* (Latin for "soothing"), and its leaf tea acts as a narcotic sedative. The plant's toxin, solanine, is responsible; it depresses digestion, circulation, and breathing. John Gerard, in his *Herbal* (1633), writes of the well known danger: "some [nightshades] cause sleeping even unto death."

Solanine also irritates the digestive tract, causing abdominal pain, vomiting, and diarrhea. Hence, nightshade was used as both an emetic and a purge. Gerard himself touted black nightshade to remedy St. Anthony's fire and shingles, conditions that were thought to be cured by driving evil humors from the body.

The Comanche and the Rappahannock drank the leaf tea to treat tuberculosis and expel worms. It was also taken for colic, asthma, rheumatism, measles, and mumps. Nightshade tea was even given to Beth March to treat scarlet fever in Louisa May Alcott's *Little Women* (1868).

The crushed leaves and berries were made into poultices to relieve burns, "cancers," inflammations, and arthritis. Some folk healers applied the leaves to insect bites and rashes.

Devil's Herb Gone Good?

Despite their medicinal utility, the nightshades connoted death and evil. The Devil himself was thought to tend deadly nightshade, and the plant was known as devil's herb. Its genus name, *Atropa*, derives from Atropos, one of the three Fates of Greek mythology, who wields the shears with which to cut the thread of life.

The nightshades are still valued medicinally. Extracts of woody nightshade (also known as bittersweet) have been found to have antitumor activity. Two constituents in deadly nightshade that calm the digestive tract, hyoscyamus and mandragora, are used in antispasmodic drugs for diarrhea, irritable colon, and peptic ulcers. A third, atropine, is used by eye doctors to dilate the pupils during examinations. Its nickname, belladonna (Italian for "beautiful lady"), is said to derive from its use by Italian women to make their eyes look more attractive.

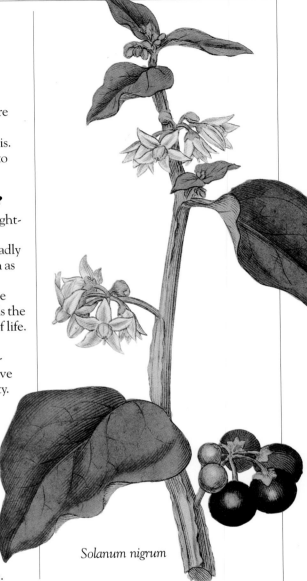

Solanum nigrum

Active plant parts Leaves
Uses Prescription drugs for diarrhea, irritable colon, and peptic ulcers
Cautions All parts of the plant are toxic, especially the leaves and the unripe berries. Symptoms of poisoning include headache, stomachache, subnormal temperature, dilated pupils, paralysis, vertigo, vomiting, diarrhea, speech difficulties, shock, circulatory and respiratory depression, and death. The unripe berries may be fatal if ingested by children.

NOSEBLEED

Dry winter air, a lingering head cold, an unlucky bounce in a schoolyard basketball game—there are many ways a nosebleed can start, and even more folk remedies to staunch the flow. Placing a cold metal object on the back of the neck—steel scissors, a silver spoon, or a butter knife straight from the icebox—has long been a favorite on the theory that the chill slows the flow of blood. Likewise, ice-water and snow are used.

The moist passages inside the nose are jammed with blood vessels, which warm cold air before it reaches the lungs. But these vessels also easily dry out in the parched, heated air of homes in winter. This drying can irritate the nasal linings and clog the sinuses: the resulting raw, tender tissue, combined with frequent nose blowing, can lead to bleeding. To prevent nosebleeds, use a humidifier, especially at night in the bedroom. Also, blow your nose as gently as possible.

Pond Slime and Charms

To help the blood to clot, Indians sniffed the dust-like spores of puffball fungi, a practice European settlers also brought with them from the Old World. The settlers also sometimes used finely powdered salt beef instead of the foul-smelling puffballs, which may cause pulmonary disorders. The dried, pulverized leaves of many species of medicinal plants—plantain and nettles among them—were used to pack bleeding nostrils.

In the Spanish Southwest, blue-green algae—the filamentous "slime" that grows in stagnant ponds—was considered a good preventive against nosebleeds. A wet, stringy handful was placed on the back of the neck and kept there until it turned dry and yellow. Folk herbalists often prescribed a tincture of yarrow. This aromatic plant also had a very different— and more curious—connection to nosebleeds. Appalachian girls of courting age

would hold a sprig of yarrow flowers beneath their noses and sing, "Yarroway, yarroway, bear a white blow/If my lover loves me my nose will bleed now." Disappointment must have been rather frequent: simply smelling a yarrow will not cause a hemorrhage in the nose. Instead, yarrow can actually stanch bleeding.

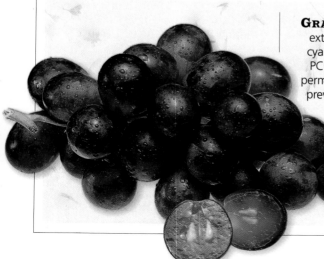

GRAPE SEED Standardized grape seed extracts contain 92 to 95 percent procyanidolic oligomers (commonly called PCOs), which reportedly decrease the permeability and fragility of capillaries. To prevent nosebleeds, take 50 milligrams of the extract daily. If a nosebleed occurs, take 150 to 300 milligrams daily for therapeutic purposes.

The seeds of red grapes contain helpful PCOs.

PLANTAIN Break a fresh plantain leaf to release the juice, then insert the leaf into the nostril until the bleeding subsides. Plantain is effective against nosebleeds because of its mucilage content. No side effects have been reported.

YARROW Yarrow has astringent properties, which help stop bleeding. To stop a nosebleed, insert a small amount of clean, fresh yarrow leaf into the nostril. Severe allergic reactions may occur in some people, although these are rare. Yarrow extracts are also available.

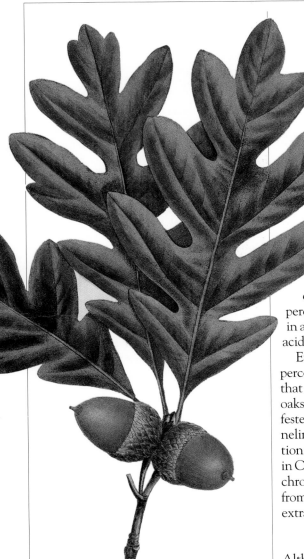

OAK

Quercus spp.

With more than 200 species to choose from, it is not surprising that the Indians used oaks as both food and medicine. Acorns were a staple of many Indian diets, and the tannin-rich bark of some species was used as a healing agent. The white oak contains so much tannic acid (8 to 10 percent) that its acorns had to be placed in a stream, which leached out enough acid to make them edible.

Even richer in tannins, at 50 to 80 percent, are nutgalls: marble-sized knobs that form on the trunk and branches of oaks as a response to insect damage. Infested trees protect themselves by channeling tannic acid to the site of the infection. The nutgalls—prized for centuries in China as a treatment for bleeding, chronic diarrhea, and dysentery—are cut from the tree, and their tannic acid is extracted for pharmaceutical use.

Gastrointestinal Aid

Although all species of *Quercus* have similar therapeutic properties, white oak is the most common source for powdered oak bark in North American products. Today, white oak bark is an ingredient in a number of prepared herbal mixtures and over-the-counter gastrointestinal remedies. Extracts and tea bags are also sold.

White oak's high tannin content makes it an effective treatment for diarrhea. With its mild astringent and antiseptic properties, tannic acid reduces intestinal inflammation by binding to the surface protein layer of the inflamed mucous membrane. Externally, extracts of oak bark are used to treat hemorrhoids, such skin conditions as eczema, and inflammation of the gums and the mucous membranes of the throat.

Home Remedies

To make a white oak decoction, break open a few capsules and add ½ teaspoon powdered bark to 1 cup cold water. Boil for five minutes, strain, and let cool before drinking. To treat diarrhea, drink two or three cups a day. (But take note: If diarrhea continues for more than two days, consult your doctor.) To make a hemorrhoid ointment, simmer the decoction until thickened, then combine it with an equal amount of vegetable shortening.

Fresh leaves plucked from an oak can also be used in home remedies. For minor wounds, make a poultice by bruising a few leaves and placing them directly on the affected area; then cover with a warm cloth and secure it with gauze or a bandage. To soothe a sore throat, pour 2 cups boiling water over six or seven bruised oak leaves and let steep for 10 minutes. Strain and let cool before using as a gargle.

Active plant parts Bark, leaves
Uses Diarrhea, hemorrhoids, sore throat, minor wounds
Cautions No contraindications for internal use are known, but do not consume large amounts. Do not use oak externally on large areas of damaged skin.

ONION

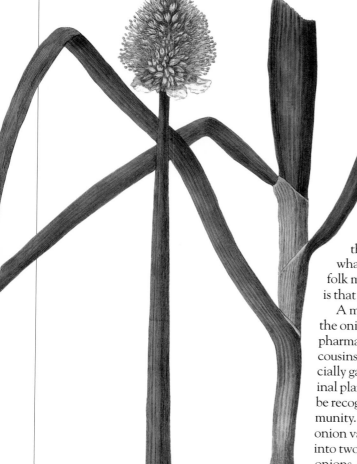

Allium cepa

It is said that George Washington's favorite remedy for the common cold was "always to eat, just before I step into bed, a hot roasted onion." Indeed, Washington was hardly alone in relying on the humble onion to cure what ailed him. In the world of folk medicine, onion's special aura is that of a panacea.

A member of the genus *Allium*, the onion has much in common pharmacologically with its cousins—leeks, shallots, and especially garlic, whose value as a medicinal plant has only recently begun to be recognized by the scientific community. The scores of different onion varieties are generally divided into two main categories: spring onions, with green tops and white bulb that are mild in flavor; and globe onions, with dry outer skins and a stronger, more pungent flavor. Shallots, with the characteristics of onions and garlic, are considerably milder than both.

Active plant parts Bulb, green tops
Uses Cuts and abrasions; anticoagulant
Cautions Eating too many onions may cause gastrointestinal distress.

Head to Toe

Many early North Americans believed that rubbing a little onion juice on the scalp and lying in the sun would cure baldness. To ease a head cold, folk healers advised putting slices of raw onion in the bottoms of socks and wearing the socks to bed. A remedy for earache called for carefully placing the heart of a roasted onion into the ear canal. In a standard treatment that has been in use for centuries, a halved raw onion was rubbed on a wound or insect bite to prevent infection.

The onion was considered equally effective when taken internally for an almost limitless range of health problems. Folk practitioners swore by a glass of milk mixed with chopped onions to cure sore throat. Some claimed that alternately ingesting a teacupful of red-onion juice and a half-liter of horsemint tea would remedy kidney stones. Even today, a syrup made of boiled onion water and honey is administered by grandmothers convinced of its power over coughs and colds.

Explorers on an 1832 expedition to chart the Missouri River basin found an altogether different use for onion. Afflicted with scurvy, they cured themselves by consuming wild onions. Today scientists know why they got better: scurvy is caused by a dietary shortage of vitamin C, of which onions are a good source.

Cultivated for nearly 6,000 years around the world, the onion is believed to have originated in Afghanistan or Persia; even now it is referred to in China as the Muhammadan onion. To the ancient Egyptians, the onion bulb was a symbol of the multilayered universe: they made offerings of onion to their gods, depicted the plant frequently in their tomb paintings, and took oaths on an onion, just as people do today on the Bible. As a food, the onion was such a staple that the Egyptians are reported to have traded eight tonnes of gold for onions to feed the builders of the pyramids.

Heart to Stomach

Although there is no scientific evidence to support some of the more outlandish claims for onions—including curing baldness and the common cold—some research has verified other long-held beliefs and suggests that the onion may be beneficial in the treatment of serious medical conditions.

Folk healers have advocated onions as a "heart tonic" for centuries. Researchers have now confirmed that an organic compound in onions, called adenosine, functions as an anticoagulating agent as effective as aspirin. This finding suggests that eating onions may be useful in preventing heart attacks, strokes, coronary thrombosis, and atherosclerosis.

Furthermore, scientists have discovered that allicin—a volatile sulfur compound contained in all the members of the Allium family—is a powerful antibacterial agent, lending credence to the effectiveness of onions in the treatment of wounds and infections. There is also evidence that eating onions may help lower blood pressure, regulate blood sugar, and raise the levels of the high-density lipoproteins (HDLs, the so-called good cholesterol), which may protect against the clogging of arteries.

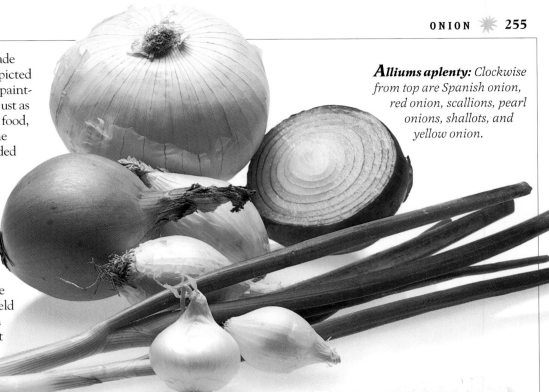

Alliums aplenty: Clockwise from top are Spanish onion, red onion, scallions, pearl onions, shallots, and yellow onion.

It has been demonstrated that cooking onions reduces or eliminates many of their healthful benefits, so most experts recommend eating onions raw as frequently as possible. There is a price to pay, of course—the resulting "onion breath" after eating onions and the unpleasant odor on the hands after chopping them. (Roll fresh lavender flowers between the fingers to mask the scent on the hands.)

Sulfur compounds in onions are responsible for the onion odor, but they may be worth the trouble. These same compounds have been found to block the cancer-causing potential of certain carcinogens. Two large-scale studies, one in China and the other in Italy, found a reduced number of deaths from stomach cancer among people who consumed large quantities of raw onions or other members of the Allium family.

Harvesting Bulbs

If you grow your own onions, ensure maximum concentration of the plant's active principles by bending the green tops over with the back of a rake once they have turned yellow; this will divert the plant's energy to the bulbs instead of the stems. In a day or so, after the tops have turned brown, lift the bulbs with a fork. Let them cure for a few days on the soil, covering them with a thin layer of straw to protect them from the sun. While you're at it, try this folk weather-forecasting trick: Count a newly harvested onion's outer layers of skin. Folklore holds that if the layers are thin and few, winter will be mild. If they are thick and numerous, the winter will be a harsh one.

PARSLEY

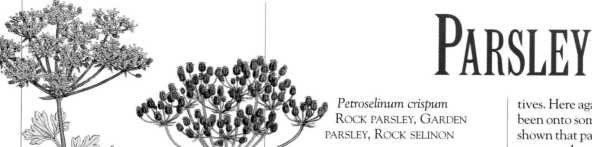

Petroselinum crispum
ROCK PARSLEY, GARDEN
PARSLEY, ROCK SELINON

Well known for its culinary use and as a dinner-plate garnish at restaurants, parsley has also enjoyed a distinguished history as a medicinal herb. More than 2,000 years ago, the Greeks and Romans employed the little green plant—its leaves, as well as the roots and seeds—for digestive, kidney, and menstrual irregularities. Although the early North Americans used parsley to treat dozens of ailments, its potency is mild at best, and today its medicinal use is limited.

Eat That Garnish!

There are three possible reasons for parsley's conspicuous place at dinner. First, parsley was once thought to help keep you sober and improve liver function, no matter how much you imbibed at the evening meal. (Not surprisingly, there is no evidence to support this claim.) Second, parsley was known as a natural breath freshener; in fact, its high chlorophyll content has been found to be mildly deodorizing. Third, the leaves and roots were used as digestive aids and laxa-tives. Here again, folk wisdom may have been onto something: Studies have shown that parsley oil, found in small amounts throughout the plant but predominantly in the seeds, has the potential to mildly relieve indigestion and gas.

Actually, the best reason to eat parsley may be its nutritional value. The herb is loaded with calcium, iron, carotene, manganese, copper, ascorbic acid, and vitamins A and C. This may help explain its elevated standing among the ancient Greeks, who associated it with Hercules, awarded parsley crowns to athletic champions, and fed the greens to their horses for strength and endurance.

Conversely, the plant was linked with death. Graves were often decorated with parsley wreaths. Corpses were sprinkled with parsley to lighten their odor. Moreover, to some Europeans in the Middle Ages, the harmless plant symbolized bad luck unless it was planted on Good Friday.

Cleansing Diuretic

Another common medicinal use of parsley was as a diuretic tea made from the leaves or roots, although the herb's diuretic effect is now thought to be slight at best. Diuretics induce urination and, in folk medicine, were thought to cleanse the body of impurities as fluid made its way through and out of the system. Thus, parsley was used to treat urinary tract infections, kidney stones, and liver, bladder, and prostate troubles.

Parsley tea's following was widespread. The Cherokee, who learned of its medicinal value from the settlers, drank the tea

Active plant parts Seeds, leaves, roots
Uses Flatulence, bad breath, delayed menstruation, urinary tract infections
Cautions Apiol and myristicin, found in the volatile oil, are uterine stimulants; therefore, parsley oil, juice, and seeds should be avoided during pregnancy. In large amounts, parsley may irritate the kidneys. It may also cause an allergic reaction, such as sensitivity to light.

Not to be confused with ...

Parsley looks very similar to two toxic and potentially lethal plants that grow in the wild. The first, water hemlock or musquash root (*Cicuta maculata*), is found in swamps and marshy places, including tidal flats. The second, poison parsley or poison hemlock (*Conium maculatum*), is native to Asia and Europe but is widely naturalized in North America, especially in waste places where the soil is moist. Both plants have white flowers, differentiating them from true parsley, whose yellow blooms appear only in the second year.

for kidney and bladder pain and dropsy, now commonly known as edema, a condition marked by the accumulation of excess fluid in the body's tissues. In the 1800s, similar uses were endorsed by the U.S. Pharmacopeia (until 1926) and the Thomsonians, a sprawling association of herbal physicians who followed the work of botanist Samuel Thomson.

Parsley tea is still used today, as many diuretics are, to help reduce high blood pressure. If you choose to use parsley or its tea medicinally, keep in mind that prolonged use of diuretics can irritate the kidneys, and any at-home treatment for high blood pressure should be strictly supervised by your doctor.

Uterine Trigger

As a treatment for late or painful menstruation, parsley was thought to stimulate menstrual flow and soothe such symptoms as cramps, fluid retention, fever, and tender breasts. Parsley may indeed be able to reduce fever and help ease bloating, but it is more potent as a uterine stimulant. Studies have shown that two constituents of parsley oil, apiol and myristicin, cause the uterine muscles to contract, prompting menstrual flow.

The herb's uterine-stimulant properties led both the Indians and the settlers to use it to induce abortion, and at one time, apiol capsules were sold for this purpose. Although eating small portions of parsley is unlikely to produce such an effect, pregnant women are advised against ingesting parsley oil, juice, or seeds and eating large portions of the leaves and roots. In large doses, parsley oil can be toxic and cause such symptoms as nausea, headache, vertigo, giddiness, hallucinations, hives, and liver and kidney damage.

Women's faith in parsley was so great that even footbaths and poultices made with parsley were thought to relieve the discomforts of both menstruation and menopause. Nursing mothers also applied parsley poultices to encourage milk production and relieve swollen breasts.

Garden Medicine

Perhaps because parsley was so abundant and easy to grow, it was used for many ailments, including anemia, arthritis, coughs, diabetes, sciatica, and lice. It was even employed as a substitute for quinine in treating the fever associated with malaria. Parsley juice, alone or mixed into salves, was applied to bruises, freckles, and insect bites. The tea was thought to remedy styes and strengthen loose teeth, and was used as a skin lotion and hair rinse. However, aside from its limited potential for reducing fever, blocking histamines, and fighting bacteria, there is no evidence that parsley can remedy most of the ailments for which it was historically used.

Nevertheless, the herb does have a pleasant aroma, and it makes a nice addition to any garden. Although it is a biennial, parsley is usually cultivated as an annual. The seeds can be sown in 6 mm (¼ in.) of moist, sandy soil (anytime from spring to fall) and may take up to six weeks to germinate. The leaves can be harvested in the first year, once the plant has grown to a height of 20 cm (8 in.) or more.

In the second year, the plant grows up to 90 cm (3 ft) and bears clusters of yellow flowers that yield small, grayish seeds. The feathery leaves are either curly or flat; the flat-leaved variety is known as Italian parsley. In spring, parsley is one of the first plants to appear—hence its use in the seder, the traditional Jewish Passover meal, as a symbol of new beginnings.

Crowns of parsley once symbolized strength. Indeed, the crisp sprigs can fortify any diet.

PENNYROYAL

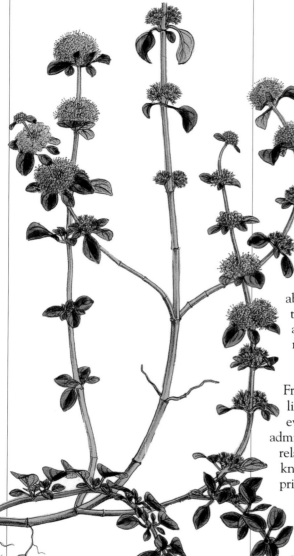

Hedeoma pulegioides
SQUAW MINT, FLEABANE

Among Indians, penny-royal was called "squaw mint" because women used it to treat menstrual problems and induce abortion. In fact, a tea made from pennyroyal leaves and flowers does help bring on delayed menstrual periods and regulate menstrual flow. But the herb's use as an abortifacient is another matter: the toxicity of pennyroyal is such that abortion is induced only at lethal or near-lethal doses.

Dangerous Oil

From 1831 to 1931 pennyroyal was listed in the U.S. Pharmacopeia, evidence that in its usual form of administration—tea—the herb is relatively safe. Today, however, we know that pulegone, pennyroyal's primary active principle, is highly poisonous. A mere teaspoonful of the oil contains enough pulegone to cause vomiting, convulsions, hallucinations, and even death. What's more, the oil is so potent that even external use is ill advised.

Benign Tea

Taken in proper amounts— one teaspoon dried herb to one cup water, drunk three times a day—pennyroyal tea can induce sweating, soothe an upset stomach, and promote menstrual flow. In the 19th century the Eclectics recommended the tea as a stimulant, fever reducer, and digestive aid and noted in their *King's American Dispensatory* that it was "an excellent remedy for the common cold."

Thomsonian herbalists packed pennyroyal leaves into their patients' nostrils to stop nosebleeds. In the West, pioneer women used aromatic garlands of pennyroyal to soothe children's coughs. Inhabitants of Appalachia made the leaves into poultices to dress wounds, and rubbed them on the skin to repel insects—hence "fleabane," one of the herb's nicknames.

Not to be confused with...

Two mint family plants are called pennyroyal. American pennyroyal *(Hedeoma pulegioides),* standing straight on fibrous stalks from 15 to 30 cm (6 to 12 in.) high, grows wild in barren fields and dry, wooded areas across North America. English or European pennyroyal *(Mentha pulegium),* native to Europe and Asia, thrives in moist, boggy spots, where it grows close to the ground. Most botanists consider American pennyroyal to be the more potent medicine.

Active plant parts Leaves, flowers
Uses Decongestant, carminative, menstrual regulator
Cautions Pennyroyal oil is not approved for sale in Canada. Never ingest; it may cause convulsions and can be lethal, even in small doses. Women using it as an abortifacient have died.

PINE

Pinus spp.

It's little wonder that our forebears found so many uses for pine. According to the pioneers, the white-pine forests of the east were so vast and pervasive that a squirrel could live its life aloft in the branches and never touch down. Of the roughly 90 species of pine, dozens grow in North America. All are cone-bearing evergreens with needle-like leaves in groups of one to five. Pines are often divided into soft, or white, pines, and hard, or yellow, pines. The needles of the soft pines are usually found in groups of five; those of the hard pines, in groups of two or three.

Some Common Pines

The wood of the white pine was unrivaled as a building material. This tree, which is found in the eastern parts of the United States and Canada, grows straight and tall and was used to make the masts of sailing ships. The twigs, bark, leaves, and pitch were valued as medicinals.

Other important pines included the yellow pines of the American South: the longleaf pine, prized for its pitch and a main source of turpentine, and its cousin the shortleaf pine, regarded for its inner bark, buds, and pitch. New Englanders and mountain dwellers in the Appalachians often utilized the pitch pine, a small, gnarled hardy tree that grows in dry, rocky soil. This is often the first tree to appear after a forest fire, because intense heat melts the resin that encloses its seeds.

In the Rocky Mountains and the American Southwest grows the ponderosa pine, a hard pine valued for its timber. But the needles of this tree, as well as those of the similar loblolly pine, are thought to be toxic. To be safe, do not consume the needles of any Western pine. Also in the Southwest are the small piñon pines; their cones contain edible seeds known as pine nuts, which are used in cooking. The medicinal value of the needles, bark, and pitch of the different pines varies widely—not only among the various species but even from tree to tree.

Piney Cough Cures

Given its penetrating aroma, it is not hard to imagine why pine was frequently used to treat coughs and colds. Pine needle teas and cough syrups were popular expectorants. When stronger medicine was called for, a decoction was made from the tree's inner bark. It was also common practice to chew a small piece of pine pitch; this was said to produce "fruitful" expectoration and alleviate sore throats. The Indians used the resin, or pitch, in teas not

Active plant parts Needles, inner bark, sap, resin
Uses Bronchial congestion, rheumatic pains
Cautions Pine oil can be toxic, especially in children. The oil from some species of pine may irritate the skin. Do not ingest the needles of any Western pine, as they may be toxic. Pregnant women should avoid pine.

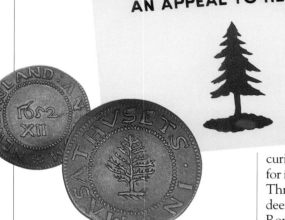

AN APPEAL TO HEAVEN

So valued was the white pine that it graced the first flag of the American Revolution as well as a 17th-century New England shilling.

only to treat colds and flu but also to relieve kidney troubles and chronic indigestion. They chewed the bark and young sprigs as expectorants for bronchial congestion, chest infections, croup, and tonsillitis. In 1927, the Eaton's Catalogue advertised Pinex as a "good cure for coughs, colds" and other maladies. Pinene, the volatile oil contained in pine, juniper, and other gymnosperms, is still believed by many to have expectorant properties. The inner bark contains a soothing mucilage and may have expectorant properties as well.

As unappealing as it sounds, pine sawdust mixed with whiskey was considered another cough cure. Even more

curious was an asthma remedy that called for inhaling the smoke of pine sawdust. Throughout the ages, pine was also deemed useful against tuberculosis. The Roman naturalist Pliny the Elder reported it useful to treat chest and lung ailments. More than a thousand years later, our settlers brewed twig tea for lung troubles. The Indians preferred pitch or bark tea.

A Sticky Wound Healer

Ancient man recognized that some trees, when injured, secrete a gummy substance that protects the wound. Thus inspired, he used the goo to heal his own wounds. Pine pitch, also commonly called pine gum or resin, remained a popular treat-

ment for open sores. The settlers applied a wad of pitch to cuts; the gum would harden, forming a seal that later became rather difficult to remove. Warmed pitch was also spread on splinters, which, with luck, came out when the tar was peeled off.

Pine pitch was also applied to swellings and broken bones. According to the 17th-century British herbalist Nicholas Culpeper, "The Rozin of Pitch-tree … being spread upon a cloth is excellently good for old aches coming of former bruises or dislocations." He also noted that "Pitch mollifies hard swellings, and brings boils and sores to suppuration [to a head], it breaks carbuncles, disperses aposthumes [abscesses], cleanses ulcers of corruption and fills them with flesh."

The Indians shared the belief that pitch helps new skin grow over wounds. They also applied warm pitch as a poultice to treat gonorrhea. Some tribes chewed and swallowed "pills" made of pitch to ward off syphilis. Indians in Alabama pulverized the bark of the piñon pine and dusted it on venereal sores. Pine pitch was used on wounds and sores for good reason: it is a natural antibiotic.

For some families the gathering of pine pitch was a yearly ritual. A V-shaped notch was made in the trunk of the tree,

From left to right is the piñon pine (which bears pine nuts), the short-leaf pine, the longleaf pine (a popular source of turpentine), and the scrubby pitch pine.

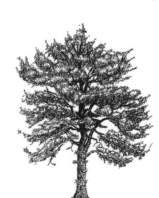

preferably in the summertime, when the pitch ran like sap. It was then stored in a jar or can for future use. The more meticulous heated the pitch until it was watery, then strained it through a cloth to remove bugs and bits of bark before storing it. The pitch was often mixed with lard or beeswax to keep it soft; in the late 19th century, petroleum jelly was used instead because it did not spoil.

Like pine pitch, pine bark was also used to heal wounds and prevent scarring. It was often ground, soaked in liquor until soft, then applied as a poultice. Some boiled it and stripped out the inner bark, which was then ground into a plaster.

Spring Tonic

Come spring, juicy young pine needles were made into a tea that was drunk as a tonic to cleanse the system; the tea, considered a pleasant diuretic, was rich in vitamin C. In fact, in the 16th century, eastern Indians administered pine needle tea to European explorers afflicted with scurvy, thereby saving their lives. Pine-top tea, made from young shoots that appear at the tips of the twigs in the spring, was also popular. The peeled shoots, eaten raw or cooked, were considered a delicacy. Settlers candied the shoots by boiling them in a heavy sugar syrup.

Probably because of its diuretic action, pine was prescribed centuries ago by the botanist John Gerard as a remedy for bladder, urinary, and kidney problems. Indeed, both the Indians and the settlers found pine products to be beneficial to the urinary tract. Indians in the Rocky Mountains used a tea made from the full-grown buds of the ponderosa pine to strengthen the urinary organs. Infusions of the resin were taken by both the Indians and the settlers to treat diarrhea, no doubt because of the resin's astringency.

Aromatic Pain Relief

Thanks to its aromatic properties, pine was also used to relieve pain. The Ojibwa Indians crushed white-pine needles and applied them to the head to relieve headaches. To cure backaches as well as headaches, many tribes inhaled the fumes of the heated needles.

Pine resin was considered an excellent remedy for rheumatism. Today herbalists recommend pine oil baths to soothe aching joints; the oil acts as a stimulant and counterirritant to distract the body from underlying pain. And, of course, pine oil is used in household cleaning products for its disinfectant properties.

Other Medicinal Conifers

Apart from pine trees, dozens of other conifers were used to heal. Among the most popular was the balsam fir, prized as a Christmas tree because of its pyramid shape and lovely scent. The tree has blisters on its bark that are filled with a resin, known as Canada balsam. It was used as an antiseptic against gonorrhea and leukorrhea, and in ointments for hemorrhoids. The Indians applied the resin as a painkiller for burns, sores, bruises, and wounds. (Note: The resin of balsam fir may cause dermatitis in some people.) Canada balsam is still used in some shampoos.

The bark of hemlock trees is so astringent that it was used not only in poultices for bleeding wounds but also to tan hides. Bark teas were used to treat colds, stomach ailments, and scurvy, as an enema for diarrhea, and as a rub for rheumatism. The leafy twig tips were brewed as a cure for kidney, bladder, and vaginal ailments.

Many conifers, including pine and spruce trees, provided a precursor to modern-day chewing gum. When the bark was bruised, the pitch would run out and eventually harden. The pitch was pried from the tree with a knife and chewed, either for pleasure or to counter indigestion. Spruce needles and twigs (below) were the source of spruce beer, popular in 17th- and 18th-century New France. Newfoundlanders mixed the beer with molasses and rum to make a beverage called callibogus. Spruce was also the origin of "burgundy pitch," which was used as a counterirritant in diseases of the lungs, stomach, and intestines.

The Indians particularly valued cedars. They chewed red cedar berries as a cure for canker sores and made teas to treat colds, worms, rheumatism, and headaches. Doctors once prescribed tinctures of the leaves for warts, hemorrhoids, ulcers, and fungal infections; leaf extracts have been shown to have antiseptic and antiviral properties. However, the oil is toxic; ingesting it can cause death.

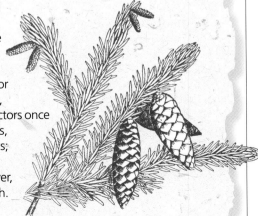

PINE TAR

The Indians and settlers noticed that injured pine trees secreted a sticky substance that formed a protective seal over the wound. They reasoned that this resin—and also the gooey pine tar that they learned to distill from the wood—might be used to heal burns, wounds, and skin problems in both humans and animals. Thus, pine tar—as well as related substances, including juniper, birch, coal tar, and tar water (a cold infusion of tar in water used as a cure-all)—became a popular folk remedy.

Making Tar

Tar is a thick, viscous fluid that is only slightly soluble in water. It is obtained through a laborious distillation process that involves slowly burning wood or coal in a closed reservoir so that it is reduced to charcoal; by-products of the charcoal are trapped and condensed into a dark, thick, smoky liquid. The darker the color and the worse the taste and smell of this tar, the more beneficial it was deemed.

Of the cedar tree, the 17th-century British herbalist Nicholas Culpeper wrote, "When it is burned comes forth that which, with us, is usually known by the name of Tar, and is excellently good for unction either for scabs, itch, or manginess, either in men or beasts, as also against leprosy, tetters, ringworms, and scald heads [a scalp disease]."

Throughout the 18th and 19th centuries, pine tar, often mixed with lard or beeswax, was used to treat wounds and such skin conditions as psoriasis, eczema, boils, wens [cysts], corns, and calluses. To heal wounds, sores, and even piles (hemorrhoids), home remedies called for boiling pine tar in water and applying the strained water, often mixed with lard, to the wound. American Civil War soldiers used these salves on the battlefield, and settlers applied them to injured farm animals. Some of these folk uses do have scientific foundation: the creosote compounds in pine tar are mildly antibacterial, antiseptic, and anesthetic.

A Sticky Cough Cure

To relieve coughs and sore throats, the settlers boiled pine, beech, or juniper tar (also known as cade oil) on the stove and inhaled the steam. This was thought to thin the mucus and promote expectoration. Pine tar cough syrups, occasionally containing other ingredients as well, were popular throughout the 19th century and well into the 20th century. The tar was also used in salves and plasters that were applied to the throat and chest to help ease congestion. One plaster formula called for a mixture of pine tar, lard, camphor, mutton tallow, soot, and turpentine.

Tar preparations were also used to treat skin conditions, dandruff, and itchy scalp. In fact, shampoos containing pine and coal tar are still found in some pharmacies today. (Note: Coal tar shampoos are quite messy and tend to stain the skin and hair.) Pine tar soaps, said to help stop itching, are available, too. Coal tar is also found in some eczema and psoriasis ointments and in "tar gels," which are far less messy than earlier coal tar preparations. These products do work, but they may make the skin more sensitive to sunlight. Long-term use should be supervised by a doctor.

Pine tar soaps and shampoos were used to combat itching.

Active plant part A sticky, brownish-black substance distilled from the wood of pine trees
Uses Congestion, skin problems
Cautions External use of pine tar may cause dermatitis in some people.

PINKEYE

Bloodshot redness, gritty discomfort, and discharges of mucus mark this common eye problem. Also known as conjunctivitis, pinkeye is the infection or inflammation of the thin membrane (the conjunctiva) that covers the eyeball and the inner eyelid. Treating pinkeye—whether in children, adults, pets, horses, or cattle—includes the use of sterile washes that are not going to worsen the condition. Unfortunately, this discounts many remedies prepared at home.

Of the most common folk remedies— diluted boric acid, yellow mercuric oxide, and cool infusions of eyebright or borage—only boric acid has withstood the test of time. Deemed mildly soothing but ineffective against bacterial infections, it should be used only in commercially sold isotonic solutions that are safe for the eyes. Likewise, a solution of sodium bicarbonate (baking soda), which is similar in composition to the eye's natural tears, can be made; follow label instructions carefully to obtain proper dilution.

Eyebright, whose flower resembles a bloodshot eye, was used by the ancient Greeks and the North American Indians to relieve a slew of eye problems. However, in his book *American Medicinal Plants*, medical researcher Charles Millspaugh acknowledged that, despite eyebright's reputation, its efficacy was not recorded in "modern times"—and that was in 1892. Recent studies have shown that it is ineffective and potentially harmful.

Nonprescription eyedrops, such as artificial tears, whiteners, and cleansers, can also irritate the eye. Only antibiotic or antihistamine drops prescribed by an eye doctor will remedy pinkeye.

Get the Pink Out

Pinkeye is usually caused by a bacterial or viral infection or an allergy. When caused by an infection, it is very contagious. To avoid spreading it, do not scratch or rub the eyes and temporarily stop using contact lenses and eye makeup. If any of the following occur—severe mucus discharge, worsening redness, pain, sensitivity to bright light, or blurred vision—or if the condition lasts more than a few days, consult a doctor. Pinkeye can be debilitating—Mark Twain's wife (and editor), Olivia Langdon Clemens, was unable to review *A Connecticut Yankee in King Arthur's Court*, an outrageous work, because of a bout with pinkeye.

Two recommended folk eyewashes are those made with goldenseal root, which contains antibacterial hydrastine, and chamomile flowers. When preparing an eyewash at home, simmer it for at least 15 minutes and properly sterilize the eyedropper or eyecup if you use one.

Aside from warm and cold compresses to soothe bacterial and allergenic conjunctivitis, using most folk remedies is merely blind optimism. Still, many things have been tried, including breast milk, rainwater that falls on Holy Thursday, mullein root tea (for a "cold in the eye"), and eyewashes made from maple bark or peach tree leaves—all of which may be bacterially unsafe.

Use only sterile eyewashes and eyecups when treating eye problems.

GOLDENSEAL To make an antimicrobial eyewash, add ½ liter boiling water and 1 teaspoon boric acid to 1 teaspoon chopped root; stir, let cool, then strain through cheesecloth into a glass. Add 1 teaspoon liquid to ½ cup cool water. Apply with a sterilized eyedropper or eyecup, three or four times a day.

CHAMOMILE To make an antibacterial and anti-inflammatory wash, pour 1 cup boiling water over 1 teaspoon flowers, steep, then strain through cheesecloth. Let cool. Apply with a sterilized eyedropper or eyecup, three or four times a day.

CALENDULA Dilute 5 to 10 milliliters commercial tincture in 2 cups hot water. Soak a clean cloth in the dilution and squeeze out excess liquid. Hold the anti-inflammatory compress against the eye until it is cool or dry, four times a day.

PLANTAIN

Plantago spp.

There are some 250 species of this common weed, several of which were inadvertently brought to North America by the European settlers. The Indians called plantain "white man's footprint" because wherever the settlers went, the weed was sure to follow. It should not be confused with the tropical plant, also called plantain, that bears greenish banana-like fruit.

Wound Healer

The leaves of such species as *Plantago major*, called common broadleaf or greater plantain, have long been valued as astringents for the treatment of wounds. In Shakespeare's *Romeo and Juliet*, Romeo suggests plantain leaves for a cut shin.

Pioneers used the leaves for bites, burns, boils, infections, stings, and splinters. The settlers bound the leaves to bruises to "draw out the infection" and applied them to sore eyes and feet. The Indians pressed the leaves to the forehead to treat headache and tied the wet leaves to snakebites. Appalachian folk healer Tommie Bass not only used the leaves to treat stings, sunburn, and poison ivy but also placed hot leaves on swollen joints, strains, and sprains. The plant's juice, mixed with water, was used as a douche for vaginitis, and a decoction of leaves and roots was used for venereal disease.

Plantain leaves remained a cure for bites and stings into the 20th century, and for good reason. The juice derived from the leaves contains astringent tannins and a soothing mucilage; it is also antibacterial. Plantain has shown some efficacy in treating hemorrhoids and irritable bowel syndrome. What's more, there is some evidence that the leaves help stop the itching and spreading of poison ivy.

Psyllium: a Laxative

Another plantain species, *Plantago psyllium*, has been used as a bulk laxative for centuries, although it didn't catch on in North America until after the First World War. The seeds are neither absorbed nor digested in the intestinal tract. Their husks, which contain cells filled with mucilage, swell when they come into contact with water, thereby providing both bulk and lubrication and making stools easier to pass. One must drink large amounts of water when taking psyllium. Today psyllium seeds, considered safe and gentle, are the main ingredient in many popular over-the-counter laxatives.

Several studies have demonstrated that psyllium seeds have the capacity to lower blood cholesterol levels. The seeds have been approved for this use in Germany but not in the U.S. and Canada.

Active plant parts Leaves, dried ripe seeds and their husks, roots

Uses Cuts, bruises, blisters, poison ivy, constipation

Cautions Psyllium seeds should not be ground or chewed, since doing so has been reported to release a pigment that collects in renal tubules. The seeds should not be used in cases of intestinal obstruction and must be taken with plenty of water. They should not be given to children under two. Excessive use should be avoided during pregnancy.

POISON IVY

The best medicine for a poison ivy rash is to avoid the vine-like plant altogether: "Leaflets three, let it be." That is easier said than done, and countless folk remedies have been used to relieve the itchy rash. In times past, the plant was even used topically to treat many conditions, including arthritis.

The rash is an allergic reaction to the plant resin, urushiol, of poison ivy, poison oak, and poison sumac (all of the *Toxicodendron* genus). Urushiol, a mixture of irritants, can cause a rash even if the skin does not touch the plant. The stubborn resin can cling to clothes, shoes, garden tools, workbenches, pet fur—anything!—for months before it is transferred to the skin. It can also penetrate lightweight clothing and, if the plant is burned, can be inhaled, affecting the respiratory tract.

Generally, the rash appears from two hours to 14 days after contact with the resin and lasts up to three weeks. Symptoms can include headache and fatigue. If the reaction is particularly severe, covers a large or sensitive area, or affects the nose, mouth, or throat, see a doctor.

Soothe or Suffer

Once the resin is on the skin, it can spread to other parts of the body and to other people. Therefore, as soon as you have been in contact with the plant, wash, dry, and treat the skin with rubbing alcohol. Also wash any clothing and shoes that may be tainted with the resin. Old remedies used to clean and dry the skin include homemade "yellow kitchen soap," laundry soap, and witch hazel water—which is still widely available. Old remedies that are now considered unsafe or ineffective include whiskey, bleach, horse urine, and mercurials (mercury-based solutions, such as Mercurochrome and Merthiolate).

Like modern corticosteroid creams, old-time over-the-counter remedies attempt to soothe the skin, keep the rash dry, and reduce swelling. Calamine lotion, aluminum acetate (also known as Burow's Solution), and baths and poultices made with oatmeal, cornstarch, or baking soda can relieve itchy, inflamed skin.

Plant-based remedies can also counter the itching and inflammation. The sap of jewelweed, ironically known also as touch-me-not, has been reported (but not proven) to clear up poison ivy in two to three days. Infusions of white oak, yarrow, and plantain can also be beneficial.

Of the more than 100 folk remedies for poison ivy, some intriguing applications are ice-cold whole milk, white shoe polish that contains pipe clay, the inside of a banana peel, and green-tomato juice.

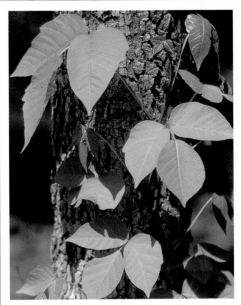

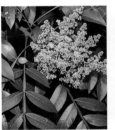
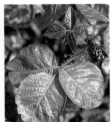

Hikers, gardeners, and nature lovers know to avoid these rash-causing plants: poison ivy (top), poison sumac (bottom left), and poison oak (bottom right).

SOAP & RUBBING ALCOHOL To prevent the rash, wash away the plant resin before it reacts with the skin—within 15 minutes of contact.

OATMEAL BATH Boil 250 to 500 grams oatmeal in 4 to 8 liters water for 30 minutes, then add to bathwater. Or apply an oatmeal poultice up to four times a day. Commercial oatmeal bath products are also available.

JEWELWEED Extract sap from the stem or leaves of fresh jewelweed (*Impatiens capensis*), or make a tea by adding any part of the herb to boiling water. Steep, then strain. Apply the sap or tea up to three times a day.

PLANTAIN Extract the plant's juice by pressing its fresh leaves. Apply the juice to the rash up to four times a day. Contact dermatitis may occur.

THE HEALING TRADITIONS OF
THE NAVAJO

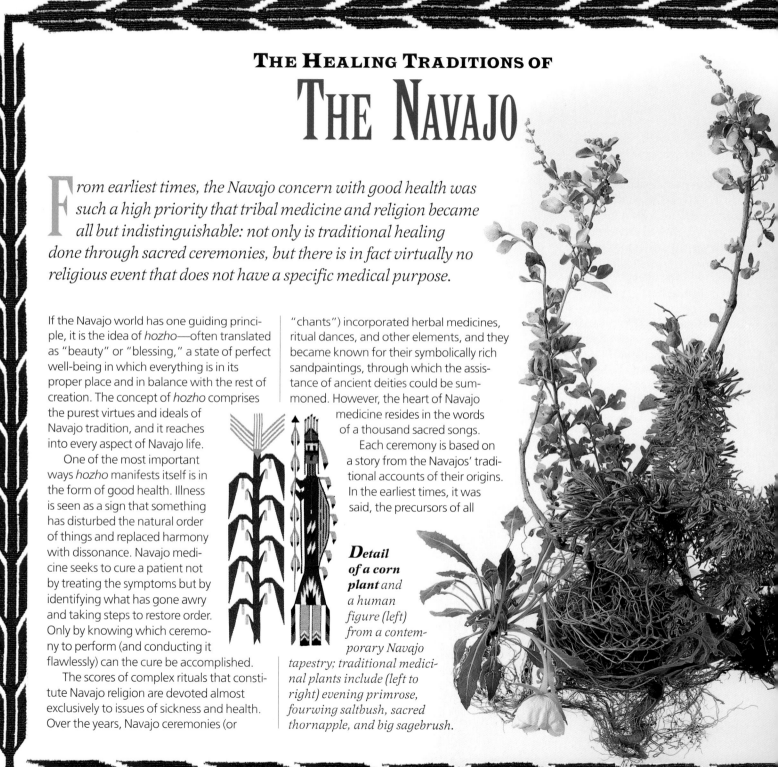

From earliest times, the Navajo concern with good health was such a high priority that tribal medicine and religion became all but indistinguishable: not only is traditional healing done through sacred ceremonies, but there is in fact virtually no religious event that does not have a specific medical purpose.

If the Navajo world has one guiding principle, it is the idea of *hozho*—often translated as "beauty" or "blessing," a state of perfect well-being in which everything is in its proper place and in balance with the rest of creation. The concept of *hozho* comprises the purest virtues and ideals of Navajo tradition, and it reaches into every aspect of Navajo life.

One of the most important ways *hozho* manifests itself is in the form of good health. Illness is seen as a sign that something has disturbed the natural order of things and replaced harmony with dissonance. Navajo medicine seeks to cure a patient not by treating the symptoms but by identifying what has gone awry and taking steps to restore order. Only by knowing which ceremony to perform (and conducting it flawlessly) can the cure be accomplished.

The scores of complex rituals that constitute Navajo religion are devoted almost exclusively to issues of sickness and health. Over the years, Navajo ceremonies (or "chants") incorporated herbal medicines, ritual dances, and other elements, and they became known for their symbolically rich sandpaintings, through which the assistance of ancient deities could be summoned. However, the heart of Navajo medicine resides in the words of a thousand sacred songs.

Each ceremony is based on a story from the Navajos' traditional accounts of their origins. In the earliest times, it was said, the precursors of all

Detail of a corn plant and a human figure (left) from a contemporary Navajo tapestry; traditional medicinal plants include (left to right) evening primrose, fourwing saltbush, sacred thornapple, and big sagebrush.

Images of Power

Traditionally, the main role of a Navajo sandpainting was to attract the Holy People to a curing rite and enlist their aid in healing the patient. The stylized images retell an episode from tribal legend during which a hero learns how certain diseases can be cured. If all goes well, the Holy People will be persuaded to restore the patient's health, just as they cured the hero in the original myth. The colored sand now becomes the medium through which their power is transferred; thus a painting must be destroyed immediately afterward so that no one can steal the power it still possesses.

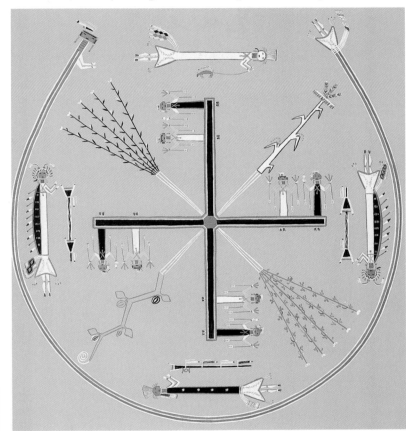

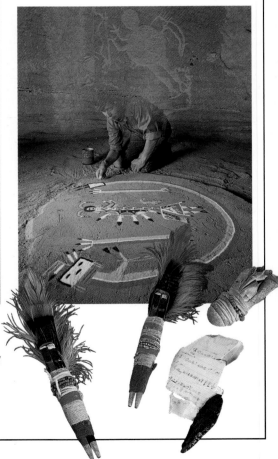

Extending a sacred tradition, Navajo sandpainter Art Etcitty (below) works on a depiction of Bi'ganaskiddi, the hump-backed Yei. Items from an aged shaman's medicine bundle (bottom) include feathered prayer sticks and fragments of notes that helped him memorize prayers and songs.

Contemporary Navajo art freely incorporates images borrowed from the Holyway ceremony and others, taking care to avoid sacrilege by adapting them in nontraditional ways. "Whirling Logs with Storm" (above), by Johnny Benally, Sr., includes such potent Navajo symbols as the four sacred mountains, the four sacred plants (corn, beans, squash, and tobacco, all rooted in a central circle of water), and four feather-bedecked Yei, or Holy People. During a curing ceremony, the same Yei would be impersonated by dancers in masks and costumes that duplicate those in the painting.

Knowledge of the Holy People

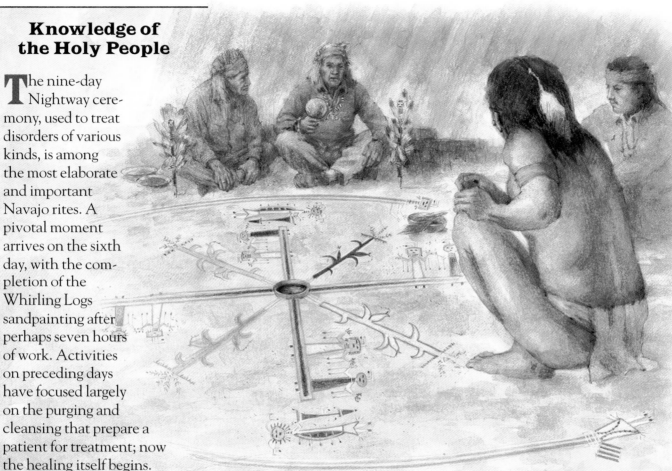

The nine-day Nightway ceremony, used to treat disorders of various kinds, is among the most elaborate and important Navajo rites. A pivotal moment arrives on the sixth day, with the completion of the Whirling Logs sandpainting after perhaps seven hours of work. Activities on preceding days have focused largely on the purging and cleansing that prepare a patient for treatment; now the healing itself begins.

The Whirling Logs sandpainting depicts the Navajo myth in which Bitahatini, the young visionary, journeys to a holy place where four whirling logs move about a sacred lake. Here he learns of the songs and medicines used by the Yei, or Holy People, and then returns to cure the Earth People's illnesses.

Before the patient is summoned, the priest sprinkles sacred cornmeal on parts of the picture and sets up plumed wands in the sand on three sides. He prepares an infusion of water mixed with corn pollen and charcoal powder in an earthen bowl, placing it in the center to represent the lake visited by Bitahatini. Lastly, he applies corn pollen to all the gods in the drawing, seeking their help.

Only then does the patient enter the hogan. Removing all his clothing except for a loincloth, he sits on the southeastern part of the painting and prepares to begin absorbing its curative power.

earthly creatures—insects, animals, and humans—had migrated upward through a series of sunless worlds where strife and disorder always forced them to move on. Finally the Navajos' ancestors emerged into the sunlight in a place that would become their tribal homeland. It was bounded by four sacred mountains, and its radiant beauty was a profound contrast to the dark chaos of the lower worlds. It was, in short, the embodiment of *hozho* in a living landscape.

Summoning the Spirits

The ancestors' emergence had been made possible by the exploits of Changing Woman, the Navajos' most beloved deity, and countless other sacred beings known as the Holy People. These spirits taught the people how to grow corn, hunt animals, and conduct their lives according to the ideals of *hozho*. The lessons were passed down in stories of ancestors who were punished by the Holy People with pain and disease for improper behavior only to be saved by the same Holy People, from whom they learned the

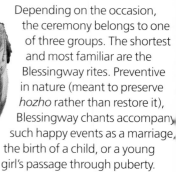

A prayer board used in certain rites bears the image of a snake-handler; snakes were believed to cause stomach ailments.

ceremony that cured each affliction. Thus, the goal of every Navajo medicine rite is to retell the creation story in a way that attracts the Holy People's attention and persuades them to restore the patient's health, just as they did long ago.

This mythical reenactment is driven by songs—hundreds of them in the course of a five- or nine-day ritual—performed from memory by a priest who learned them during years of apprenticeship. Each chant must be word-perfect: a single mistake can undo everything—indeed, it may bring on greater suffering.

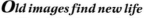

Old images find new life in Navajo basket art (left), as with this turtle and four-sided maze. The past is evident in the ruins of the Pueblo del Arroyo (below left), while a solid and still occupied hogan (below) evinces the present.

Depending on the occasion, the ceremony belongs to one of three groups. The shortest and most familiar are the Blessingway rites. Preventive in nature (meant to preserve *hozho* rather than restore it), Blessingway chants accompany such happy events as a marriage, the birth of a child, or a young girl's passage through puberty.

More elaborate are the Evilway chants, designed to exorcise and purify someone who has been contaminated by contact with the malevolent power of ghosts. The third and largest group are the Holyway chants, used to cure most illnesses and injuries. A skilled diagnostician can usually find the source of a disease, but some diseases may be triggered by numerous things—plants, animals, storms, or dreams. Only trial and error determine which ceremony will work best.

Most Holyway chants include a cleansing bath, a purifying sweat-and-emetic ritual, preparation of one or more sandpaintings, and, near the end, a nightlong cycle of songs in which priest and patient are joined by participants, spectators, and family. If it succeeds, the chant will guide the patient on a journey that parallels the ancestors' upward migration—from the chaos that breeds disease and death toward the healing light of *hozho*. After the final night, a patient often takes time to walk outside and "breathe in the dawn." And the ceremony usually closes with a prayer that affirms the patient's recovery: "Beauty has been restored."

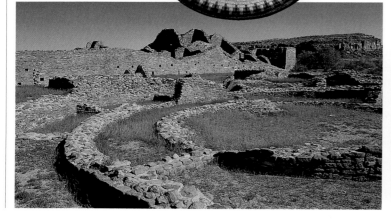

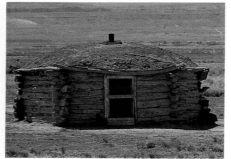

POKE

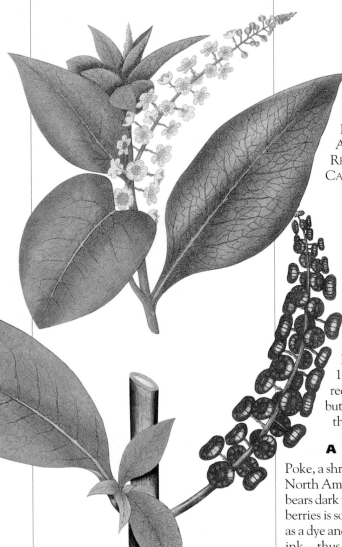

Phytolacca americana
POKEWEED, POKEROOT,
POKEBERRY, INKBERRY, SCOKE,
AMERICAN NIGHTSHADE,
RED-INK PLANT, CROWBERRY,
CANCER JALAP, CANCER ROOT

It is remarkable that our forebears not only used this poisonous herb to treat all manner of ailments, but also seemed aware of the plant's toxicity. In the 19th century scores of people died after consuming the roots as a treatment for rheumatism, yet poke was listed in the U.S. Pharmacopeia as recently as 1947. Some herbalists still recommend it for countless ills, but reputable sources agree that the plant should not be ingested.

A Poisonous "Cure-all"

Poke, a shrub-like weed native to eastern North America, California, and Hawaii, bears dark purple berries. The color of the berries is so rich that the fruits were used as a dye and also as an early source of ink—thus one of the plant's many nicknames, red-ink plant. One of poke's other monikers was cancer root, because poultices of the root were thought to cure cancer, especially of the skin and breast. The plant was also used as an emetic and purgative, hence a third sobriquet: cancer jalap (jalap is the name of another purgative). Poke, because of its toxicity, probably does act as a purgative, but it may also cause severe abdominal cramping, nausea, diarrhea, and difficulty breathing.

Among poke's supposed powers was its ability to stimulate the lymphatic system; therefore, it was used in cases of swollen glands, tonsillitis, laryngitis, mumps, and thyroid conditions. It was also highly popular for treating various skin ailments, including poison ivy, ringworm, scabies, running ulcers, sores, and "the itch" (a condition caused by mites).

The most common use for poke was as a treatment for rheumatic pains, often in the form of root tinctures and berry teas. Some "cured" themselves by eating the fresh or dried berries. Others soaked the berries in brandy, whiskey, or wine.

Although some parts of the poke plant are more dangerous than others (the roots are the most poisonous), it is wise to avoid the herb altogether. One woman suffered severe poisoning from drinking a cup of tea made with ½ teaspoon of the powdered root. Some say that it is safe to consume the fresh berries in small numbers (fewer than 10), and the cooked berries are edible. Young poke shoots, harvested before they produce leaves and cooked through two changes of water, are sometimes eaten in "hot salads." Recently, however, a group of campers fell ill after ingesting the properly cooked greens.

Active plant parts Roots, leaves, berries
Uses Poke is unsafe for medicinal use.
Cautions Ingestion of this plant is not recommended; it may cause severe stomach cramps, diarrhea, nausea, vomiting, difficulty breathing, weakness, spasms, hypotension, severe convulsions, and death. Wear gloves when handling the plant to avoid skin irritation.

PSORIASIS

Imagine your skin cells reproducing at a rate 10 times faster than normal— so quickly, in fact, that the skin is growing faster than it is shedding, becoming thicker, inflamed, and uncomfortable. Patches of dead skin—dry silvery scales—stubbornly cling to your trunk, back, knees, elbows, or scalp. This is psoriasis, a condition that affects about 2 percent of the population, usually between the ages of 10 and 30.

Shed Some Skin

The best folk remedies are anti-inflammatories and astringents that soothe the affected areas and help the dead skin fall away. Early settlers commonly turned to evening primrose oil and external washes made from St. Johnswort, goldenseal, and yellow dock. Evening primrose oil, taken internally, may help control inflammation when taken over several weeks; it is a source of gamma linolenic acid, which may have anti-inflammatory properties. St. Johnswort and goldenseal (a favorite among Indians for a variety of skin problems) have anti-inflammatory and astringent constituents. Yellow dock, which is strongly astringent due to its tannin content, was used by Indians and settlers to treat "scabby eruptions."

Lesser known but potentially effective remedies included a poultice of papaya leaves, which are said to soften skin, and jojoba oil. Jojoba is a desert shrub native to Arizona, California, and northern Mexico, and its oil, said to mimic the skin's natural sebum, has been used as a leather softener and skin moisturizer.

Today Australian tea tree oil, Indian neem tree oil (found in commercial creams), and an extract of milk thistle seeds are gaining popularity.

Other applications that may provide some benefit include lemon oil, comfrey ointment, and washes of sage, burdock, and yarrow. Studies suggest that capsaicin (a derivative of red pepper), applied topically, and diets supplemented with fish oils or vitamin D may reduce discomfort. Last, sedative teas, such as skullcap, vervain, and chamomile, can help reduce stress, a possible trigger of psoriasis.

Let the Sun Shine In

Although the exact cause of psoriasis is unknown, the condition tends to run in families. The skin changes may be accompanied by joint stiffness and pain, nail damage, itching, and small pustules. Psoriasis is chronic, but single attacks— typically provoked by stress, skin damage, or a physical illness, such as sore throat— can be effectively managed. Orthodox treatments include over-the-counter emollients, coal-tar lotions, and hydrocortisone ointments, some of which contain derivatives of *Dioscorea* species (wild yam). Also, a widely prescribed warm-weather cure is a trip to the beach: exposure to sunlight and the unique benefits of saltwater can speed healing.

GOTU KOLA Used in traditional Eastern medicine, gotu kola (also called hydrocotyle) has shown promise in clearing up psoriasis. Commercial extracts or creams containing TECA (titrated extract of *Centalla asiatica*), administered topically, have wound-healing and anti-inflammatory properties. Apply the diluted extract (5 parts water to 1 part extract) or the cream directly to the skin three times a day. Ingesting commercial capsules that contain the leaves may also help. Internal or external use may cause dermatitis.

BURDOCK To make a tea, place 1 teaspoon chopped fresh or dried root in 1 cup cold water, let stand for 5 minutes, bring to a boil, then strain. Drink 1 cup three times a day. Internal use of burdock may interfere with medications that regulate blood sugar levels. Do not use during pregnancy and lactation.

EVENING PRIMROSE To relieve itching, take the standard daily dose of the oil, available in extracts and capsules— 6 to 8 grams for adults, 2 to 4 grams for children. A minimum of 12 weeks of use may be required to see benefits.

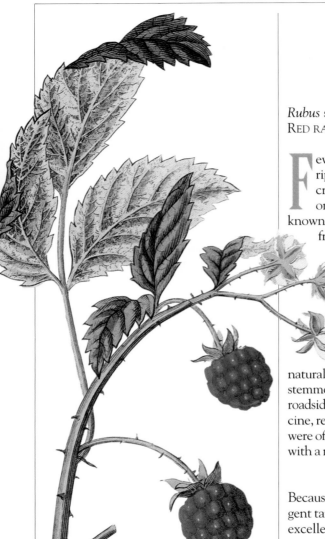

RASPBERRY

Rubus spp.
RED RASPBERRY, HINDBERRY, BRAMBLE

Few summer pleasures surpass that of ripe red raspberries, bathed in fresh cream or simmered into jams, jellies, or syrup. However, the shrub—best known for its delicate jewel-like fruit—has also been tapped for its medicinal virtues. Many uses have been ascribed to the plant over the years—most notably, against diarrhea; in recent years, though, its role as a "women's herb" has eclipsed all others.

Native to Europe and naturalized in North America, the prickly-stemmed raspberry shrub grows wild along roadsides and in thickets. In folk medicine, red raspberry and black raspberry were often used interchangeably, along with a related plant, the blackberry.

Diarrhea Remedy

Because raspberry leaves are rich in astringent tannins, they were considered an excellent remedy for a number of ailments. The 17th-century British herbalist Nicholas Culpeper described the plant as "very binding," and recommended it for piles, sores, and excessive menstrual flow.

In 17th-century Europe a syrup was made from the berries to prevent vomiting, and the berries were used to dissolve tartar on the teeth. They were later deemed beneficial against heart disease.

Above all, raspberry was recommended for bowel troubles. North America's 19th-century Eclectic physicians paid more heed to the blackberry plant than to the raspberry, but they noted in *King's American Dispensatory* that either the bark of the blackberry root or the leaves of the raspberry were useful as astringents and were "an excellent remedy in diarrhea, dysentery (chronic), cholera infantum, relaxed conditions of the intestines of children, passive hemorrhage from the stomach, bowels, or uterus, and in colliquative [watery] diarrhea." It was also said that the fruit, "when eaten freely, promotes the actions of the bowels."

The Omaha scraped and boiled the roots of red and black raspberry and gave the tea to children with bowel disorders. The Pawnee, Omaha, and Dakota used decoctions of black raspberry roots to remedy dysentery. Scientific studies support the use of raspberry as an astringent in the treatment of diarrhea.

Even more popular than raspberry for bowel troubles was blackberry. Blackberry or dewberry jam or syrup was given to children to counter dysentery. In some households blackberry jam was reserved as a medicine. American botanist W. P. C. Barton wrote in 1817 that blackberry tea, made from the root, was viewed as a "general corrective of all vitiated humours, a strengthener of the stomach

Active plant parts Leaf, root bark, fruit
Uses Menstrual cramps, diarrhea
Cautions Pregnant women should consult their obstetrician before taking raspberry leaf tea or a tea made with any other herb.

and bowels, in short as a perfect panacea." Several decades later, another botanist, R. E. Griffith, wrote that "no article of the materia medica is more relied upon in domestic practice" than blackberry.

The Eclectics recommended a decoction of blackberry root bark or raspberry leaves to act against gonorrhea, gleet (inflammation of the urethra), leukorrhea (vaginal discharge), and prolapsed uterus. They also advised that "the leaves of raspberry, in decoction with cream, will allay nausea and vomiting," and that raspberry syrup with water was "a refreshing and beneficial beverage for fever patients." The fruit juice was gargled to soothe inflamed tonsils. Some Indians made an infusion of the root bark and applied it to sore eyes.

Women's Herb

The Eclectics believed that raspberry leaves strengthened uterine contractions during labor and helped relieve postpartum pains. Raspberry leaf tea was commonly taken during the last days of pregnancy—the period formerly known as confinement—to lessen the duration and pain of childbirth.

Today, raspberry's reputation as a women's herb is stronger still, thanks in part to a 1941 study performed on isolated tissues of guinea pigs and frogs. The study demonstrated that the leaf extract was a smooth-muscle stimulant and also an antispasmodic (a substance capable of relieving spasms). Another animal study showed that raspberry leaf extract relaxed the uterus if it was "in tone" and caused contractions if it was relaxed. This would explain the use of raspberry leaves both in inducing labor and in easing menstrual cramps. However, according to modern researchers, the clinical evidence for this is scant and inconclusive. No chemical

A Bevy of Brambles

Raspberries, blackberries, and dewberries are all known as brambles and were used somewhat interchangeably, although many expressed belief in the greater relative value of one or another. Blackberry was long the best-known bramble; today raspberry leaves occupy the limelight.

Raspberries include the red and the black raspberry (also known as thimbleberries or blackcaps). Raspberries separate from a core that remains on the plant. The cores of blackberries, on the other hand, are part of the fruit. Blackberries are particularly abundant in the East and along the Pacific Coast. There are several different species, including the low or creeping blackberry (*Rubus canadensis*) and the coveted dewberry (*R. trivialis* and other species), also called the ground blackberry because it grows along the ground.

Blackberry syrups and jams were preferred over those of raspberries for use against dysentery because they were thought to be more astringent. The leaves were preferred by the aging for another reason: according to the 17th-century herbalist Nicholas Culpeper, the leaves, boiled with lye, was a rinse that "maketh the hair black."

Raspberries, blackberries, and bicolored hybrids are good eating, but the leaves may also heal you.

constituent of the leaves capable of inducing such activity has yet been identified.

Some herbalists now recommend infusions of raspberry leaves during pregnancy to increase muscle tone in the uterine wall and help prevent miscarriage. They suggest taking an infusion during childbirth to both relax and stimulate the uterus and to lessen postpartum bleeding. (Pregnant women should be aware that no data about potential long-term toxicity are available for raspberry. Check with your doctor before taking any herb during

pregnancy.) Raspberry leaf tea remains a popular treatment for painful menstrual periods and for premenstrual syndrome.

Raspberry may prove to have still other uses. Antiviral activity against herpes simplex type 2, influenza, and other viruses has been demonstrated in cell cultures. One animal study showed that raspberry helps reduce blood sugar, suggesting a possible role in the management of diabetes. Another study showed that tannins in the plant's root may be of value in treating a rare form of cancer.

RED CLOVER

Trifolium pratense
MEADOW CLOVER,
PURPLE CLOVER,
TREFOIL

Like the shamrock, red clover was considered a talisman against witches and evil in the Middle Ages. As such, medieval herbalists advised their patients to drink three to four cups of red clover tea daily to ward off sickness.

Indeed, red clover is one of many botanicals that were traditionally believed to improve overall health. In both Eastern and Western cultures, the dried flower heads were used to make a tea that relaxed the muscles, "purified" the blood, and cleared the chest of phlegm. Red clover cigarettes were prescribed for asthma patients, and red clover tea was a common draft for babies with whooping cough. A red clover salve was a popular treatment for chronic skin diseases—especially eczema and psoriasis.

Although the plant's chemistry is well documented (red clover contains many biologically active compounds, including estrogens and coumarin, which has an anticoagulant effect), studies of its pharmacological proper-ties are limited. Accordingly, no evidence has been found to justify its use in folk treatments, and red clover was dropped from the U.S. National Formulary in 1946. Despite this, today red clover compounds are regularly advertised in catalogs and sold in natural products stores.

Trifolium Compounds

In the early 20th century, medicines that included red clover as a primary ingredient enjoyed an unwarranted reputation as cures for venereal disease. A number of major pharmaceutical companies manufactured and sold these "trifolium compounds" (named after the plant's genus), even after the American Medical Association reported in 1912 that the preparations "possess no medicinal properties."

Such merchandising paled, however, beside the claims of one Harry Hoxsey, a naturopath who in 1924 began to treat cancer patients with a red clover–based herbal formula inherited from his great-grandfather. Even though the medical establishment was outraged, thousands of people tried the formula, and by the 1950s Hoxsey's Texas clinic had branches in 17 American states. (Among Hoxsey's other cancer "cures" were eating raw liver and giving coffee enemas, which at times proved lethal.) The product was later banned, leading "Hoxsey formula" therapists to move their operations to Mexico.

More benignly, extracts of red clover's naturally sweet blossoms—a familiar treat for children who live in the country—are used as a flavoring ingredient in foods, including baked goods, candy, and jams.

Active plant parts Flower heads
Uses Traditionally for bronchitis, whooping cough, and skin conditions
Cautions Because of the plant's estrogenic components, excessive ingestion of red clover should be avoided. Pregnant women and nursing mothers should avoid the herb. Large doses may interfere with anticoagulant and hormonal therapies.

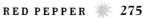

RED PEPPER

Capsicum spp.
CAPSICUM, CAYENNE PEPPER, CHILI
PEPPER, HOT PEPPER, TABASCO PEPPER,
AFRICAN PEPPER, BIRD PEPPER,
LOUISIANA LONG PEPPER

In 1492 Columbus sailed in search of the Spice Islands but stumbled upon the New World instead. The local Arawak Indians fed him stews flavored with what he later termed (in Spanish) "red pepper"; thus, he became one of the first Europeans to taste capsicum. Columbus transported the fiery fruits back to Spain, and from there they spread throughout Europe. The Spanish and Portuguese explorers carried them along the maritime trade routes to India and Africa, so that soon the peppers virtually spanned the globe.

Now cultivated by nearly every society in the world, "red pepper" refers to about 20 species of capsicum—spreading, shrubby perennial herbs that are indigenous to tropical America. The species most common in North America are *Capsicum frutescens* and *C. annuum*; the mild bell peppers belong to the latter. A mild variety of *C. annuum* yields paprika, also known as sweet pepper, which contains few pungent principles. The searing tabasco pepper, a variety of *C. frutescens*, grows along North America's Gulf coast; the highly pungent fruits, when used as a spice, are harvested when fully ripe, then dried and ground. All red peppers are a good source of vitamins A and C.

Red-hot Tonic

The hottest spice yet discovered, red pepper has been prized by many cultures for its effects on the body. Not all of the plant's applications, however, have been medicinal. After Columbus brought red pepper to Europe, some men mixed it with snuff for a stronger "kick." One herbalist warned against this practice, claiming that the combination caused sneezing so violent it might break blood vessels in the head. As a stimulant, red pepper was thought to benefit the circulatory, nervous, and digestive systems.

According to the 17th-century British herbalist Nicholas Culpeper, red pepper was so hot that too much "might prove dangerous to life." However, in modest doses, he believed it to "help digestion, provoke urine, relieve toothache, preserve the teeth from rottenness, comfort a cold stomach, expel the stone from the kidney, and take away dimness of sight." To bring on menstruation, he advised a mixture of red pepper, gentian, and bay laurel, inserted vaginally (no doubt a highly painful proposition).

One of the first North Americans to advocate red pepper as a remedy was Samuel Thomson, the father of Thomsonian medicine. Thomson believed that

---

Active plant parts Fruit
Uses Arthritis, rheumatism, neuralgia, lumbago, frostbite, chilblains
Cautions Red pepper is highly irritating to the eyes and other mucous membranes and to tender skin. Flush with water any area that comes into contact with it. Do not ingest capsicum tinctures and alcoholic extracts, which may be toxic. When capsicum was fed to laboratory rats as 10 percent of their diet, it was shown to produce liver tumors.

most diseases are caused by cold and cured by heat; consequently, red pepper was one of his favorite treatments. The Thomsonians even prescribed red pepper enemas for the sick.

Later in the 19th century the Eclectic physicians recommended red pepper externally for arthritis and muscle soreness, and internally as a digestive stimulant as well as a treatment for fever, nausea, diarrhea, constipation, hemorrhoids, and toothache. It was thought especially worthwhile as a general tonic. According to the Eclectics, it was "particularly useful in old people when the body-heat is low, vitality depressed, and reaction sluggish." Capsicum mixed with salt, vinegar, and water was recommended to ease nausea and prevent vomiting. Capsicum was also used to treat flatulent dyspepsia and colic.

The Appalachian folk healer Tommie Bass prescribed red pepper as a stimulant tonic

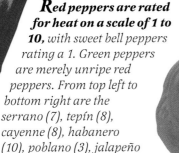

Red peppers are rated for heat on a scale of 1 to 10, with sweet bell peppers rating a 1. Green peppers are merely unripe red peppers. From top left to bottom right are the serrano (7), tepín (8), cayenne (8), habanero (10), poblano (3), jalapeño (5.5), tabasco (9), and Anaheim (2-3).

(in fact, it was one of his favorites). Bass maintained that the pepper would "go around" the body faster than anything else—and take any other medicines with it. Red pepper may indeed be a boon to circulation; it is thought to help dissolve blood clots and to reduce the risk of atherosclerosis by lowering blood cholesterol and triglyceride levels.

Fiery Cold Medicine

Not surprisingly, red pepper was used to "break up" a cold, and it was often brewed into a three-alarm tea to treat the flu. The Cherokee valued red pepper for colds and also applied poultices to the soles of the feet to treat low, or "nervous," fevers.

Red-pepper gargles were used to numb sore throats, and plasters were applied to the chest to loosen congestion. Research has confirmed that nose sprays containing capsaicin, the pungent principle in red pepper, desensitize the nerves that cause running, sneezing, and congestion.

Red pepper was also sprinkled in socks to keep the feet warm. To treat chilblains (itchy, red swellings caused by exposure to cold), the Eclectics advised sprinkling a piece of flannel with red pepper and rubbing it on the skin "until a strong tingling and electrical feeling is produced." The pepper does indeed stimulate peripheral circulation and prevent chilblains— although it should be used only sparingly—and today

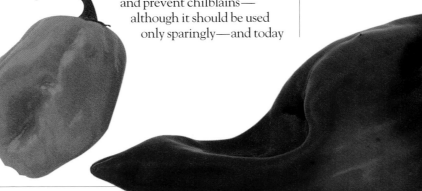

heat plasters that contain red pepper and other herbs are available.

Because it was believed to sustain the nervous system, red pepper was especially valued by the Eclectics for treating delirium tremens (also called the D.T.'s), the delirium and tremors often experienced in the advanced stages of alcoholism. "It enables the stomach to take and retain food, and the best form of administration is a strong beef tea, or strong soup made hot with red pepper," they wrote. They also recommended it for the "atonic dyspepsia of drunkards" and for dipsomania (uncontrollable craving for alcohol), believing that it "takes the place of alcoholic stimulants, removing the craving for alcoholics and sense of sinking at the pit of the stomach, prevents the morning sickness and vomiting, restores gastric tone and promotes the digestion of wholesome food." One modern study has shown that red pepper may protect against alcohol-induced stomach damage.

Some cultures believe that red pepper causes or exacerbates ulcers. Yet in such places as India, the East Indies, Africa, Mexico, and the Caribbean, it has a long history as a digestive aid. Recently, scientific research has provided new information on the subject: one study found no difference in the healing rate of duodenal ulcers among patients who ingested three grams of capsicum daily and those who ate none. Another study, in which participants were examined with a fiber-optic device, found that eating the peppers does no damage to the stomach walls.

Arthritis Relief

Because it creates a soothing sensation of heat, red pepper has long been popular with those suffering from rheumatism and arthritis. Some mixed tallow with red pepper tea and rubbed it on aching joints; others mixed the pepper in alcohol and applied it with a piece of flannel.

Scientists have discovered that red pepper is in fact an excellent treatment for the pain of arthritis, and not only because it creates a feeling of warmth. An application of red pepper causes the body to release a compound known as substance P, which transmits pain signals to the spinal cord and ultimately the brain. As the applications are repeated, the stores of substance P are depleted and pain signals can no longer be sent. Capsaicin may also trigger the release of a natural anti-inflammatory. Red pepper has been approved for use in prescription and over-the-counter topical products.

Creams containing red pepper work in a similar fashion against

pain associated with herpes zoster, commonly called shingles. Patients with shingles often feel excruciating pain around the infected nerve tracts for months or even years. Studies have shown that repeated use of capsaicin decreases the pain, although some patients find the initial burning sensation intolerable.

Moreover, intranasal application of a special capsaicin ointment has been shown to relieve "cluster headaches," migraine-like headaches that tend to occur one to three times a day for several days. Red pepper is also used to relieve psoriasis, a skin disease characterized by itchy red patches and linked with excessive levels of substance P.

Handle With Care

Red pepper is so irritating that it is found in some self-defense sprays. When sprayed into an attacker's eyes, it causes an intense burning sensation and temporary blindness, but no permanent damage.

Wear rubber gloves when peeling or chopping red peppers, and keep your hands away from your nose and eyes. If you do touch a sensitive area with red pepper, flush it with water or milk. Note that the pungent principle in red pepper is virtually insoluble in water, so even if you've washed your hands, traces of the oil may remain and irritate sensitive areas several hours later. To avoid

this, dunk your hands in a solution of one part bleach to five parts water, then rinse them in plain water; or, bathe them in vinegar. When cooking with red peppers, remove the seeds, which contain the most heat. To tame a spicy meal, eat rice, bread, or bananas along with it. Finally, drink a glass of milk; the protein is said to wash away the red pepper's capsaicin.

Pepper Nomenclature

Columbus mistook the fiery fruits of the New World for peppers because their pungency reminded him of black pepper, so coveted that it helped him win royal sponsorship for his journey to the Spice Islands. However, capsicums are unrelated to black peppercorns. In another confusion, the spice they yield is commonly called "cayenne," but cayenne is actually a specific variety of capsicum. Therefore, "red pepper" is the preferred term for the commercial spice, which is often a blend of several of the hottest types.

Red peppers are often called "chile" peppers (also spelled "chili" or "chilli"), whereas "chili" refers to the dish made with meat, beans, and spice. Most chili powder bought in North America is made from two rather mild varieties of capsicum (the Anaheim and a New Mexico variety called 6-4) and other spices.

RHUBARB

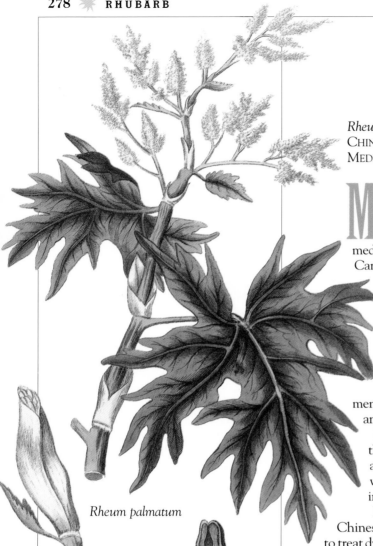

Rheum palmatum

Rheum palmatum, R. officinale
CHINESE RHUBARB, PIE PLANT,
MEDICINAL RHUBARB

More than 2,000 years ago in China, rhubarb was called *tahuang*, or "great yellow," because of its medicinal yellow rhizome. Caravans trekking along ancient trade routes brought the prized rhizome from its native soil, in the mountains of western China and Tibet, westward into the hands of Greek physicians. Used to promote menstruation, treat jaundice and internal bleeding, heal burns and sores, and clear the bowels, rhubarb earned a reputation as a medicinal wherever it traveled, including North America.

In the early 20th century, Chinese rhubarb was widely used to treat dysentery, but its medicinal use steadily subsided—a decline that historians attribute to World War I, during which the English were advised (wrongly) to eat rhubarb leaves to increase their vegetable intake and, as a result, became sick because of the leaves' severe toxicity. Today, Chinese rhubarb (not to be confused with garden rhubarb, which is nonmedicinal) is found mainly in "natural" laxatives and antidiarrheals.

Unique Dual Action

Chinese rhubarb's uniqueness is illustrated by the ailments it was used to treat. Diarrhea (abrupt, watery stools) and constipation (irregular, dry stools) are often thought of as "opposite" ailments. Yet rhubarb root, which contains both astringent and laxative properties that act on the gastrointestinal tract, was historically used to treat both. This dual effect is unusual among medicinal plants and modern medicines alike.

In folk medicine, small amounts of rhubarb root were taken to relieve diarrhea, and studies have shown that such doses can be effective. Rhubarb's diarrhea-fighting capability derives from its astringent tannins, which can help reduce the water content of the stool. However, rhubarb's effects on the intestines are considered too harsh, and it is no longer recommended for treating diarrhea.

Larger amounts of the root were taken to remedy constipation. Anthraquinones provide a "stimulant" laxative effect (they promote a bowel movement by slightly irritating the intestinal walls). Today, however, rhubarb is recommended to relieve constipation only as a last resort.

Active plant parts Roots, rhizome
Uses Constipation, diarrhea
Cautions Prolonged ingestion of the roots and rhizome may reduce the body's water and salt content. Although no side effects are attributed to rhubarb, it may irritate the intestines and cause abdominal cramping. Rhubarb and its extracts should not be used by pregnant or lactating women, or in cases of intestinal obstruction, ulcers, or colitis. The leaves contain poisonous levels of soluble oxalates; ingesting them may cause burning of the mouth and throat, stomach pain, vomiting, liver or kidney damage, or death.

Chinese rhubarb can still be found in both raw and commercial forms. In the U.S. and Canada, the raw root or rhizome is rarely used medicinally. However, herbalists endorse rhubarb extract and tea as mild laxatives. Rhubarb tea is made by steeping ½ to 1 teaspoon powdered root in a cup of boiling water—a pinch of cinnamon or ginger is commonly added for flavoring. Tablets are also available.

Studies of Chinese rhubarb and its derivatives have shown potential antimicrobial, anti-inflammatory, and diuretic

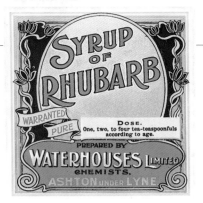

***Rhubarb syrups,** like this one from the early 20th century, were taken as mild laxatives.*

effects. Extracts have been used in studies to treat bleeding of the upper digestive tract. The plant also contains aloe-emodin, which has shown anticancer activity. Despite this, beware of "slimming cures" and "blood-cleans-

ing" teas that contain rhubarb; neither the plant nor its extracts provide these effects.

"Pie Plant"

Dr. John C. Gunn, in his *Gunn's Domestic Medicine* (1830), remarked on Chinese rhubarb's dual action for both diarrhea and constipation: "In this it certainly differs from almost every other purgative of the same class known in medicine." A strong advocate of medicinal rhubarb, Gunn encouraged people to grow the imported plant in their gardens. In North America today, most commercially-grown rhubarb comes from the region of the Pacific Northwest, near Mount Rainier, where the climate is mild but rainy—conditions that rhubarb loves. Gardeners prefer garden rhubarb (R. x *cultorum*), which grows only 91 cm (3 ft) high, over the taller Chinese rhubarb.

Although rhubarb is cultivated around the world and is still used medicinally, the plant is best known for its edible stalks. The stalks are low in calories; however, because they are so sour, they are usually cooked with sugar or other high-calorie sweeteners when used in such traditional desserts as preserves, puddings, and, most commonly, strawberry-and- rhubarb pie. Rhubarb pie, also known as "springtime pie," has become a symbol of spring in many communities across North America. Every spring, many towns hold a rhubarb festival to celebrate the season and the year's first harvest.

The leaves, however, should be avoided by all—they contain high levels of soluble oxalates, which, if ingested, can cause toxic effects on the body, including kidney damage.

The Peculiar Associations of "Rhubarb"

What do the ancient Greeks, Shakespeare, and the Brooklyn Dodgers have in common? Rhubarb. The word "rhubarb" has taken on three distinct meanings, each with an unusual origin. The first-century Greek physician Dioscorides named the Chinese plant *rha barbarum*, meaning "plant grown by the barbarians who live beyond the Volga River." The name was eventually shortened to rhubarb.

In a practice that has been traced to stage productions in Shakespeare's England, a small group of actors would say "rhubarb, rhubarb" over and over again to simulate the rabble of an angry crowd. Introduced to colonial North America (like the plant itself), this device may survive on some small-town stages.

Rhubarb has also come to mean a heated argument. This usage is said to have originated in England, but it has taken on an association with the uniquely North American sport of baseball. The use of "rhubarb" to describe a nose-to-nose dispute between an umpire and a manager—or a bench-clearing tangle of arms and legs of opposing players—is commonly attributed to Red Barber during his days as a Brooklyn Dodgers broadcaster. Reportedly, Barber himself credited that use of the word to a local sportswriter, who in turn claimed that he had heard a Brooklyn bartender use it to describe a bar fight. Today "rhubarb" remains part of baseball's lexicon. For whatever reason, the plant remains eternally linked with barbarians, angry mobs, and brawlers.

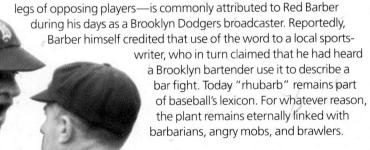

***Legendary baseball manager Casey Stengel** (left) often engaged the umpire in a rhubarb.*

RINGWORM

Once upon a time, some folks believed that ringworm was an actual worm curled up just beneath the skin's surface. (An old remedy from southern Appalachia advised, "Put turpentine and pure hog's lard on the ringworm and pop it right out.") This was, of course, a misconception: Ringworm is a red, itchy fungal skin infection characterized by blister-like ring-shaped inflammations.

Ringworm that is not controlled can be contagious—a ringworm "epidemic" among children in the 1940s was attributed in part to unsanitized barbers' shears and upholstered seats in movie theaters.

Fungus Fighters

The best treatment for ringworm is to keep the skin clean and dry and apply antifungal ointments or oils. Earlier this century, pharmaceutical mixtures, some of which are still available in pharmacies, were popular ringworm remedies. Castellani's paint (a carbolfuchsin solution) is a proven antifungal, but some doctors consider it too harsh for home use. Potassium permanganate (crystals that are added to a solution or a bath) is a superior disinfectant and drying agent, but it can produce a burn-like irritation. Such old standbys, as well as sulfur and coal tar preparations, have now been eclipsed by modern drugs.

Plant-based antifungals, such as garlic, have also been used to treat ringworm. Garlic was even listed in John Wesley's *Primitive Physick* (1747), one of the first medical guides used by North Americans. Angelica, thyme, and cinnamon, all with antifungal properties, have also been tried. Today Australian tea tree oil is gaining popularity as an effective antifungal treatment.

Extracts or juice from the nut casing of black walnut, when applied to the skin, can effectively fight fungal infections. The latex from the stems of milkweed (*Asclepias* spp.), which was utilized by both Indians and Americans of African descent, may also work. (Note that black walnut extracts and milkweed should be used with caution: they can be toxic when ingested.) As for borage and calendula, both were traditionally used as ringworm remedies, but only their concentrated oil is antifungal.

Unique treatments for ringworm, also known as "tetter," included placing old newspapers or a penny soaked in vinegar on the rash. Blue fountain-pen ink and antibacterial wild indigo, sometimes mixed with urine or tobacco ashes, were also applied to the affected skin. Mildly antifungal dyes and "stains" made from gentian violet were painted on infections, too, leaving the skin soothed and blue.

The leaves of black walnut are valued for their antifungal effect.

BLACK WALNUT To make an astringent, mildly antifungal wash, pulverize 5 teaspoons dried leaves. Add to 1 cup water, bring to a boil, then strain. Alternatively, crush the green rind of the unripe fruit to yield its pulp. Apply the wash or pulp to the skin up to four times a day. Using a commercial extract (one part extract diluted in five parts water) may also help. The wash, pulp, and extract may be toxic if ingested.

TURMERIC Although turmeric's antifungal action may be news to North Americans, the spice is a traditional ringworm remedy in Asia. Mix 1 or 2 teaspoons powdered root with enough water to make a paste. Apply to the affected area, cover with a bandage, and leave on for 20 minutes to one hour. Repeat three or four times a day. Turmeric may irritate sensitive skin.

GOLDENSEAL To make an antimicrobial wash, pour 1 cup boiling water over 2 teaspoons powdered root. Let stand until cool. Apply to the skin up to four times a day. After each application, dust a little powdered root on the skin.

ROSE

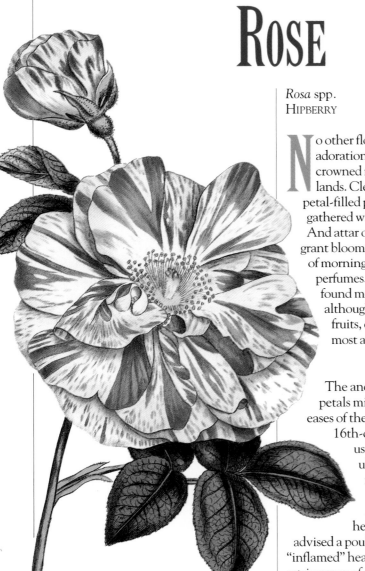

Rosa spp.
HIPBERRY

No other flower has garnered such adoration as the rose. The Romans crowned newlyweds with rose garlands. Cleopatra laid her head on petal-filled pillows. Indian braves gathered wild roses for their brides. And attar of roses, derived from fragrant blooms plucked in the wee hours of morning, scents the world's finest perfumes. Over the years the rose has found medicinal uses as well, although today it is the flower's fruits, or hips, that attract the most attention.

Pretty Petals

The ancient Greeks used rose petals mixed with oil to treat diseases of the uterus. John Gerard, the 16th-century English botanist, used honey of roses to cure ulcers and old wounds, and rose-petal conserve to strengthen the heart.

A century later, the British herbalist Nicholas Culpeper advised a poultice of rose petals for an "inflamed" heart. Culpeper, noting the astringency of the rose, wrote that it "strengthens the stomach, prevents vomiting, stops tickling coughs," and counters diarrhea. He suggested rose petal decoctions in wine for headaches and pains in the eyes, ears, throat, rectum, and uterus. Europeans made teas from the dried petals to treat headache, dizziness, menstrual cramps, and mouth sores.

The Indians applied rose petals mixed with bear grease to mouth sores and made a powder from the dried petals to heal fever blisters. The 19th-century Eclectic physicians described red-rose petals as tonic and mildly astringent and thought them beneficial for bowel disorders and as a poultice for the eyes. However, they preferred the hips, which they ground into a pulp as a base for other medicines. The settlers liked the bitter taste of the hips and made them into jellies and teas.

Vitamin-Rich Hips

In the 1930s rose hips gained sudden popularity when researchers discovered that they contain high concentrations of vitamin C—far more than oranges do. However, because much of this valuable vitamin is lost in the drying process, most commercial rose hips tablets contain added synthetic vitamin C. Moreover, only a portion of the herb's vitamin stores is extracted by the water in rose hip teas.

Most hips come from the dog rose (*Rosa canina*). They consist of the opened, dried hypanthium (the base of the flower), and contain "true" fruits (sometimes called "pips"); these should be removed before the hips are used.

Rose hips are said to be mildly diuretic and laxative; their pectin and citric acid content may account for these reported effects. Rose hip tea—made by steeping 2 teaspoons finely chopped rose hips in 1 cup hot water for 10 minutes, then filtering through cheesecloth—is advised as an eyewash by some herbalists; it can also be used in a compress for tired eyes.

Active plant parts Petals, hips, root bark
Uses Nutritional supplement and antiscorbutic, or scurvy preventive

ROSEMARY

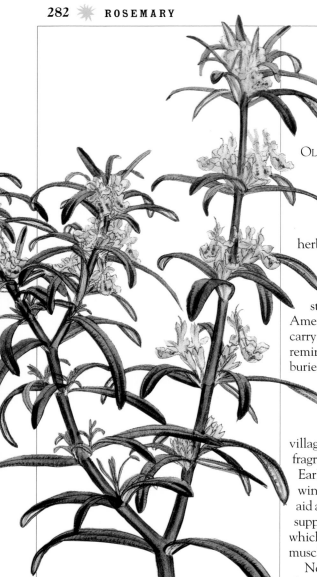

Rosmarinus officinalis
OLD MAN, ROSEMARINE, INCENSIER

Says Ophelia in Shakespeare's *Hamlet*, "There's rosemary, that's for remembrance," voicing what the herb had symbolized for centuries. In ancient Greece, students put sprigs of rosemary in their hair to help improve memory when they studied. Brides in pioneer North America kept the European tradition of carrying rosemary in their bouquets as a reminder of their families. The dead were buried with rosemary to show that they would always be remembered.

The herb was also used as a medicinal. When deadly diseases swept towns and villages, people burned branches of the fragrant, piney plant as a disinfectant. Early herbalists recommended rosemary wine or extract of rosemary as a digestive aid and to relieve gas. This practice is supported by modern scientific research, which shows that rosemary relaxes the muscles of the digestive tract.

Nervous tension and headaches were also treated with rosemary preparations. The herb was thought to be good for the outer head as well: it was made into a hair tonic to prevent baldness. Although there is evidence that the herb can ease some types of headaches, the promise of a full head of hair was purely wishful thinking.

Extracts of the volatile oil were used as an abortifacient, or abortion inducer, and to promote menstruation. Today there is disagreement over whether rosemary induced abortions or merely brought on menstruation in women who were actually not pregnant. Still, doctors caution pregnant women to avoid this herb.

Active Principles

Few clinical studies have been done with rosemary, but some of its components have shown medicinal qualities. The volatile oil, containing camphor, borneol, and cineole, appears to fight bacteria. Studies have also isolated principles in the oil that soothe the digestive system. Another principle, rosmarinic acid, works rather like aspirin to relieve headaches.

Rosemary is a natural preservative, as effective as the synthetic antioxidants BHA and BHT; its extracts are sometimes used in the preparation of meat, alcoholic beverages, condiments, candy, and baked goods. The antioxidant effect may also extend to fighting disease. In studies on lab animals, those fed rosemary oil had a significantly lower incidence of cancers.

Rosemary oil is used as a fragrance in soaps and perfumes. For a refreshing bath, put 1½ cups dried rosemary and ½ cup dried lavender in 2 liters water and bring to a boil. Steep, covered, for 10 to 15 minutes; strain and add to bathwater.

Active plant parts Leaves, flowering tops
Uses Gas, upset stomach, headache; menstruation promoter
Cautions Rosemary leaves are safe to use as a culinary herb, but undiluted rosemary oil should not be taken internally: in large quantities, the oil can cause stomach and intestinal irritation and kidney damage. Toiletries containing rosemary extract can cause dermatitis in some people. Pregnant women should not use this herb medicinally.

RUE

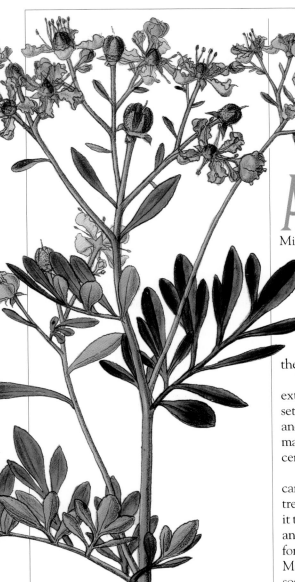

Ruta graveolens
GARDEN RUE,
HERB-OF-GRACE

As one of the most ancient Old World herbs, rue carries a pedigree that has as much to do with mysticism as with medicine. By the Middle Ages, the herb was considered to be a valuable antidote to all manner of poisons and witchcraft, and was also strewn about to ward off the plague. Brushes made of rue were even used to sprinkle holy water before Catholic High Mass—a practice that may account for one of the plant's nicknames, herb-of-grace.

Belief in the mystical qualities of rue extended to North America as well. Many settlers held that a gunflint boiled in rue and vervain would ensure good marksmanship. The Navajo drank rue tea after ceremonial war dances to gain bravery.

Until the 20th century, North Americans used the herb, most often as a tea, to treat many complaints. Doctors prescribed it to remedy gas pain, colic, and epilepsy, and to expel intestinal worms. Treatments for snakebite almost always included rue. Many called for the bruised leaves to be soaked in beer and ice and then pressed against the wound; the remaining liquid was to be drunk by the patient.

Be Forewarned

Despite the plant's documented toxicity, rue also earned widespread renown as an inducer not only of menstruation but also of abortion. Today doctors agree that the potentially lethal risks attached to ingesting this herb outweigh any medicinal benefits it may offer. Pregnant women should avoid rue at all costs.

Rue's volatile oil contains several active constituents, including rutin (a vitamin C derivative similar to compounds found in citrus fruits) and the alkaloids arborine and arborinine, which account for many of the plant's muscle-relaxant properties. Rue also secretes photosynthesizing substances that cause significant skin irritation, especially when the skin is exposed to sunlight. For this reason, it is wise to avoid even simple topical remedies that call for rubbing the leaves of rue directly onto the skin to treat headache and insect bites.

Not to be confused with ...

The sharp-smelling, blue-leaved, yellow-flowered shrub that most people know as garden or medicinal rue is often confused with a benign plant called meadow rue. Meadow rue (*Thalictrum* spp.) has attractive gray-green or blue-green leaves with loose sprays of tiny flowers. The plant has no medicinal uses and poses none of the dangers of garden rue.

Active plant parts Leaves, oil
Uses Rue is considered unsafe for medicinal use.
Cautions Handling rue may cause contact dermatitis; pregnant women should avoid it.

SAGE

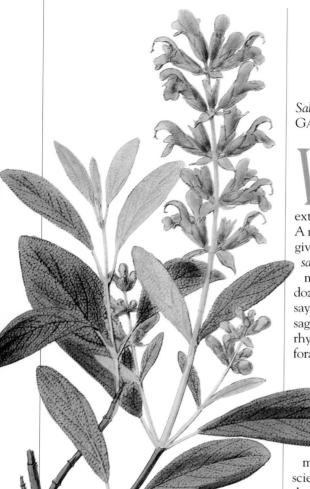

Salvia officinalis
GARDEN SAGE, MEADOW SAGE

With its pleasant aroma and distinctive taste, garden sage has earned an honored place in the kitchen. Yet this herb's reputation extends far beyond roasts and stuffings. A member of the mint family, sage was given the name *Salvia*, from the Latin *salvere*, "to heal." The doctors of medieval Italy used the herb to treat dozens of illnesses and had a common saying: "Why should a person die when sage grows in his garden?" An English folk rhyme declared that "He that would live foraye [forever], must eat sage in May."

Although early settlers hardly expected sage to make them immortal, they used it to treat more than 60 different complaints, from poor memory to intestinal worms. Modern scientists, however, have been skeptical of the herb's medicinal value; instead, they warn of sage's potential dangers.

Native to Mediterranean Europe, garden sage thrives in dry soil and full sun, which makes it ideal for dooryard herb gardens across North America. A rugged, bushy perennial 60 to 90 cm (2 to 3 ft) in height, it has paired, opposite leaves, each one a long, narrow oval cloaked in dense green-gray fuzz. The stem is square—a characteristic typical of the mint family—and its tubular, deep blue flowers are borne at the top of a tall spike. Rub a plucked leaf and a delightful fragrance fills the air, the product of volatile oils.

Another sage used for food and medicine is Spanish sage (*S. lavandulifolia*). It is also the source of the distilled sage oil that is often used to adulterate oil of lavender, which it resembles in smell and chemistry. Other *Salvia* species abound, but most are grown only as ornamentals.

Historical Uses

Sage once had a reputation as an herbal cure-all, but it was most often used as a gargle for sore throats, to reduce the drenching "night sweats" associated with tuberculosis and fevers, and to restrict the flow of bodily fluids—especially a mother's breast milk when it was time to wean her infant. Moreover, sage tea has a long history as a reliever of upset stomachs—not surprising, since volatile oils often help to expel gas from the digestive tract.

Sage tea was used by German immigrants to "break up" a cold. Rural North Americans of many ethnic backgrounds used it to relieve headache, to fight insomnia, and to curb flatulence, diarrhea, and various digestive complaints. Some herbals claimed that sage would speed the course of a measles rash, bringing a patient relief—although the herb's reputed ability to reduce sweating would seem counterproductive in that case.

Active plant parts Leaves
Uses Gargle for mouth or throat inflammation
Cautions Because the thujones in sage are toxic, do not ingest sage oil or apply it externally. Sage extracts, too, should be used with caution. Pregnant and lactating women should avoid the herb altogether.

Not to be confused with ...

Brought to North America by the first settlers, garden sage should not be confused with native sagebrush (*Artemisia tridentata* and other closely related *Artemisia* species). Sagebrush is a woody shrub that dominates much of the arid land of North America's intermountain West. Although it has a pungent, vaguely sage-like odor, its leaves taste terrible and cannot be used as food. Nevertheless, some Indian tribes used sagebrush for many purposes — as fuel, as a yellow dye, as a topical disinfectant, and as a purifying smoke for sweat lodge rituals. While sagebrush was sometimes used medicinally, it is toxic even in small doses, and should be avoided entirely.

Also do not confuse garden sage with the ornamental sages, the most popular of which is scarlet sage *(Salvia coccinea),* prized for its brilliant red flowers. The leaves of ornamental sages have no medicinal properties. In fact, the species name *officinalis* was given to garden sage to distinguish it from the nonmedicinal sages.

Among descendants of Africa, sage tea was traditionally used to treat menstrual cramps and high blood pressure, along with the more widespread applications against colds and sore throat. The crushed fresh leaves were used to destroy warts and to heal cuts and abrasions. To stimulate hair growth, the head was rinsed with a sage–rosemary tea; the tea was also said to maintain the sheen of dark hair.

Use With Caution

Sage may have impressed early healers, but modern tests have shown remarkably little pharmacological activity for this much-vaunted herb. Salvin, an acid found in tiny amounts in sage, may suppress microbes, especially certain forms of *Staphylococcus*. And sage oil, derived from the leaves by steam distillation, has shown an antispasmodic effect on the digestive tract and may help expel gas.

In spite of these potential benefits, scientists have raised red flags about sage's safety. The tea can cause mouth irritation, and substances called alpha- and beta-thujones, which constitute 50 percent of sage's volatile oil, are toxic. Thujone does act as an antiputrification agent, but sage tea should be used routinely only as a mouthwash or gargle; to make a tea, add 2 teaspoons of chopped leaves to boiling water, steep for 10 minutes, then strain. If you decide to drink sage tea, avoid consuming large doses at one time or small amounts over long periods; otherwise, you may experience rapid heartbeat, hot flashes, and dizziness. In the kitchen, however, you needn't worry: heat drives out the thujones, making sage safe to use.

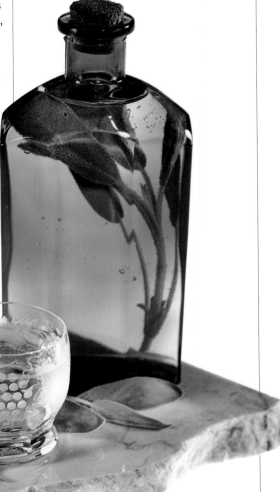

An aromatic mouthwash *made with sage freshens the breath and is safe to use.*

Despite sage's lackluster performance in the laboratory, some surprises may be hiding within its cells. Research by the United States Department of Agriculture has turned up some interesting clues, suggesting that sage tea taken by people with type 2 diabetes may enhance the effects of insulin. If these findings are borne out by further clinical trials, sage may finally live up to its traditional reputation as a valuable medicinal herb.

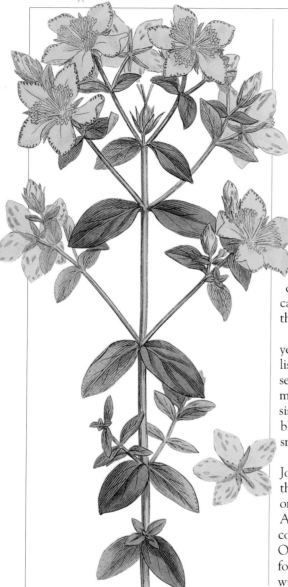

St. Johnswort

Hypericum perforatum
GOD'S GRACE

There is irony in the early North American pioneer custom of hanging sprigs of St. Johnswort in the doorways of homes in midsummer to ward off "evil spirits." Today scientists know that this perennial, which grows in meadows across much of North America, has chemical properties that are indeed capable of deterring negative "spirits"—those of mild depression.

Used medicinally for thousands of years, St. Johnswort ("wort" is Old English for "plant") was employed by early settlers to treat many ailments. Indians made a tea and drank it to fight tuberculosis; they also used the herb to staunch bleeding, reduce fever, and treat snakebites, diarrhea, and skin problems.

The Pennsylvania Dutch called St. Johnswort "the blessed herb" and valued the protection they believed it bestowed on their newborn babies. During the American Civil War, the plant was a common treatment for gunshot wounds. One early recipe, still in use today, called for packing a wide-mouthed jar loosely with the fresh leaves and flowers of St. Johnswort and covering them with olive oil. The jar is sealed, left in a sunny window, and given a good shake daily for three weeks. The resulting blood-red oil is then strained. It is said to promote the healing of any skin wound and, when rubbed on stiff joints, to bring relief from the pain of rheumatism and sciatica.

St. Johnswort is now known to be a rich source of tannins—chemicals with astringent properties that were undoubtedly responsible for the plant's reputation as a wound-healer, dermatological aid, antidiarrheal, and hemorrhoid treatment. One German study of the plant's burn-healing activity found that an ointment made from St. Johnswort substantially reduced the healing time of burns and resulted in less scarring.

Nature's Tranquilizer

It is the plant's growing reputation as "nature's own tranquilizer" that has been the focus of most recent interest in St. Johnswort. A variety of studies have lent credibility to the long-standing claims of folk healers that it is an effective antidepressant. Findings show that certain compounds in the herb—particularly hypericin, which is believed to exert a tranquilizing effect by increasing the blood flow through capillaries—act in tandem to prevent the enzyme monoamine oxidase (MAO) from breaking down serotonin, dopamine, and other amines that elevate mood and emotions. The relationship between the inhibition of MAO and depression is not clear to scientists; still, MAO inhibitors were one

---

Active plant parts Leaves, flowering tops
Uses Mild to moderate depression, cuts and abrasions, burns, diarrhea, hemorrhoids
Cautions St. Johnswort can cause photosensitivity: when taking the herb, allow yourself only minimum exposure to sun. People with high blood pressure, pregnant women and nursing mothers, and those who are taking MAO inhibitors should avoid the herb. However, it is advisable to take the plant only under the supervision of a physician.

of the earliest types of pharmaceutical antidepressants and many are still in use.

In Germany, where research on St. Johnswort has been most extensive, preparations of the herb are sold in pharmacies as an over-the-counter treatment for people suffering from mild depression, nervousness, and sleep disturbances. The results have been so positive that St. Johnswort has become Germany's leading antidepressant, outselling even Prozac.

In 1997 an analysis of 23 clinical trials worldwide—most comparing the herb to placebo and antidepressants—showed St. Johnswort significantly superior to the placebo in treating depression. Compared to antidepressants, it showed promise in being equally effective and had fewer side effects, although more research is needed. Moreover, the herb has no effect on major, as opposed to mild, depression.

In recommended amounts, St. Johnswort is not as powerful as pharmaceutical MAO inhibitors, but anyone who uses either should avoid certain substances. These include cold or hay fever medications, amphetamines and narcotics, the amino acids tryptophan and tyrosine, asthma inhalants, alcohol, coffee, chocolate, and pickled foods. Ingesting these products or foodstuffs in tandem with MAO inhibitors may cause blood pressure to rise dangerously.

A cup of St. Johnswort tea can be safely drunk up to three times a day. Commercial capsules are also available where herbal products are sold. But take note: in some people even the tea has been shown to cause delayed photosensitivity—an abnormal reaction to sunlight that usually results in a skin rash.

Modern Findings

It appears that the ancients weren't far wrong in their belief in St. Johnswort's powers. Many of the properties early folk healers ascribed to the plant have stood up to scientific scrutiny, and new medicinal applications are still being found. Laboratory experiments have demonstrated activity against the bacterium that causes tuberculosis, lending support to the Indians' use for that illness. And the folk remedy that called for treating "hysteria" and the symptoms of menopause with St. Johnswort is now seen in a new light, thanks to the herb's antidepressive activity. Furthermore, certain compounds in the plant have more recently shown antiviral activity against herpes simplex virus types 1 and 2, influenza types A and B, and hepatitis C.

The leaves and flowers of St. Johnswort are traditionally steeped in vegetable oil.

The Blood of St. John

There are many explanations of how St. Johnswort was named. One ascribes the name to the plant's yellow flowers, which are said to be in particular abundance on June 24, the birthday of John the Baptist. Another, perhaps more credible, explanation arises from the fact that glands found on the leaves of the plant exude a red oil when pinched. Early Christians believed that St. Johnswort released the oil on August 29, the anniversary of John the Baptist's beheading. According to the medieval Doctrine of Signatures, which said that an herb's physical appearance revealed its healing powers, the plant's blood-red oil indicated that it should be used for healing wounds—a medicinal application with a centuries-long history, but little scientific support.

Researchers at New York University found in 1988 that St. Johnswort exhibited action against a group of viruses that includes AIDS, noting that hypericin did not exhibit the extreme toxicity to normal cells that had been manifest in other compounds previously used against this virus group. Trials were conducted but were later dropped. Sadly, hypericin showed no efficacy against such viruses.

SALT

Sodium chloride

Salt might be called our lifeblood: it permeates us, bathing every cell in a weak saline solution. Sodium—the unifying element in table salt (sodium chloride), baking soda (sodium bicarbonate), and other common compounds—is critical to the proper functioning of the body. It regulates the body's water balance, thereby allowing muscles to work, maintaining an even heartbeat, and helping to initiate nerve impulses.

Our ancestors were aware of the importance of salt. Mankind has made it a symbol of life, honor, and trust for millennia, from its ceremonial use in binding covenants in Biblical days to the tradition of giving newlyweds bread, wine, and salt to ensure a happy life. To this day, a person of good character is said to be "the salt of the earth," while the opposite sort "isn't worth his salt."

Saltwater Treatments

Little wonder, then, that a substance so intimately associated with life, both biologically and culturally, should have myriad uses in folk healing. The most common form is simple salt water. Because higher concentrations of sodium chloride draw water from surrounding tissues by osmosis, salt water was often used by early North American folk healers to soothe swollen gums or relieve the pressure of an abscess; dentists still recommend rinsing with a solution of warm salt water to ease gum irritation and speed healing. For generations, people suffering from head colds have relied on warm, diluted salt water, sniffed gently up the nostrils, to clear mucus from the nasal passages. Likewise, a salt water gargle relieves a sore throat. But not all folk uses worked: bathing "weak eyes" with a salt solution did nothing for poor vision but it did sting ferociously.

Still, salt water is as popular as ever. Two teaspoons of salt in a half-liter of tepid water make a footbath that helps curb fungal infections by softening and cleansing the skin. Similarly, a salt-water soak makes it easier to remove a stubborn splinter. Salt water heated to body temperature may relieve earaches by loosening wax. In stronger doses, salt can induce vomiting—but large amounts are toxic.

Salt was sometimes used alone (licking a small quantity was thought to cure headaches, and a spoonful thrown in the back of the throat was said to stop seizures), but it was most often mixed with other ingredients. Bruises or sprains on both people and livestock were doctored with a thick paste of egg white and salt, while an egg yolk with a pinch of salt was claimed to cure indigestion. Salt and brandy were used against rheumatism and dysentery. Some folks gave children with the croup a dose of equal parts honey and salt; they also used salt with nutmeg, flour, and sugar to help alleviate diarrhea.

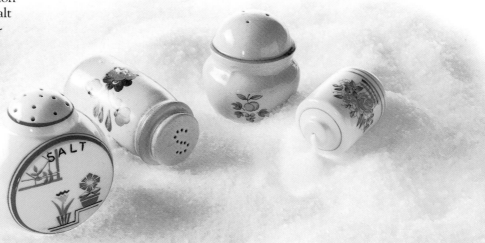

A kitchen essential, table salt has been used in a multitude of home remedies.

Uses Sore throat, irritated or swollen gums, earaches, skin infections
Cautions Overconsumption is linked to hypertension, which can cause heart attack, strokes, and kidney failure. Very large doses can have toxic, even fatal, effects.

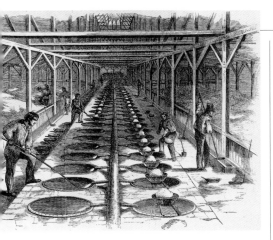

The saltworks at Syracuse, New York, was one of many such 19th-century establishments.

When these remedies worked, it was because high concentrations of salt are antimicrobial and anti-itch. Salt may, in fact, have an external germicidal effect; evidence comes from the fact that high concentrations of salt were used as preservatives in the days before refrigeration.

Valuable Yet Risky

Salt has been one of our most valued resources for millennia (the word "salary" comes from *salarium*, the allowance of salt paid to soldiers in ancient Rome). On the frontier, natural salt licks and springs attracted people who boiled down the brine to obtain salt. Today, while some salt is still produced by evaporation, much of the commercial supply comes from deep mines. Mined salt is actually sea salt, albeit very old; the great underground salt domes near Chicago, Illinois, for example, were originally formed hundreds of millions of years ago when seawater, trapped behind ocean reefs, evaporated.

As with many foods, too much or too little sodium can be hazardous to health. Signs of sodium deficiency include muscle cramps, weakness, and headaches. (These

A Vital Preservative

In the bone-deep cold of January, 1778, Daniel Boone led a party of 30 men north from Boonesborough in Kentucky to the Blue Licks, a group of natural salt springs along the Licking River. For more than a month, the men worked at boiling down the brine into more than 300 bushels of coarse salt—until their capture by the Shawnee brought the labor to an abrupt end. While Boone later escaped from the Indians, the episode shows the dangerous lengths to which settlers were willing to go in order to get salt. The mineral was necessary for tanning hides into leather, and it was absolutely vital for preserving food in the days before refrigeration.

Because salt is hygroscopic, it draws moisture from meat, drying it while at the same time creating an environment inhospitable to the microorganisms that cause spoilage; this process can be reinforced by hanging a piece of salted meat in a smokehouse for several weeks, further "curing" it. As the fall butchering season approached, a farm family had two choices for salting their winter meat supply—burying the meat in layers of finely powdered salt, or the less expensive method of brine-curing, in which the food is laid up in barrels or crocks with a strong solution of salt and water. Salt was used as a preservative not only for meat and fish, but for vegetables— turning cabbage into sauerkraut and cucumbers into pickles.

For searching out salt, Daniel Boone paid a high price: four months in captivity.

symptoms can also occur when vomiting, diarrhea, or a diuretic depletes sodium.)

Most North Americans consume far too much salt, usually in the form of sodium chloride. Canadian guidelines advise that an average, healthy adult ingest no more than 2,400 milligrams of sodium each day. Most people need no more than 500 milligrams, but the average person in Canada consumes 3,100 milligrams daily—not just in so-called salty foods, like chips and pretzels, but also in soft drinks, fast foods, and products containing such sodium preservatives as sodium benzoate and sodium propionate. Too much sodium has been linked to hypertension, a condition that can lead to kidney failure and stroke—a powerful reason to closely watch your intake of this important mineral.

SARSAPARILLA

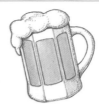

Smilax spp.

A bit of trivia for root beer lovers: sarsaparilla, a key ingredient in this tasty brew, has a 500-year history as a remedy for a certain social disease—namely, syphilis. Even pirates and cowboys took the "cure," say historians, often in the form of tonics and "blood purifiers." But despite such wishful thinking, periods of wild popularity, and controversy over its efficacy, there has been surprisingly little scientific research on the herb. In fact, sarsaparilla remains an enigma to experts.

Among many cultures, from the ancient Chinese to the North American Indians, sarsaparilla boasts a long, rich history of use as a long-term tonic and treatment for skin diseases, rheumatism, and urinary tract infections. According to Roman legend, the maiden Smilax was slighted in love and subsequently transformed into the flowering plant—hence the genus's Latin name. The group of medicinal plants called sarsaparilla derive their common name from the Spanish *zarza* ("bramble") and *parrilla* ("small vine"). A member of the lily family, the herb is found in eastern North America and Central America; related *Smilax* species grow worldwide.

Sarsaparilla was introduced to European medicine in the mid-16th century by Spanish explorers of New Spain (Mexico), who valued the locally grown "zarza parrilla" as a cure for syphilis, which they believed to be a New World disease. Its use extended through the 17th century to cure the common cold and other ills. In later years, statements by leading physicians that the herb was worthless did not stop the influx of the vine into England.

North American Use

In the Americas, Indians used native species of *Smilax* in ways remarkably similar to those of the Europeans and the Chinese, including that of a tonic "to make one young." Many tribes in eastern North America also used other plants that are called sarsaparilla—species of the genera *Aralia* and *Menispermum*.

Early settlers relied on imported sarsaparilla and related local species of *Smilax* for the same ailments that the Europeans did, notably syphilis. The herb would remain listed in either the *U.S. Dispensatory* or U.S. Pharmacopeia for a span of 145 years. By the early 1900s, sarsaparilla patent remedies had swept the continent. Most celebrated was Ayer's Sarsaparilla, which euphemistically "made the weak strong." In Canada, Eaton's sold Peerless Sarsaparilla Compound for "purifying blood and toning up the system."

Smilax regelii

Active plant parts Rhizome and roots
Uses Skin conditions; digestive aid, diuretic
Cautions Use sarsaparilla in medicinal amounts only under a doctor's supervision. Discontinue use if you experience a burning sensation in the mouth or stomach. Sarsaparilla should not be used by pregnant women or children under the age of two.

A legendary patent medicine did not shy from proclaiming its worth. Fever blisters, indigestion, headache, flatulence, and "that tired feeling" were but a few of the ailments Ayer's Sarsaparilla promised to remedy.

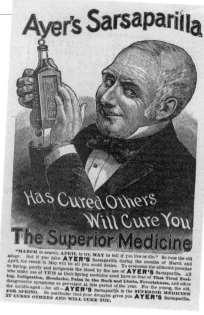

Ayer's Sarsaparilla

Has Cured Others Will Cure You
The Superior Medicine

"MARCH to search, APRIL to try, MAY to tell if you live or die." So runs the old adage. But if you take **AYER'S** Sarsaparilla during the months of March and April, the result in May will be all you could desire. To overcome the ailments peculiar to Spring, purify and invigorate the blood by the use of **AYER'S** Sarsaparilla. All who make use of THIS as their Spring medicine need have no fear of That Tired Feeling, Indigestion, Headache, Pains in the Back and Limbs, Feverishness, and other disagreeable symptoms so prevalent at this period of the year. For the young, the old, the middle-aged—for all—**AYER'S** Sarsaparilla is the SUPERIOR MEDICINE FOR SPRING. Be particular that your druggist gives you **AYER'S** Sarsaparilla. IT CURES OTHERS AND WILL CURE YOU.

Sarsaparilla-flavored drinks were also popular. People of African ancestry made "a very pleasant beer" from sassafras, maize, molasses, and the tuber of a local *Smilax* species—hence the name "root beer." Today sarsaparilla is still utilized as a flavoring agent in foods and beverages, and Europeans continue to use the herb as a tonic for skin disease (especially psoriasis), rheumatic complaints, kidney disease, and as a diuretic and sweat-inducer. The Chinese use a local *Smilax* species for similar ills, as well as for syphilis. Many also still believe that the herb has an aphrodisiac effect, although no such effect has been proven.

Sarsaparilla's most controversial usage today is as a "natural" way to build muscle. Many herbal body-building products claim that the herb is a reliable source of the anabolic steroid testosterone.

Promise Unfulfilled

Despite sarsaparilla's rich history of use, scientists say that there is little sound research to back up the many claims for the herb. The only clinical studies on sarsaparilla are almost 50 years old, and they do not meet today's rigorous research guidelines. These studies showed improvement in appetite and digestion, beneficial effects on certain skin diseases, and diuretic effects. More recent studies, using laboratory animals, have found liver-protective, diuretic, and anti-inflammatory properties in sarsaparilla. However, its value for humans has not yet been demonstrated. Accordingly, the German Commission E—the world's most respected authority on the efficacy of herbal medicines—does not recommend it as a remedy.

As for the muscle-building claims, they, too, are without merit. Sarsaparilla does contain several steroids, which have been used to produce various synthetic steroidal drugs. But these compounds cannot convert to anabolic steroids, including testosterone, in the body.

Nevertheless, many scientists are not ready to write off sarsaparilla. Some suspect that the rise and fall of the herb's popularity may be due to the use of inferior-quality roots, substitutes, and adulterants. Even though there are some 350 species of *Smilax* worldwide, only a few plants known as sarsaparilla are sold for their medicinal properties: Honduran (*Smilax regelii*), Mexican (*S. aristolochiaefolia*), Jamaican (*S. ornata*), and Ecuadorian (*S. febrifuga*). Substitutes or adulterants include American sarsaparilla (*Aralia racemosa*), Bullbrier (*Smilax rotundifolia*), and Indian and European sarsaparillas.

History suggests that sarsaparilla is not a quick fix and may be effective only with long-term use. Even so, until many questions are answered, the efficacy of sarsaparilla remains in doubt. Some leading herbalists maintain that there is no scientific basis for the medicinal use of sarsaparilla and that the herb's only legitimate use is as a flavoring and foaming agent in foods and such drinks as root beer.

Not to be confused with ...

Three other plants go by the name sarsaparilla. The first, spikenard (*Aralia racemosa*), is also known as American sarsaparilla (below). A member of the ginseng family, it was used by the Micmac as a salve for cuts and wounds; the Ojibwa used the root in a poultice to heal broken bones. Closely related to spikenard is wild sarsaparilla (*A. nudicaulis*), which was used not only medicinally but, like the *Smilax* species, as a flavoring for root beer. A third plant, *Menispermum canadense*, is known as yellow sarsaparilla, Texas sarsaparilla, and Canada moonseed; like spikenard, it is also called American sarsaparilla. Some still use it to treat both high and low blood pressure, arthritis, and bladder and kidney problems.

SASSAFRAS

Sassafras albidum
SASSAFRAC, SAXIFRAX TREE,
AGUE TREE, CINNAMONWOOD,
SALOOP, SMELLING-STICK

Before North America's luxuriant furs reached the markets of Europe, before its eastern white pines were coveted for ships' masts, and before its tobacco was craved by London's pipe smokers, sassafras was the first commercial bonanza of the New World. Indians had been using the fragrant bark and reddish root wood of this small, scrubby tree for centuries, and they passed on the knowledge to French colonists in Florida in the late 1600s. The French, soon overrun by the Spanish, told their adversaries about sassafras root, which was said to have extraordinary medicinal properties. From there the word spread across Europe, thanks to a Spanish physician named Nicholas Monardes.

"… Of Great Vertues"

Monardes's 1574 book, *Joyfull Newes Out of the Newe Founde Worlde*, hailed the wonders of sassafras: "A woodd and roote of a tree that groweth in those partes, of greate vertues, and great excellencies, that thei heale there with greevous and variable deseases." This marvelous new drug, he claimed, cured malaria and other fevers, stomach and liver ailments, dropsy (edema), kidney stones, and "griefs of the breast caused by cold humors."

Such unstinting acclaim set off what was, in 16th-century terms, a sassafras rush. The English sent a ship to scour the coast of North Carolina in 1584 and another to New England in 1602, when the dried bark was bringing £336 sterling per ton—a princely sum in those days. A year later, a two-ship expedition to "Virginia" (actually, the coast of Connecticut) returned to England with full loads, despite intermittent Indian attacks. The English at Jamestown were even required to provide the colony's backers with sassafras as a condition of their charter.

The imported North American root was used by Europeans to treat, among things, syphilis—an application they may have learned from the Iroquois, who used it for the same purpose. It later became clear, however, that the plant was useless against any kind of venereal disease.

The boom went bust in the early 17th century when buyers realized that sassafras, despite its pleasant smell and taste, was not the cure-all Monardes and others had claimed. Nevertheless, the bark continued to play a central role in folk medicine right through the 20th century in North America. In the Appalachian and Ozark mountains, sassafras tea was a "good for what ails you" standby and the root bark was a main ingredient of spring

---

Active plant parts All parts, especially the root bark
Uses No significant therapeutic effects have been documented.
Cautions Safrole, the aromatic ether in sassafras, is carcinogenic in humans. Safrole-free sassafras extract has also caused malignant tumors in laboratory animals.

tonics. Like sarsaparilla, sassafras oil served as the flavor foundation for traditional root beer, as well as a number of other foods, and sassafras leaves were a staple of country cooking—not for their medicinal qualities but because their mucilage served as an especially effective thickening agent when added to soups or stews. Its reputation for healing notwithstanding, many mountain dwellers continue to drink sassafras tea simply because they like the taste. Its use extends even to the vegetable garden: some use the dregs of the tea as a fertilizer for tomatoes.

Many Parts, Many Uses

Although closely associated with mountainous Appalachia, the native species of this tree grows in the wild in North America, from Ontario south to Florida and Texas and as far west as Missouri. Before the dangers of sassafras were recognized, North Americans attributed a variety of healthful effects to every part of the tree. A root-bark decoction was often used on the frontier to fight fevers, known as "ague"; indeed, sassafras is still sometimes called by its old name, "ague tree." In New England, sassafras

Often put up with herbs like yellowroot or wild cherry bark, sassafras is still seen on pantry shelves in the Appalachian range, even though the safrole in the plant has been shown to be dangerous.

root chips boiled in beer were said to be "excellent to allay the hot rage of feavers." The Pennsylvania Dutch called the plant "fiewerbaum" (fever tree) and boiled the flowers in water to make a medicinal tea.

Crushed sassafras leaves were applied topically to relieve the itch of insect bites and stings, while some folk practitioners swore it worked against rheumatism, gout, and kidney problems. The oil of sassafras was also credited with medicinal properties. Peter Kalm, an 18th-century naturalist, reported that a woman cured chronic, crippling pain in her foot by rubbing it with oil extracted from boiled sassafras berries. Even the twig pith, which is mucilaginous, was used as an eyewash or poultice. Some added the pith to lye soap to soothe skin rashes. The pitch from the tree was thinned and drunk for digestive complaints.

Furthermore, like cedar, the pungent wood was believed to repel insects. Bedsteads were made of the fragrant timber to drive away bedbugs, and cabin floors and henhouses were built of sassafras to keep termites at bay. In fact, scientific research has found that safrole, the aromatic (if dangerous) substance in sassafras oil, protects against insect infestation by mimicking the juvenile growth hormones of some insect pests, thereby stunting their development and curbing reproduction.

The Safrole Question

Only in recent years was sassafras discovered to be hazardous. Experiments showed that safrole, a phenolic ether in sassafras oil, causes liver tumors in laboratory animals. Accordingly, in 1961 the U.S. FDA banned the use of safrole and oil of sassafras in food and beverages, including root beer. In 1976 the agency banned the interstate sale of sassafras root bark, used to make tea; a single cup may contain up to 200 milligrams of safrole, several times the amount at which humans are believed to be at risk. Even safrole-free sassafras extract was found to cause malignant tumors in two-thirds of the laboratory animals that received it.

In Canada, the Food and Drugs Act prohibits the use of safrole in food products, and only allows sassafras to be added as a food flavoring if it is safrole-free. Therapeutic products containing safrole are subject to severe scrutiny by Health Canada; only products labeled with a Drug Identification Number (DIN) have been authorized for sale by Canada's Health Protection Branch.

Safrole does occur in much smaller, safer amounts in many other plants, including nutmeg, black pepper, mace, bay leaves, and camphor. Furthermore, not everyone is convinced that it is dangerous. A Swiss study—in which humans given tiny doses of safrole showed no sign of the carcinogenic metabolite in their urine—is often cited as evidence that humans may metabolize safrole differently than rats do.

Other skeptics argue that the safrole in a can of old-fashioned root beer is less carcinogenic than the alcohol in a similar quantity of beer. Regardless of the degree of danger, however, experts caution that sassafras has no proven medicinal value and is not worth even a slight risk.

SAW PALMETTO

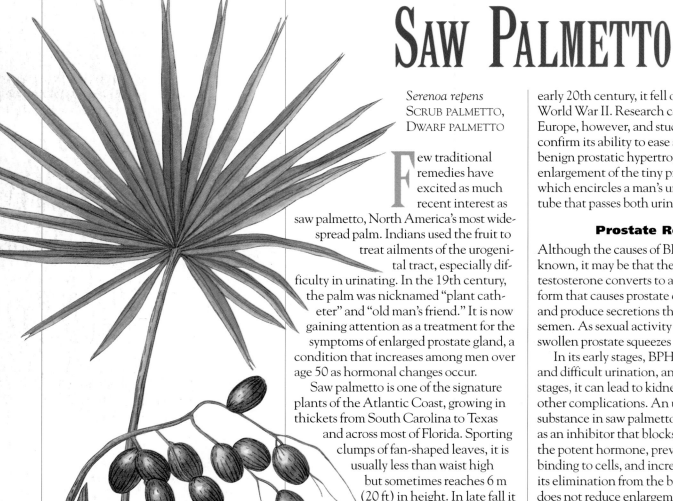

Serenoa repens
SCRUB PALMETTO,
DWARF PALMETTO

Few traditional remedies have excited as much recent interest as saw palmetto, North America's most widespread palm. Indians used the fruit to treat ailments of the urogenital tract, especially difficulty in urinating. In the 19th century, the palm was nicknamed "plant catheter" and "old man's friend." It is now gaining attention as a treatment for the symptoms of enlarged prostate gland, a condition that increases among men over age 50 as hormonal changes occur.

Saw palmetto is one of the signature plants of the Atlantic Coast, growing in thickets from South Carolina to Texas and across most of Florida. Sporting clumps of fan-shaped leaves, it is usually less than waist high but sometimes reaches 6 m (20 ft) in height. In late fall it bears oily blue-black fruits. Although saw palmetto was prescribed in North America for prostate problems in the early 20th century, it fell out of favor after World War II. Research continued in Europe, however, and studies seemed to confirm its ability to ease symptoms of benign prostatic hypertrophy (BPH), an enlargement of the tiny prostate gland which encircles a man's urethra—the tube that passes both urine and semen.

Prostate Relief

Although the causes of BPH are not known, it may be that the hormone testosterone converts to a more potent form that causes prostate cells to multiply and produce secretions that are added to semen. As sexual activity declines, the swollen prostate squeezes the urethra.

In its early stages, BPH causes frequent and difficult urination, and in advanced stages, it can lead to kidney damage and other complications. An unidentified substance in saw palmetto extract serves as an inhibitor that blocks formation of the potent hormone, prevents it from binding to cells, and increases the rate of its elimination from the body. The extract does not reduce enlargement of the prostate but relieves some of the symptoms.

The tea is of little value; the active ingredients in the fruit are fat-soluble and do not dissolve in water. Although preparations containing the extracts are widely sold in North America, Health Canada only permits their sale as diuretic products; it is prohibited to market them as treatments for BPH. Saw palmetto should be taken only under the guidance of a physician, since it may interfere with prescription drugs that combat BPH.

Active plant parts Ripe fruit
Uses Treatment of symptoms stemming from enlarged prostate
Cautions Consult a doctor before taking; men should have regular prostate exams to check for cancer. The tea made from saw palmetto has little medicinal value. In rare cases, saw palmetto may cause stomach disorders. It may also interact with prescription drugs taken to treat enlargement of the prostate.

SCABIES

Known simply as "the itch," scabies is a notorious skin condition caused by mites (*Sarcoptes scabiei*) that infest the skin; it is characterized by severe itching, especially at night. Since antiquity, countless stories have been told of scabies afflicting large groups of soldiers and crippling armies. Today the condition is estimated to affect 300 million people worldwide each year.

Some of the safest and most effective remedies used today have their roots in folk tradition: these include permethrin (a synthetic derivative of the pyrethrum plant), sulfur, and calamine lotion.

Debugging Remedies

To kill the mites, folk medicine commonly employed natural insecticides, such as dried chrysanthemum flowers that were first imported to North America for this purpose in the late 19th century. One particular chrysanthemum, pyrethrum, has been found to contain an insecticide called pyrethrin. A pyrethrin-like chemical, permethrin, is approved by Health Canada for the treatment of scabies.

Other plant-based insecticides—toxic for mites but safe for humans when used topically—are washes made from alder, tobacco, and common indigo. European derris root extract contains rotenone, which is now used in pesticides today.

Whatever treatment is chosen, there are certain measures that should be taken. First, see a family doctor or dermatologist to confirm the diagnosis. Second, because of the contagious nature of the disease, have all members of the affected person's immediate family treated simultaneously. Third, wash all bedding and clothing in hot water—at least 49°C (120°F). An old folk remedy advised wearing the same clothes for a week, but the mites can live on your clothes and escape treatments that are applied to the skin. Also, because itching can last for up to two weeks after the mites have been eradicated, itch-fighting treatments, such as calamine lotion, should be kept close at hand.

Sulfur and Springs

Folk wisdom wrongly associated scabies with uncleanliness; in fact, scabies can be acquired only by contact with another affected person. Scabies washes were made with strong rum, lemon juice, yellow dock, and sweet gum (also called liquidambar), or American laurel leaves. Ill-advised folk remedies included a preparation of toxic pokeroot and "red precipitate ointment," or mercury oxide, which was known to potentially "bring a worse evil than it cures."

To relieve the itching, plantain leaves and wild yams were applied, although a dip in a natural spring may have been more soothing. The Indians favored many natural sulfurous springs, including those in Casco, Maine; Palm Springs, California; and Radium Hot Springs, British Columbia. Sulfur preparations, which are messy and leave stains, are still in use, and are said by some doctors to be safe and effective; others consider them too weak.

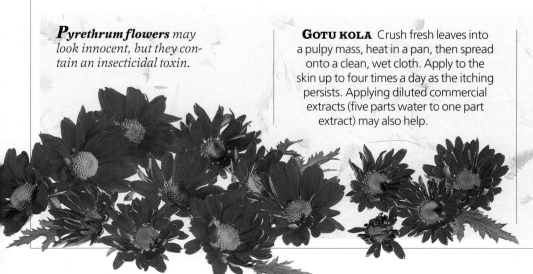

Pyrethrum flowers may look innocent, but they contain an insecticidal toxin.

GOTU KOLA Crush fresh leaves into a pulpy mass, heat in a pan, then spread onto a clean, wet cloth. Apply to the skin up to four times a day as the itching persists. Applying diluted commercial extracts (five parts water to one part extract) may also help.

PERMETHRIN CREAM Apply a 1 percent cream or ointment (available commercially) to the skin for 10 minutes. A second application may be required. Permethrin, a toxic insecticide, is a synthetic derivative of the pyrethrum plant. Tingling and irritation may occur.

ALDER Boil the inner bark of *Alnus glutinosa* in vinegar for 10 minutes. Use 1 teaspoon bark for each cup of vinegar. Strain, then apply to the skin up to four times a day. Note that alder may color the skin and should not be ingested.

WAGON TRAIN & PRAIRIE MEDICINE

Medicine on the prairies of the frontier West can be best summed up as an exercise in self-sufficiency. Whenever illness or accident struck, the pioneers usually had to rely on their own ingenuity and whatever meager resources were on hand, whether they were rolling west in wagons or were settled in their new homesteads.

Early explorers extolled the healthfulness of the West, and many of the pioneers who emigrated to this promised land reported that they had "never felt better in their lives." The air itself was believed to improve health, for it was thought to be pure and dry. Yet such optimism was too often shattered. Devastating diseases—cholera, malaria, smallpox, typhoid, and dysentery—were a constant threat. Thousands of emigrants died of cholera on the westward migration of 1849–50. One terrified wagoner wrote that along the Platte River he was "scarcely out of the sight of grave diggers." Facing vast distances, sometimes hostile Indians, and a scarcity of doctors, pioneers made do with their often inadequate

supplies and all the resolve and courage they could summon.

The Medicine Bag

Along with their provisions of foodstuffs, clothing, and tools, most pioneer families carried a bag or chest full of medicines from home. These might include "physicking pills," castor oil, and essence of peppermint—a medicine one manufacturer claimed "would cure anything that ailed you, from colic in newborn babes to aches and pains accompanying old age." (This

was just one of many medicines and foodstuffs pitched to the emigrants; another was the "meat biscuit"—an early forerunner of the beef stock cube.) The journal of one pioneer traveler records that he brought quinine for malaria and tormentil in case of snakebite. Some foods, too, were thought to be medicinal: many emigrants stocked up on pickles, believing that these would help prevent scurvy. Unknown to the travelers, the pickling process actually destroys the store of vitamin C in food.

Whiskey was considered another necessity for maintaining good health. Besides using it to disinfect wounds and as an anesthetic, the settlers believed that bad water (a recurring problem) could be purified with the addition of the spirit. Other plant-based substances, too, were used.

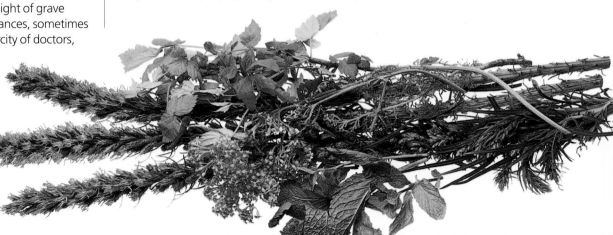

Medicinal plants
useful to the pioneers included (from left) gayfeather (Liatris punctata), *raspberry leaf, yarrow, and species of mint.*

Treating Sick Livestock

When it came to staying healthy, early prairie settlers had more than their families to worry about. Also of concern were the livestock—essential to their livelihood. Horses supplied the power to plow the fields and haul wheat to market. Cattle and oxen, first kept to supply westbound travelers with fresh livestock, were by the mid 1860s part of a new beef industry.

From the mid-19th century, two of the most dreaded animal diseases on the prairie were Texas fever (a tick-borne cattle disease) and hog cholera. Unfortunately, veterinarians were virtually unknown in the North American West at the time. Answering the call were self-proclaimed practitioners, known as "cow leeches" by some because of their propensity for "relentless bleeding, burning, and blistering." Not until the late 1800s were these quack veterinarians put out of business by trained, college-educated veterinary surgeons.

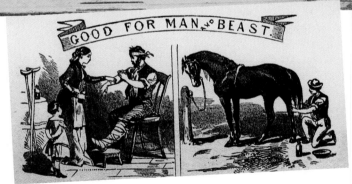

As this 1896 photograph attests, veterinarians were in demand. By the late 1800s, 30 percent of Canada's veterinary surgeons were based out West.

After graduate veterinarians arrived, quacks dismissed them as having "learned their business" in college, not on the land. In the end, the veterinarians' successful techniques and new equipment (right) rendered cruel treatments obsolete.

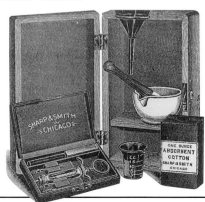

Medical care was so scarce on the prairie—for people and livestock alike—that dual-purpose patent medicines were common. Medical books, too, were often designed for both humans and animals. With progress and the advent of licensed veterinarians, such all-in-one health aids disappeared from the scene.

in two & apply one half to the wound like a poultice and it will draw out the poison."

Such self-reliance and reciprocity continued until the turn of the century. As life on the prairie changed with the times, the region's few doctors—many of them drawn westward by a lack of success back East, others untrained but equipped with medical books and homeopathic remedies— were replaced by qualified physicians. In the modern day, the home remedies once so necessary to health care on the prairie have become a matter of choice.

The Pioneer Woman

If men performed the heavy work required of life out on the western plains, women took charge of health matters. Home remedies were most often prepared from plant material and medicines from back East, but women were quick to make use of whatever was at hand. Freshly dug echinacea root made a tea for a child with whooping cough; mashed raspberry leaves became a poultice for sores. Household items, too, were called upon. Mothers rubbed goose grease and turpentine on their children's chests whenever they had a cold. "It was all you could smell in a classroom," one settler recalled.

On the journey west, a pioneer wife attends to her husband, his feet rubbed raw by day after day of walking. Having learned of the medicinal plants of the prairie through her correspondence with earlier emigrants, she and her young son have scouted the open fields and have come upon native yarrow. With the aromatic flowers and fernlike leaves in hand, they prepare a healing bath. The son adds more stalks to the steaming soak as his mother begins the bandaging.

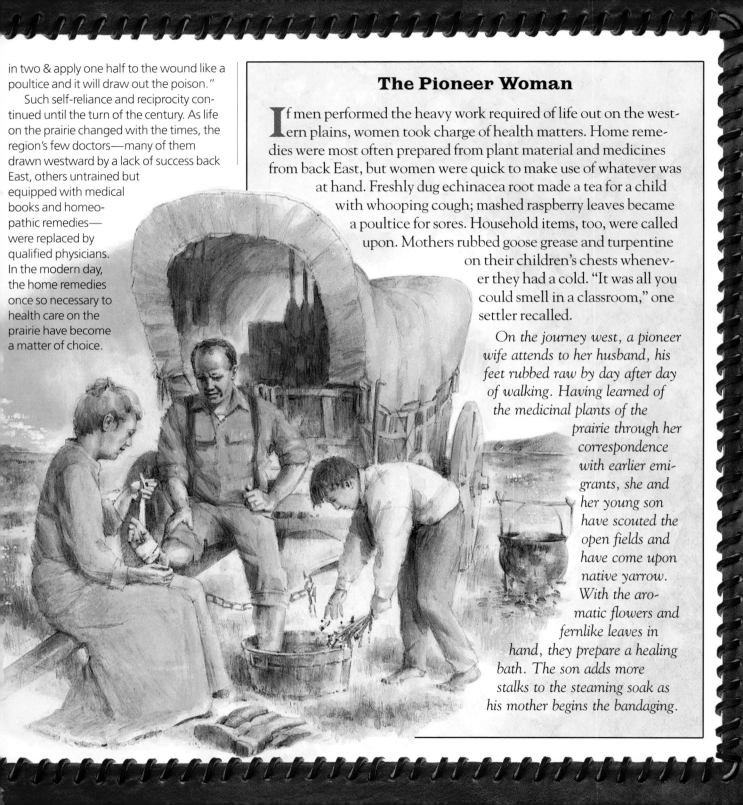

One family, rightfully fearful of contracting cholera from contaminated water, was told by a mountain man they encountered that red-pepper sauce would work as a water purifier. For the rest of their months-long trek, the family would not take even a sip of water without adding a dash of the fiery sauce.

Accidents were a constant worry; the most common were accidental shootings, drownings, injuries from handling livestock, and being crushed beneath wagon wheels. Even feet were at risk: astonishingly, many emigrants walked the entire trek, either striding alongside the family wagon to lighten the oxen team's load or—as was common in the Mormons' westward journey—pushing their belongings in a handcart. In a time when shoes were usually ill-fitting, the feet were often rubbed so raw that they bled.

Shared Wisdom

Contrary to popular belief, the westbound travelers learned little about medicinal plants from the Indians they encountered. Instead, they picked up medical advice from one another and from those already familiar with the western landscape. When illness struck, they shared supplies. In a letter to a friend, one man offered the following advice on outfitting a wagon: "Get double the quantity of butter crackers that you do of flour. Ours lasted all the way through. These and our large cheese made our wagon the frequent resort on behalf of the sick."

Childbirth was common on wagon treks west, and often occurred without benefit of professional medical help. Sometimes the wagons or ox-driven carts would stop for a day or two of rest, but often settlers would pause only briefly for the birth before setting off again. Tending to infants was rigorous, and required imagination. If new mothers found themselves unable to nurse their babies, they turned to other nursing mothers. One woman suffering from painful nipples resorted to the use of a bottle and cow's milk. The only problem was finding a useful nipple. "Have obtained a mare's tit," she reported. "Hope to succeed in using it." Even after settling, pioneer women helped one another. When children were sick or a baby was born, friends and neighbors gathered at the house to prepare meals and perform the chores.

On the Homestead

Once established on far-flung ranches and farms, pioneer families supplemented the medical supplies that were shipped to the region with home remedies culled from the land. Herbs, prairie plants, and tree roots were brewed into potent teas and used to combat specific ailments—buttercup for asthma, sassafras root for fevers, alfalfa for kidney disorders. In some parts of the West, the rootlets of gayfeather were burned and the smoke inhaled to ease headache and nosebleeds. Just as essence of peppermint had been a common item on the trek, the various species of mint were made into teas to relieve insomnia, upset stomachs, and colds.

Trial and error was the rule, and if a remedy succeeded, it was eagerly passed on to others. "I must give you this prescription for rattle snake bites," one woman wrote to a friend. "Please tell all the men on your ranch… Cut a cactus

*"**Electrical**" gadgets* and patent medicines found a ready market in a region with a scarcity of doctors. Dr. Blackburn's No. 1 Electric Galvanic Body Battery (below) was worn to bed to build strength for next day's toil. Dried herb kits for wagoners (below right) first appeared in the mid 1800s.

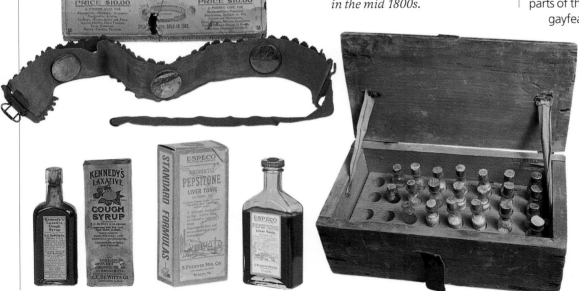

SENNA

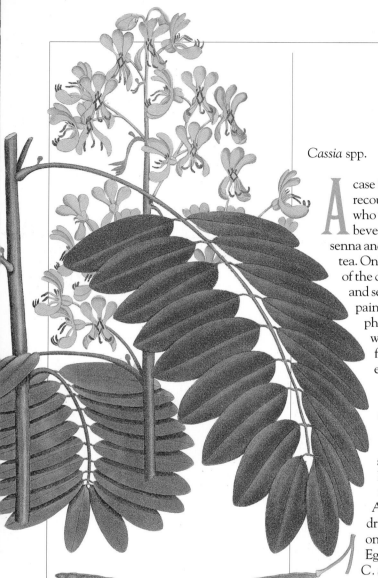

Cassia spp.

A case in the medical literature recounts the story of a housewife who wanted to try a new hot beverage. She chose a packet of senna and drank several cups of the tea. Only after suffering for most of the day with diarrhea, nausea, and severe gripes (spasmodic pain in the bowels) did she phone her doctor and learn what herbalists have known for centuries: senna is a powerful laxative—one that must be used with care.

The senna usually employed for medicinal purposes comes from the dried leaflets of two species. *Cassia senna* (also known as *C. acutifolia*) is native to the Nile region of Africa. It is called Alexandrian senna because it was once imported from the Egyptian city of Alexandria. *C. angustifolia* comes from India and is called Tinnevelly senna. A somewhat milder *Cassia* species, *C. marilandica*, dubbed wild senna or American senna, grows in the eastern and southern United States.

A Potent Laxative

Named by the Arabs, senna has been used as a laxative by that culture since ancient times. They turned to the herb because it was actually gentler than the standard purgatives of the day (a concept difficult to grasp, given senna's strength). Europeans started using senna sometime in the 11th century, and it is still popular today.

In England, Methodist leader John Wesley recorded in his *Primitive Physick* (1747) a recipe for a potion called Daffy's Elixir. It included senna, guaiacum (the resin of a tropical evergreen), licorice, aniseed, coriander seed, elecampane root, and raisins. All these were mixed into a liter of the best brandy, which was then to "stand by the fire a few days" before being strained. The elixir was said to relieve colic. As a purge, he recommended an infusion made with three drams (about 2 teaspoons) of senna and a scruple (about ¼ teaspoon) of salt of tartar in a quarter-liter of river water.

The settlers were well versed in the virtues of senna. Dr. William Barton, an eminent physician and professor of botany in the 1830s, advised, "When you inquire for Senna as a medicine at a Doctor's shop, always ask for a dose of Senna and Manna, because these two medicines are always given together." (Today herbalists consider manna—a dried exudate of the European ash—so mild as to be

---

Active plant parts Dried leaflets, seed pods
Uses Constipation
Cautions Take only the recommended dosage; larger amounts may cause diarrhea, nausea, and severe abdominal cramps. Do not take senna for more than two weeks; prolonged use of laxatives can impair normal bowel function and cause dehydration. Do not use laxatives if you have abdominal pain, nausea, vomiting, or intestinal obstruction or inflammation unless instructed by a doctor. Do not give senna to children under the age of two. Note that so-called weight-loss teas containing laxatives have caused several deaths.

possibly inactive.) "Sometimes," he went on, "a little Salts is mixed with the Senna and Manna, especially if you wish to make the operation sure and active." Salts were often used to help make senna's active principle more soluble.

Barton also noted a side effect of the herb and suggested a way to counteract it: "Senna has but one fault; it is apt to give gripe during operation: this can always be prevented, however, by adding a little ginger." In fact, senna was combined with a host of different herbs to prevent intestinal cramps—and to disguise its taste, which is described as disgusting.

Nineteenth-century Eclectic physicians included in *King's American Dispensatory* a recipe for a syrup of senna that contained bruised senna leaves, oil of coriander, alcohol, sugar, and water. This they described as a "mild purgative"—a misnomer, since the word "purgative" implies strong action. They also included an aromatic syrup recipe that contained senna, jalap (the dried root of *Ipomoea purga*, a Mexican plant popular as a purgative), rhubarb, cinnamon, cloves, nutmeg, lemon oil, sugar, and alcohol.

The settlers created their own recipes using senna. A simple tea was made with ¼ to ½ teaspoon of the dried leaves. One recipe called for figs baked in senna tea. Another called for an infusion of senna mixed with syrup of buckthorn. A third was a tea made of pulverized senna, jalap, and peppermint, to be fed to the fasting patient. This was said to be an excellent remedy for "serious and bilious diseases."

Although senna was used mainly against constipation—and especially in cases of chronic constipation—it was also employed to prevent illness or to "flush" an illness out of the system. The plant's pods were said to be milder than the leaves, and this has been confirmed.

Wild Senna

North America's native species of senna, *Cassia marilandica*, was deemed virtually equivalent to the so-called European senna, although somewhat milder. John Gunn, author of *Gunn's Domestic Medicine*, wrote about it in his 1830 medical guide: "I have used them both, and can discover no difference. This affords another proof of a bountiful Providence, in bestowing on this people, a plant of so much value, and one which, before its discovery here, we were compelled to import from Egypt."

The Indians used the native senna plant in a number of ways, although not primarily as a laxative. Instead, the Cherokee drank senna tea to reduce fevers and applied poultices of the root to sores. The Mesquakie soaked the seeds in water to release their mucilage and ate them to soothe sore throats.

Wild senna was also believed to expel worms and counteract bad breath. Blacks in the American South used the leaves mixed with grease as an ointment for abscesses. In the absence of Alexandrian senna or wild senna, the Eclectics recommended another species, prairie senna (*C. chamaecrista*), which grows on the North American and Mexican prairies.

An Herb of Last Resort

Senna is a powerful laxative; it contains chemicals known as anthraquinone glycosides, which stimulate contractions of the large intestine. It should be used only after other measures have been tried—such as increasing your intake of fiber and liquids and taking bulk laxatives; even then, use only with caution. Senna is recommended primarily for those with loose stool constipation, who need only to increase the frequency of bowel movement. Overuse may deprive the body of fluid and electrolytes, and long-term use has resulted in severe clubbing (enlargement of the ends of the fingers and toes). Also note that prolonged use of any laxative, senna included, may cause dependence on them.

Taken orally, senna and other stimulant laxatives generally work within 6 to 12 hours. Be aware that they may turn the urine reddish or brownish. Senna teas can be made by mixing the dried leaves with honey, lemon, and sugar, along with such aromatic herbs as anise or peppermint to improve the taste and prevent intestinal cramping. Over-the-counter syrups and tablets may be preferable to home brews because they provide a standardized dosage of the active principle. Many senna products also contain bulk laxatives, although there is no evidence that a combination of bulk and stimulant laxatives is more effective.

Senna is more popular today than the milder cascara sagrada (which also has a long folk history as a laxative), mainly because it costs considerably less. It is one of the herbs approved for use as a drug by Health Canada, when it is prescribed therapeutically as a laxative.

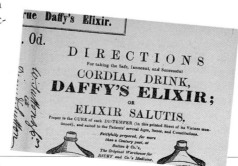

Senna was an ingredient in *Daffy's Elixir, an imported English patent medicine. The brew was said to cure colic and gripes.*

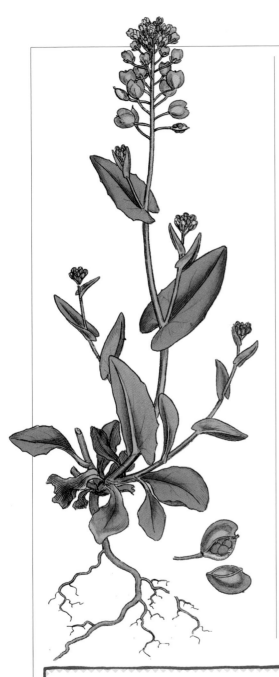

SHEPHERD'S PURSE

Capsella bursa-pastoris
CASEWEED, MOTHER'S-HEART,
SHOVELWEED

The unique shape of the seed pods of shepherd's purse inspired nicknames that included the words "heart" and "shovel." But the name that survives comes from the pod's similarity to the leather pouches once worn by European shepherds. Until the early 1900s, the herb was used to remedy cuts, bruises, excessive menstrual flow, nosebleeds, and internal bleeding—even though it was considered by some practitioners to be little more than a foul-smelling weed. Today researchers have found the medical effect of shepherd's purse to be insignificant.

Blood Stopper

Although the medicinal use of the plant dates back to ancient Greece, its styptic (astringent) properties were not known until the 16th century, when Italian physician Pietro Mattioli discovered that shepherd's purse tea helped slow excessive bleeding. Ever since, the herb has been used in countless remedies for internal and external bleeding.

The herb tea, made from the seeds or leaves, was taken to relieve heavy menstrual bleeding and pain, blood in the urine, and internal hemorrhages. Herbalist John Gerard (1545–1612) advocated shepherd's purse—taken as a tea, applied as a poultice, or added to a bath—to "stay bleeding in any part of the body." In both World Wars, German and Allied medics administered extracts of the plant to reduce internal bleeding.

Like the thousands of seeds that each plant can produce, the astringent uses of shepherd's purse were seemingly limitless. It was applied to cuts, bruises, and inflammations. An infusion was snuffed—or used to soak cotton balls that were inserted into the nostrils to stop nosebleeds. A salve made from its leaves relieved hemorrhoids. Famed 17th-century herbalist Nicholas Culpeper espoused applying the plant's juice to head wounds.

Research has confirmed that the plant does have properties that cause bleeding to stop, stimulate uterine contractions, and help prevent certain ulcers. It has also shown anti-inflammatory, antiseptic, astringent, and antitumor potential. Yet these effects are negligible when the plant is ingested. Greater benefits may occur with moderate, long-term use, a course of treatment that requires further study.

The wide-ranging potential of shepherd's purse is illustrated by its folk use. As a tonic, it was used to help the heart, kidneys, stomach, and liver. The plant, "bruised and bound to the wrists and soles of the feet," was thought to cure jaundice. It was also taken to ease labor pains and to remedy diarrhea, gout, and bedwetting. Drops of its juice were even put in the ear for earaches and toothaches.

Active plant parts Leaves, seeds
Uses Nosebleeds, cuts, excessive blood loss during menstruation
Cautions Seed powder or tincture may irritate the skin. Effects of excessive or long-term use are unknown. Do not administer to children under the age of two.

SHINGLES

Like many conditions that cause pain, blisters, and itching, shingles can be relieved with topical applications that are anti-inflammatory, antiseptic, and analgesic. For this reason, folk remedies can help. In fact, one of the most effective treatments for the pain and itching of shingles is traditional capsaicin (a constituent of red pepper). Before shingles emerges on the skin's surface, it attacks underlying nerves, causing pain that can last long after the skin condition clears up. Not only does capsaicin produce a soothing heat on the surface of the skin, it interferes with the local nerves' ability to send pain messages to the brain. Hence, it is included in many over-the-counter ointments used to treat shingles.

Blisters All in a Row

Shingles, also known as herpes zoster, is caused by the varicella-zoster virus—which also causes chicken pox. It may lie dormant for decades before emerging as shingles, which is often triggered by stress or a breakdown in the immune system. Although shingles is less contagious than chicken pox, both can be passed on to susceptible people.

The virus infects the nerves of certain areas of skin. The first symptoms can be chills, fever, tingling or prickly sensations on the skin, and nerve pain. Then the rash emerges, bringing with it small, crusting blisters, itching, and more pain. The blisters often appear in rows, usually on one side of the face or body (along a rib). In *Primitive Physick* (1747), John Wesley described shingles as encircling the body "like a belt of a hand's breadth." He treated it with freshly crushed garlic, a proven anti-inflammatory.

If you suspect you have shingles, see a doctor immediately. When the condition strikes the elderly, it is debilitating. When it affects the eyes, it can damage vision. A folk myth held that death would result if the rash reached around the body, but this is not true—shingles can be extensive, but it is very rarely fatal. While the virus runs its course, analgesics, special creams, and antiviral drugs may help. Scratching the blisters can promote bacterial infections and should be avoided.

Take a Bath

An old-fashioned bath prepared with oatmeal, baking soda, or Epsom salts can relieve itching and improve the affected person's spirits. These ingredients can be used in pastes and applied directly to the blistered skin. Applications of chaparral, common purslane, yellow dock, yarrow, and apple cider vinegar (used particularly in New England) may also help. Catnip tea may calm the ailing body and promote sweating. Folk remedies that are not going to work include drinking celery juice or applying—believe it or not—the blood of a black cat to the skin.

The purslane growing in your backyard may soothe the shingles rash.

RED PEPPER Capsaicin, found in red pepper, may relieve the nerve pain associated with shingles. Apply a commercial cream four to five times a day for up to four weeks. Avoid contact with the eyes and nose.

PURSLANE This common weed contains norepinephrine, which reduces hemorrhaging on the skin's surface. To make a wash, pour boiling water over the aerial parts (collected in summer or early fall), let cool, then strain. Apply the wash or juice pressed from its leaves to the skin up to four times a day.

GOTU KOLA Crush fresh leaves into a pulpy mass, heat in a pan, then spread onto a clean, wet cloth. Apply three to four times a day as needed. Commercial creams and extracts (one part extract per five parts water) also help but may produce a burning feeling.

SKIN RASHES

For many years, folk treatments have been used successfully to treat skin rashes, commonly called eczema or dermatitis. The best folk remedies have shown the ability to cleanse and soothe the skin and help reduce inflammation. Some even mimic antihistamines and can interfere with the spread of rashes caused by allergic reactions. Today many of these old plant remedies live on, as herbs and herbal derivatives continue to be used widely in commercial skin care products.

The word "rash" is a generic term. Eczema (or dermatitis) is characterized by skin that turns red, itchy, and scaly; the skin may even become slightly raised and blistery. In general, these rashes can appear anywhere on the body, including the scalp (causing dandruff). Urticaria is an inflammation with wheals or hives—itchy, slightly reddened bumps—that occur mainly on the

Calendula flowers are traditionally used in soothing salves.

limbs and torso. Skin rashes can frequently be attributed to stress, physical irritants—including insect bites, scratches, cosmetics, and the weather—or allergies, especially those caused by food.

Tannin-Rich Herbs

Orthodox treatments for irritated skin include antihistamines and cooling, anti-inflammatory lotions that contain such ingredients as zinc oxide, glycerin, and calamine. Providing similar effects, the strongest (and safest) folk remedies are plants that contain astringent tannins. Tannins promote healing by helping to reduce swelling and cleanse, dry, and soothe the skin. The most popular tannin-rich plant remedies are goldenseal root, witch hazel extract, white oak bark, and calendula flowers—all of which were used by the Indians and the first settlers. Applied as cool washes or ointments, these remedies provide comfort and healing effects that remain useful today.

Almost anything that could soothe the skin and help curb the inflammation has been tried in folk medicine. Valid treatments included baths made with colloidal oatmeal, cornstarch, and psyllium as well as an abundance of herbal extracts and washes with mild healing properties. Papaya and plantain leaves, burdock tea (ingested or applied to the skin), pineapple juice (which contains bromelain), the resin of balm of Gilead buds and the acacia plant, and poultices of houseleek (*Sempervivum tectorum*), tobacco, and chickweed have all been claimed to be mildly antiseptic and anti-inflammatory. (Note that sensitivity to contact with some plants, including plantain, can

GOLDENSEAL To make an astringent wash, pour 1 cup boiling water over 2 teaspoons powdered root. Let cool. Apply four times a day. After each application, sprinkle a little powdered root on the rash.

WITCH HAZEL Make a nondistilled extract by soaking ½ cup leaves in 1 cup water for 24 hours. Add 2 tablespoons alcohol as a preservative. Or use a standardized commercial extract. Apply up to four times a day.

CALENDULA To make a soothing wash, pour 1 cup boiling water over 1 heaping teaspoon dried petals, steep, then strain. Apply up to four times a day.

WHITE OAK For an astringent wash, add 2 teaspoons powdered bark to ½ liter cold water. Bring to a boil, let cool, then strain. Apply to the skin up to four times a day. Do not use over a large area; excessive use can be toxic.

actually cause dermatitis.) Such handy applications as mud (soothing but unsanitary) and milk of magnesia have also been used to treat itching and burning. Aloe vera gel, long popular, has been used to treat a variety of skin conditions.

Salves, made with combinations of herbs, often differed from community to community and household to household. Mixed with glycerin or boric acid, these family salves would be used for a variety of skin conditions, including burns, "cancers," and eczema. (It was believed, sometimes illogically, that anything that would heal one type of rash would heal another.)

A Healing Diet

Although folk treatments for rashes included such fanciful remedies as washing with "the water from a point where three boundaries meet" and wearing asafetida (a smelly glob of hardened resin), a simple course of treatment was a proper diet, fresh air, and plenty of sunlight. A diet consisting of fruits, vegetables, seeds, nuts, and greens provides a healthy amount of quercetin, a bioflavo-

ENGLISH WALNUT Put 5 teaspoons dried leaves of *Juglans regia* in 1 cup water, bring to a boil; strain and let cool. Apply to the skin up to four times a day. Or use one part black walnut extract (*J. nigra*) in a dilution with five parts water.

CHAMOMILE To make a salve, melt petroleum jelly in a double boiler. Stir in flowers (at a ratio of one part flowers to eight parts jelly). Heat for two hours or until flowers are crisp. Squeeze the hot mixture through a jelly bag that is tightly fitted atop a glass jar. Apply to the skin up to four times a day. Commercial chamomile creams are also available.

noid that acts like an antihistamine and that is said to work best when combined with vitamin C. Extracts of quercetin are available in health food stores.

Folk Sense

For many, the skin was, and still is, considered "an index to health." In this way, a rash was thought to be symptomatic of a deeper health problem. Thus, remedies not only had to remedy the itchy and painful skin but also had to restore health to the entire body. To this end, remedies were tried both internally and externally.

There are many examples of folk remedies that were used with dual aims. The juice of the nettle plant was applied directly to the skin and ingested; today freeze-dried extracts of nettle (taken internally) have been found to contain anti-inflammatory and anti-allergenic properties and are used to treat chronic hives. (Remember that nettle and other plants can also cause allergic dermatitis.)

Tannin-rich yellow dock, jewelweed, and psyllium (also known as papago) were used topically to cleanse the skin and internally to move the bowels; today jewelweed's astringent resin is thought by some herbalists to be effective against rashes, such as poison ivy, that are caused

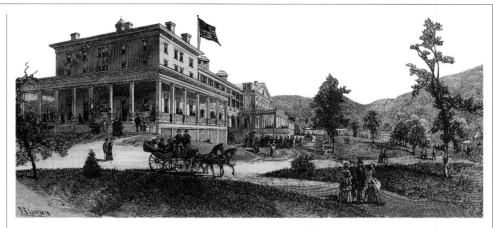

Spas, such as the Greenbrier in White Sulphur Springs, West Virginia (pictured in 1884), have traditionally benefited the skin—and the soul.

by plant allergies. Many species of alder were used by the Indians as both astringents and purges. Chamomile oil was applied to repair damaged skin, while chamomile tea was taken to reduce stress.

Anxiety, simply known as "nerves," was correctly thought to often result in a rash, and a variety of sedative teas—including catnip, valerian, passion flower, and peppermint—have been used to treat hives that are brought on by stress.

Poisoning was thought to cause rashes marked by "sore skin." Although several poisons, including arsenic, can induce a rash, relief will not come from traditional "blood-purifying" teas, such as those made from sassafras (now known to be a potential carcinogen), sarsaparilla, boneset, and wild cherry bark. Similarly, buttermilk and brewer's yeast served as "blood tonics" and topical applications.

For an infant with hives, midwives endorsed echinacea tea to boost the immune system and catnip tea to induce sweating and "clear the liver." Echinacea, however, is no longer advised for infants.

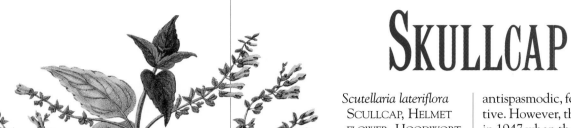

SKULLCAP

Scutellaria lateriflora
SCULLCAP, HELMET
FLOWER, HOODWORT,
QUAKER BONNET,
MAD-DOG WEED,
BLUE PIMPERNEL

Since the 1700s, skullcap's medicinal use has been alternately praised and discounted. In 1773 Dr. Lawrence Van Derveer spurred renewed interest in the plant when he claimed that it helped cure hundreds of patients of hydrophobia, now commonly known as rabies. Although neither skullcap nor its derivatives have been proven to remedy rabies, one of the plant's surviving nicknames, mad-dog weed, derives from this former use.

The increased focus on skullcap stirred a divided chorus of medical opinions. Its backers advised the plant as a sedative for a variety of ills, including insomnia, nervousness, and epileptic seizures. Its detractors claimed that the plant lacked potency. Skullcap was listed in many drug references as an effective antispasmodic, fever reducer, and sedative. However, that changed dramatically in 1947 when the U.S. National Formulary deemed the plant to have no medical value. Today the debate continues.

Sleep on It

Both the Indians and the early settlers used the native herb to calm spasms and anxiety. In the 1800s Thomsonian herbalists advised it to relieve teething pain in babies and to ease the symptoms of St. Vitus' dance (a disorder characterized by jerky spasms) and delirium tremens (confusion and trembling associated with alcohol withdrawal). Eclectic physicians endorsed skullcap for restlessness caused by "excessive study" or "over-exercise."

The herb was used to treat rheumatism and menstrual cramps, because it was believed (incorrectly) that they were nervous conditions. Old herbals also touted skullcap for curing the "explosive headaches of school teachers" and "excessive sexual desire." Its usefulness even made the plant a cash crop in the southern Appalachians, particularly in North Carolina in the late 1800s.

The mixed findings on skullcap may be a result of adulteration and substitution in commercial products. Still, the plant has shown potential anti-inflammatory and antimicrobial activity; its extracts may also help inhibit viruses. Skullcap contains scutellarin, an antispasmodic glycoside, which may help reduce blood pressure; its extracts are used in sleep aids. Skullcap tea may also help relax the uterus and reduce the risk of heart disease.

Active plant parts Leaves, root, stem, flowers
Uses Anxiety, insomnia
Cautions Large doses may cause giddiness, confusion, muscle twitching, and seizures. Skullcap is not recommended for pregnant women, nursing mothers, or children under age 3. Medicinal use and use by the elderly should be supervised by a doctor.

SLIPPERY ELM

Ulmus rubra
RED ELM, MOOSE ELM, INDIAN ELM

Few medicinal plants have stood the test of time as well as slippery elm. Once commonly used by Indians throughout its range in the eastern U.S. and southern Canada, the tree remains one of the most widely used wild plants whose extracts are approved for over-the-counter sale in North America.

The slippery elm tree is smaller than its relative, the American elm; its leaves, which are shorter on one side than the other, have a lopsided look and are covered with rough, fuzzy hairs on the lower surface.

A Good Chew

It is the tree's inner bark—collected when the leaf buds swell with sap in the spring—that is of medicinal interest. When chewed, a sliver of the bark produces a mucilaginous substance that tastes of licorice. This quality made slippery elm bark a favorite "chewing gum" and thirst quencher in frontier days and one of the most popular remedies for sore throats and coughs in North American history.

When dried, powdered, and mixed with water, the bark forms a thick paste to use externally on wounds, boils, burns, and cold sores. One 1830 herbal recounted its use during the American Revolutionary War: "Surgeons used it with the happiest effects. They applied poultices of it to fresh wounds, and always produced ... a quick disposition to heal."

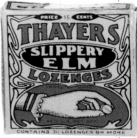

Slippery elm *was sold in lozenge form by the 19th century.*

Slippery Tea

Mixed with milk or water, the ground bark of slippery elm was given to newly weaned infants and others who needed easily digestible food. A tea was brewed to quell gastrointestinal ailments and for use as a laxative. Today the bark is a popular folk treatment for stomach ulcers.

Many Indian tribes made slippery elm tea to ease labor. They were also known to insert pieces of bark from the tree into the cervix to induce abortion—a practice that often led to infection and death. In more common Indian practice, the tea was taken internally to ease fevers, colds, and bowel complaints such as diarrhea.

When they weren't brewing or eating slippery elm bark, both Indians and settlers used it to make ropes and baskets. Powdered bark was added to rendered animal fat to keep it from getting rancid.

Modern medical science recognizes the gentle action of slippery elm bark, which is commercially available in several forms, including throat lozenges and powder. Slippery elm bark can also be collected in the wild, but beware: some people develop a skin rash from touching the leaves of this elm.

Active plant parts Inner bark
Uses Sore throat, coughs, stomach ulcers, digestive disorders, wounds, and boils
Cautions Some people develop contact dermatitis from this and other elm species.

SMOOTH SUMAC

Rhus glabra
RED SUMAC, SUMACH

Smooth sumac suffers by association. It is a member of the same genus as poison ivy and poison oak, and its close cousin—poison sumac—produces severe, itchy rashes. But smooth sumac itself is harmless and, in fact, has a long history of medicinal uses. It is also the source of a refreshing beverage—"sumacade."

Common from southeastern Quebec and New England to the Gulf Coast and west into the plains, smooth sumac grows in sunny locations, where it forms tight clumps that may reach 4.5 m (15 ft) in height. Its compound leaves are long, tapered, and serrated, and in autumn they blaze with color, turning a brilliant scarlet. In midsummer the plant bears upright clusters of red berries that are covered with short, velvety hairs. (Poison sumac, by contrast, grows mostly in swampy locations and has smooth-edged leaves and white berries.)

Although it has been little studied by modern science, smooth sumac was often used by both Indians and settlers. Extremely high in tannic acid, the bark is a useful astringent. Bark tea was also used as a gargle to remedy sore throats and mouth ulcers, and it was drunk to treat diarrhea and fevers.

As they still do, many Indian tribes used smooth sumac to treat urinary tract disorders. An extract of a related species, the sweet or fragrant sumac (*Rhus aromatica*), was used by doctors in the 19th century to stop bedwetting among children.

A Bracing Drink

In addition to its medicinal uses, smooth sumac can offer one of summer's most invigorating beverages—"pink sumacade," a tart lemonade substitute that also contains a healthy dose of vitamin C.

Although the plant bears clusters of fuzzy berries for much of the year, collect them only in late summer or early autumn. Crush the clusters slightly and add to cold water—about 1 cup fruit to each liter of water. (Note: do not use hot water; it will leach tannin out of the stems and make the drink taste bitter.)

Allow the mixture to soak for 15 to 20 minutes, stirring occasionally; it will turn pinkish-red. Strain through cheesecloth to remove the tiny hairs. Sweeten with sugar or honey and serve iced. Because it may cause an allergic reaction in some people, drink "sumacade" in moderation.

This lemonade substitute was a favorite drink of many eastern Indian tribes. In winter, they would hang sumac seed heads in the rafters of their longhouses for use as a scurvy preventive.

Active plant parts Fruit, leaves, bark
Uses Diarrhea, sore throat, mouth and throat ulcers, urinary and kidney problems, dysentery. The berries make a tart beverage called sumacade.
Cautions Related poison sumac has white, not reddish, berries. Some people may have an allergic reaction to sumacade; drink it in moderation.

SNAKEBITE

Of the nearly 120 species of snakes in North America, only about 25 are venomous. Still, they have inspired fear for centuries, much of it misplaced. Although snakebite is a potentially life-threatening emergency, few people in North America die from it—less than 2 percent of snakebite cases result in death if proper medical care is given. Bee stings, by contrast, kill four times as many North Americans.

Scores of plants have been touted as snakebite cures, and many of them were named for their supposed value—snakeroot, rattlesnake master, rattlesnake plantain, rattlesnake root, rattlesnake weed, and many others. Yet not one has been proven effective against snakebite. The best advice for victims of snakebite is to get to a hospital for medical treatment with antivenin as quickly as possible.

Snake Families

Two families of venomous snakes are found in North America. The pit viper family (named for the tiny, heat-sensing pits between the eye and the nostril that allow the snake to track rodents and other warm-blooded prey in the dark) includes rattlesnakes, copperheads, and water moccasins. In this family are the three most dangerous snakes in North America—the eastern and western diamondback rattlesnakes and the Mojave rattlesnake of the American southwestern deserts. The smaller coral snake family, found in the American South and Southwest, has three species: brightly colored snakes called elapids, close relatives of the cobras and sea snakes. These snakes pack potent venom, but because they are so reclusive and have short fangs, few people are bitten by them each year.

Pit vipers have what is known as cytolytic venom, which attacks the body's tissues, producing tremendous swelling and internal hemorrhaging that may lead to death. Coral snakes, on the other hand, have neurotoxic venom, which causes little pain or swelling; this venom quietly interferes with the functioning of the nervous system, leading (in severe bites)

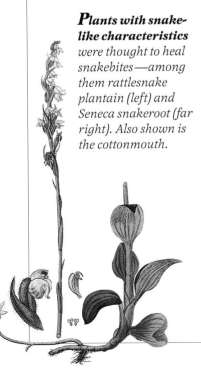

Plants with snake-like characteristics *were thought to heal snakebites—among them rattlesnake plantain (left) and Seneca snakeroot (far right). Also shown is the cottonmouth.*

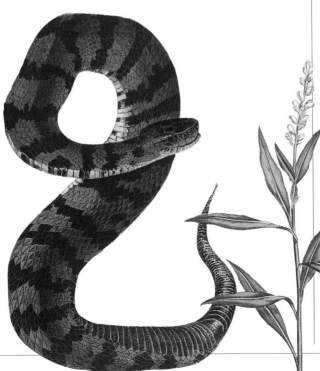

Avoiding Snakebite

◆ Use common sense in snake country. Stay on trails and out of places where visibility is limited, such as thick brush and tall grass.

◆ If you see a snake, just back away. Many snakebites occur because people try to catch or kill the snake. Snakes will not chase people or attack unless they are frightened.

◆ Don't believe the old myth that rattlesnakes always give a warning before striking; they do not. Likewise, many nonvenomous snakes make their tails vibrate, which in dry leaves may sound like the buzz of a rattler.

◆ Don't do foolish things when drinking. In an Arizona study, 50 percent of snakebite victims had been consuming alcohol.

to a fatal paralysis of the lungs and heart. Fortunately, coral snakes are usually reluctant to bite, and they lack the large, folding fangs of the pit vipers. A coral snake must grab a flap of skin and chew (difficult because its mouth is so small), as venom trickles down its stubby fangs.

To the Hospital!

Medical authorities agree that the best first aid is to get to a hospital immediately. Unfortunately, there is much less agreement on the proper first aid if medical help is more than half an hour away. The approach used in Westerns—a tourniquet, lots of alcohol, and cutting Xs over the fang marks—is the worst thing you can do. Nor should you use ice packs; venom makes the tissue sensitive to cold, and ice may do more damage than the bite.

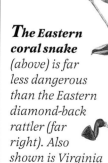

The Eastern coral snake *(above) is far less dangerous than the Eastern diamond-back rattler (far right). Also shown is Virginia snakeroot.*

The venom of the prairie rattlesnake *(right), of the American West, is stronger than that of the copperhead (far right), of the eastern and southern United States.*

The Canadian Red Cross advises getting the victim to a hospital as quickly as possible—within 30 minutes. Keep him immobilized and at rest in a semi-seated position; the injured arm or leg should be held immobile and lower than the heart. Also wash the wound with soap and water. Give the victim plenty of reassurance as he awaits treatment. As for suction, applying it over the fang marks during the first 30 to 60 minutes following the bite is helpful. The best suction device is the Sawyer Extractor, sold at sporting goods stores. (Sucking the bite with the mouth will introduce undesirable bacteria.)

Snakebite Herbs

Because snakebite can be a gruesome way to die, people have long sought natural antidotes to the venom. They have tried to "draw" the poison from the wound by packing it with mud (which merely introduces contaminating bacteria) or holding half an onion against it. Most remedies, however, focused on native plants, especially those known as snakeroot—several unrelated plants used by the Indians and quickly adopted by frightened settlers. Virginia snakeroot (*Aristolochia serpentaria*), a spindly woodland flower of the birthwort

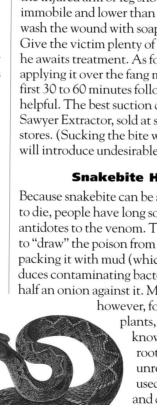

family, was a "much used antidote against the bite of the rattlesnake or ... adder or viper, whose bite is very deadly," according to one 1633 physician. The rattlesnake plantain (*Goodyera pubescens*), a wild orchid, was thought to be a cure because its leaves have markings that resemble scales and its small flower spike looks like a string of rattles. "It grows plentifully near dens. Wherever these dangerous serpents haunt, nature seems to have provided an effectual antidote against the venom," wrote one physician in 1785. Similarly, Seneca snakeroot (*Polygala senega*) was named for its hard, crooked, snake-like rootstock and rattle-like flower spikes.

Many people believed that snakes used a special herb to fight the effects of their own venom; the way to find it was to provoke a rattler into biting itself, then follow the serpent to its stash. Actually, pit vipers are almost immune to their own venom and need no help from plants.

Over the years, desperate people tried many folk treatments. Some of these—soaking the bite in coal oil or splitting a live chicken or frog in half and applying the bloody carcass to the wound—could only be called bizarre. None of the traditional remedies for snakebite have been shown to work; the only effective treatment is antivenin, which is made from the blood serum of horses that have been injected with tiny amounts of snake venom.

Bite Variables

If the old herbal remedies for snake venom are worthless, why did so many of them seem to work? Even in the past, most people bitten by poisonous snakes survived. The answer lies in a number of variables: body size (children are at much greater risk than adults), the victim's general health, and the location of the bite (the closer the bite is to the abdomen, the greater the risk of serious injury or death). Remarkably, when a snake bites, it does not always inject venom. Pit vipers have a surprising degree of control over how much venom they release with each bite; roughly half the time, little or none is injected. What's more, not all venomous snakes are equally dangerous. The bite of a 1.8-m (6-ft) Eastern diamondback rattlesnake can be deadly, while the 30-cm (12-in.) pygmy rattlers of the American South have caused few, if any, deaths.

Harmless nonvenomous snakes, such as garter and water snakes, will also bite. They leave a curving row of small puncture wounds, which should be washed with soap and water; follow with a tetanus booster shot if needed.

"They Shall Take Up Serpents ..."

Because of their sinister role in Genesis, snakes have been stigmatized. But for a handful of Fundamentalist congregations in the central and southern Appalachians, venomous snakes are a vivid way to demonstrate their faith. Snake handling began in 1909 in eastern Tennessee. George Hensley, a local farmer, had a revelation after reading two Bible verses from Mark 16:17–18. "And these signs shall follow them that believe: In my name shall they cast out devils; they shall speak with new tongues; they shall take up serpents." Following Hensley's example, the practice of handling venomous snakes spread to neighboring states by the 1930s.

Participants use a variety of venomous snakes, particularly timber rattlesnakes and copperheads, holding handfuls of them as they dance in ecstasy and pass the snakes through the congregation. Bites are not infrequent—some adherents say they have been bitten more than 100 times—and many, believing the bite is a test of their faith, refuse medical treatment. Herpetologists believe that the high survival rate is related to the snake handler developing his or her own toxin after a few bites. But not all bites are mild. Since the movement began, at least 78 people have died—including Hensley, who succumbed in 1955 after being bitten by a rattler. Snake handling is illegal in all Appalachian states but Georgia and West Virginia, although authorities are often reluctant to prosecute.

Ecstatic, an Alabama snake handler feels the spirit of the Lord.

YARROW As the Okanagan Indians of the Pacific Northwest knew, a yarrow poultice can aid the healing of a snakebite. Use yarrow to alleviate the painful symptoms, but only after you have been treated by a physician. Wash, then crush, enough yarrow leaves to cover the wound. Apply, then cover with a bandage. Replace the poultice every two to four hours.

GARLIC Garlic has broad-spectrum antimicrobial activity. Apply a cut clove to the bite two to three times daily.

PLANTAIN The Cherokee pressed the juice from plantain leaves and applied it to snakebites. Anti-inflammatory acids in plantain aid wound healing. After undergoing emergency treatment for snakebite, press the juice from fresh plantain leaves and apply to the bite two to three times a day. Discontinue use if skin irritation occurs.

ALOE VERA GEL Aloe vera gel penetrates injured tissue and dilates capillaries, increasing blood supply to the injury. After emergency treatment, scoop fresh gel from a split aloe leaf and apply to the bite as often as desired.

Sore Throat

The nose and throat are the body's first lines of defense against colds and flu. Their mucous lining traps viruses and bacteria on their way into the body, and microscopic hairs sweep them into the stomach, where they are destroyed. Occasionally, however, intruders overwhelm this defense system and infect the throat cells. In response, white blood cells flock to the area, along with an increased blood supply, which cause the throat tissue to redden and swell.

A potentially serious condition is strep throat, a bacterial infection requiring treatment with antibiotics; symptoms include a sudden fever and white spots on or around the tonsils. Also potentially serious is tonsillitis, caused by a viral or bacterial infection; it is usually accompanied by a fever. Tonsillitis was once treated by removing the tonsils; today surgery is usually reserved for cases of recurring infection. If a sore throat lasts for more than three days, see a doctor. (Note: If a child under 18 has a virus, never give him aspirin, which increases the risk of Reye's syndrome, a potentially fatal disease.)

Sweet-and-Sour Folk Cures

Early settlers relied on teas and gargles that paired soothing demulcents, such as honey or sugar, with astringents, such as lemon or vinegar. Combinations often included sage, thyme, myrrh, alum, witch hazel, goldenseal, or red pepper—a wise array indeed, as all of these have astringent or anti-inflammatory effects. Sage and thyme are also antiseptic, and goldenseal acts as a mild local anesthetic. In addition, the steam from hot tea helps loosen mucus. Red pepper, irritating though it seems, was sometimes swabbed directly on the throat, as was peppermint oil, a mild local anesthetic. Whiskey also has anesthetic and antiseptic properties, and was used in gargles. Salt was popular in gargles, too; it is mildly antiseptic and helps clear away phlegm, as do baking soda and brewer's yeast, other folk cures.

Finally, to coat the throat, slippery elm, mullein, flaxseed, marsh mallow root, and glycerin were called into action. Some people ate butter coated with sugar; a spoonful of honey works equally well.

Wise folk remedies included thyme, red pepper, sage, myrrh, and tea with honey and lemon.

HONEY Honey coats a sore throat and has mild antibacterial properties that may fight certain infections. Add 1 to 3 teaspoons to 1 cup of hot water. Do not give honey to babies under one year old.

SALT WATER Salt is mildly antiseptic. Better still, it draws water out of the mucous membranes to dilute the mucus and also acts mechanically to cleanse the throat of phlegm. Gargle with ½ teaspoon salt in a glass of warm water three to four times daily.

SLIPPERY ELM The inner bark of the slippery elm tree contains a mucilage that soothes a sore throat. Slippery elm lozenges are available. Or you can make a tea by steeping 1 heaping teaspoon pulverized inner bark in 2 cups boiling water. Strain, then drink.

HOREHOUND Horehound curbs inflammation and thins mucus, making it easier to expel. To make a tea, steep 2 heaping teaspoons chopped herb in 1 cup boiling water for 10 minutes. Strain and drink. Lozenges are available.

PEPPERMINT To dull sore throat pain, take one lozenge containing 2 to 20 milligrams menthol every two hours, or gargle with a few drops peppermint tincture in 1 cup hot water. This herb is not for children under the age of two.

SPLINTERS

One can easily imagine that in the days when people built their homes of rough-hewn logs and split enough wood to keep the home fires burning, splinters were a common vexation. To remove these "slivers," the settlers devised countless poultices. Most of these either softened and lubricated the skin around the splinter or exerted an astringent, or "drawing," effect; the best did both.

Poultices and Pine Pitch

To soften the skin around the splinter, some people bound the area with strips of raw bacon, salt pork, or pork fat, sometimes sprinkled with white sugar to increase their drawing power. Others moistened crabgrass with hot water and mixed it with a tablespoon of bacon drippings and ½ cup salt. (Salt was popular as an effective drawing agent.)

Other poultices used to soften the skin included one made with oatmeal, banana, and water, and applied alternately with olive oil compresses. This treatment was said to enable the patient to squeeze out the splinter by day's end. Another called for a mixture of brown laundry soap, sugar, and water. (Soap and sugar are mildly antiseptic.) Bread soaked in milk was said to bring splinters to a head, but it was difficult to bind to the wound and often developed a sour smell once it hardened. Some people advised heating the ingredients before applying them; heat does help soften skin and bring sores to a head.

The Indians favored plantain leaves for removing splinters and thorns because of the plant's combination of softening mucilage and astringent tannins. Plantain also has antibacterial properties. Other substances once employed for their ability to coax splinters out of the skin included melted rosin, turpentine, and agrimony (a plant long used against skin irritations), which was dried, ground into a powder, and mixed with hot water.

Woodcutters had their own way of removing splinters: they spread warmed pine pitch on the skin and then peeled it off after it dried—hopefully taking the splinter with it. Repeated applications were often necessary, and the crude process was potentially painful—which may have added to its appeal. Similarly, it has been said that if adhesive tape is placed over a splinter at night, the offending particle will most likely be stuck to the tape by morning.

If the area around the splinter was sore, a slice of raw onion was often applied to reduce the swelling; onions do have a mild antiseptic effect. To treat infections caused by thorns or slivers, some people bathed the skin with a tea made by boiling the leaves of the mucilaginous "cheese plant," or mallow. Soaking the area in hot water to which any skin-softening agent is added is beneficial. An Epsom salts solution has long been used for this purpose.

One of the most common home remedies is also the simplest: sticking the point of a needle briefly into a flame, then using it to gently work the splinter out.

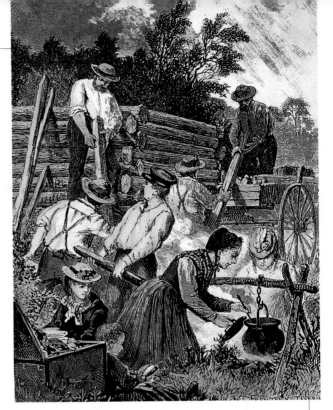

Wood pervaded the lives of the pioneers—and so, no doubt, did irksome splinters.

CHICKWEED Ointments made with *Stellaria media* are used to draw boils and splinters. The plant softens the skin and speeds healing. To make your own ointment, melt 1 cup petroleum jelly in a double boiler. Stir in 2 tablespoons chopped herb and heat for two hours, or until the chickweed is crisp. Strain through a cheesecloth, let cool, then apply. Store in a glass jar.

PLANTAIN Plantain has the ideal elements for treating splinters: softening mucilage, astringent tannins, and antibacterial agents. To make a poultice, soak chopped dried leaves in a bit of water. Place over the affected area. Replace every two to four hours.

SPRAINS

You turn your ankle in a weekend basketball game. You trip over your cat and land hard on your hands. You twist your knee while moving furniture. In each case a sprain can result. A sprained joint (which most commonly occurs in the ankle, wrist, or knee) is the result of a sudden injury in which the ligaments that bind the joints to the ends of the bones are stretched or torn. The condition ranges from mild swelling and pain, only when the joint is moved, to severe ligament damage that can render the entire limb useless until it heals.

Folk remedies included wraps, splints, soaks, and salves—anything that soothed the pain or immobilized the joint.

R-I-C-E Spells Relief

Rooted in common sense and practiced by our forebears, the best treatment for mild sprains is known today as RICE, which stands for Rest, Ice, Compression, and Elevation. Rest—not using the injured appendage—helps reduce pain and prevents aggravating the injury. The 18th-century reformer John Wesley suggested standing on, or "testing," an injury, but this should be done with caution. A sprained knee or ankle should not be "walked on" without the aid of a crutch. Once the pain has subsided (usually in a few days), the joint should be gently exercised. Massage may also help.

Ice—either a commercial ice pack or ice cubes wrapped in a cloth—should be applied immediately to a sprain; doing so effectively relieves pain and curtails swelling. Apply ice for 20 minutes, every two hours, for up to 48 hours after the injury. Similarly, many folk treatments called for soaking a sprain in cold water for the first day. After the swelling subsides, heat may be applied. But use caution: Although heat can be soothing, it can also promote inflammation and interfere with the healing process.

Compression involves wrapping a towel or an elastic bandage tight enough to immobilize the joint but not so tight that it cuts off circulation. Folk wraps included flannel, linen, rawhide, and eel skin.

Elevation is to raise the injury to heart level; this helps prevent fluid from accumulating in the damaged tissues. One remedy called for elevating the limb and applying a poultice of mud and chopped walnut bark until it dried and fell away.

Ideally, the RICE procedures should be used together. To treat a sprained ankle, the patient should lie on his or her back with the ankle propped up, wrapped in a bandage, and iced every two hours. Analgesics may be taken to alleviate the pain.

Plants for Pain

Dozens of herbal applications were used to treat sore muscles and joints. Most simply provided warmth and stimulated local circulation. Others had mild analgesic and anti-inflammatory properties. The most beneficial ingredients included the leaves of comfrey, mullein, and wintergreen, and the bark (called "silver bark") of young oak twigs—all of which can help repair damaged tissue.

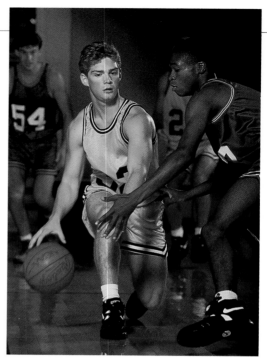

Studies of athletes *show that wearing high-top sneakers and taping the ankles help prevent ankle sprains.*

See a doctor if ...

Joint sprains and muscle strains can range from mild to severe. Severe injuries may require a cast or surgery to heal properly. Consult a doctor if any of the following occur.

◆ Pain in the joint or muscle, swelling, or spasm is severe or continues for more than two days without subsiding.
◆ Pain is centered in a bone or joint.
◆ Stiffness or pain prevents the joint from being moved at all.
◆ Pain is stabbing or radiating.
◆ The joint tingles, feels numb, or appears dislocated.
◆ The skin is discolored.

Liniments, such as those made with lavender flowers, gingerroot, or dissolved cakes of camphor, often included vinegar, whiskey, and lard to enhance their soothing effects. A straight camphor–whiskey mixture was used in Wisconsin to treat injuries from falling off a horse. Kerosene and turpentine were also employed, but they are known to irritate the skin.

The Indians were the first North Americans to use splints on injured limbs. The Ojibwa bound dressings of wild ginger and spikenard with splints made from cedar branches. The Pima made splints out of the flat, elastic ribs of the giant cactus. The Creek washed sprains with the boiled bark water of cottonwood and made splints from the inner bark.

Regional remedies included wormwood in Wyoming; salted cornmeal in Appalachia; and, in Indiana, oil derived from "melting" common earthworms in a glass jar left in the sun. Well-known Indian poultices included yucca root, used by the Blackfeet and the Nanticoke, and red clay, prized by the Rappahannock.

Renowned Salves

Some salves became famous. The "Red Lead Sear Cloth Salve" was popular in Kentucky. Made with linseed oil and lead oxide, it allegedly healed a 20-year-old injury from the American Revolutionary War. Another popular liniment was balsam, a resin that contains benzoic acid and salicin (an aspirin-like substance). Balsam was the active ingredient in one of Parke-Davis's earliest commercial liniments in the late 19th century.

The active ingredients in Ben-Gay, North America's most famous commercial rub, are camphor and methyl salicylate (found in wintergreen and other plants), both of which were widely used in folk medicine.

YUCCA Grate enough of the fresh roots of *Yucca glauca* to cover the affected joint. Place the pulpy gratings on a clean cloth and apply, root side down, to the skin. Change the poultice every two to four hours until the swelling and pain begin to subside. The roots contain saponins, which exert anti-inflammatory and analgesic effects.

ARNICA Arnica helps curtail the inflammation of sprains and bruises; it may also be mildly analgesic. Use only in commercially prepared ointments. Apply up to three times a day every two hours. Arnica is severely toxic if taken internally and should not be used on sensitive or broken skin.

THYME To make a soothing compress, add 10 drops of thyme oil to 4 teaspoons water. Soak a clean cloth and apply to the joint three or four times a day. Thyme causes minor irritation on the skin, thereby stimulating local circulation and encouraging repair.

SPIKE LAVENDER To make a massage oil, add a few drops of the oil of spike lavender (*Lavandula latifolia*) to 5 teaspoons olive oil. Massage directly onto the sprain, but not until at least 24 hours after the injury has occurred; otherwise, massage may be harmful.

COMFREY Apply a commercial ointment three times a day. Do not use for more than four to six weeks in a year. Comfrey is toxic if ingested and should not be used on broken skin or by pregnant or lactating women.

MULLEIN Mullein's main components—saponins, tannins, flavonoids, and iridoids—may soothe joint pain and swelling. To make an astringent poultice, mash the fresh or dried leaves and apply directly to the sprain; change every two to four hours. Or apply an infused oil as a salve.

OAK To make a poultice, mix 20 grams commercial chopped bark with 2 liters water and apply directly to the skin. Replace poultice every two to four hours as needed. Or add 5 grams of chopped oak bark to 2 liters lukewarm water and soak the affected joint for 20 minutes twice a day, for up to three weeks.

TURMERIC To make an anti-inflammatory paste, mix 2 parts powdered root and 1 part salt with just enough water to get consistency. Apply to the sprain once a day for 20 minutes to one hour and cover snugly with cotton or muslin. Turmeric can stain clothing and skin (temporarily) and irritate mucous membranes and sensitive skin.

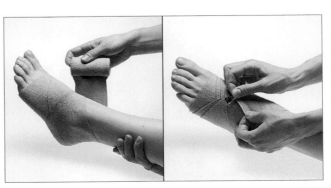

To wrap a sprained ankle, wind the bandage around the foot twice and then around the ankle (far left). Continue in a figure eight pattern, moving the bandage slightly higher on the leg with each turn, until the foot, ankle, and lower leg are covered. Secure the end (left).

STOMACH ULCERS

A peptic ulcer is an open sore in the lining of the gastrointestinal tract, usually in the duodenum (upper part of the small intestine) or the stomach. It is the result of erosion by acid and by pepsin, a digestive enzyme that gives peptic ulcers their name. The main symptom is a burning upper-abdominal pain, especially when the stomach is empty and the ulcer is thus more likely to come into contact with stomach acid. The pain is often relieved by antacids.

Many people with peptic ulcers have no symptoms. Others experience nausea, vomiting, belching, a bloated feeling, and weight loss. The pain of a duodenal ulcer is often relieved by eating, although it returns after a few hours. Conversely, the pain of a large ulcer in the stomach is often actually provoked by eating.

Anyone with a suspected peptic ulcer should have a screening evaluation with a doctor. Diagnosis involves threading a fiber-optic tube down the throat and into the intestinal tract, or an X ray in conjunction with a barium swallow. If an ulcer is left untreated, complications may develop. These include bleeding from the ulcer (which may result in vomiting of blood) and a perforated ulcer (one that breaks through the intestinal wall). Both require emergency medical treatment.

What Causes Ulcers?

Stress was once thought to be the primary cause of ulcers. However, scientists have discovered that most ulcers are associated with a bacterium called *Helicobacter pylori*, which compromises the ability of the stomach lining to protect itself from being digested. An antibiotic program heals the ulcer and prevents it from recurring.

Today doctors often treat ulcers with antibiotics in conjunction with other drugs, such as sucralfate (believed to form a protective barrier over the ulcer) and histamine-2-receptor antagonists (which reduce acid secretion). Before antibiotics became part of ulcer treatment, such drugs often had to be used continually at low dosages to prevent recurrence.

Just as ulcers were thought to be caused by stress, they were also said to be exacerbated by spicy food. Doctors prescribed bland diets and plenty of milk, which was believed to soothe the ulcer. But recent studies have shown that spices have no effect on the healing rate of ulcers, and milk, although it has a mild antacid effect initially, later produces a rebound effect whereby more acid is produced.

Wise Folk Treatments

To treat ulcers at home, many people took baking soda in a glass of water after meals. This may relieve the symptoms, but it does nothing to cure the ulcer. In fact, excessive use of baking soda may, like milk, cause a rebound effect, in which

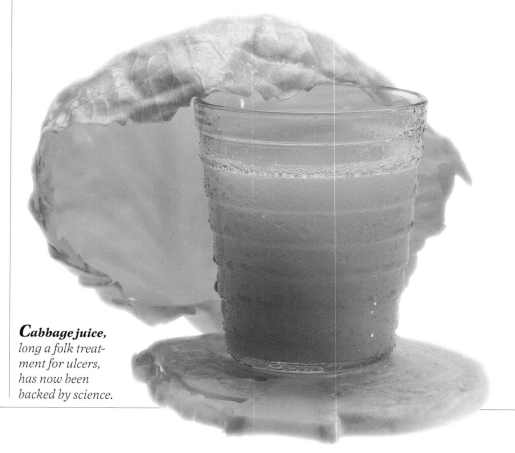

Cabbage juice, *long a folk treatment for ulcers, has now been backed by science.*

more acid is produced. At least one misguided soul recommended aspirin for ulcer pain; aspirin actually makes ulcers worse, as do alcohol, coffee, and tea.

Yet many folk treatments did hold up, including one of the most popular: slippery elm bark. The tree's inner bark is valued for its mucilage, which coats not only sore throats but inflamed stomach linings, too. The powdered bark was usually taken in milk or water. Some filled capsules with slippery elm, ginger, and goldenseal—a winning combination indeed. Animal studies show that ginger inhibits gastric secretions and blocks the formation of gastric lesions. No studies of the effects of goldenseal on ulcers have been conducted, but the herb contains a compound called berberine, which has anti-inflammatory, antiseptic, and immunostimulant properties. Other herbs that contain berberine include yellow-

Stress may exacerbate an ulcer, but a bacterium is the primary cause.

root, used by Indians and inhabitants of Appalachia to treat ulcers, and barberry roots, once a popular ulcer treatment in Europe.

Like slippery elm, marsh mallow was used to coat ulcers. It and other demulcents, such as flaxseed, were mixed with tonic herbs—notably goldenseal, strawberry leaves, and raspberry leaves—to promote healing.

Licorice root tea was also called into action, and wisely so: root extracts stimulate the defense mechanisms of the stomach lining that prevent ulcers. Studies

show that licorice is even more effective in healing ulcers than the histamine-2-receptor antagonists often prescribed.

The Cabbage Cure

In the 1940s an eminent physician fed fresh cabbage juice to guinea pigs and found that it discouraged the formation of ulcers. Clinical trials have since confirmed that the juice protects the gastrointestinal lining from stomach acid. Drinking a liter a day of the raw juice for three weeks has been said to cure most peptic ulcers. Potato juice has also been tried, but it does not promote healing and may cause side effects.

Other natural treatments that show promise include garlic, turmeric, and very ripe bananas. Gentian and bilberry may also be useful, but clinical studies are needed. Aloe may help ulcers heal, too.

ASTRAGALUS This herb (*Astragalus membranaceus*) stimulates the immune system and works as an antibacterial and anti-inflammatory agent. Take one to two grams in capsule form daily. Or make a tea by adding 1 teaspoon powdered root to 1 cup boiling water. Steep, then strain. Drink after each meal.

SLIPPERY ELM The inner bark of the slippery elm has long been valued for its mucilage, which forms a protective layer over ulcers. To make a decoction, add 1 heaping teaspoon crushed bark to 1 cup water. Steep for 30 minutes, stirring occasionally, then strain. Drink one cup (or take one or two 350-milligram tablets) after meals.

GOLDENSEAL Goldenseal has a reputation for healing ulcers. The herb acts as an antiseptic and also stimulates

the immune system; however, no specific studies have been done to confirm its efficacy. To make a tea, add 1 teaspoon powdered rootstock to 1 cup boiling water. Steep, then strain. Drink one cup after every meal.

GINGER Animal studies have shown that extracts of fresh ginger inhibit gastric secretions and the formation of ulcers. Dissolve ⅛ to ¼ teaspoon powdered root in 1 cup water or juice. Drink after meals. Do not exceed ½ to 1 teaspoon of ginger daily; large doses can cause gastrointestinal irritation.

LICORICE The anti-inflammatory activity and mucilage content of licorice root team up to make a soothing ulcer treatment. To make a decoction, pour ½ cup boiling water over 1 teaspoon dried rhizome and roots. Simmer for five

minutes, cool, then strain. Drink after meals. Do not use licorice for more than four to six weeks. The elderly and those with cardiovascular disease or liver or kidney problems should avoid licorice.

CHAMOMILE More than a stomach soother, chamomile exerts mild wound-healing and anti-inflammatory actions. To make a tea, pour ½ cup boiling water over 2 teaspoons chopped flowers. Steep, then strain. Drink after meals.

PEPPERMINT Peppermint has shown anti-inflammatory and anti-ulcer properties in laboratory animals. To make a tea, pour one cup boiling water over 1 tablespoon chopped leaves. Steep, then strain. Drink after meals. Capsules of peppermint oil are also effective when taken three times daily after meals; however, they are difficult to obtain in standardized form.

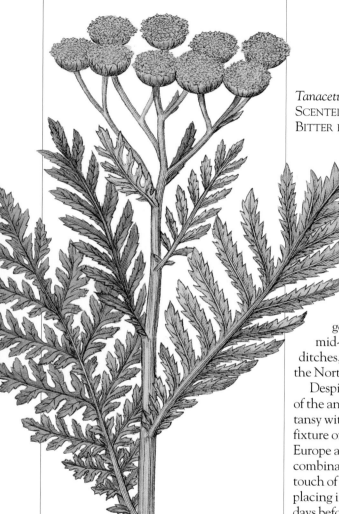

TANSY

Tanacetum vulgare
SCENTED FERN, STINKING WILLIE,
BITTER BUTTONS, PARSLEY FERN

Among the plants brought by the earliest European settlers to North America was this tough and dangerous garden perennial. But as it had in Europe, the plant escaped cultivation. Today tansy, with its fern-like leaves and tight clusters of button-like, golden flowerheads that bloom in mid- to late summer, grows wild in ditches, open fields, and roadsides across the North American continent.

Despite its known dangers (even some of the ancient herbals suggested using tansy with great care) the plant was a fixture of herb and medicinal gardens in Europe and Asia. Its pungent aroma—a combination of pepper, camphor, and a touch of citrus—led to the custom of placing it in coffins and shrouds. In the days before bathing was commonplace, tansy was used as a "strewing herb": when scattered on the floor and trampled underfoot, it exuded a scent that made social gatherings more pleasant. The plant also kept pesky insects at bay; the stems were piled up in closets or cabinets, hung in bunches from rafters, and packed between bedsheets and mattresses to prevent infestations of fleas, lice, ants, moths, and many species of flies.

Given tansy's potency, it is not surprising that the herb was also used medicinally. Its leaves and flowers, often combined with pomegranate or black cumin, were a common ingredient in worm-expelling medications. Tansy tea was regarded as a carminative (an agent that helps expel gas), a stimulating tonic, and an antispasmodic. As an emmenagogue, tansy helped to bring on delayed menses and also relieved menstrual cramps.

Plant of the Past

The perils of using tansy have long been known, but only recently has the reason for the plant's toxicity come to be understood. The active principle in tansy oil, thujone (which is also found in sage), is potentially lethal if taken in too large a dose; it may cause rapid and feeble pulse, severe gastritis, convulsions, hallucinations, and even death. One of tansy's more common applications was to induce abortion, and the herbal literature abounds with horrific descriptions of the last throes of women who had taken strong doses of tansy tea for this purpose.

Part of the danger inherent in consuming tansy is that the concentration of thujone varies so much from plant to plant—as does an individual's response to it. It is impossible to know, without chemical analysis, how powerful a tansy tea or

Active plant parts Leaves, flowers
Uses Tansy should not be used medicinally.
Cautions Tansy's essential oil, thujone, is potentially toxic. Health Canada has concerns about its safety; the sale of tansy or its oil is prohibited in the United States.

extract is, or what effect it will have. For these reasons, the sale of the tansy plant and the oil derived from it is now prohibited in the United States. Although no prohibition exists in Canada, Health Canada has concerns about its safety.

Tansy's hazards notwithstanding, its astringent properties have long given it a reputation as an external skin treatment. In the late 17th century, Englishman Nicholas Culpeper's *Complete Herbal* recommended boiling the leaves and flowers in water and salt: "The distilled water cleanses the skin of all discolorings, as morphew, sun-burns, pimples, freckles, etc. Dropped into the eyes, or cloths wet therein and applied, [the water] takes away their heat and inflammation." The leaves were also placed in shoes to ease sore and swollen feet, and tansy footbaths were popular among settlers and Indians alike. However, many people suffered allergic reactions to the oil in tansy, developing severe contact dermatitis.

Family pets, too, were subjected to applications of tansy. A regular rubdown with a handful of the fresh leaves was regarded as an effective way to prevent fleas on dogs; however, the practice was not recommended for cats, since the animals were likely to ingest the toxic oil during their regular self-groomings.

Boon Companions

Interestingly, our ancestors grew tansy in their flower, vegetable, and herb gardens for another reason. They were aware that the plant's extremely aromatic foliage, so repellent to insects, helps to protect nearby plants from infestation. As a companion plant, tansy can perform the same service for today's gardeners.

Among the insects that dislike tansy are ants. By repelling ants, tansy also controls the gardener's bane, the aphid.

Herbs and Pregnancy

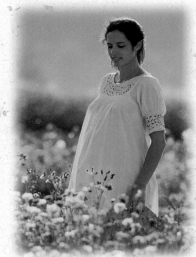

If you have a baby on the way, caffeine, alcohol, and chemically based drugs are not the only taboos; be wary of most "natural" remedies, too. Many of the herbs that are considered safe as tonics for general health or as treatments for specific ailments can be harmful when taken during pregnancy. In some instances, the very chemicals that make a botanical an effective stimulant or muscle relaxant also make it a potential abortifacient.

Tansy, for example, is drunk as a tea to relieve menstrual pain, but it is listed among the most dangerous herbs for pregnant women; it contains alkaloids that cause liver damage in adults if used regularly over time and may damage a fetus's developing liver as well. Another example is pennyroyal. This herb is used in teas to induce menstruation, but when taken in large doses by a pregnant woman it can cause convulsions, miscarriage, and even death—as cases in California and Colorado have shown. In general, pregnant women should avoid herbs known to affect female hormone levels or the uterus. Of these, there are dozens, from angelica to skullcap, black cohosh to raspberry; even seemingly innocuous culinary herbs like parsley, rosemary, and thyme fall into this category when they are used medicinally.

During pregnancy and the breastfeeding period, consult with your doctor before using any medicinal herb. Frankly, it may be wise to forgo herbal remedies altogether while you are pregnant and nursing: the fact is, there is insufficient research on most herbs (including those used in preparations that are often recommended by modern herbalists for pregnant women, such as raspberry leaf tea) to determine what effect they may have on a developing fetus and what dosages are safe.

Some species of ants actually farm aphids, gathering their eggs in the fall, tending them over winter, and then placing the newly hatched sapsuckers on the stems and leaves of certain plants—all for the sake of honeydew, the sweet substance exuded by aphids. To control the pests, interplant tansy with plants that are attractive to aphids—especially fruit trees and roses, which will not be overgrown by this aggressive plant. Tansy also makes a good companion for those plants that are often attacked by grubs and larvae, including such cane fruits as raspberry and blueberry, members of the cabbage (brassica) family, and fruit trees in general.

TARRAGON

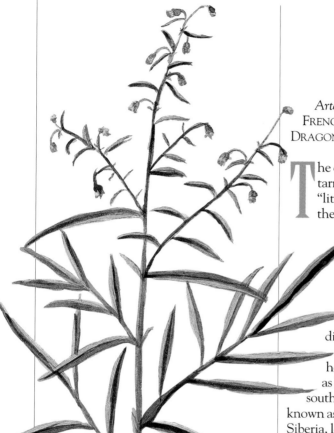

Artemisia dracunculus
FRENCH TARRAGON, ESTRAGON,
DRAGON'S MUGWORT

The darling of French kitchens, tarragon is known in France as the "little dragon," probably because of the plant's serpentine root system. Like most plants with snaking roots, it was once believed to cure snakebite as well as the bite of mad dogs. Tarragon's pungent flavor is reminiscent of licorice; it lends béarnaise sauce its distinctive taste and is often used in vinegars, dressings, and herbed butters. The herb is known as French tarragon and is native to southern Europe. Another variety, known as Russian tarragon and native to Siberia, looks similar but has paler leaves and is all but tasteless; this is the tarragon that grows in the wild in North America. Unlike Russian tarragon, the so-called French plant rarely produces seeds and is propagated from cuttings or root divisions.

Outside the kitchen, French tarragon was used not only to treat snakebite but also to impart stamina. The Roman naturalist Pliny the Elder believed it to prevent fatigue on long journeys, and, during the Middle Ages, pilgrims walked with sprigs of the herb in their shoes. The ancient Greeks chewed tarragon to numb toothache pain (the herb contains eugenol, a local anesthetic). It was also recommended as an appetite stimulant, along with its bitter botanical cousin, wormwood. In England tarragon was said to benefit the head, heart, and liver. In the New World, however, its medicinal role was scant. North America's 19th-century Eclectic physicians found no use for tarragon whatsoever, although some Indians used the Russian variety to treat colds, dysentery, diarrhea, and headaches.

An Impotent Herb

Despite tarragon's abundance of taste, its medicinal virtues are meager. Some herbalists view it as a diuretic, an appetite stimulant, and a digestive aid. A cup of tarragon tea is said to help induce sleep, and some recommend the herb for easing the pain of rheumatism. However, none of these uses is backed by science. Tarragon is also said to induce menstruation, and there is some evidence that it may do so. Like many aromatic herbs, tarragon has also been used to treat flatulence and colic, and it is said to sweeten the breath.

Drying tarragon largely destroys the active component in its volatile oil, so it is best to store the herb in vegetable or olive oil. Place a layer of washed and dried tarragon leaves in a jar, then pour a layer of oil over it. Continue layering herb and oil, finishing with a layer of oil. When stored this way, the herb will keep in the refrigerator for up to nine months.

Active plant parts Leaves, root
Uses Traditionally used to treat toothache, flatulence, and colic
Cautions Tarragon's volatile oil contains a substance that is toxic and potentially carcinogenic in large doses. Do not take tarragon tea during pregnancy, and do not take it for more than four successive weeks.

TEETHING

What doctors call the "cutting" or the first "eruption" of teeth is commonly known as teething—the time when a baby's first set of teeth grows through the gums. As the teeth come in, the gums become inflamed and sore. Signs of teething often include irritability (crying and fidgeting), dribbling (because more saliva is produced), and troubled sleep. The little one will also become more clingy when held and try to chew on anything within reach.

Folk remedies sought to calm the baby and soothe the gums; most common were weak sedative teas or simply something to chew on, like a finger or a wet cloth.

"Children's Remedies"

Although some babies are born with their lower front teeth already showing, teeth usually begin to show in the sixth month, and the first set of 20 deciduous teeth are fully in place sometime during the baby's third year. Therefore, teething can come and go for two years or more—a long time to listen to a fretful baby's whining.

Accordingly, sedative teas, often sweetened with honey or sugar, were used to ease a child's distress. Teas made from chamomile flowers and catnip leaves were known to be effective—and safe. In the 1800s both were employed as "children's remedies" to allay not only teething pain but also colic and other childhood ills.

Remedies also included things safe to chew on, such as a slice of apple, crushed ice wrapped in a cloth (called by some a "magic remedy" for teething), or even the wet cloth itself. Rubbing a finger gently over the child's gums can also help—some mothers used their wedding-ring finger. Chewable remedies included licorice, marsh mallow root, and assorted objects that were hung around the neck, including a dime, a mole's paw, or a dog's tooth.

Small doses of analgesics were also tried, and whiskey was used as a gum-soothing rub. (Some teasingly advised drinking a shot if the child kept crying.) Magical remedies also existed. Putting a woolen cap on the baby was supposed to help, whereas a man's hat was thought to make teething more difficult. One folk belief held that teething would be easier if the baby did not see himself in a mirror.

No matter how fussy a baby gets, teething will not—as many people believe—cause diaper rash, fever, vomit-

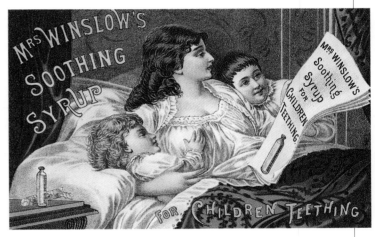

Mrs. Winslow's Soothing Syrup, sold in the 1880s, was aptly named: it was, in fact, laced with morphine.

ing, diarrhea, prolonged loss of appetite, earache, coughing, or convulsions; all of these are symptoms of illness and should be evaluated by a physician.

CHAMOMILE To make a soothing tea, steep 1 teaspoon minced flowers in 2 cups boiling water, then strain. Give the baby warm chamomile tea in a baby's bottle before meals—but no more than twice a day. Alternatively, place one to two drops of chamomile oil on a wet cotton swab and apply to the gums twice a day.

CATNIP To make a calming tea, steep 1 teaspoon leaves in 2 cups boiling water, then strain. Sweeten with sugar. Give warm tea in a baby's bottle before meals, no more than twice a day.

WASHCLOTH Let the child chew on a clean cloth that has been run under cool water. Or wrap crushed ice in a soft cloth and rub it on the gums to ease the pain. Keep moving the ice over the gums so as not to damage the tissue.

LEMON BALM To make a mildly sedative tea, steep 1 teaspoon leaves in 2 cups boiling water, then strain. Give warm tea in a baby's bottle before meals, no more than twice a day.

THRUSH

Pity the poor pioneer baby who came down with thrush, a condition made evident by a whitish tongue and throat and painful swallowing. One remedy called for having a stranger blow into the infant's mouth. Frontier mothers were also advised to let their babies chew on their wet diapers. (Urine does contain medically useful biochemicals, but they must be extracted and refined.)

A Common Fungus

Thrush, or candidiasis, is an infection of the mucous membranes of the mouth, vagina, or digestive tract. Occasionally, it even infects the skin around the fingernails. Its cause is *Candida albicans,* a yeast-like fungus that lives in the body unnoticed under normal circumstances. When the infection occurs in the mouth, it is commonly known as thrush. When it occurs in the vagina, it is called vaginitis. The method of treatment depends on where the fungus occurs.

Flavorful cinnamon
has been shown in German and Japanese studies to be an effective killer of fungi.

Thrush is a common childhood affliction, but it can also occur in adults, when the body's chemistry is thrown off balance and the candida fungus proliferates. This can happen after a regimen of antibiotics has destroyed too many of the normal bacteria that keep the fungus in check, or in women who take birth control pills.

People with iron-deficiency anemia, diabetes, or hormone-related disorders—as well as those suffering from obesity or who are on long-term corticosteroid treatment—are at particular risk of developing thrush. For HIV patients and others whose immune systems have been compromised, the ailment can present especially serious problems.

GARLIC Garlic is reported to be more effective than many antifungal pharmaceuticals against *Candida albicans.* Let four garlic cloves stand in water for six to eight hours, then strain. Alternatively, put four cloves through a garlic press and mix ½ teaspoon of the paste in ½ cup water. Rinse the mouth or gargle with either mixture three or four times daily.

CINNAMON Mix up to 1 teaspoon of a tincture of cinnamon oil in 1 cup water. Or prepare your own solution by mixing ½ to 1 teaspoon powdered cinnamon bark in 1 cup water. Rinse the mouth or gargle with either mixture three or four times

Beneficial Eats

Studies indicate that yogurt is a double-barreled prevention aid against thrush in the mouth or digestive tract. To treat vaginitis, yogurt is best applied externally. (Note: Do not apply yogurt to bacterial infections.) Not only is yogurt rich in *Lactobacillus acidophilus,* bacteria that keep the fungus in check, but it is a source of zinc, which boosts the immune system.

Garlic, too, has demonstrated antifungal properties, and eating a couple of raw cloves each day—peeled and chewed, swallowed whole, or chopped into foods—may prevent fungus overgrowth. One hospital study has indicated that garlic has anti-fungal properties superior to nystatin, one of the most prescribed medicines for thrush. Cinnamon has also been shown to be effective against fungus, as have the essential oil and flavonoids in chamomile flowers and the hydrastine and berberine in goldenseal.

daily. Do not swallow: taken internally, cinnamon oil can cause nausea, vomiting, and kidney damage.

GOLDENSEAL This herb is known to be effective against the candida fungus. It not only alleviates the painful sore mouth caused by thrush but promotes healing as well. Mix 2 teaspoons powdered rootstock (available commercially) in 1 cup boiling water. Let stand for ten minutes, then strain. Rinse or gargle with the mixture three or four times daily. Do not eat fresh goldenseal: it may cause further ulceration and inflammation of the mouth. Also, do not ingest high doses of the herb; doing so can be fatal. Pregnant women and people with high blood pressure should avoid using goldenseal altogether.

THYME

Thymus vulgaris
COMMON THYME, GARDEN
THYME, RUBBED THYME

Best known as a culinary spice, thyme is used to enhance the flavor and aroma of sauces, soups, stuffings, salads, and meat dishes. Since ancient times, the popular herb has also been employed in a variety of folk remedies—most successfully as a cough suppressant, a use that is still highly regarded.

Cough, Be Quiet

One of the first herbs brought by European settlers to the New World, thyme was commonly cultivated in pioneer gardens, and a tea made from its leaves and flowers was used to relieve cold symptoms, including fever, congestion, cough, and poor sleep. Thyme has expectorant, antiseptic, and antispasmodic properties that work together to suppress coughs, loosen congestion, and fight infections in the throat and lungs. The tea was also used to remedy bronchitis and whooping cough, and in modern Germany, commercial thyme products are approved for these specific uses. Sweetening the tea with honey, a demulcent, can enhance its ability to quiet a cough.

Another reason for thyme's effectiveness is thyme oil: when ingested, it is removed from the body through the lungs; as a result, its healing constituents can work directly where they are most needed. Today thyme oil is an ingredient in commercial cough syrups and lozenges. Although thyme oil can be toxic, it is safe to ingest in very small amounts.

Fairies were thought to sleep on beds of the herb; perhaps that is why people slept on pillows stuffed with thyme to lift depression. The mildly sedative tea was taken to prevent nightmares.

Thyme infusions were also added to baths to relieve sore joints, and diluted thyme oil was massaged into the skin to loosen chest congestion and relax tense muscles. Thyme oil must be diluted in a reliable carrier oil, such as olive oil—not water—before it is used. It is an effective counterirritant and antiseptic, but in its pure form it can easily burn the skin.

Thyme Heals All Wounds?

Thyme's chief constituent, thymol, is a strong antiseptic; hence, gargling the tea can soothe sore throats and rubbing the crushed leaves or diluted oil on the skin can clean minor cuts. Thyme oil has also been used to fight tooth decay, prevent molding, and embalm the dead. Listerine, invented by Missourian Joseph Lawrence in 1879, contains thymol, as do many skin and hygiene products.

Active plant parts Leaves, flowering tops
Uses Coughs, chest congestion, indigestion, gas, minor cuts and scrapes
Cautions Medicinal (not culinary) amounts are contraindicated in cases of enterocolitis and cardiac insufficiency and should not be taken by pregnant women, nursing mothers, or anyone with an overactive thyroid. Excessive use may cause gastrointestinal distress. Pure thyme oil should not be ingested and should be used externally only after it has been sufficiently diluted in a carrier oil. Taken internally, thyme oil may lower blood pressure and cause abdominal pain and shock. Thymol, the active principle of thyme and thyme oil, can be toxic. Thymol poisoning may cause nausea, vomiting, gastric pain, headache, dizziness, convulsions, coma, or cardiac or respiratory arrest.

TOBACCO

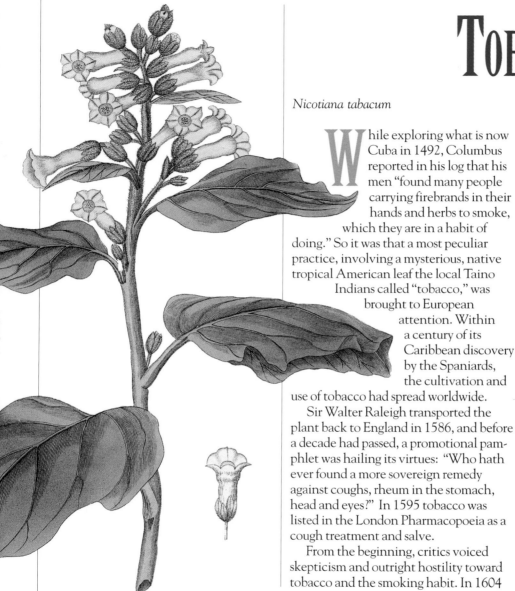

Nicotiana tabacum

While exploring what is now Cuba in 1492, Columbus reported in his log that his men "found many people carrying firebrands in their hands and herbs to smoke, which they are in a habit of doing." So it was that a most peculiar practice, involving a mysterious, native tropical American leaf the local Taino Indians called "tobacco," was brought to European attention. Within a century of its Caribbean discovery by the Spaniards, the cultivation and use of tobacco had spread worldwide.

Sir Walter Raleigh transported the plant back to England in 1586, and before a decade had passed, a promotional pamphlet was hailing its virtues: "Who hath ever found a more sovereign remedy against coughs, rheum in the stomach, head and eyes?" In 1595 tobacco was listed in the London Pharmacopoeia as a cough treatment and salve.

From the beginning, critics voiced skepticism and outright hostility toward tobacco and the smoking habit. In 1604 King James condemned the plant as "a custome … daungerous to the Lungs, and in the black stinking fume thereof, neerest resembling the horrible Stigian smoak of the pit that is bottomlesse." Later, the New England clergyman Cotton Mather asserted that the "caustick Salt in the Smoke … may lay foundations for Diseases in Millions of unadvised People."

Nevertheless, to the Jamestown colonists in what would become Virginia, the marvelous plant had magical properties. The smoke, they believed, was especially effective when inhaled and cleared the lungs of impurities. It was John Rolfe, husband of Pocahontas, who crossed the harsh local variety of tobacco with a milder strain from the West Indies, creating a strong, but sweet, new hybrid. As "Virginia tobacco," it became an addictive luxury to the English upper classes.

Gotta Light?

By the 19th century, all across North America the consumption of tobacco was an accepted way of life. Both sexes dipped snuff and smoked pipes. Gentlemen also indulged in smoking cigars and chewing tobacco; the brass spittoon became a fixture in virtually every public building.

Medically, the plant was considered a virtual panacea. "Tobacconists" were a majority of the medical profession, and doctors prescribed tobacco as poultices, in pills, chewed, snuffed, and drunk in teas for aches, pains, swellings, snake-bite, gunshots, and even bad breath. Tobacco became one of the 10 most commonly used plants in North American folk

Active plant parts Leaves, seeds
Uses Tobacco products
Cautions Tobacco is narcotic and highly addictive. It is well-documented that the use of tobacco products, especially when smoked, poses a high risk for cancer, emphysema, and heart and artery disease.

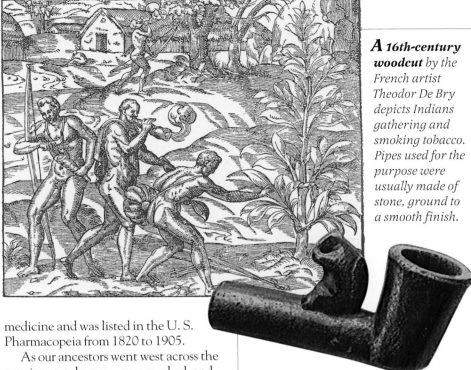

A 16th-century woodcut by the French artist Theodor De Bry depicts Indians gathering and smoking tobacco. Pipes used for the purpose were usually made of stone, ground to a smooth finish.

medicine and was listed in the U. S. Pharmacopeia from 1820 to 1905.

As our ancestors went west across the continent, tobacco—raw, smoked, and as "ST" (smokeless chewing tobacco and snuff)—even played a minor role in the expansion drama as explorers and settlers made their way from the Laurentians to beyond the Rockies. In their journals, Lewis and Clark reported tobacco's importance in their dealings with the often hostile Indians they met.

For household medicinal use, Dr. John Gunn, author of *Gunn's Domestic Medicine*, one of the major medical primers of the early 19th century, recommended "tobacco leaves pounded and mixed with vinegar, and applied as a poultice to the breast and belly" as a vermifuge to expel worms. Gunn also found the tobacco plant "very serviceable" in cases of tetanus, as a diuretic and enema, and for constipation, dropsy, and colic "where all other medicines have proved ineffectual." Presciently, the renowned physician felt it necessary to proffer this warning as well: "The tobacco plant is an active and pow-

erful medicine, and dangerous when used to injudicious excess."

In some rural communities, the smoke itself is still used medicinally today. In Appalachia, tobacco smoke blown into the ear is thought to ease the pain of earaches, and colicky babies are said to benefit from smoke being blown onto their faces or into their formulas—practices more dubious than effective.

Many Cons ...

Nicotine is a powerful compound that stimulates the central nervous system, taking only eight seconds after inhalation to be circulated to the brain. Pure nicotine is so toxic that cigarette tobacco contains only 1 to 2 percent. Still, when the leaf is ignited and begins to smoke, the nicotine decomposes into an assortment of lethal substances, including hydrocyanic acid and carbon monoxide. The result?

A higher risk of heart disease and cancers of the lungs, cervix, esophagus, larynx, bladder, and pancreas. And while the risks from exposure to secondary smoke are lower than those from active smoking, a 10-year study of 32,000 nonsmoking women found in 1997 that regular exposure to passive smoke almost doubled the rate of heart disease. Moreover, smoke is not the only hazard inherent in the use of tobacco. A resurgence of the popularity of snuff and chewing tobacco among young men of all social classes has resulted in a marked increase in cases of oral cancer.

Smoking is especially dangerous during pregnancy. Carbon monoxide in the blood depletes available oxygen, stunting fetal growth. Statistics have shown that babies born to smoking mothers weigh on average half a kilogram less than those born to nonsmoking mothers.

... and Some Pros?

As strange as it may seem—especially after Health and Welfare Canada confirmed the link between tobacco smoking and lung cancer in a 1963 report—scientists in the late 20th century are discovering positive medical uses for tobacco. The plant has shown potential benefit for such varied conditions as Parkinson's and Alzheimer's diseases, glaucoma, and such inflammatory bowel diseases as ulcerative colitis and regional ileitis, or Crohn's disease. It also may have potential for treating the neurological condition called Tourette's syndrome.

With new medical uses being explored, might tobacco someday be thought of again as a miracle plant? Probably not. But as the smoking habit wanes and a new century dawns, it is possible that future generations may view nicotine not as an addictive drug but as a medicine with specific, if limited, benefits.

THE HEALING TRADITIONS OF
THE INUIT

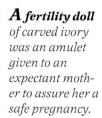

To its early inhabitants, the vast landscape of Alaska and the Canadian North was a realm teeming with spirits, supernatural beings that assumed many forms and influenced every aspect of life. It was clear, therefore, that the well-being of humans depended on maintaining proper relations with the invisible world—never an easy task—as well as preserving more tangible knowledge and skills.

*A **fertility doll** of carved ivory was an amulet given to an expectant mother to assure her a safe pregnancy.*

For innumerable generations, the providers of medicine among the Inuit were, in effect, amateurs—working men and women drawn to medicine by a special aptitude. Everyday maladies were often treated by members of the community whose only qualification was familiarity with traditional healing—herbal or other empirical cures that had been found effective in the past. Most families included at least one female elder with a working knowledge of medicinal plants—for instance, the leaves of Labrador tea were mixed with fried seal oil and water as an ointment to relieve pain, fever, sore throats, and nosebleeds. Mountain sandwort (the "lettuce of the Inuit") was eaten raw to cure diarrhea, and cloudberry leaves were drunk as a tea to ease kidney ailments and stomachaches. Many animal products were also versatile. Seal oil, in particular, was used to treat ailments ranging from constipation (drinking a small amount usually relieved it) to pneumonia (the oil was applied to the underside of a rabbit skin, which was placed overnight on the patient's chest).

Inuit medicine included basic surgery as well. Whales, seals, and caribou were dangerous prey: hunters faced constant risk of injury, and when it occurred, quick treatment could mean the difference between life and death. Large cuts were sutured with human hair or sinew from caribou legs; an infected wound was covered with a compress of whale blubber or caribou fat held in place with grass string. Broken limbs were set as carefully as possible, then immobilized in a wrapping of thick, hard animal skin. Bloodletting was also often used. Some traditional healers practiced a massage technique called organ manipulation that is still used today.

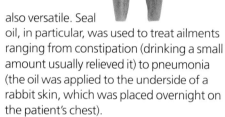

*A **carved stone oil lamp** bears a relief of a hunter in his kayak, watched over by a protective spirit. Such lamps held seal oil, which was burned to provide light and heat on ceremonial occasions.*

Invisible Power in Tangible Form

Healing rites used by shamans involved dancing, chanting, and other elements, and in such dramatic ceremonies masks played a key role. A mask was based on a shaman's vision or dream, and it represented a spirit or being whose power entered the shaman's body while he was wearing it. Masks were made either by the shamans themselves or by carvers working under their direction. Driftwood was the most common material, with fur, feathers, caribou hair, and other items added to achieve a particular symbolic effect. Inuit tradition also ascribed great importance to amulets—objects imbued with powers that could help bring success in the hunt, ensure good health, and propitiate the spirit world. They were usually small objects—stones, teeth, miniature knives, pieces of animal skin—that could be attached to clothing or worn dangling from a special belt. Amulets were of benefit only to their rightful owners, and each had a specific function—one to ward off headaches, for example, another to make its owner invisible when stalking caribou.

In an early photo, women dancers exhibited the playfulness inherent in their society. The empty mask frames would be held to the face as the dancers contorted their features, mimicking a mask.

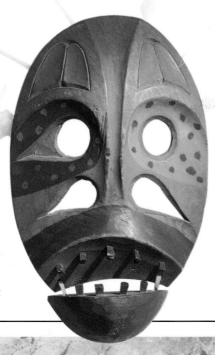

A mask of painted wood, with a hinged jaw piece and a corona of feathers, evokes the powerful spirit of a bear. As with many ceremonial masks, its anthropomorphic features suggest the intimate links between mankind and the invisible forces populating the spirit world.

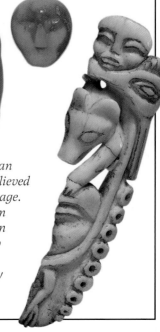

Amulets of polished stone (above right) may have been gifts from a shaman or family elder; they were believed to grow more powerful with age. A healing charm carved from ivory (right) shows a shaman astride a raven perched atop a bear—an alliance potent enough to deal with virtually any illness the shaman was likely to encounter.

Harmony in Diversity

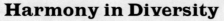

Contemporary health clinics in many Inuit communities see no conflict in blending traditional and Western medical treatments. Indeed, Inuit medicine long made use of both spiritual and empirical methods. In the past, healing arts were carried on by an eclectic group of practitioners—surgeons, masseuses, herbalists, and others whose roles could be likened to those of specialists today.

Illustrated here is a famed healer, the late tribal doctor Della Keats, who worked in cooperation with Western physicians in northern clinics in the 1950s and 1960s. Doctor Keats and other traditional healers—predominantly older women—specialized in a form of deep abdominal massage, known as organ manipulation, that has been practiced for centuries. The technique was developed to treat stomach, bladder, uterine, and other internal disorders. It usually involves "softening" the patient's abdomen first with a precise and increasingly forceful massage, then stretching or moving the affected organ with a kneading or raking motion of the fingers. The process usually takes no more than 10 minutes, and it often produces remarkable improvement.

The Inuit also heat rocks or sand and place them strategically on the body— like a hot-water bottle—to treat stomachaches, bladder ailments, infection, and delayed menstruation. Cold stones are placed on the back of the neck to stop a nosebleed.

Shamans and Spirits

Some kinds of disease, however, had supernatural origins and had to be dealt with differently. Of all the spirits inhabiting the earth, sea, and sky, none was more important than the human soul—the vital inner force that breathed life into each person's body. Serious illness was often taken to mean that the soul had been attacked in some way.

Over the centuries, a complex of rituals and taboos had become part of the fabric of life, governing conduct in virtually every kind of situation. Failure to comply with any of them could lead to injury, disease, or worse. When a hunter killed an animal, for instance, rituals of respect had to be performed and taboos strictly observed lest the animal's spirit wreak vengeance on the entire community.

When someone fell ill and did not respond to empirical treatments, a shaman was consulted. Shamans were not a separate, priestly class in Inuit societies; they worked, raised families, and outwardly were like everyone else in the community. However, it was clear that they possessed special powers, for which they were respected and feared—powers to predict the weather, discover why animals were scarce, inflict harm on enemies, and restore health to friends.

The best shamans were intensely theatrical in their healing rituals. The patient's soul may have been attacked by a malevolent spirit or stolen through sorcery; it may have gone astray for some other reason and become lost. The shaman would enter a trance-like state, through which he made contact with the supernatural world and set about discovering and correcting whatever had caused the patient's affliction. The process was likely to be dramatic and suspenseful process, performed in dim light before an audience of the patient's family and friends. Chanting, dancing, ventriloquism, and legerdemain, accompanied by the beating of drums, might all be used. In a trance, the shaman might search the labyrinth of sea and sky for the lost soul and lead it on a tortuous journey home or expel hostile spirits from the patient's body after a fierce struggle that ends dramatically with his hands covered with blood—all this as objects fly about in the semidarkness, guided on unseen strings by his assistants.

A shaman's reputation rose or fell on his ability to perform such seemingly impossible feats. But if these "power displays" were actually works of stagecraft and illusion—techniques mastered during years of apprenticeship—their effects were no less real. A convincing display could be powerful indeed: many patients who were sick when a shamanic ritual began felt well when it was over. In this regard, Inuit tradition reflected a knowledge that has only gradually become accepted by Western physicians— that healing is as much art as science, and faith can be a uniquely potent medicine.

A rare miniature mask of beaten copper may have been used to cover a doll's face during a healing ceremony.

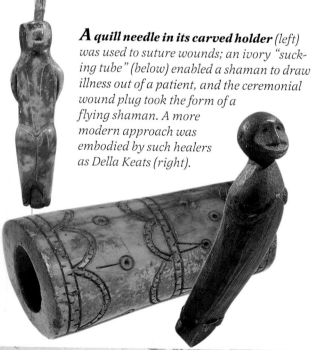

*A **quill needle in its carved holder** (left) was used to suture wounds; an ivory "sucking tube" (below) enabled a shaman to draw illness out of a patient, and the ceremonial wound plug took the form of a flying shaman. A more modern approach was embodied by such healers as Della Keats (right).*

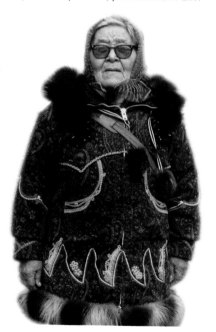

TOOTHACHE

Medical guidebooks used by early North Americans could be counted on to include not one but many cures for the excruciating pain associated with an aching tooth. Well over 70 different herbs, many introduced by the Indians to the settlers, were prescribed in the form of poultices, fillings, chews, and mouth rinses. Other treatments included placing one's own earwax or the fat of a grey squirrel on the tooth—practices that have long been discarded.

Root Causes

Toothaches remain a common ailment today, second only to the common cold. Symptoms vary from a stabbing pain whenever one bites down to an intermittent "burst" to a throbbing of the face. A toothache is often a tip-off that serious tooth decay is present: bacteria penetrate tissue at the center of the tooth, and the subsequent inflammation and pressure cause pain. Tooth pain can also be an early indicator of more serious problems, such as gum disease or an abscess—a localized area of infection at the root tip. Less commonly, lost fillings, tooth fractures, sinus conditions, and even heart ailments can cause toothache.

Even if the pain disappears, see a dentist as soon as possible; gum disease can progress for months without any hint of trouble. Your dentist will look for the telltale signs of a cavity (a soft or brown spot on the tooth), infection (a red or yellow bump at the base of the tooth), or gum inflammation. In most cases, X rays will be taken to determine the seriousness of the problem.

Early Herbal Aids

Some of the pioneers' medical guidebooks endorsed tobacco as a toothache remedy. One advised smoking it through a wad of cotton stuffed in a pipe, to obtain the tobacco "oil," then applying the soaked cotton to the cavity. Surprisingly, this was not an Indian remedy: the medicinal use of tobacco for toothache by the Indians was rare at this time. Only later did the Indians utilize tobacco to relieve toothache, stuffing a plug of chewed tobacco into the cheek and blowing pipe smoke onto the affected tooth.

Yet settlers did adopt other medicinal plants and practices relied upon by the Indians. Bark, berries, roots, or leaves were chewed to release mild astringent compounds that fought infection—a practice learned from the Comanche, who chewed echinacea root for its numbing and healing effects, and the Plains Indians, who used calamus, or sweet flag, to reduce gum inflammation and to ease tooth pain.

One remedy esteemed by various tribes was a tincture of the root bark or the berries of the prickly ash, also known as the toothache tree. One 19th-century North American medical textbook explained that the plant "powerfully stimulates secretion from mucous surfaces." Prickly ash, called

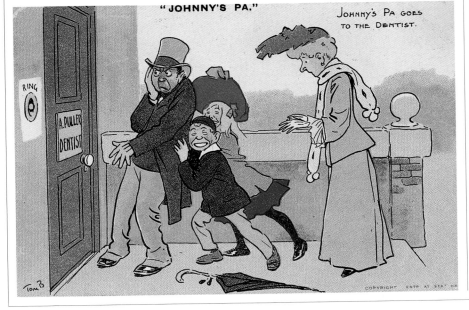

"JOHNNY'S PA."

JOHNNY'S PA GOES TO THE DENTIST.

RING

A. PULLEM DENTIST

Children weren't the only ones to fear the dentist, as this turn-of-the-century cartoon shows.

Hercules's club by people of African descent, continues to be used for toothache by modern herbalists for its anti-inflammatory and analgesic effects.

All kinds of substances—among them herbs (powdered, burned, or in tea form), whiskey, clove oil, and salt water—were held in the mouth to ease tooth pain. The Seneca Indians scooped sticky, black petroleum from oily pools and applied it to the painful tooth and gums. Later, they sold oil to the settlers to treat a plethora of ailments. North American doctors apparently had little to say about this so-called wound healer, although the 19th-century Scottish physician William Cullen decried petroleum "in every form ... a very disagreeable remedy."

Poultices and Charms

Herbal poultices were another approach for easing the pain. John Wesley, in his *Primitive Physick* (1755), recommended "[laying] roasted parings of turnips, as hot as may be, behind the ear." Also employed were rubefacients, including cayenne

pepper and black mustard. Applying a cold pack to ease pain and reduce inflammation became widespread only after refrigeration had become common.

Various verbal charms and special rituals were used against toothache as well. In his 1820 Pennsylvania Dutch "pow-wow" manual, John George Hohman offered this intriguing cure: "Cut out a piece of greensward [sod] in the morning before sunrise, quite unbeshrewdly from any place, breathe three times upon it, and put it down upon the same place from which it was taken."

First Aid for Toothaches

Prevention is the best defense: brush with a fluoridated toothpaste, floss, and see your dentist twice a year. If your jaw feels like a pounding jackhammer and the dentist cannot see you right away, ease the pain with one or more of these steps.

◆ Try rinsing with lukewarm water first; sometimes an irritating piece of food is the source of the ache and can be dislodged. Electric gum-cleaning devices are especially helpful. Avoid hot or cold water, which can aggravate an already sensitive tooth. A saltwater rinse is also recommended: it not only cleanses the area around the tooth but also draws out some of the fluid that causes swelling.

◆ Apply an ice pack to the jaw. Ice has the dual effect of reducing swelling and shutting down sensitive superficial nerves.

◆ Take an analgesic for temporary relief. However, contrary to some folk beliefs, never put an aspirin directly on a tooth—its acids will burn the gums.

CLOVE A volatile oil in clove, eugenol, has anesthetic properties. Lightly crack a clove between the teeth to release a tiny amount of oil, then hold it between the cheek and the gum of the affected area. If using clove oil (sometimes sold as eugenol), follow the directions on the label. Repeated use of the undiluted oil causes gum damage.

PRICKLY ASH The bark of the prickly ash (*Zanthoxylum* spp.), or toothache tree, remains a popular remedy today; it has analgesic and anti-inflammatory properties. Chew a piece of the fresh bark and pack the moist mass around the painful tooth. Leave

it on for no more than a few minutes and do not swallow the bark, which contains potentially toxic alkaloids. If pregnant, lactating, or taking anticoagulant drugs, do not use prickly ash.

THYME Thyme oil applied locally can ease the pain of a toothache. Soak a clean cotton ball in water and squeeze out any excess liquid. Then put 2 to 4 drops thyme oil on the cotton ball. Apply to the surface of the aching tooth and surrounding gums for no more than a few minutes. Repeat the procedure up to two to three times a day. Thyme oil should always be diluted and should never be ingested.

GINGER Ginger's anti-inflammatory and rubefacient effects aid pain relief. To ease a toothache, apply a fresh slice of ginger or a cotton swab wetted with 2 drops of its essential oil to the affected area. Remove when the burning sensation becomes intolerable. In general, ginger oil is safe, although some people may be sensitive to it.

MYRRH The astringent and antimicrobial effects of myrrh make it a good mouthwash for toothache. Simmer 1 teaspoon powdered myrrh in 2 cups water for 30 minutes. Strain and cool. Rinse with 1 teaspoon of the solution in ½ cup water five to six times daily.

TURPENTINE

We think of it as a paint solvent, but to our forebears turpentine was potent medicine, used as a liniment for aches and pains and ingested with a spoonful of sugar to clear congestion. Yet when taken internally, turpentine is toxic; children have been fatally poisoned by as little as 15 milliliters (½ oz). If turpentine is swallowed, call a poison control center immediately.

Turpentine is an oleoresin, a plant substance that contains both volatile oil and resin. However, the word "turpentine" normally refers to the oil that is distilled from this oleoresin, also called turpentine oil or spirits of turpentine. It is usually obtained from the longleaf pine, but it may also derive from other conifers. (So-called Canada turpentine comes from the balsam fir; Venice turpentine is derived from the larch tree.) Today most turpentine is made from by-products of the lumber and paper industries.

Turpentine was once a popular rub for rheumatism; it was often mixed with lard or vegetable oil to keep it from burning the skin. As anyone who has touched or even smelled the substance knows, it is an irritant. When applied externally, it causes increased blood flow to the area and a tingling sensation that distracts the patient from underlying muscle or joint pain. Turpentine was also frequently applied to sprains.

Although the treatment was no doubt torturous, Indians used turpentine extracted from the white pine to heal, in the words of one 17th-century British observer, "desperate wounds." The settlers applied the substance to hemorrhoids despite the intense pain it must have caused, and also to cuts and stings. A somewhat more soothing salve combined rosin (another word for pine resin) with beeswax, tallow, and turpentine.

A Vaporous Cold Cure

Turpentine was considered so essential that it figured among the medicinal supplies George Washington requested be brought back from London in 1767. It was used not only against wounds and aches but also as a cure for colds and congestion. Doctors prescribed a few drops on a spoonful of sugar. It was also mixed with lard and rubbed on the chest, then covered with a piece of flannel. If left on overnight, such poultices occasionally caused severe blistering, but this hardly discouraged their use. To treat croup,

WHITE CLOVERINE BRAND
REG. U.S. PAT. OFF.
Active Ingredient : White Petroleum Jelly compounded with physiologically inactive amounts of Rectified Oil of Turpentine, White Wax and perfume.
THE ORIGINAL WHITE CLOVERINE BRAND
SALVE
Compounded from a Physician's Prescription
MFD. SINCE 1895 BY
THE WILSON CHEMICAL CO., INC.
TYRONE, PENNA.
(SEE BACK)
NET. WT. 1 OZ.
PRICE 25¢

A touch of turpentine enhanced household products such as White Cloverine Salve, formulated in 1860.

some parents made a vaporous (and unsafe) steam inhalation by adding a few drops of turpentine to a kettle of water on the stove. A popular method of "dislodging" tapeworms called for a dose of turpentine and castor oil. One mother, after administering this cure, claimed to have extracted a worm several meters long. Mixed with hog's lard, turpentine was said to make ringworms "pop out"; actually, ringworm is not a worm but a fungus. To treat pinworms, turpentine was dabbed onto the child's navel, where the parasites were thought to gather.

No doubt because of its tingling action, turpentine was also used to treat frostbite. One remedy called for a mixture of olive oil, peppermint oil, turpentine, and ammonia to be rubbed on the frostbitten skin. (This may have helped restore circulation to the area, but it is inadvisable.) A salve made of resin, beeswax, and turpentine was utilized to cure "scald head," an infectious scalp condition. Proponents of this remedy warned that it permanently removed one's hair, causing the head to resemble a peeled onion.

Today some people still use turpentine in liniments to soothe aches and pains. However, since turpentine is absorbed into the bloodstream even when applied topically, excessive use may cause toxic side effects. In some people, any amount of turpentine may cause skin irritation.

Uses Rheumatism, aches, pains
Cautions Turpentine is toxic if taken internally; it may produce headache, insomnia, coughing, vomiting, bloody urine, coma, and death. Pregnant women should avoid turpentine fumes. In some people, any amount of turpentine used externally may cause redness of the skin or a blistering rash.

URINE

It is hard to imagine a less palatable medication than urine, yet this human waste has been used to treat ailments, both minor and serious, down through the centuries. While researchers dismiss its folk uses as worthless and potentially dangerous, some of the biochemicals urine contains—including urea and dihydrourea—have beneficial applications once they are extracted and refined. (Both of these chemicals have a softening effect, which has led to their inclusion in skin lotions and hair conditioners.)

Urine is produced in the kidneys, which filter and secrete the waste products from the bloodstream. On average, humans produce ½ to 2 liters of it per day—the low end if they are in a hot environment or exercising and don't drink enough fluids, the higher end if they consume a lot of water. Barring a urinary tract infection, urine is essentially sterile when first excreted. Nevertheless, it can quickly blossom with bacteria, creating the noxious "stale urine" smell of ammonia; this is true especially among women, whose urine is more likely to be contaminated by bacteria and yeast.

Urine mixed with vinegar and applied to the skin was a folk treatment to lighten freckles (the "unpolluted" urine of an infant was favored). A few drops of warm urine was reputed to relieve earache, perhaps by softening wax deposits—although folk wisdom held that only urine from someone of the opposite sex would work. In World War I, soldiers sometimes resorted to dipping their handkerchiefs in urine and wearing them over their faces if they were caught without their gas masks.

A Gauge of Health

Remarkably, drinking one's own urine as a daily tonic was once believed to be a panacea. Such "urine therapy" is not a thing of the past; it is enjoying a modest resurgence in New Age circles, even though physicians and researchers are virtually unanimous in condemning it as foolhardy and useless. They note that urine contains the very toxins one's body has gotten rid of and that drinking the fluid merely forces the kidneys to do the same job twice. Likewise, injections of urine, a weight-loss fad some years back, were proved worthless.

Urine can be a useful gauge of health; a change in its color or odor may be a symptom of a serious condition. Cloudy urine may signal a urinary tract infection, and cloudy, tea-colored urine can be a sign of internal bleeding—a disorder that requires immediate medical attention. (Note, however, that some food dyes and drugs can turn urine red.) Hepatitis can cause urine color to change to a deep orange or brown. Odor, too, can be a clue: sweet-smelling urine is a possible sign of diabetes, while an acrid smell may be caused by nothing more serious than having eaten a plate of asparagus, which, when metabolized, produces methyl mercaptan, a sulfur compound.

Among the biochemicals medical researchers have isolated in urine are erythropoietin, a hormone formed in the kidneys that regulates red blood cells, and chorionic gonadotropin, which stimulates ovulation. Another hormone, human menopausal gonadotropin (hMG), used to treat infertility, is extracted from the urine of postmenopausal women. Researchers are also investigating potential tumor-fighting and appetite-controlling compounds in human urine.

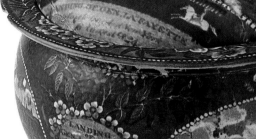

The chamber pot was not replaced by toilets until the late 1800s.

Uses No home remedies based on urine are recommended.
Cautions Consumption is considered inadvisable and worthless.

VAGINAL PROBLEMS

Vaginitis is a general term for inflammation of the vagina. It is usually caused by a disturbance of the delicate acid-base balance, which is maintained by naturally occurring, acid-forming bacteria. The bacteria check the growth of a yeast-like fungus called *Candida albicans,* which is also normally present. A lack of bacteria allows the fungus to overgrow, causing a so-called yeast infection. Occasionally, the opposite problem occurs: the bacteria multiply, causing a bacterial infection.

Symptoms of vaginitis include itching and abnormal vaginal discharge. Yeast infections were once known as "the whites" for the thick white discharge they produce. Unlike yeast infections, bacterial infections cause an odor. A foamy greenish-yellow discharge may indicate the parasite *Trichomonas vaginalis,* which requires treatment with an antiprotozoan drug; both sexual partners should be treated. Yeast infections are treated with antifungal suppositories, creams, or ointments, available in prescription and nonprescription strength. Vaginitis can sometimes be a symptom of a more serious sexually transmitted disease, such as gonorrhea, which requires a doctor's care.

Preventing Vaginitis

Yeast and bacteria prefer a warm, moist environment. Therefore, to discourage infections, avoid nylon underwear (which doesn't allow air to circulate) and tight-fitting clothing, especially pantyhose. Change promptly out of a damp bathing suit, and dry carefully after bathing. Also, change tampons often, and wipe from front to back after a bowel movement. Other factors that increase the risk of yeast infections include lack of sleep, poor diet, diabetes, oral contraceptives, and broad-spectrum antibiotics, which kill off the bacteria that keep the yeast in check.

If you must take antibiotics for an infection elsewhere, some herbalists recommend taking acidophilus supplements (which inhibit the growth of yeast) at the same time. Alternatively, eat yogurt that contains *Lactobacillus acidophilus* cultures; this has been shown to reduce the recurrence of yeast infections.

While you have an infection, it is best to abstain from sexual intercourse, which can aggravate the inflammation and cause the yeast or bacteria to spread to your partner, who may reinfect you later. If the problem doesn't respond to self-treatment within two or three days, see a doctor.

Another common problem is vaginal itching in postmenopausal women. As estrogen levels plummet, the lining of the vagina becomes thinner, drier, and more prone to inflammation. Hormone replacement therapy may solve the problem, as may the use of a vaginal lubricant during intercourse. Vaginal itching may also be caused by allergic reactions to strong soaps, bath oils, douches, spermicides, and perfumed or dyed toilet paper.

Herbal Folk Cures

Before the days of antibiotics and antifungal creams, astringent and tonic herbs were used in external washes and douches to treat leukorrhea, or abnormal vaginal discharge. White-oak bark was popular, as were ragweed, ragwort, and plantain.

Yeast infection treatments include yogurt with acidophilus cultures; echinacea, which stimulates the immune system; and garlic, tea-tree oil, and the oil of calendula, all antifungal.

Nylon pantyhose, *introduced in 1940, trap moisture and encourage the growth of yeast.*

Yarrow, used as a wound healer since ancient times, was recommended by the 16th-century British herbalist John Gerard for treating the "swelling of those secret parts." Settlers used infusions of yarrow as a douche and also took it internally as a tea or syrup.

Goldenseal was an obvious choice, given its reputation as an antiseptic and an anti-inflammatory, as was chamomile, which some herbalists still prescribe. Trillium (*Trillium erectum*), also called bethroot, was popular with Indians and settlers alike because of its astringent and

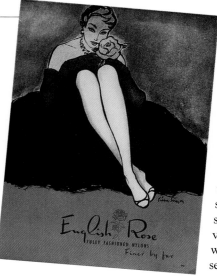

English Rose
FULLY FASHIONED NYLONS
Finer by far

tonic properties; some people drank the root tea every night before bed. Wild geranium (*Geranium maculatum*), also called alumroot or cranesbill, was used as an astringent wash by the Indians and the settlers. Infusions of slippery elm bark, valued for its mucilage, were used to soothe severe irritation.

The Douche Debate

Pennsylvania farm wives made an acidic douche of two teaspoons alum or two tablespoons white vinegar per liter of lukewarm water; this was used twice daily for one week. Others used a strong infusion of tea or one tablespoon witch hazel

in two liters warm water. Vinegar-and-water douches remain popular with some women prone to yeast infections, but most doctors advise against them, since douching upsets the natural vaginal flora and may actually promote infection.

Plain water was also a popular douche. In *Gunn's Domestic Medicine* (1830), Knoxville physician John Gunn recommended "bathing well those parts in cold water, three or four times a day; and injecting up the birth-place, frequently, the same thing, cold water." Others advised hot douches. Water, preferably lukewarm, is the mildest of douches.

Because leukorrhea was said to strike on the heels of a "run-down condition," patients were advised to follow a diet similar to that recommended for anemics. Lowered resistance due to fatigue or poor diet may indeed increase one's susceptibility. Echinacea, which stimulates the immune system, may prevent and cure yeast infections, but more study is needed.

YOGURT Yogurt that contains active *Lactobacillus acidophilus* cultures (usually found in low-fat or nonfat varieties) inhibits the growth of the fungus that causes most vaginal infections. A 1992 study showed that eating 1 cup of yogurt daily reduces the recurrence of yeast infections. To treat an infection, yogurt may also be applied directly twice daily, although this approach is messy. Acidophilus tablets are available. Note that yogurt works only for yeast infections; treating a bacterial infection with yogurt will aggravate the problem.

TEA TREE AND CALENDULA PESSARIES Tea tree is one of the best herbal antiseptics, effective against the fungus *Candida albicans* and the parasite

Trichomonas vaginalis. Calendula is useful too as an antifungal and antiseptic. Although no clinical studies have been conducted, herbalists recommend using either essential oil in pessaries (vaginal suppositories). To prepare, shape aluminum foil into 24 molds that are 19 mm (¾ in.) long and 9 mm (⅜ in.) in diameter, tapering to 6 mm (¼ in.). To form the lubricant, combine 2 teaspoons soft soap, 45 ml (1½ oz) glycerin, and 45 ml (1½ oz) denatured alcohol. Pour this mixture into the foil, then pour it off after a few seconds. Next, melt 20 g (⅔ oz) cocoa butter and remove from heat. Add 30 drops tea tree or calendula essential oil. Pour this mixture into the molds. After three hours, remove the foil. Insert one pessary at night and repeat in the morning, while

the infection persists. Store the pessaries in a cool place in a container lined with waxed paper. Alternatively, add 30 drops essential oil to 2 tablespoons vegetable oil; dab onto a tampon and insert. Discontinue use if burning or irritation occurs.

GARLIC Garlic is a highly effective antibacterial and antifungal agent, and garlic extract has been reported to be more effective than the prescription antifungal drug nystatin against *Candida albicans*. Peel a garlic clove, crush it lightly, wrap it in gauze, then insert it into the vagina. Insert garlic twice daily, using a fresh clove each time. Documented adverse effects include burning and irritation. If either effect occurs, discontinue use.

VALERIAN

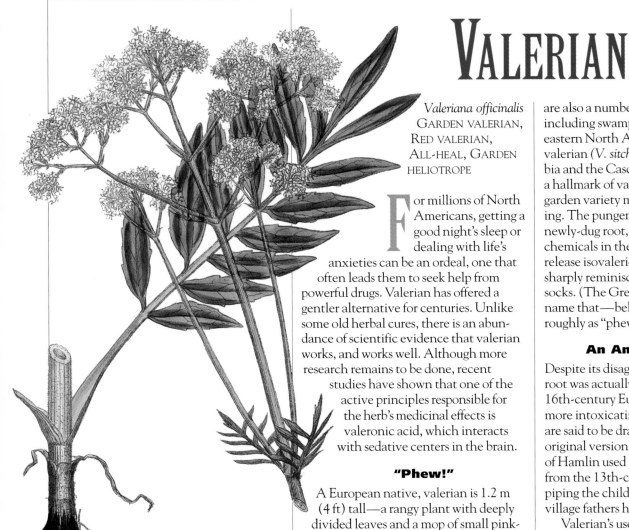

Valeriana officinalis
GARDEN VALERIAN,
RED VALERIAN,
ALL-HEAL, GARDEN
HELIOTROPE

For millions of North Americans, getting a good night's sleep or dealing with life's anxieties can be an ordeal, one that often leads them to seek help from powerful drugs. Valerian has offered a gentler alternative for centuries. Unlike some old herbal cures, there is an abundance of scientific evidence that valerian works, and works well. Although more research remains to be done, recent studies have shown that one of the active principles responsible for the herb's medicinal effects is valeronic acid, which interacts with sedative centers in the brain.

"Phew!"

A European native, valerian is 1.2 m (4 ft) tall—a rangy plant with deeply divided leaves and a mop of small pinkish flowers massed at the top. One of the first plants brought to the New World, it escaped cultivation and now grows wild in many parts of North America. There are also a number of native species, including swamp valerian (*V. uliginosa*) in eastern North America and mountain valerian (*V. sitchensis*) in British Columbia and the Cascade Range. Its foul odor is a hallmark of valerian, including the garden variety most often used for healing. The pungent smell is absent from the newly-dug root, but as the root dries, chemicals in the plant break down and release isovaleric acid—a compound sharply reminiscent of unwashed gym socks. (The Greeks called the herb *phu*, a name that—believe it or not—translates roughly as "phew!")

An Ancient Remedy

Despite its disagreeable odor, valerian root was actually the basis of perfumes in 16th-century Europe. Cats find it even more intoxicating than catnip, and rats are said to be drawn to it. In fact, in the original version of the tale, the Pied Piper of Hamlin used valerian to lure the rats from the 13th-century German town, piping the children away only after the village fathers had refused to pay his fee.

Valerian's use as a medicinal plant dates to ancient Greece. The Roman naturalist Pliny the Elder stated that the root "helps all stoppings and stranglings in any part of the body." Others credited it with improving the flow of urine, easing menstruation, and counteracting poisons.

The great second-century Roman physician Galen was the first to record valerian's use against insomnia. Still, for the larger part of the past millennium, valerian was used mostly to treat ailments

Plant parts used Dried rhizome and roots
Uses Mild sedative and sleep aid, antispasmodic
Cautions Valerian may magnify the effects of other central nervous system depressants; avoid long-term use and consult a physician before administering the herb to children under the age of six. Pregnant women and nursing mothers should avoid valerian.

other than sleeplessness. It gained an apparently unwarranted reputation as a remedy for epilepsy after a 16th-century Italian botanist and physician, Fabius Columna, claimed he cured his own bouts of "falling sickness" with the herb. In the mid-1600s, English physicians prescribed valerian "boiled with liquorice, raisins and anniseed" for short-windedness, and boiled with wine as an antidote to venomous bites and stings. In the 18th century, it was a popular treatment for asthma, convulsions, and disorders of the uterus.

Nature's Sleeping Pill

Today it is valerian's use as a sedative and sleep aid that attracts the most attention. Long before the arrival of powerful synthetic sedatives, this garden plant exerted a gentle, calming effect; it was widely used in Europe during both world wars to treat those suffering from shell-shock and so-called "bombing neurosis." These uses faded with the advent of synthetic benzodiazepine tranquilizers like Valium—which, despite its similarity in name, is not made from valerian and has no close chemical relation to it. Such synthetic drugs are now controlled substances; not only can their use lead to chemical addiction but they may also interfere with desirable dream-producing, rapid-eye-movement (REM) sleep. What's more, even over-the-counter sleep aids can cause a hangover-like drowsiness that lasts through the following morning.

Valerian, on the other hand, seems to have no such side effects. Although it binds with the same neurotransmitter sites in the brain as benzodiazepines, it does so weakly and is not addictive—in fact, it may even provide a therapy for those trying to break an addiction to the more powerful drugs. Furthermore, its effects are not magnified by alcohol, as are

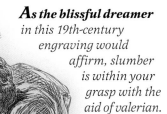

As the blissful dreamer *in this 19th-century engraving would affirm, slumber is within your grasp with the aid of valerian.*

those of most commercial tranquilizers. (Valerian does, however, act in concert with other sedatives to depress the central nervous system; anyone using a sedative should consult his doctor before taking the herb.) Several studies have confirmed that valerian does help people fall asleep, and allows for deeper, more restful slumber, especially among chronic insomniacs.

How It Works

Valerian is not a hypnotic—that is, it does not produce sleep directly but calms the body and brain enough to allow sleep to come on its own. All of the active principles responsible for its medicinal effects have yet to be identified. However, at least one recent study has found that the plant's valeronic acid interacts with the gamma-aminobutyric acid, or GABA, receptors in the brain, which are associated with sedative-type activity.

Scientists express some concern about other compounds in valerian, including the valepotriates, which have been shown to damage cells. However, valepotriates decompose rapidly in the prepared root and are not easily absorbed by the body. While experts caution against the long-term use of valerian, no side effects have been reported. (Valerian is a well-regarded treatment in Europe, where it is an ingredient in scores of over-the-counter preparations.) Still, parents should consult a doctor before giving valerian to children under the age of six; pregnant women and nursing mothers should avoid the herb, as its safety during pregnancy and lactation has not been proved.

One or two cups of tea or a full teaspoon of valerian tincture can be taken before bed to help bring on sleep. Researchers advise that a mere few drops—the usual dosage with tinctures—does not provide enough valerian to be effective.

VARICOSE VEINS

In the early 19th century, Knoxville physician John Gunn advised rest in a "lying posture" with tight bandages wrapped around the legs—"which will give due support to the vessels"—and moderate exercise for what he called "sore legs of long standing." Today, the best measures for varicose veins have been only slightly updated: sitting down with the legs elevated, wearing elastic support stockings, and regular walking.

Although varicose veins in the legs are the most familiar, they also form in the anal area, where we know them as hemorrhoids. Yet unlike hemorrhoids, varicosities in the legs were rarely treated by folk healers, who more often attended to the leg ulcers that developed in the later, more serious, stages of the condition.

Hidden Damage

For ages, varicose veins in the legs have been considered nothing more than unsightly embarrassments to be covered up by long petticoats and slacks. However, the bulging, contorted blue veins that lie just below the skin are more than just a cosmetic problem. They can lead to painful cramps, itching, and more serious conditions, such as edema and blood clotting. In addition, a large varicosity can rupture, causing severe bruising or bleeding.

Special valves in veins are responsible for pushing blood back toward the heart. When the valves fail, blood seeps back into the veins and pools in them, causing them to bulge. In cases affecting the legs, the ankles and feet may also swell from edema. During the day, when a person spends more time standing, symptoms can worsen and will be relieved only by sitting with the legs raised. Self-help includes taking rutin and vitamins C and E. Serious cases may require sclerotherapy, which involves

See a doctor if ...

In most cases, varicose veins are benign and manageable. However, they can become severe and lead to more serious conditions. Consult a doctor if any of the following occur.
◆ A varicose vein ruptures, causing severe bleeding or bruising.
◆ Pain is severe and unabating, even after sitting and elevating the legs.
◆ Lumps are visible or palpable (a sign of blood clotting).
◆ Varicosities do not decrease in size, even after sitting and raising the legs.
◆ The skin becomes ulcerated.
◆ If itching and a cord-like swelling occur—signs of thrombophlebitis, an inflammation of a vein that can cause a fatal pulmonary embolism.

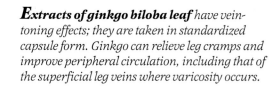

Extracts of ginkgo biloba leaf *have vein-toning effects; they are taken in standardized capsule form. Ginkgo can relieve leg cramps and improve peripheral circulation, including that of the superficial leg veins where varicosity occurs.*

injections, or stripping, a surgical procedure that removes the affected veins.

Factors that increase the likelihood of varicose veins include a family history of the condition, smoking, inactivity, and hormonal changes during pregnancy or menopause. Birth control pills, hormone replacement therapy, and pressure on the abdomen caused by obesity or pregnancy can also increase the risk.

Vein Toners

The best folk remedies for "sore legs" are those that strengthen the veins and soothe the skin. Horse chestnut extracts have shown the ability to reduce edema (fluid retention) and are used in Germany to improve circulation. Although the nuts and husks were once chopped and applied to varicosities, they are toxic and should not be used in home remedies.

In the 19th century, extracts of witch hazel were applied topically to treat varicose veins; witch hazel has shown astringent and hemostatic properties when used topically. Another traditional remedy was the fruit of bilberry—taken as a tea or applied directly to the veins; it contains anthocyanosides, which have vein-toning and anti-edemic potential.

Treating "Leg Ulcers"

Left untreated, varicose veins hamper circulation and deprive the skin of nutrients, causing thin skin and sometimes, the formation of ulcers. In the past, varicose veins rarely garnered medical attention, but leg ulcers did. Calendula flowers and oak bark, used in washes, ointments, and poultices, have shown the potential to help heal varicose ulcers. The astringency of apple cider vinegar and various species of *Rumex* (dock or sorrel) may also help. Other folk remedies with scant or unproven benefits include washes of tansy or sage, tinctures of redroot (*Ceanothus americanus*) or St. Johnswort, and poultices of fern roots, blackberries, or carrots.

Many of these same natural ingredients were used in footbaths. For a bath that cleanses and soothes the ulcers and promotes circulation in the lower legs, use a deep pot or tub that holds enough warm or cold water to cover the calves.

Help From Leeches?

Once used in the early practice of bloodletting, leeches are again being looked at by the medical community. One reason is the anticoagulant effect of leech saliva—first noted in 1884 by Welsh scientist John B. Haycraft. He saw that the blood stored inside of a leech did not coagulate and wounds where leeches had been attached bled for abnormally long periods. In the 1950s German scientist Fritz Marquardt isolated the active principle in the medicinal leech (*Hirudo medicinalis*)—a protein he called hirudin. Hirudin was found to inhibit the action of thrombin, a chemical that plays a major role in the clotting of blood. Today ointments containing hirudin (or the synthetic version, hirulog) are used in Germany to prevent clotting in varicose veins.

BUTCHER'S BROOM Saponins provide the health benefits of butcher's broom (*Ruscus aculeatus*). Take up to 33 milligrams three times a day of tablets; each butcher's broom tablet should contain 9 to 11 percent ruscogenin.

GRAPE SEED Extracts containing procyanidolic oligomers (PCOs), which help tone blood vessels, are available commercially. Take 150 to 300 milligrams a day for at least four weeks.

WITCH HAZEL The high concentration of tannins in witch hazel is responsible for its astringent, antiseptic, and vein-toning action against varicose veins. Apply nondistilled hydroalcoholic extracts up to four times a day.

BILBERRY Take standardized commercial extracts of bilberry (*Vaccinium myrtillus*) in tablet form—250 to 480 milligrams a day. The tablets should contain 25 percent anthocyanidin, a compound that tones the veins.

GINKGO A stalwart of Chinese medicine, ginkgo helps improve peripheral circulation in the legs. Take ginkgo biloba extract in standardized commercial capsules—either 40 milligrams three times a day or 60 milligrams twice a day for at least six weeks.

GOTU KOLA The commercial standardized extract of gotu kola may tone the veins and improve blood flow. Take 60 to 120 milligrams a day for at least two weeks. Sensitivity to light, dermatitis, and itching may occur. Avoid using during pregnancy, lactation, and hypoglycemic therapy.

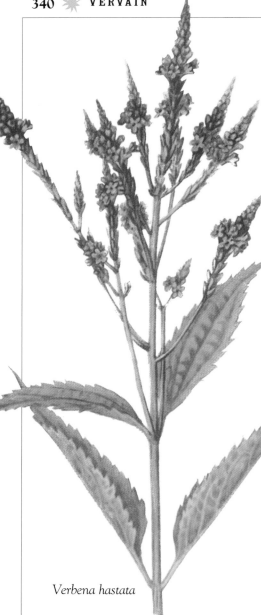

Verbena hastata

VERVAIN

Verbena hastata, V. officinalis
BLUE VERVAIN, SIMPLER'S-JOY

If even a fraction of the claims that early North American folk healers made for humble vervain were true, the herb would qualify as one of the world's most magical medicines. It was, healers insisted, a good stimulant for the liver, a relaxing nerve tonic, and a palliative for a range of digestive problems and skin conditions. It was also claimed to eliminate worms, treat scurvy, and alleviate the common cold.

Long regarded with awe, the plant was valued in ancient Rome, where it was used to cleanse the altars of Jupiter before sacrificial feasts and to purify Roman homes and temples. The name "vervain" derives from the Celtic word *ferfaen*, which means "to drive away a stone," a reference to one time-honored use—that of treating kidney stones.

Blue vervain, a perennial that grows up to 1.2 m (4 ft) tall, is native to North America. A European species, *Verbena officinalis*, was imported by the settlers; now almost as widespread as the native species, it is the source of many of the commercial vervain products found on the North American market.

Tarnished Reputation

Not everyone has been as enamored of vervain's cure-all status as North American folk practitioners once were. One prominent early herbalist referred to it as "Clownes all-heal of New England," dismissing many of the claims that were being made for the plant's powers.

The native species was listed in the U.S. National Formulary from 1916 to 1926, but it fell out of use because of its weak action. Likewise, modern studies focusing on vervain's medicinal properties have lent little scientific support to the many claims made on its behalf.

Nevertheless, there are indications that the European species of vervain is an effective diuretic and treatment for painful menstruation. Decoctions of the plant have also been shown to increase lactation in nursing mothers. As research continues, only time will tell whether vervain can regain its former status as a valued medicinal herb.

Vermouth Flavorer

One of the herb's common names, simpler's-joy, dates back to medieval times, when single-herb preparations were known as "simples" and herbalists as "simplers." This is but one of vervain's many connections to ancient times: The Roman naturalist Pliny the Elder suggested that if "the dining room be sprinkled with water in which the herbe hath been steeped, the guests will be merrier." In a contemporary parallel, vervain is an ingredient in vermouth, the wine that gives martinis their distinctive flavor.

Active plant parts Leaves, roots
Uses Painful menstruation; diuretic, lactation stimulant
Cautions Because vervain is known to cause mild uterine contractions, pregnant women should avoid taking the herb. In high doses, vervain causes vomiting.

VINEGAR

With its sharp, nose-twisting tang and agreeably sour taste, vinegar has been a cooking staple since time immemorial—and a staple of folk medicine for just as long. Over the past 5,000 years, it has been considered proof against everything from headaches and sore muscles to the Black Death.

Vinegar is the result of a two-step process that starts when yeasts or molds are added to a sugary liquid and allowed to ferment, producing alcohol. Bacteria then convert the alcohol to acetic acid, creating vinegar—not only distilled white vinegar but apple-cider and malt vinegars, molasses and honey vinegars, and a cornucopia of wine vinegars. (The name itself comes from the French word *vinaigre*, or "sour wine.") Most home remedies call for the more potent distilled white vinegar, although many practitioners of traditional medicine swear by apple-cider vinegar, which has an acetic acid content of only 4 to 6 percent.

Vinegar, which kills some fungi and a wide variety of bacteria, was one of the first effective topical antibiotics used by man. It destroys the fungus that causes athlete's foot; in fact, one of the oldest treatments

for this itchy, burning condition is to apply vinegar to the toes and soak one's socks in it regularly to prevent reinfection. Vinegar was also mixed with either the leaves of European dock or the native wildflower bloodroot to treat

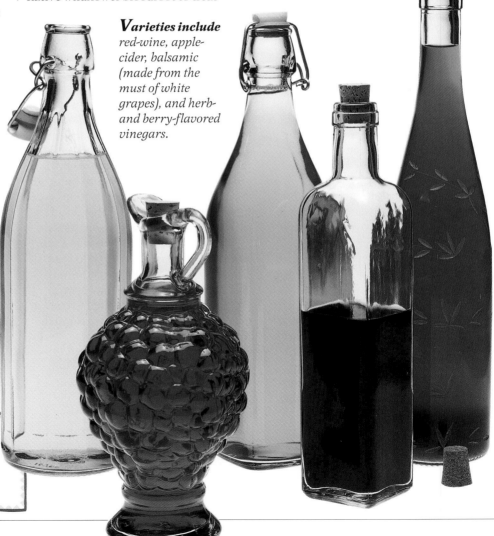

Varieties include *red-wine, apple-cider, balsamic (made from the must of white grapes), and herb- and berry-flavored vinegars.*

the fungal infection known as ringworm. In the days before synthetic antibiotics, infected wounds, even those that had developed gangrene, were often bathed with vinegar—a practice that was no doubt extremely painful.

Vinegar was one of the most common all-around folk medicinals. Some of its uses—including pouring it on iron door

---

Uses Sunburn, swimmer's ear, athlete's foot
Cautions Too much vinegar may cause stomach upset. People who are allergic to molds may develop a reaction to nondistilled vinegar.

hinges to cure a headache—were dubious at best. A more widely used headache remedy involved soaking a kerchief in vinegar and wrapping it tightly around the head. As the cloth dried and tightened, it was believed to take away the pain. Bands of brown wrapping paper, similarly soaked and allowed to dry, were thought to have the same effect. For toothache, a cheek-sized piece of brown paper was drenched with vinegar, then covered on one side with black pepper and applied to the face over the swelling. (A variation on this treatment called for using a piece of the gray, absorbent wall of a hornets' nest instead of brown paper.)

To ease headaches and nasal congestion, a cup each of water and vinegar were brought to a boil in a saucepan. Using a towel as a hood—and taking care not to get burned—the patient would breathe in the pungent, head-clearing fumes.

A Soothing Rub

Bandages soaked in vinegar were used to treat sprains in both livestock and people, and vinegar—often mixed with turpentine—was used in liniments for sore muscles. Both vinegar and turpentine are counterirritants—substances that increase blood circulation near the skin's surface and relieve deep muscle pain. In the days before penicillin, when rheumatic fever struck children and left them with severe joint pain, cloths dipped in hot apple-cider vinegar were often used to relieve the ache. Some arthritis sufferers claimed that a daily tonic of vinegar and honey eased the pain in their joints; others preferred a mixture of two parts apple-cider vinegar to three parts water.

Vinegar mixed with honey was one of the great standbys of folk medicine, and it was used for a panoply of complaints, particularly colds, coughs, sore throat,

fatigue, heartburn, and indigestion. The usual recipe was a spoonful each of vinegar and honey taken in a cup of warm water; this combination was also used as a gargle in rural Vermont. The Pennsylvania Dutch utilized straight apple-cider vinegar as a mouthwash. Mixed with a splash of water, a spoonful of baking soda, and a bit of sugar to improve the taste, the sour liquid was sometimes also drunk as a bubbly remedy for upset stomach.

Before commercial smelling salts were available, vinegar was combined with camphor, clove oil, lavender, and other aromatic herbs to "produce a powerful excitant impression," as one old recipe put it. Vinegar was also mixed with ground horseradish root and sniffed to stop the sneezing caused by hay fever.

Diluted with water, vinegar has also long been used as a douche. (Although vinegar mimics the body's natural acidity, it has not been proven to encourage the growth of beneficial bacteria in the vagina and thereby prevent yeast infections; moreover, most doctors say that douching isn't necessary and that excessive douching can lead to dryness.) A sponge soaked in diluted vinegar and inserted like a tampon was also employed as a primitive, and often ineffective, contraceptive.

Externally, vinegar was used to combat head lice and was mixed with garlic juice to fight pimples. Amazingly, it was even used to treat mental illness. John Wesley, the 18th-century reformer and author of a popular book of home remedies, claimed that a mix of vinegar and ground-ivy leaves, rubbed on the head several times a day, would cure "lunacy." Failing that, he recommended drinking two tablespoons of distilled white vinegar daily.

On the frontier, doctors tried to flush out intestinal worms by applying a poultice of tobacco leaves and vinegar to the

stomach, with uncertain results. (A diluted vinegar-and-water enema, however, is said to expel threadworms.) For painful corns, doctors advised taping a piece of mashed bread—soaked in vinegar for half an hour—over the corn overnight; this softened the skin so that the corn could be peeled away.

For Skin and Hair

Vinegar was also applied to itches or stings caused by mosquito bites, diaper rash, prickly heat, or poison ivy. Hawaiians rubbed it on wounds caused by stingray and jellyfish. Indeed, two cups of vinegar added to bathwater will often soothe itchy skin, and some people still dab vinegar on sunburns to cool the skin.

In the days when people washed their hair with harsh, alkaline soap, women would rinse with a cup of vinegar, which loosened the dulling scum left behind, gave the hair a brilliant luster, and tamed

Making Vinegar

Flavored vinegars, prepared by infusing store-bought vinegar with herbs or berries, are easy to make at home. But creating vinegar from scratch is another matter. In order for alcohol to be converted to acetic acid, bacteria from the genus *Acetobacter* must be present. Cultures of these bacteria, known as mother of vinegar, are added to wine or cider to induce fermentation. They are available from many winemaking suppliers. Once you make your first batch of vinegar, some of the liquid may then be used as a culture or "mother" for your next batch.

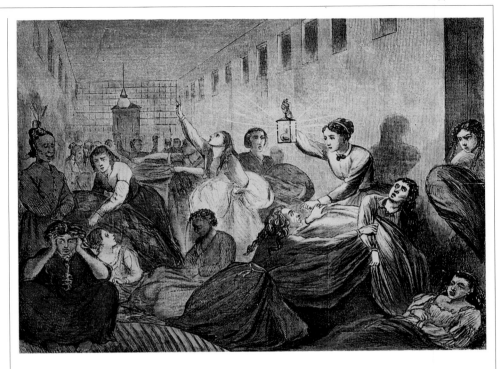

Vinegar's powers, thought John Wesley, extended to quieting the terrors of lunacy—evidence of the misunderstood nature of mental illness in early days. This 1868 engraving depicts a night scene at an asylum on Blackwell's Island, New York.

unmanageable hair. Blondes, however, were advised to stick with lemon juice, which accomplished much the same thing without darkening the hair, as vinegar may do. (Note: Because today's shampoos are usually pH-balanced, a vinegar rinse is rarely necessary.)

"Ill Humors" Fighter

Perhaps because of its acrid smell, vinegar was considered good against "ill humors" in the air, which were thought to cause disease. It was sometimes sprayed in sickrooms or on the pillows of patients. Vinegar even developed a reputation as a defense against bubonic plague, the fearsome "Black Death" that periodically ravaged Europe. In 1720, the so-called Great Plague hit France, decimating the population of Marseilles and providing rich pickings for a ring of thieves who robbed the homes of the dead and dying. Caught and sentenced to death, the four men supposedly struck a bargain: their lives in exchange for the secret that kept them from contracting the fatal disease.

The recipe they gave became famous as the Vinegar of the Four Thieves, and it was widely accepted by physicians of the time. John Wesley repeated the directions: "Infuse rue, sage, mint, rosemary, wormwood, of each a handful, into two quarts of the sharpest vinegar, over warm embers for eight days: then strain it through a funnel, and add half an ounce camphire dissolved in three ounces of rectified spirits of wine." He suggested washing the loins and face with the mixture and snuffing it up the nose before going outside. "Smell to a sponge dipped therein when you approach infected persons or places," he cautioned. Bubonic plague, however, is not transmitted through the air but through the bite of infected fleas, carried by rats. Unless the aromatic vinegar acted as an insect repellent—a possibility—its value would have been entirely psychological. In later years, there were many variations on the recipe, incorporating several different aromatic herbs; it was used mostly to dispel foul odors in sickrooms and hospital wards.

Preventing Swimmer's Ear

Although many people have sworn by vinegar as a treatment for everything from arthritis and heart problems to cancer, scientists have found very little to back up such claims. One medicinal use that does have the support of most doctors is as a treatment for swimmer's ear, a bothersome infection that can develop when water is trapped in the inner ear. Swimmer's ear makes the ear feel itchy and plugged and may interfere with hearing.

To prevent a waterlogged ear from becoming infected, doctors recommend placing a mixture of half isopropyl alcohol and half white vinegar into the ear with a dropper. To open the ear canal, tilt the head so that the clogged ear is facing upward and pull the ear toward the top of the head and back. Then add the mixture, massaging the outside of the ear. Tilt the head so that the ear is facing downward, allowing the fluid to drain out. The alcohol, a mild antibiotic, will help dry the ear canal, and the vinegar's antifungal properties may help prevent an infection. Note that people with perforated eardrums should avoid this treatment.

WARTS

Perhaps no ailment except the common cold has inspired more folk remedies than warts, no doubt due to their stubborn nature and unseemly appearance. Most of the remedies—such as tying a white string around the wart, then burying the string in a hole in the ground—stemmed more from magic than from science. Nonetheless, because of the power of suggestion, they may have worked as well as or better than anything modern medicine has to offer.

Raised growths on the skin or mucous membranes, warts are caused by the papilloma virus. The virus enters the skin through a cut or a scratch, then incubates for several months before blossoming. Warts are contagious, but they most often reinfect the same person instead of spreading to someone else. They come in several varieties. Common warts infect the hands, face, knees, or scalp, especially those of young children; they are hard,

grayish, and rough-textured. Flat warts are flat-topped, flesh-colored growths, sometimes itchy; these occur mainly on the wrist, the backs of the hands, and the face. Particularly stubborn are plantar warts, which grow on the soles of the feet. These warts are flat because of the pressure put on them, and they are often very painful. A fourth variety is genital warts, pink cauliflower-like areas that require immediate treatment. In women, warts may infect the cervix and cause a greater risk of cervical cancer. Condoms generally prevent the spread of genital warts.

Modern Wart Weapons

Doctors have several ways to treat warts, but none are perfect. Liquid nitrogen is used to freeze the wart; as the wart thaws, a blister forms, which often lifts the wart off. Alternatively, a blister-producing

liquid may be used. In either case, several treatments may be required. The doctor may apply a corrosive acid in liquid or plaster form or he may remove the wart with a scalpel, electric needle, or laser. Most of these methods leave scars; what's more, even with treatment, there is a 25 percent chance that the wart will grow back. (Fifty percent of warts disappear in 6 to 12 months with no treatment.)

Over-the-counter remedies include plasters that contain salicylic acid, which has a peeling effect. These plasters expose

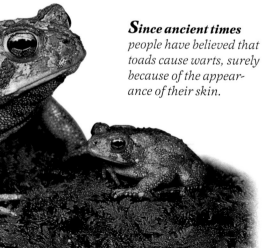

Since ancient times *people have believed that toads cause warts, surely because of the appearance of their skin.*

The Theory of Transference

Because of their belief in the unity of all things, folk healers around the world have long subscribed to the notion that ailments can be transferred from a person to a tree, animal, or object. For instance, one could get rid of warts by counting the growths, then cutting the same number of notches in a stick and burying the stick. A common cure involved cutting a lock of hair from the patient's head and plugging it into a hole bored in a tree.

A toad placed on the head was said to stop a headache when the toad died. People with rheumatism were advised to follow a deserted path in the woods; on reaching the foot of a tree, they were to dig up a root with their left hand and say, "Rheumatism, I leave you here and will take you back when I pass this way again," then bury the root with their left hand—and never go back.

the hidden virus colony, which may then be attacked by the immune system. Herbs that stimulate the immune system, such as echinacea, may also be of use.

An Arsenal of Folk Cures

In the annals of folk medicine, wart remedies could fill a book. People applied castor oil, corrosive lemon or pineapple juice, sheep sorrel, crushed marigold flowers, and milkweed or dandelion sap to the pestiferous growths. They also washed them with the rainwater that pools in old tree stumps. Today some people suggest squeezing the contents of a vitamin E capsule on the wart every night.

Still, the preponderance of folk cures involved more magic than medicine. It was widely believed that a wart would disappear if someone who wasn't a relative spit on it. There were also countless ways to "transfer" the wart to another person, an animal, or an object. For instance, one could draw blood from the wart, place the blood on a grain of corn, then feed the grain to a chicken. Or one could count the warts, tie that many knots in a string, then tie the string to the end of a downspout, where rainwater would flow over it; the warts would disappear when the knots rotted. A wart could also be rubbed with a rock that was then placed in a box; whoever opened the box would get the wart. Warts could even be "sold" for a penny to a "wart charmer." Other cures involved rubbing sliced potatoes, raw meat, or a dirty dishrag on the wart, then burying or hiding the item—preferably in secrecy.

As far-fetched as these remedies seem, so many success stories have been documented that some doctors now believe that the body may indeed be able to rid itself of warts through the power of hypnotic suggestion; in fact, this has been confirmed by at least one study. And doctors have seen it for themselves. One physician who had been unsuccessful in treating a man with warts all over his body put the patient in an X-ray room and explained that he was going to bombard him with powerful radiation. Although the man was in fact given no radiation at all, his warts fell off the next day.

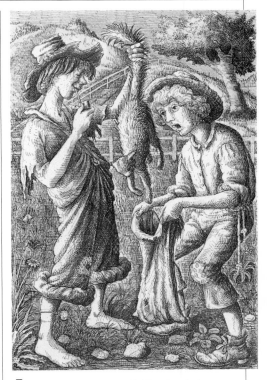

In **Tom Sawyer,** *Huck Finn's advice for curing warts was to leave a dead cat in the cemetery at midnight.*

CELANDINE The sap of this plant has been shown to inhibit the growth of the virus that causes warts. Apply the fresh juice from the leaves, stems, and flowers to the wart daily and allow to dry. Handle the fresh plant with caution, and take care to apply the juice only to the wart and not to the skin surrounding it. Internal use of the juice is toxic.

PAPAYA Papain, the enzyme in papaya, is a popular meat tenderizer and may be used against warts because it digests dead tissue. Make shallow cuts on the surface of the unripe green fruit, collect the sap that runs out, and let it coagulate. Mix with water to make a slurry, then apply morning and night. Papain is available as a powder; add enough water to form a paste and apply. (Protect the surrounding skin with petroleum jelly or talcum powder.) Do not use the sap or powder internally. Papain can be a severe skin irritant.

WHITE CEDAR LEAF Available as a tincture, the oil distilled from the leaves and twigs of the white cedar (*Thuja occidentalis*) is a popular wart treatment in Europe. Antiviral activity has been demonstrated in laboratory tests. (It is said to work better against small warts.) Paint the tincture on the wart morning and night. Because of its high thujone content, white cedar oil is toxic and should not be ingested.

GARLIC Because of its general antiviral activity, garlic is widely reported to cure warts even when other methods have failed. Slice a fresh clove and place it on the wart. Bind it with gauze and allow it to sit for as long as possible; do this morning and night. Garlic is especially useful against warts on the hand.

TEA TREE The oil of tea tree (*Melaleuca alternifolia*) may be useful against warts. It is available as an oil or a cream. Apply morning and night. Skin irritation may occur in some people.

WHITE CLOVER

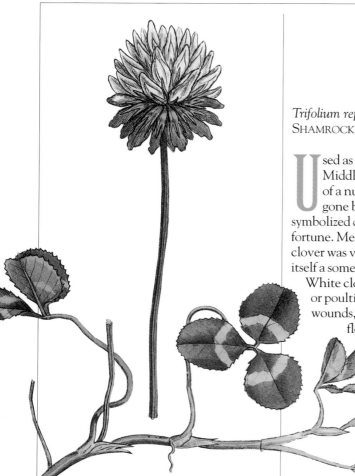

Trifolium repens
SHAMROCK, DUTCH CLOVER

Used as a charm against evil in the Middle Ages, white clover—one of a number of plants that have gone by the name shamrock—also symbolized domestic harmony and good fortune. Medicinally, however, white clover was valued less than red clover—itself a somewhat weak plant remedy. White clover was applied as a wash or poultice to clean skin ulcers and wounds, and extracts of the leaves and flowers were taken as teas or tinctures to purify the blood. Indians drank the tea for cold symptoms, rheumatism, gout, and vaginal discharge. Early settlers used white clover as a tonic for venereal disease and in enemas to relieve abdominal pain.

Sweet Cousins

Clovers of another genus, *Melilotus*, include white sweet clover (*Melilotus alba*). It has long been grown as forage crops in North America but has also been employed medicinally. In the 1920s cows

The True Shamrock?

According to legend, the man who would become St. Patrick preached to the pagan natives on the Hill of Tara in County Meath shortly after his arrival in Ireland in A.D. 432. To illustrate the doctrine of the Holy Trinity, he plucked a three-leafed plant from the sod at his feet—the shamrock, later to become Ireland's revered national emblem.

Scholars have long speculated about the identity of the plant that St. Patrick made famous. In the course of time, contenders for "true shamrock" status were narrowed to white clover and the yellow-flowered small hop clover (*Trifolium procumbens*). Today it is believed that the latter is St. Patrick's plant—a theory based on doubt about white clover's native origin and the fact that the small hop clover is known to colonize rocky soil, much like that of the Hill of Tara.

feeding on spoiled white sweet clover silage began hemorrhaging—the result of ingesting coumarin, a substance also found in white and red clovers. This eventually led to the discovery of the anticoagulant called dicoumarol, created after the clover is cut and then incubated in storage. From dicoumarol was synthesized warfarin, now a very popular anticoagulant drug on the market.

Active plant parts Flowers, leaves
Uses Skin ulcers; tonic
Cautions Large doses may affect normal levels of estrogens, or female hormones, due to the plant's isoflavones. Pregnant women and nursing mothers should avoid the herb.

WILD CHERRY

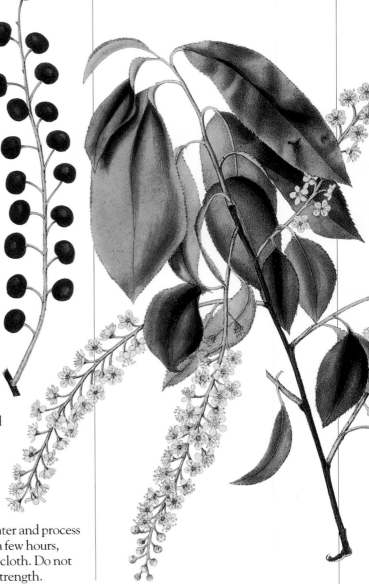

Prunus serotina
WILD BLACK CHERRY, RUM CHERRY

The cherry flavor of many of today's cough syrups and lozenges has its origin in a centuries-old folk cure. When Indians had a cough or a lung ailment, they made a tea from the bark of the wild cherry tree and drank it to loosen phlegm. Early settlers followed suit, treating bronchitis and whooping cough with the bark of either the wild cherry or the chokecherry *(Prunus virginiana)*. The bark was steeped in boiled water and the liquid was strained and sweetened with honey. Other ingredients might be added, including onions to promote coughing and loosen congestion, and whiskey to ease the pain of sore throats.

The Mesquakie used the root bark to make a sedative tea, and the Cherokee gave it to women during childbirth to dull labor pain. Other tribes used it for intestinal complaints. During the Lewis and Clark expedition, Captain Meriwether Lewis attested that when he was stricken with abdominal cramps and fever, he dosed himself with chokecherry bark tea and recovered by the next day.

Patent Medicine Favorite

In the 19th century wild cherry bark became one of the most popular botanical medicines in North America, and was found in many patent medicines. It was sold until the 1940s in over-the-counter cough syrups; although both the tree and the root bark were used, the root bark was considered more potent. The bark contains the glycoside prunasin, which is broken down by the enzyme prunase into two substances: hydrocyanic acid, which is related to the poison cyanide, and benzaldehyde. Hydrocyanic acid appears to have a slightly sedating effect, and benzaldehyde loosens phlegm.

Today pharmacologists credit wild cherry with only mild expectorant activity. It is, however, still commonly used as a flavoring agent in medicine. A cup of wild cherry bark tea can also be drunk for digestive complaints. Bark gathered in the fall is said to be the most potent, but it should not be stored for more than a year. Young, thin branch bark is preferred. Add 1 tablespoon finely chopped bark to 2 cups water and process in a blender; let stand for a few hours, then filter through cheesecloth. Do not boil; doing so lessens the strength.

Active plant parts Tree bark, root bark
Uses Coughs, respiratory illnesses, digestive disorders
Cautions Wild cherry bark should not be consumed by pregnant women or children under age two. Because hydrocyanic acid is toxic in large doses, others should limit consumption of wild cherry bark tea to three cups a day.

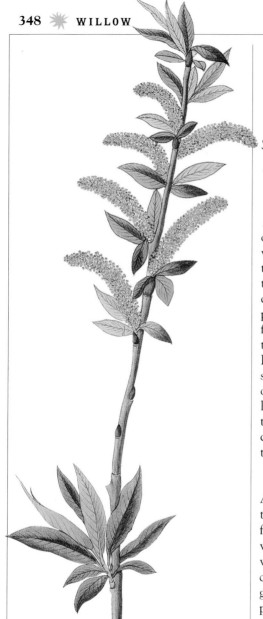

WILLOW

Salix spp.

Many of the medicinal plants of North America were unknown to European settlers, who eagerly learned from the Indians which ones were useful. Willow, however, was valued in the healing traditions of both the Old and the New World for its ability to reduce fevers and ease pain. The 1st-century Greek physician Dioscorides praised the plant's effectiveness against fevers, while North American Indian tribes from the Atlantic Coast to the Pacific made frequent use of native species. The Paiute and Shoshone tribes of the Great Basin used the sandbar willow as a laxative, and the Chickasaw of the South boiled black willow root with cottonwood to treat dysentery—a remedy that was soon adopted by white settlers.

Fever and Pain Treatment

Almost every native tribe used a decoction of willow bark, leaves, or root to treat fevers. However, the species of choice varied greatly—the scores of willow varieties in North America range from a dwarf Arctic species that hugs the frozen ground to the majestic black willow, perhaps the largest willow in the world, which grows as high as 36.5 m (120 ft).

Why willow is effective against fever and pain is well known. The plant contains a family of chemicals called phenolic glycosides, of which salicin is a member. When these compounds are ingested and metabolized, they form salicylic acid, a drug that blocks pain and lowers fevers.

Salicin was first extracted from the white willow (*Salix alba*) in 1828. Ten years later an Italian professor discovered salicylic acid. In 1899 the German company Bayer produced acetylsalicylic acid, a synthetic version of the chemical that reduced such side effects as stomach irritation. Today this synthetic chemical is sold as aspirin, one of the most successful drugs in the history of medicine.

Despite their commonalities, willow is by no means as effective as aspirin. The bark of white willow, the species most often sold medicinally, contains less than 1 percent salicin; to get an effective dose of salicylic acid would require drinking up to 144 liters of tea—an absurdly large and potentially toxic amount. Chewing the bitter twigs "until your ears ring," an old headache remedy used by the Indians and the pioneers alike, is also dangerous: tinnitus (ringing in the ears) is a sign of salicylic acid poisoning.

Nonetheless, because of willow's similarity to aspirin, the same cautions apply. Aspirin can cause Reye's syndrome (a potentially fatal condition) in a child with a cold, the flu, or chicken pox. Willow should not be given to a child with these illnesses or any child under two years of age. Also, willow's safety during pregnancy has not been established.

Active plant parts Leaves, bark, roots
Uses Mild fevers, inflammation, general aches and pains
Cautions Avoid willow if you are sensitive to aspirin or have peptic ulcers, gout, asthma, diabetes, hemophilia, or kidney or liver disease. Avoid taking with other salicylate drugs, including aspirin. Do not give to children suffering from a cold, the flu, or chicken pox.

WINTERGREEN

Gaultheria procumbens
TEABERRY, CANADA TEA, GROUND
HOLLY, GAULTHERIA OIL

Near the end of the last ice age, great mastodons stalked the bogs of the northern United States and Canada. Scientists believe that the beasts perished because of the changing climate. But in the mythology of the Lenape Indians of the mid-Atlantic, the mastodons were killed in a great battle with animals that resented their destructive ways. Drops of mastodon blood scattered across the bogs were turned into the red berries of wintergreen—a beacon for the Lenape and other tribes, who used the aromatic evergreen to relieve the aches and pains of daily life.

A Powerful Scent

Wintergreen is a low-growing plant that bears glossy green leaves with a particularly heady scent. Like willow bark, it contains a pain reliever related to aspirin—methyl salicylate, which is toxic if taken internally but which eases aches when applied topically. The natural oils of wintergreen and the chemically-similar sweet birch oil are used in tiny amounts as a flavoring for everything from toothpaste to root beer, while the synthetic oil of either is a component of commercial liniments and ointments for muscle pain.

The Indians enjoyed wintergreen tea, which they introduced to the settlers. During pioneer days, the brew served American patriots as a substitute for the heavily taxed Oriental tea. Medicinally, the leaves were used in poultices to treat rheumatism and muscle aches.

Use With Care

Wintergreen oil, although once used internally, is extremely toxic; as little as 2.6 milliliters can be fatal. Excessive topical use can be dangerous, too, because the oil is easily absorbed through the skin, especially after vigorous exercise or when used in conjunction with a heating pad. Nausea, vomiting, and ringing in the ears are signs of salicylate poisoning.

Not to be confused with ...

Several species of low-growing evergreen plants are sometimes called by the name wintergreen. Partridgeberry (*Mitchella repens*) has pairs of tiny, glossy leaves and red berries. Pipsissewa (*Chimaphila umbellata*) and spotted wintergreen (*C. maculata*) have flat, waxy white flowers. One-flowered pyrola (*Moneses uniflora*), also called one-flowered wintergreen, bears a rosette of tiny leaves and one waxy white flower.

Active plant parts Leaves
Uses Aches and pains
Cautions Wintergreen oil is highly toxic and should not be taken internally. Use caution even when using the oil externally because it can be absorbed through the skin; fatalities resulting from external use have been reported. Rubs or poultices of the crushed leaves are safe if used no more than once or twice a day for short periods.

WITCH HAZEL

Hamamelis virginiana
HAMAMELIS, WINTER BLOOM

In 1744 New York physician Cadwallader Colden wrote to a friend about witch hazel: "I shall tell you what I learn'd of the use of the Hamamelis from a Minister of the Church of England who officiates among the Mohawk Indians. He saw allmost total blindness occasioned by a blow cur'd by receiving a Warm Stream of a Decoction of the Bark of this Shrub ... I have since experienc'd the benefit of it used in the same manner in an Inflammation of the eye from a blow."

For centuries, witch hazel has been prized for its medicinal properties—a reputation that went far beyond the treatment of black eyes. Popular among many eastern North American Indian tribes, the leaves and bark of this native shrub were made into a tea to cure various maladies, mashed into a poultice to reduce inflammation or control the bleeding of skin sores, or applied as a liniment to soothe aching joints and muscles. The Iroquois drank a bitter witch hazel tea, sweetening it with maple sugar, to treat diarrhea; farther south, the Cherokee concocted a mixture of witch hazel bark, Virginia pine needles, and leaves of spicebush (*Lindera benzoin*) to fight colds and fevers. As time passed, European settlers learned about the powers of witch hazel from Indian healers. An early pioneer folk treatment for sores called for a poultice made from a handful of witch hazel bark steeped in a half-liter of water, then mixed with wheat bran.

The name witch hazel refers not to Indian or even Anglo-Saxon witchcraft but to the Old English word *wych*, which meant "pliable"—a reference to the plant's supple limbs, which were used by North American Indians to make bows. Still, witch hazel does boast a supernatural association: its bendable branches remain a favorite with dowsers, who claim to be able to find underground sources of water by using a forked branch of wood.

"Witch Hazel Water"

In autumn, when other deciduous trees and shrubs are shutting down for winter, witch hazel's bare branches erupt in squiggly, scented yellow flowers. Yet it is the plant's bark and leaves, which contain relatively high proportions of naturally astringent tannins as well as an equally aromatic volatile oil, that are the source of its medicinal properties.

Originally, witch hazel was used medically in the form of a strong decoction. But in the mid-19th century North Americans began producing commercial

Active plant parts Leaves, bark, twigs
Uses Skin rashes and sores, hemorrhoids, diarrhea
Cautions Because of the plant's high tannin content, do not ingest witch hazel tea or extracts in large doses; do not take internally for more than a two-day period. Excessive internal use may cause stomach irritation and, in rare cases, liver damage.

Straight from the Garden

Cultivating witch hazel and preparing your own nondistilled product puts you in touch with a time when self-sufficiency was a way of life. Keep a bottle of homemade witch hazel in the medicine cabinet and use it to soothe skin irritations, cuts, and scrapes more effectively than distilled witch hazel products do.

To start, buy *Hamamelis virginiana* seedlings at a nursery or garden center. The plants can also be grown from seed, but germination usually does not occur until the second spring after sowing. In either case, choose a spot in well-drained, humus-rich, slightly acid soil that receives full sun or partial shade.

Leaves and bark can be harvested after the plant grows 91 cm (3 ft) tall. Cut the leaves at the stem base, then rinse. To harvest bark, lop off a branch and scrape off the bark. To dry, place the plant material on paper towel-lined trays, then store it in a dark place at 20 to 30°C (70 to 90° F) for a week or so.

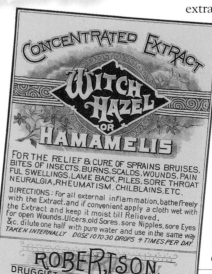

Although lovely, *witch hazel blooms possess none of the powers of the leaves and bark.*

There are many ways to prepare witch hazel for use against skin rashes and other external complaints (see recipes on pp. 47, 65, 93, and 304). One method is to use a blender to process the dried leaves and bark. After processing, combine with water, using 1 tablespoon plant matter for each cup of water. Pour into a saucepan, bring to a boil, and simmer for 20 minutes; remove from heat, then steep for 2 hours. Strain through cheesecloth into sterilized jars and store in the refrigerator.

Nevertheless, to this day witch hazel water remains one of the most popular over-the-counter remedies on the market. It is used to treat insect bites, itching, rashes, acne, sprains, bruises, headaches (when rubbed on the temples), and arthritis. It is also an ingredient in many cosmetics, skin lotions, and shaving creams. Perhaps its most common use is as a hemorrhoid treatment; some commercial hemorrhoid pads contain up to 50 percent witch hazel water.

Drinkable Tea?

The internal use of witch hazel is less common than it once was. Its high tannic acid content (up to 10 percent) can lead to stomach irritation, nausea, and constipation. Witch hazel has also been linked, in rare cases, to liver damage when taken in large doses. Still, a witch hazel tea made from the leaves and bark is generally regarded as safe when taken in proper doses and for brief periods. Avoid drinking more than three cups a day and do not take for more than two days at a time. (This also applies to tea made with commercial witch hazel tea bags.) Liquid extracts containing 45 percent alcohol can be taken after being diluted in water.

As for distilled witch hazel products made for external use, they may be used topically as often as needed with no ill effects—but should never be ingested.

Many purveyors *of witch hazel products referred to the plant as hamamelis.*

witch hazel products, using steam distillation. The result was so-called witch hazel water—the product found on drugstore shelves today. Herein lies an irony almost unparalleled in the annals of medical merchandising: steam distillation removes almost all the plant's tannins, which account for its astringency. In fact, it is witch hazel water's 14-percent alcohol base that provides its astringent action. (Some experts have pointed out that red wine would make a more effective astringent, given that it contains not only the same amount of alcohol but tannins, too.)

Doctors began questioning the value of distilled witch hazel water as early as the turn of the 20th century. According to *The Dispensatory of the United States of America* in 1947, "Hamamelis is so nearly destitute of medicinal virtues that it scarcely deserves official recognition."

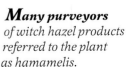

WORMS

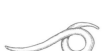 

Few thoughts are as unsettling as that of worms living inside the human body—for days, months, or years—without telltale symptoms. Worms affect about 10 percent of the North American population (mostly children) at any one time, but countless others host the parasites unknowingly. Worldwide, the incidence of worms is more common, particularly in developing countries.

Folk treatments were plentiful, ranging from natural anthelmintics (medicines that expel worms) and laxatives to magical chants. In general, modern drugs have made traditional remedies obsolete, in part because many folk cures are now considered ineffective or toxic.

Uninvited Guests

Parasitic worms most commonly enter the body in one of two ways. First, eating infested, undercooked meat (especially pork) can carry worms or their eggs directly into the digestive tract. Second, eating with fingers that carry microscopic worm eggs picked up from contaminated soil or water—most often in areas with poor sanitation—will also cause an infestation. Worms can be particularly upsetting and cause physical distress, but most cases can be taken care of with modern anthelmintic drugs, among them mebendazole, pyrantel, and thiabendazole.

Roundworms, one of two classifications of worms, resemble small earthworms and include the pinworm and the hookworm. Pinworms, which often affect children, are the most common intestinal worm in the U.S. and Canada. They typically cause anal itching at night, when the female worm emerges from the anus to lay her eggs. The eggs can then be spread via toilet seats, bedding, and clothing.

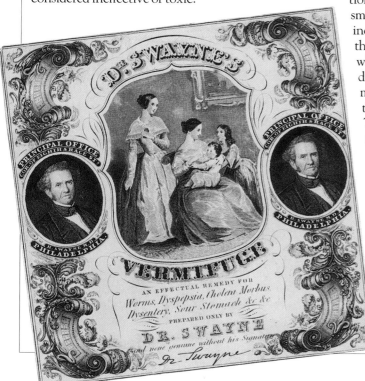

The laxative effect of many worm remedies, like this one from 1840, was also helpful in treating indigestion.

Hookworms are the most common parasitic worms worldwide, but they are rare in North America, with the exception of the rural American South. They enter the body directly through the skin (usually, bare feet) and settle in the small intestine, where they can cause abdominal pain and iron-deficiency anemia. Other roundworms are ascarids, whipworms, and trichinae.

The second classification of worms is the flat-bodied platyhelminth, which includes tapeworms and liver flukes. Tapeworms, which are most common in developing countries, are perhaps the most notorious type of parasitic worm. Ingested as larvae (in undercooked meat), tapeworms mature in the intestines and may grow to 9 m (30 ft) or more. They are able to grow so long when no symptoms are felt. Still, tapeworms can cause abdominal pain, diarrhea, and anemia.

Natural Expellers

Natural anthelmintics and vermifuges were often combined with laxatives to paralyze and remove worms from the digestive tract. In Canada, the T. Eaton Co.'s catalogue sold worm bonbons and powders for many years. Such remedies are now considered either too mild or too toxic in comparison to modern drugs.

Of the milder remedies, the fruits and leaves of papaya (*Carica papaya*) and pumpkin seeds were ingested to treat worms. Papaya contains papain, which is safe and potentially effective against mild infestations in children. The seeds of the pumpkin (*Cucurbita pepo*) were boiled to make a tea, ground up into a porridge, roasted, or eaten raw to treat worms in livestock and humans. Some people even ate the seeds every day to prevent worms. Although pumpkin's active principle, cucurbitin, varies in concentration from seed to seed, it has shown the ability to paralyze and expel intestinal worms. In fact, extracts of the seed have been patented for use as an anthelmintic.

A study in which garlic decoctions were used as enemas to treat pinworms in children showed promising results. Folk healers advised eating garlic raw, drunk in a tea, and worn around the neck to stop the worms from "coming up the throat."

Ineffective folk remedies included drinking cabbage juice or tea made from thyme leaves. Traditional remedies that are now considered too harsh include chinaberry, male fern, and wormseed.

Teases and Chants

Folklore perpetuated misconceptions about worms. Symptoms were thought to include paleness, bad breath, teeth grinding, and nose picking. The parasites were thought to steal food from the digestive tract; thus, fasting was encouraged to "starve" worms. (In fact, worms live off the host's blood.) Worms were also said to get hungry, so some people tried to lure them out through the nose by holding raw meat or warm milk in front of the face.

When children were affected, sweets were recommended after fasting in order to "trick" the worm: the candy would tease the worm away from where it had attached, making it susceptible to expulsion in a quick, laxative-induced bowel movement. Some healers advocated Epsom salts rather than sweets.

Worms caused folk healers to resort to other unusual remedies. A bag of dried tansy worn around the neck was thought to keep worms from choking the victim. Some even tried incantations, like this one used by the Cajun *traiteurs* of Louisiana: "Worm of the heart ... I conjure you in the name of God of Jesus Christ and by the force of tears."

What's in a Name? "Worm" Plants

A few plants that were used to treat worms acquired telltale nicknames: wormseed, wormwood, wormifuge, and worm grass. Wormseed (*Chenopodium ambrosioides*) is the source of chenopodium oil, which became so popular in the 19th century as a remedy against worms that the plant was cultivated to satisfy the needs of the pharmaceutical industry. In the American South, it was grown by slaves who, because they often went barefoot, were prone to hookworms. Because of the oil's debilitating toxicity, using it often necessitated bed rest. Although studies have shown the oil to be effective, it can cause dizziness, nausea, paralysis, and death. It should not be used in home remedies.

Teas made from two species of Artemisia, wormwood (*A. absinthium*) and sweet wormwood (*A. annua*), were taken to expel worms, but their alleged anthelmintic action has not been proven. Wormwood extract was also the main ingredient of absinthe, a green liqueur that was stylish into the early 20th century. Absinthe, now outlawed, produced a toxic high that could cause hallucinations, psychosis, and brain damage.

In the late 1800s, worm grass (*Spigelia* spp.), also known as pinkroot, was nearly harvested to extinction, and cultivating the toxic plant brought significant income to the Creek and Cherokee Indians.

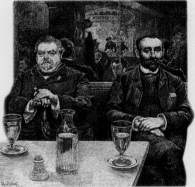

Absinthe drinkers, *likely on the road to ruin, were depicted in* Harper's *magazine in 1889.*

PUMPKIN SEEDS To paralyze worms, mix the crushed, unpeeled seeds with milk (or water) into a porridge. Eat ½ to 2 cups of the mixture three times a day on an empty stomach. To expel the worms, take a laxative two to three hours later. Cucurbitin, pumpkin's active principle, varies from plant to plant, so dosages cannot be precise.

CARROTS Children should eat 1 to 2 carrots or drink 1 cup fresh carrot juice a day for two days. Repeat two weeks later. Carrots are toxic to threadworms; in the past, a child would be fed only carrots until the worms were gone.

ELECAMPANE Add one part liquid extract to one part 25 percent alcohol solution. Take ½ to 1 teaspoon of the mixture three times a day for five days. In the United States, alantolactone (the active principle of elecampane) is sold in tablet form. However, the use of alantolactone tablets is not advisable during pregnancy or lactation. Prolonged use of the tablets is also not recommended; use may be allergenic or hypotensive.

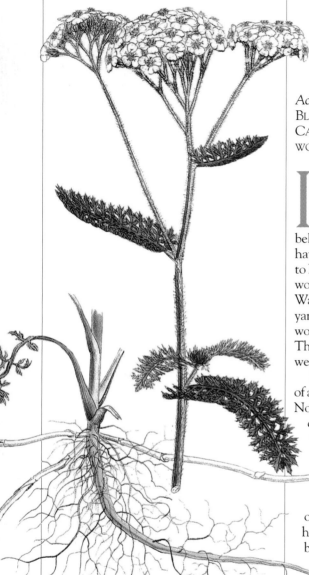

YARROW

Achillea millefolium
BLOODWORT, MILFOIL, THOUSAND-LEAF, CARPENTER WEED, SOLDIER'S WOUND-WORT, NOSEBLEED, SQUAW-WEED

It is not hard to divine, given yarrow's nicknames—"bloodwort," "soldier's woundwort," and "nosebleed"—what the herb was used for. The plant belongs to the genus *Achillea*, which may have been named for Achilles, who is said to have employed yarrow to stanch the wounds of his soldiers during the Trojan War. Thousands of years later, crushed yarrow leaves were applied to bleeding wounds during the American Civil War. The leaves, inserted into the nostrils, were also a popular remedy for nosebleed.

Botanists once thought that this "plant of a thousand leaves" was brought to North America by British settlers, who considered the herb so valuable that they called it "all-heal." However, most strains of yarrow that grow in North America are indigenous.

Among the Indians, yarrow was one of the most highly valued medicinal herbs. They used the plant to check bleeding and applied leaf poultices to swellings or bathed them with yarrow infusions. They also drank yarrow teas to induce sweating and break fevers, and they made decoctions of the roots to cleanse the kidneys. Indians and settlers alike drank yarrow tea to check excessive menstrual bleeding and to relieve painful periods—hence the nickname squaw-weed. A strong infusion of the leaves was even used as an abortifacient (one reason that yarrow should not be ingested by pregnant women). No doubt because of the plant's astringency, North America's 19th-century Eclectic physicians recommended yarrow to treat hemorrhoids and diarrhea. The herb was also used as a tonic for upset stomach, probably because of its bitter components.

Modern Knowledge

Two chemicals are responsible for yarrow's blood-clotting action: achilletin and achilleine. Another chemical, chamazulene (also found in chamomile), accounts for the plant's anti-inflammatory and pain-relieving action. In animal studies, chamazulene has also been shown to stimulate the flow of bile from the gallbladder, which helps to protect the liver from damage by toxic chemicals.

Yarrow also contains tannins, terpineol and cineol, which explain its traditional use as an antiseptic. Note, however, that there are many varieties of yarrow, and their chemical constituents vary. For example, chamazulene is not found in the yarrow variety most common in Europe.

Yarrow is also useful in the garden. It is a potent insect repellent and is believed by some gardeners to boost the amount of aromatic oils in vegetables planted nearby.

Active plant parts Leaves, flowers
Uses Wounds, bruises
Cautions Because yarrow's active principles vary from variety to variety, reaction to the plant is difficult to predict. Discontinue use if you experience skin irritation or cramping. Pregnant women should not ingest yarrow.

YOGURT

Although it is nothing more than curdled milk, yogurt is considered a wonder food today. It originated in the Mediterranean and Indo-Himalayan cultures as a means of preserving milk and has long been used as both a culinary staple and a folk remedy. Early North Americans had their own versions: those from the British Isles made "bonny-clabber," and the Pennsylvania Dutch, their *dicke-millich* ("thick milk").

Beneficial Bacteria

Yogurt is beneficial because of the helpful bacteria it hosts. It is typically made with two active cultures—*Lactobacillus bulgaricus* and *Streptococcus thermophilus*. These bacteria work to transform raw milk sugar, or lactose, into lactic acid, which has both antibacterial and antispasmodic effects on the intestinal tract. Lactic acid is also responsible for giving yogurt its tangy flavor and thick texture. In fact, since the lactose in this dairy product is largely converted to lactic acid, many people who suffer from lactose intolerance can digest yogurt with no ill effects.

Recent studies indicate that *Lactobacillus acidophilus*, a third type of bacteria often added to yogurt, shows promise in countering infection, immune system failure, and perhaps even colon cancer. Although *L. bulgaricus* and *S. thermophilus* do not survive exposure to the digestive juices in the stomach, *L. acidophilus* passes through the digestive tract alive; it is thus a potentially viable agent of healing, as it helps to replenish the balance of the intestinal flora (good bacteria) that are often killed off during illness or prolonged courses of antibiotics. At this time, however, no commercial yogurt possesses a high enough count of live bacteria to make it an effective medicine on its own.

Current evidence points positively to yogurt's preventive, rather than curative, qualities. Many doctors and herbalists advocate yogurt or powdered *L. acidophilus* supplements as preventives. Yogurt is also a valuable source of calcium and phosphorous, as well as vitamin A and several B vitamins. Low-fat and nonfat varieties represent an excellent low-cholesterol substitute for ice cream

Traditional sources of yogurt are the milks of cows, goats, mares, and even buffalo.

A Cure for Yeast Infections

Folk healers have long touted plain yogurt as a vaginal suppository for yeast infections. Lactic acid and *Lactobacillus acidophilus* are thought to combat *Candida albicans*—the fungus known to cause yeast infections. Before you use this home remedy, however, it is important to have a doctor diagnose the infection: bacterial vaginitis will simply worsen in the hospitable yogurt medium, ultimately causing more serious infection and distress.

in the diet. When choosing a brand of yogurt, review the nutritional information on the package to learn about calorie and fat content and about which active cultures have been used. As for frozen yogurt, be aware that its bacteria counts are not regulated; as a result, other than its lower fat content, frozen yogurt offers no measurable benefits over ice cream.

Uses Diarrhea, gastrointestinal disorders, vaginitis
Cautions Despite its low lactose content, dairy yogurt may produce symptoms in some lactose-intolerant people. When choosing yogurt as part of a healthy diet, look for low-fat or nonfat varieties low in sugar. Also check the product label to make sure that the brand contains live active cultures.

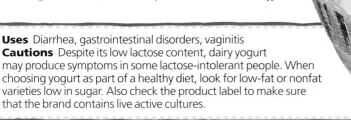

THE HEALING TRADITIONS OF
THE HAWAIIANS

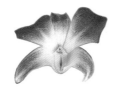 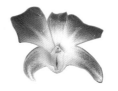

By the time of Christ, Polynesian voyagers had begun the settlement of Hawaii, and they brought with them some two dozen essential plants—species that would provide much of their food and medicine. Once established in their new home, they found that many of the islands' indigenous plants also had healing powers.

The men who discovered how to use the medicinal plants of the islands were the *kahuna lapa'au*—healers better referred to as "doctors" because their profession was every bit as specialized as that of physicians today. Each kahuna learned his art by living with and observing an already established practitioner, following him on his rounds. In this way, the apprentice mastered a vast body of knowledge—about the gods and their dealings with humans, about diseases and how to diagnose them, and about the islands' medicinal plants and minerals.

Causes of Illness

In ancient Hawaii, illness was perceived as either internal or external. Internal illness was believed to arise from wrongdoing within the family, a group so bound together (including even the ancestral spirits, or *'aumakua*) that a misdeed by one member was seen as one committed by all. Such transgressions—not keeping a promise, for example—caused a loss of *mana* (spiritual power) and, in turn, illness. If the patient or

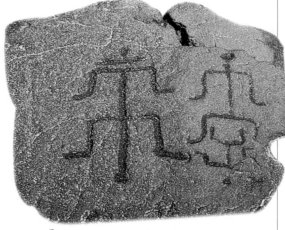

An ancient petroglyph *from the island of Hawaii is thought to depict childbirth. Such rock carvings were the only "written" records left by early Polynesians.*

his family recognized the nature of the problem and took action, internal illness might be cured by acknowledging the wrong and attempting to rectify it.

External illness, on the other hand, was caused by malevolent spirits sent by someone outside the family. In this case, uttering a phrase—perhaps *Ho'ino 'ai kou kahu* ("Go back; eat your keeper")—might send the spirits back to those who had brought them forth. But if the illness had become more serious or there were doubts about its origin and how to deal with it, the family sought the help of a kahuna lapa'au.

Spiritual Diagnosis

After questioning the family, observing various signs, and invoking the guardian 'aumakua, the kahuna diagnosed the patient's spiritual problem. If it was internal but had not been resolved, either the kahuna or a family elder conducted a *ho'oponopono,* a comfortable ritual of exploring relationships within the family; their concerns and grievances were discussed until solutions were agreed upon. By resolving hidden strife within the family and its 'amakua, the ritual alone sometimes cured the ailment.

If evil spirits were sent by someone who had been wronged, the patient could seek forgiveness from the one offended; if the patient acted to set things right, the harmful spirits would be recalled. However, if the spirits were sent for reasons of envy or greed, the patient, his family, and the kahuna would begin the process of returning the attacking spirits to the sender by using prayers, offerings, and rituals. Whatever the source of illness, treatment of the body itself could not proceed until the underlying problem had been identified.

Gifts from the Soil

Different kahunas often used different herbs. Traditionally, medicinal herbs were gathered by the kahuna and his apprentice very early in the morning on the day they were to be prepared. If the medicine was for a man, the first gathering was taken from the right side of the plant; if for a woman, from the left side. In most cases the herbs would be thoroughly pounded, steeped in hot water in a calabash, strained through a fibrous plant bundle, and served in a coconut-shell cup as a warm tea. If the kahuna saw little improvement, there were other medicines that might prove effective, many derived from the plants on this page.

Kukui, or Candlenut Tree (Aleurites moluccana), *today the state tree of Hawaii, produces oil that was burned in stone lamps (kukui means "light") and used to make candles. The meat of the nut was pounded and used medicinally as* 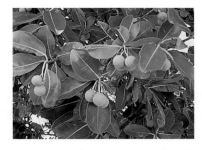 *a purgative; kukua nuts were also compounded with other plants to heal skin ailments, and the crushed leaves were applied to bruised or swollen areas.*

'Olena, or Turmeric (Curcuma domestica), *was prized for its root, which has astringent qualities. Juice extracted by pounding and pressing the root was used to treat ear and sinus problems; topically, the juice was used to stop bleeding. When cooked slightly and eaten, the root was said to ease the discomfort of bronchitis, colds, and asthma.*

'Awa, or Kava (Piper methysticum), *the root of which is pulverized and mixed with water, was an important offering to the 'aumakua and the gods. Medicinally, it was drunk to ease the pain of rheumatism and other disorders. Today it is used mainly to induce relaxation and sleep. 'Awa also provides stimulation and refreshment— but excessive amounts can lead to muscle weakness and photosensitivity.*

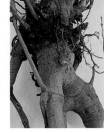

Ki, or Ti (Cordyline terminalis), *was considered sacred to the god Lono. It was thought to be a barrier, and kahunas traditionally draped the leaves around their necks as protection from evil spirits. A feverish patient was covered from the neck down with ki leaves and given hot drinks to initiate sweating. Clammy leaves were then replaced with fresh ones until the fever broke.*

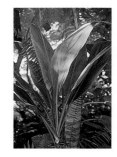

Noni, or Indian Mulberry (Morinda citrifolia), *had a variety of medicinal uses based chiefly on its fruit. The mashed berries were blended with salt and applied on wounds to cleanse and promote healing. The ripe fruit was mashed and put in a poultice to treat boils or infected sores; juice from the ripe fruit was also used to treat such internal conditions as heart disease, high blood pressure, and diabetes.*

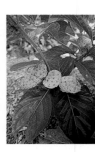

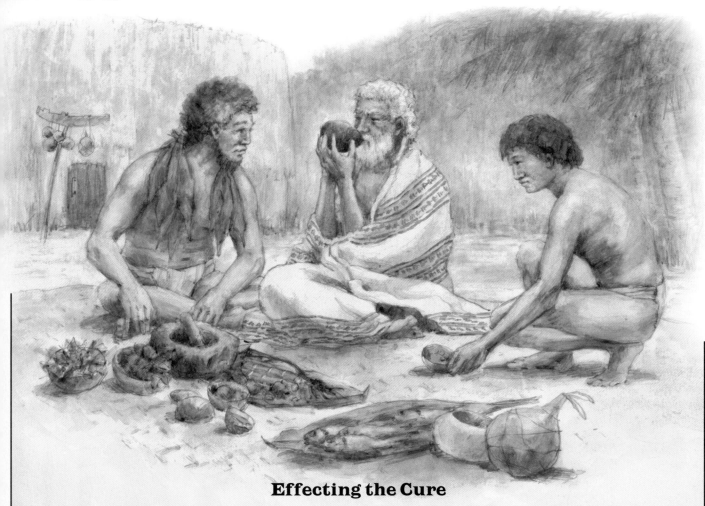

Effecting the Cure

The kahuna and his apprentice used calabashes to collect the water needed for medicines and ritual sprinklings, taking it from special sources. Water from a spring was used in medicines made to treat the childhood disease called 'ea, similar to thrush. For love-related problems, water in the folds of a taro leaf might have been used for a failed love affair or even impotence. Another special source was the sea, its salt water used for its emetic effect.

The family of an elderly man who is suffering from stomach pains has sought the aid of a kahuna lapa'au. Having diagnosed the cause, the kahuna has prescribed various medicines and foods of the same color—in this case, red—to strengthen their effect. As the kahuna watches, the patient takes a dose of medicine while the young apprentice gets ready to hand the healer the iron-rich mineral 'alae, which will be mixed with the patient's poi.

Healing the Body

The kahuna's diagnosis involved questioning the patient and noting his appearance, movements, and body odors. He may also have felt the patient's body, taking stock of skin texture, muscle tension, and irregularities. During the examination, the kahuna frequently consulted guardian spirits—his own and those of his patient's—in prayerful conversation. Then the actual treatment began.

First, "openings" (emetics, enemas, or both) were given to cleanse the system so that the kahuna's medicines would take hold. The purgatives were made from one ingredi-

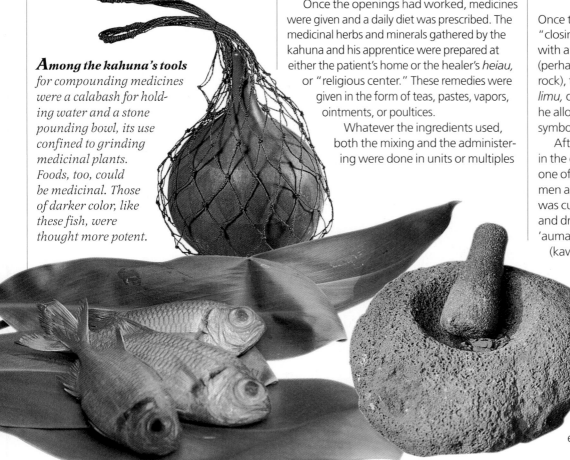

Among the kahuna's tools for compounding medicines were a calabash for holding water and a stone pounding bowl, its use confined to grinding medicinal plants. Foods, too, could be medicinal. Those of darker color, like these fish, were thought more potent.

With the arrival of coded law in 1840, kahunas were formally outlawed. But in the 1860s, the Hawaiian kingdom began issuing licenses to these traditional healers, partly because of the dearth of Western doctors.

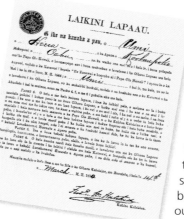

ent or more and were compounded in various formulations, depending on the patient's condition.

Once the openings had worked, medicines were given and a daily diet was prescribed. The medicinal herbs and minerals gathered by the kahuna and his apprentice were prepared at either the patient's home or the healer's *heiau*, or "religious center." These remedies were given in the form of teas, pastes, vapors, ointments, or poultices.

Whatever the ingredients used, both the mixing and the administering were done in units or multiples

of five—5, 10, or 15 pinches of a mineral, pieces of stem or bark, doses per day, or days of treatment. At times, a kind of spiritual "clean-up" might be performed before the medicine was given. One involved dipping ti (or *ki*) leaves in water to which pounded *'oleana,* or turmeric, had been added, then sprinkling it onto the patient's bed or around the inside or outside of his house.

Thanking the Gods

Once the patient was healed, a *pani,* or "closing ceremony," was held. This began with a ritual sea bath. Swimming offshore (perhaps around a tiny island or a standing rock), the patient wore a lei, often made of *limu,* or seaweed. Before returning to shore, he allowed the lei to slip into the water, symbolizing his freedom from illness.

After the swim, the patient's family joined in the closing feast. However, in keeping with one of the strongest of all *kapu* (taboos), the men and women did not eat together. As was customary, the "essence" of the food and drink was shared with the gods and the *'aumakua.* One might dip a finger into *'awa* (kava), for example, then flick the liquid over the shoulder as an offering. The color and names of various foods and drinks once had symbolic meanings, but most of these have been lost to time.

When the feast was finished and the celebrants took their leave of one another, a fitting proverb was likely to be heard: *I ola no ke kino i ka ma'ona o ka 'opu:* "The health of the body is enjoyed when the stomach is full."

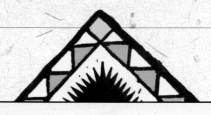

ADDENDUM

✳ 52 More Herbs ✳
You Should Know About

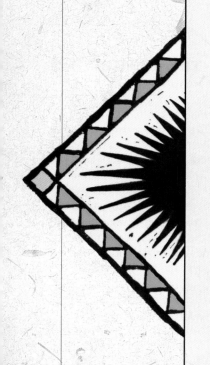

Used in conjunction with the A to Z section of this book, the information on the next 13 pages will help you make sense of the dizzying array of herbal products now found not only in health-food and natural-products stores but even drugstores and discount marts. Many of these botanicals, including ginkgo and tea tree, are newcomers to North American folk medicine, reflecting a new interest in healing traditions from other parts of the world. Others, such as gentian root, agrimony, and pipsissewa, were once popular on these shores; although used less often today, they are still to be found.

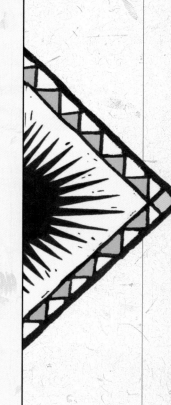

AGRIMONY
Agrimonia eupatoria

Active plant parts Leaves, flowers, root
Uses Intestinal problems, skin rashes, sore throat; anticoagulant
Cautions Consult your doctor before using agrimony. Do not treat conditions you suspect might be serious with this herb. Agrimony may cause photodermatitis after exposure to sun, and high doses may interfere with anticoagulant and blood-pressure medications.

Because of agrimony's throat-soothing properties, bottles of the herb's diluted extract are often found in dressing rooms of singers and speakers, to be used as a gargle before taking the stage. The herb is widely used in Europe as a mild astringent (both externally and internally), particularly against inflammation of the throat, gastroenteritis, and intestinal catarrh. The plant's tannins provide astringent and anti-inflammatory effects, which help remedy diarrhea and, when used topically, stop bleeding. The herb is used in compresses to treat skin rashes and is added to various bath preparations. In North America it is most often sold as a liquid extract.

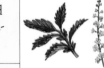

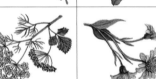

ANISE
Pimpinella anisum

Active plant parts Seeds
Uses Colic, gas, indigestion; expectorant
Cautions Anise is generally regarded as safe, but the anethole chemical in the oil may cause dermatitis in some people.

While lifting their glasses in a toast, world-travelers have probably enjoyed sweet anise without being aware of it: such beverages as Greek *ouzo* and French *pastis* are flavored with the herb. The licorice-flavored oil of anise also accounts for the flavor of many candies sold as licorice. The Romans served anise-flavored *mustaceum* cakes—ancestors of the traditional wedding cake—to help digest their copious feasts. Today the same indigestion-fighting benefits can be obtained from drinking a cup of tea made with diluted anise oil or the ground seeds, called aniseed. The oil of anise has been used traditionally as a carminative and is still found in some cough and cold remedies. Anise should not be confused with Chinese star anise (*Illicium verum*), which is primarily used as a flavoring for foodstuffs.

ALFALFA
Medicago sativa

Active plant parts Leaves, flowers, sprouting seeds
Uses Tonic, nutritional supplement
Cautions Excessive use of alfalfa sprouts, seeds, or extracts may cause unwanted side effects, including reactivation of dormant lupus and interference with blood clotting and diabetes therapies.

A legume, alfalfa was called by the Arabs of the Mediterranean region "the father of all foods," or *al-fasfasah*—hence its name. Indeed, alfalfa has long been touted as an appetite stimulant and diuretic and as a cure for such ailments as diabetes and arthritis. No human studies have been done to validate these claims, but alfalfa does have a rich store of vitamins (A, B_1, B_6, B_{12}, C, E, and K_1) as well as calcium, iron, phosphorus, potassium, and zinc, lending support to its longtime use as a tonic.

Recent animal studies hint that alfalfa may lower cholesterol levels. It is safe when eaten in small quantities, such as alfalfa sprouts in a salad, but excessive ingestion of sprouts, seeds, and alfalfa products should be avoided.

ARNICA
Arnica montana

Active plant parts Flowers
Uses Skin irritations, bruises, sore muscles, sprains
Cautions Internal use is toxic. External use may cause serious allergic reactions in some people. Do not apply to broken skin.

Despite its pretty flowers, arnica is poisonous if ingested. Health Canada has serious concerns about its safety: the aqueous and alcoholic extracts of the plant contain two unidentified substances that can produce violent gastroenteritis, nervous disturbances, change in pulse rate, muscular weakness, collapse, and death. However, topical application of diluted arnica tincture or commercial ointments containing no more than 15 percent arnica oil is generally regarded as safe for the treatment of skin irritations, bruises, and sprains. Do not apply to broken skin, and discontinue use if irritation occurs. Arnica has a long history of use, but few studies suggest that it is clinically useful, even when used topically. Still, its slight anti-inflammatory and mild analgesic effects may aid healing.

ASTRAGALUS
Astragalus membranaceus

Active plant parts Roots
Uses Wounds, fatigue, stomach ulcers; immune-system stimulant
Cautions Some North American species of astragalus, called "locoweed," have been known to poison livestock. Do not confuse these with the medicinal Chinese species described here.

Native to China, where it is called *huang qi* for its yellow-centered roots, astragalus has been used for more than two centuries as a stimulant tonic. The Chinese utilize the herb to combat fatigue, enhance the body's resistance to disease, and strengthen *qi*, or one's vital life force. Modern studies have shown that astragalus restores normal immune-system functioning following chemotherapy and radiotherapy. The herb is available as the crude dried root, the processed root (which looks like a tongue depressor), capsules, tablets, tinctures, and extracts. For maximum benefit, herbalists often combine astragalus with foods and other herbs in personalized therapeutic programs for patients.

BARBERRY
Berberis vulgaris

Active plant parts Bark of stem and root
Uses Bacteria-induced diarrhea
Cautions Use only for short-term treatment, except under the advice of a physician. Do not use during pregnancy. Large doses of barberry may have a cathartic effect.

Barberry contains an alkaloid called berberine, which is effective against bacteria-induced diarrhea. Berberine salts, derived from barberry and other plants, were once used as astringents in commercial eyedrops. Note, however, that berberine is toxic in large doses. Because of barberry bark's sour taste, the plant was traditionally used as a bitter tonic and appetite stimulant as well as a treatment for chronic diarrhea and dysentery. Inspired by the Doctrine of Signatures, medieval physicians used the yellow root bark to treat jaundice. Early North Americans took small doses of the bark to treat heartburn, stomach ulcers, and digestive problems, but today the plant is rarely used. Barberry's edible berries are rich in vitamin C.

BILBERRY
Vaccinium myrtillus

Active plant parts Berries, leaves
Uses Diarrhea, varicose veins, mild inflammations of the mouth and throat
Cautions Excessive doses of bilberry extracts are potentially toxic due to the high content of tannic acid. Use the extracts medicinally only in moderation and for no longer than three weeks.

Already popular in Europe, bilberry extract is becoming known in the U.S. and Canada as an antioxidant and is said to help prevent degenerative diseases and signs of aging. (The plant is also called Rocky Mountain blueberry.) The dried berries and leaves, both of which are astringent, have been used to treat diarrhea. Bilberry has also been recommended for treating varicose veins, hemorrhoids, and weak capillaries, as well as gastrointestinal, kidney, and urinary tract disorders, although its efficacy has not been clearly established. Moreover, it should be used only for the short term. British World War II pilots ate bilberry jam to improve their night vision, and the fruit, rich in vitamin A, is still found in some vision-enhancing remedies.

BIRCH
Betula lenta

Active plant parts Bark and twigs
Uses Muscle pain, sprains, arthritis, neuralgia
Cautions Pure birch oil is toxic and should not be ingested. The oil should be applied topically only in diluted form. Because the oil is absorbed through the skin, do not exceed four applications per day and do not use after strenuous exercise or with a heating pad.

The medicinal species of birch is called sweet birch or black birch. Sweet birch, like wintergreen, has a high content of methyl salicylate, a close chemical relative of aspirin. Its oil is so prized as a topical pain reliever (when diluted) that herbalists in Appalachia, where this birch flourishes, nearly wiped out the trees when they went into the business of distilling the oil; only the development of synthetic wintergreen oil stopped the destruction. Pure birch oil is toxic if taken internally. The bark, from which the oil is derived, is astringent and antiseptic. It was used in teas to treat fevers and stomachaches; in poultices to treat wounds; and as a mouthwash. Other birch species do not have the same medicinal properties as sweet birch.

BLOODROOT
Sanguinaria canadensis

Active plant parts Rhizome, roots
Uses Bloodroot is considered unsafe for use in home remedies.
Cautions Bloodroot is poisonous except in very small amounts. Use only under a doctor's supervision. Pregnant women, nursing mothers, and people with glaucoma should avoid the herb under all circumstances.

Probably because of its expectorant, antiseptic, and anesthetic properties, bloodroot was once used to treat fever, rheumatism, sore throat, and burns. However, the alkaloid responsible for these actions, sanguinarine, is toxic; therefore, bloodroot should not be used in home remedies. One of its common names, Indian paint, recalls the Indians' use of the rhizome's red juice as body paint. Early settlers utilized the plant, steeped in vinegar, as a wash for ringworm. Today anesthetic and antimicrobial derivatives of the herb are added to some commercial mouthwashes to control bacteria-induced sulfur buildup in the mouth, a cause of bad breath.

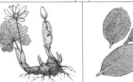

BUCHU
Agathosma spp.

Active plant parts Dried leaves
Uses Mild diuretic and urinary antiseptic
Cautions Avoid buchu if you have a kidney infection, are pregnant, or are breastfeeding.

Long valued as a diuretic and urinary antiseptic, buchu is recommended by herbalists today for treating cystitis (inflammation of the inner lining of the bladder), urethritis (inflammation of the urethra), and inflammation of the prostate gland. Animal studies have documented the plant's anti-inflammatory activity. Two species of the shrub are employed medicinally: *Agathosma betulina* and *A. crenulata*, both native to South Africa and used historically to treat a variety of conditions. In 1847 Helmbold's Compound Extract of Buchu was promoted as a cure for everything from diabetes, kidney stones, and bladder infections to venereal disease. Today buchu is found in herbal diuretics and also in herbal laxative and stomachic preparations.

BUCKTHORN
Rhamnus frangula

Active plant parts Bark, fruit
Uses Constipation, indigestion, skin irritations
Cautions Toxic when fresh, buckthorn is safe to ingest only after it has been properly dried. Use with caution (it is a powerful laxative), and do not take for more than two weeks. Do not use during pregnancy or lactation or if suffering from ulcers, colitis, or hemorrhoids.

Usually called alder buckthorn or frangula bark, this European cousin of cascara sagrada has naturalized in the northeastern U.S. It and other species of *Rhamnus*, including common buckthorn (*R. cathartica*), contain anthraquinone, a chemical that stimulates the colon and has a powerful laxative effect. George Washington reportedly ordered buckthorn juice from England, and an inventory of one pioneer pharmacy indicates that imported buckthorn syrup was a big seller. Today, a related species is included in over-the-counter laxatives. The powdered bark is also available in some herbal products stores; if using the powder to make a tea, combine it with fennel or chamomile to guard against gastrointestinal irritation.

BUTCHER'S BROOM
Ruscus aculeatus

Active plant parts Aerial parts, rhizome
Uses Varicose veins, hemorrhoids, circulatory problems of the legs
Cautions People with high blood pressure should avoid this herb.

Butcher's broom was so named because European butchers used its tough stems and rigid leaves in brooms. The shrub was valued nearly 2,000 years ago as a laxative and diuretic, but otherwise it was little used medicinally until the middle of this century, when scientists discovered that extracts of the rhizome constrict blood vessels. Accordingly, it came to be considered a specific treatment for veins, and today European herbalists use it to treat circulatory problems of the legs. It is also valued in treating varicose veins and, because of its anti-inflammatory properties, hemorrhoids. An evergreen native to the Mediterranean region, butcher's broom should not be confused with common, or Scotch, broom (*Cytisus scoparius*), a yellow-flowered plant that has naturalized in the Pacific Northwest.

CALENDULA
Calendula officinalis

Active plant parts Flowers
Uses Skin conditions, throat and mouth infections, delayed menstruation, stomach ulcers, abdominal cramps
Cautions Avoid during pregnancy. The pollen may be allergenic.

Although little scientific evidence supports calendula's medicinal use, the plant has withstood the test of time. Its daisy-like flowers have been valued for centuries, most commonly as a topical treatment for minor sores, wounds, and first-degree burns. In Germany, calendula is approved as an anti-inflammatory and wound-healing agent, and homemade or commercial calendula ointments can help soothe eczema, bruises, and dry skin; it is also used as an antifungal douche, a sitz bath for hemorrhoids, a gargle for sore throat, and a remedy for stomach disorders. The plant is commonly called pot marigold. The name marigold, which echoes that of the Virgin Mary, is thought to derive from calendula's reputation for healing sore nipples and promoting menstruation.

CAT'S CLAW
Uncaria tomentosa

Active plant parts Inner bark
Uses Arthritis, asthma, stomach ulcers, gastrointestinal disorders; immune-system stimulant
Cautions No side effects have been documented.

Also known as *uña de gato* (Spanish for "cat's claw"), this woody jungle vine grows to 30 m (100 ft) and gets its name from the two sharp, curved thorns at the base of its leaves. Dubbed the "miracle herb from the rain forest of Peru," it purportedly has immunity-boosting, antioxidant, and anti-inflammatory effects. Used historically for arthritis, asthma, irregular menses, and gastrointestinal disorders, the herb is also touted for herpes, chronic fatigue syndrome, and depression. Scientific evidence, however, has yet to support these hyperbolic claims. Cat's claw is also being researched for its potential to fight AIDS, viruses, and the so-called superbacteria that have developed an immunity to antibiotic drugs. To promote its conservation, use the inner bark, not the roots.

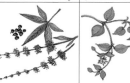

CHASTE TREE
Vitex agnus-castus

Active plant parts Seeds, fruit
Uses Menstrual problems, menopausal symptoms; lactation stimulant
Cautions Use may cause an itchy rash in sensitive individuals. Excessive use may cause a sensation called formication—the feeling that ants or insects are crawling under the skin.

In Europe the fruits of the chaste tree, or chasteberry, have long been used to regulate female hormonal imbalances and promote lactation in nursing mothers. Studies have confirmed that the fruit has a progesteronic effect that helps regulate the menstrual cycle. Today doses of the fruit extract, usually 20 milligrams a day, are taken to reestablish a normal menstrual cycle after going off the Pill, reduce water retention during menstruation, and soothe the discomforts of menopause. For centuries the plant has symbolized chastity. One nickname, monk's pepper, derives from its reputation for diminishing the male sex drive. In monasteries, the seed powder was used as a condiment and the flowers were strewn in the paths of novices.

CHICKWEED
Stellaria media

Active plant parts Leaves, stems
Uses Eczema, psoriasis, dry skin, dermatitis, skin ulcers, boils, splinters, wounds
Cautions No side effects have been documented.

Chickweed's name derives from its use as a barnyard food for domesticated fowl, but some herbalists claim that it is more than mere bird feed. Yet even though it has been used historically to treat colds, coughs, and all sorts of inflammations (both internal and external), chickweed's therapeutic value is largely limited to soothing the skin. The herb was most commonly used in a tea to suppress coughs and in ointments, poultices, and baths to soothe itchy skin inflammations, such as eczema and nettle burn. It is still sold in tea bags and extracts, although it may be easier to find the weed growing in your yard. Even those who discount the plant's benefits can enjoy it: the young shoots, which have long been thought to boost one's strength, make tasty salad greens. Its flowers also put on a good show: they tend to open on sunny days and to close when it rains.

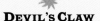

DAMIANA
Turnera diffusa

Active plant parts Leaves
Uses No effective uses have been verified.
Cautions Damiana may irritate the urethral mucous membranes.

In 1874 a druggist in Washington, D.C., began selling a tincture of damiana, a Mexican shrub, for $2 a bottle, claiming that it would enhance "the sexual ability of the enfeebled and aged." Stories of virile elderly Mexican men fathering children accompanied the imported herb. Although the claims made for damiana were soon found to be fraudulent, the herb continued to be marketed into the 20th century in such products as Nyal's Compound Extract of Damiana, the effects of which most likely came from the alcohol, cocaine, and nux vomica (strychnine) used in their preparation. The alleged aphrodisiac or hallucinogenic effects of the leaves, smoked or made into a tea, are unfounded. Likewise, claims of damiana's diuretic and laxative potential have not been verified.

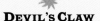

DEVIL'S CLAW
Harpagophytum procumbens

Active plant parts Secondary roots, tuber
Uses Arthritis, loss of appetite, indigestion, skin rashes
Cautions Avoid during pregnancy or if suffering from heart problems or stomach ulcers. Use may lower blood pressure.

Native to Africa, this tuberous perennial—also called grapple plant and wood spider—gets its distinctive common names from the appearance of its gnarled, barbed fruit. Used internally and topically for several ailments, including kidney problems, headache, heartburn, and boils, the tuber of devil's claw was perhaps best employed to soothe sore joints and muscles. Limited European studies have pointed to its potential anti-inflammatory and analgesic effects; the herb may also help reduce blood pressure and levels of uric acid and cholesterol.

Devil's claw is available in many forms: the dried tuber and commercial (but nonstandardized) tablets, capsules, and extracts. In Germany devil's claw products are approved for the treatment of arthritis and indigestion.

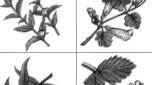

EUCALYPTUS
Eucalyptus globulus

Active plant parts Leaves
Uses Nasal and chest congestion, asthma, sore muscles, minor cuts and abrasions
Cautions Do not ingest pure eucalyptus oil; it is toxic. Internal use should be limited to a few drops of the diluted oil; also dilute the oil for topical use. Do not ingest during pregnancy. Keep the oil away from eyes. Topical use or inhalation may cause an allergic reaction.

Inhaling the steam from a few drops of eucalyptus oil (or a handful of fresh or dried leaves steeped in a liter of hot water) is an effective way to open nasal passages and clear the lungs of phlegm. The oil of this Australian tree is also valued for its counterirritant, antiseptic, antibacterial, and mild insecticidal effects and is used in commercial cough and cold preparations (as a decongestant and expectorant), liniments, and mouthwashes. Eucalyptus was introduced into North America shortly before the American Civil War; groups of trees were often planted as windbreaks and, because the huge roots absorb water so quickly, as a means of draining malarial swampland.

EYEBRIGHT
Euphrasia officinalis

Active plant parts Leaves, flowers, stems
Uses Not suitable for use in home remedies.
Cautions Homemade eyebright preparations present a risk of infection and should not be used on the eyes.

Eyebright has been used since the Middle Ages for treating eye infections and conjunctivitis (pinkeye), no doubt because the tiny plant's white petals, tinged with red, resemble irritated eyes. Lotions and infusions of eyebright were applied to the eyes, and the plant was also taken internally as a treatment for colds, allergies, and nasal congestion. Despite the fact that eyebright is used in Europe and is sold in the U.S. and Canada in capsules, tinctures, and other forms, modern studies reveal no therapeutic value. Moreover, using eyebright as an eyewash in such homemade nonsterile solutions as teas or tinctures poses a risk of infection and is not recommended. According to some botanists, the name *Euphrasia officinalis* is one that encompasses some four different species; the name most often refers to plant material harvested from the species *E. rostkoviana*.

GENTIAN ROOT
Gentiana lutea

Active plant parts Dried root and rhizome
Uses Appetite stimulant, digestive aid
Cautions Large doses of gentian extract may cause headache, nausea, and vomiting. Because gentian may stimulate gastric secretions, people with stomach ulcers should avoid it.

One of the most popular "bitters," this native of the mountains of southern Europe and western Asia is a perennial with orange flowers. Its roots contain highly bitter compounds, notably amarogentin, one of the bitterest known. Because bitters are thought to increase the flow of saliva and stomach secretions, they have long been used as appetite stimulants and digestive aids. Gentian has also been used to relieve stomachache, heartburn, and nausea, and it has been shown to increase the secretion of bile. The herb is sold in the form of the crude root, tinctures, and teas and is an ingredient in herbal digestive formulations. Another species of gentian, *G. acaulis*, is used to make the cocktail flavoring Angostura Bitters.

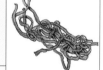

GINKGO
Ginkgo biloba

Active plant parts Leaf
Uses Circulatory problems, frostbite, skin rashes, vertigo, high blood pressure, arteriosclerosis, peripheral vascular disease
Cautions May cause mild stomach upset, restlessness, and allergic skin reactions. Use with caution if taking anticoagulant medication.

In Germany a standardized extract of ginkgo is the leading prescription and over-the-counter medication; millions of Europeans reportedly use it to prevent memory loss and stroke. Studies have shown that the concentrated leaf extract (the only form of ginkgo that has been proven effective) increases blood flow to the brain and lower body parts and combats certain conditions related to aging, including short-term memory loss. The standardized extract is used to treat high blood pressure, arteriosclerosis, phlebitis, and peripheral vascular disease, as well as certain dementias and cognitive disorders. Because it increases blood flow to the ears, the extract is also used to relieve vertigo and tinnitus.

GOLDENROD
Solidago spp.

Active plant parts Aerial parts
Uses Diuretic, anti-inflammatory
Cautions Do not use diuretics to treat cardiac or renal insufficiency.

The genus *Solidago* includes more than 100 species of yellow-flowered herbs. The species *S. virgaurea* is widely used in Europe, primarily as a diuretic to treat inflammation of the urinary tract and to flush out kidney and bladder stones. Probably because of its astringency, goldenrod was also used historically to treat wounds and to aid digestion. Indians chewed the flowers of one North American species, Canadian Goldenrod (*S. canadensis*), to ease sore throats. (This species, along with other goldenrods that bloom in late summer, are often blamed for seasonal allergies, but most reactions at this time of year are caused by the less conspicuous ragweed.) Goldenrod is still used in gargles to treat inflammation of the mouth and throat. The crude herb is available commercially, but goldenrod is rarely seen in capsule or tablet form.

GOTU KOLA
Centella asiatica

Active plant parts Leaves, root
Uses Wounds, skin conditions, varicose veins
Cautions This herb may produce a skin rash. Large doses may have a sedative effect.

Gotu kola, or hydrocotyle, is prized in Asian and African medical traditions for its ability to revitalize the body and the brain. When elephants in Sri Lanka were observed eating the plant, it developed a reputation for promoting longevity. It was also used to improve the functioning of the nervous system and the brain and to treat leprosy. The leaf extract has been shown to accelerate the healing of wounds and to improve circulation. Some studies suggest that it may have a beneficial effect on memory and learning. There is also evidence that the herb, used in India to increase fertility, may in fact reduce it. In North America gotu kola is often touted as promoting brain function, especially memory; as an energizer; and as a remedy for wounds and skin ailments. It also has a reputation as an aphrodisiac. The herb is available in a variety of forms.

HORSETAIL
Equisetum spp.

Active plant parts Dried stems
Uses Mild diuretic
Cautions The species *E. palustre* is toxic and should not be ingested.

Horsetail, sometimes called horsetail rush, is a primitive plant group of some 30 species of jointed, hollow-stemmed herbs. The stems are impregnated with silica. Early settlers and Indians used handfuls of the stems as scouring pads, hence the plant's nickname, scouring rush. The two species used most often in herbal medicine are *Equisetum hyemale* and *E. arvense*. Marketers of the herb must ensure that the plant matter is properly identified. *E. palustre*, which looks similar to *E. arvense*, contains a toxic alkaloid and has been responsible for poisoning among livestock. Horsetail, traditionally considered a mild diuretic, has been used in Germany to treat edema and inflammation of the urinary tract and in a poultice for wounds. However, there is little data to support these uses.

JEWELWEED
Impatiens capensis

Active plant parts Leaves, juice
Uses Traditionally used as a treatment for poison ivy rash
Cautions The safety of internal use has not been established.

Jewelweed is part of a plant group whose members are sometimes called "touch-me-nots" because the seedpods contain spring-like devices that project the seed up to 3 m (10 ft) from the plant when the pods are disturbed. Two common North American species are the orange-flowered *Impatiens capensis* and the yellow-flowered *I. pallida*. Jewelweed often grows in the same moist habitats as poison ivy, and it has been widely used in herbal folk medicine to treat or prevent skin rashes, especially those related to poison ivy. The fresh leaves are rubbed between the hands until the juice is extracted; the juice is then rubbed on the skin to prevent the rash or to help it heal. Jewelweed is an Indian plant remedy of long standing, although research has yet to confirm its efficacy.

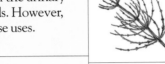

KAVA
Piper methysticum

Active plant parts Dried rhizome and root
Uses Anxiety, insomnia, fatigue
Cautions Excessive use can lead to skin problems, muscle weakness, double vision, and sensitivity to light. Do not take with alcohol.

Imbibed by Pacific Islanders for more than a thousand years, a beverage made from the pulverized root of the kava plant remains an important part of ceremonial and social occasions in Oceania today. The plant's Latin name translates as "intoxicating pepper," a clue to kava's growing—and potentially dangerous—reputation as a "feel good" herb. Used in moderation, kava is a smooth-muscle relaxant, aiding sleep and calming anxiety. It may also produce mild euphoria, but claims that kava offers a "legal high" are exaggerated. Furthermore, overconsumption of the herb can lead to serious side effects. Because of serious concerns about the safety of the herb, Health Canada has not permitted the sale of any therapeutic products containing kava. Pregnant and lactating women are advised to avoid the herb.

KHELLA
Ammi visnaga

Active plant parts Fruits
Uses Asthma, angina, hay fever
Cautions Overconsumption may cause constipation, nausea, appetite loss, headache, itching, insomnia, and photosensitivity.

Khella is a perennial herb native to the Mediterranean region of Europe and North Africa. The dried fruits, which resemble caraway seeds, have been used in folk medicine since ancient times. Made into a tea, they have been employed as a diuretic and to relieve pain caused by urethral stones. In Egypt the stems of the fruiting flower heads are sometimes sold as toothpicks. The plant contains a substance called khellin, which has been shown to relieve bronchial spasms, making it useful against asthma. It also helps prevent hay fever. Khellin may also ease intestinal, renal, and biliary colic. A component known as visnadine has been shown to have coronary vasodilating action, making it useful for preventing angina and coronary arteriosclerosis. Khella is used primarily in Europe and Africa. It is rarely sold in North America.

KOLA NUT
Cola nitida, C. acuminata

Active plant parts Dried seed, commonly called "nut," from which the seed coat has been removed
Uses Headache, asthma, fatigue
Cautions Do not take this substance if you have high blood pressure, a peptic ulcer, or heart palpitations.

"It's the real thing!" goes the Coca-Cola jingle, but the real thing is actually a seed found within the woody pods of a tropical evergreen. With a caffeine content about three times higher than that of coffee beans, the dried seeds were formerly used as a central-nervous-system stimulant and to treat headaches and diarrhea. In Africa the fresh seeds were chewed to promote digestion. Today natural-products suppliers sell it as an ingredient in tablets said to boost energy. The seed extracts are also a caffeine source in weight-loss products. Caffeine is known to increase the effects of such analgesics as aspirin and acetaminophen. Because it opens the bronchial airways, it can also be useful during an asthma attack.

KUDZU
Pueraria lobata

Active plant parts Root
Uses High blood pressure, alcoholism, colds, migraines
Cautions No side effects have been documented.

Residents of the southeastern United States who spend hours trying to eradicate the tenacious kudzu vines from their property may be surprised to learn that the plant is native to China, where it has been recommended for 2,000 years as a remedy for measles, muscle ache (especially stiffness of the neck and shoulders resulting from colds and the flu), and headache and numbness caused by high blood pressure. The plant is also used to treat hangovers, alcoholism, and drunkenness. Studies reported in 1993 found that kudzu may in fact suppress the craving for alcohol. Kudzu has been shown to increase coronary and cerebral blood flow. The root is sold as dried blocks and slices; more rarely, it is sold in formulations for allergies, colds and flu, hangover, and cardiovascular disorders.

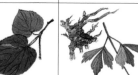

LINDEN
Tilia spp.

Active plant parts Leaves, flowers
Uses Sweat-inducer, sedative
Cautions Excessive use may result in cardiac toxicity.

Several species of linden tree, also known as lime or basswood tree, are used medicinally, including the European *Tilia cordata* and the American *T. americana*. The flowers (and, to a lesser extent, the leaves) have traditionally been made into a tea to promote sweating and "flush out" colds with fever. They have also been used to treat tension headaches, indigestion, diarrhea, and coughs. Components of the flowers and leaves have been shown to have a mild sedative effect. In Europe, where the plant is called lime flower, linden is a common ingredient in herbal preparations marketed for the treatment of colds, chills, fevers, and coughs; it is also used as a food flavoring. In France the flowers, which contain mucilage, are used to make a soothing lotion for itchy skin. The flowers and leaves are found in crude dried form, teas, tinctures, and fluid extract.

LOVAGE
Levisticum officinale

Active plant parts Roots, fruits
Uses Menstrual problems, urinary tract complaints
Cautions May cause sensitivity to sunlight.

Lovage, a member of the carrot family, is native to Europe and grows in many North American herb gardens. The stems have a flavor reminiscent of celery, although much stronger. In China lovage is sometimes called "European dong quai" because both herbs are used to treat women's conditions. In fact, whenever dong quai (*Angelica sinensis*) was in short supply in China, lovage was the substitute. The root is used to induce sweating, bring on menstruation, and ease menstrual pain. In Europe the roots and fruits (also called seeds) are used as aromatic stimulants and as carminatives for treating indigestion, flatulence, and colic. The root contains a component reported to have sedative effects in mice, and the extract is reported to have strong diuretic and antispasmodic activity. The dried roots and fruits are available commercially.

MILK THISTLE
Silybum marianum

Active plant parts Seeds, flower heads
Uses Cirrhosis, hepatitis, jaundice
Cautions Anyone suffering from a liver problem should be under the care of a physician. Milk thistle may have a mild laxative effect.

Milk thistle is best known for its effects on the liver. Silymarin, a substance contained in the seeds, prevents toxins from penetrating the liver and stimulates the regeneration of liver cells. It also increases the production of bile, which breaks down fats. Milk thistle has been used successfully to help treat hepatitis, cirrhosis, and jaundice and to detoxify people suffering from liver damage caused by infection, alcohol poisoning, and poisoning by death-cap mushrooms, whose toxins attack the liver. The herb is found in preparations marketed as liver-cell regenerators and in antioxidant capsules said to purify the system by eliminating toxins. Concentrated seed extracts are the most beneficial; teas are ineffective because the seed's active principles are not water-soluble.

MYRRH
Commiphora molmol

Active plant parts Bark
Uses Inflammations of the mouth and throat, canker sores, bad breath, indigestion, bronchial congestion
Cautions Do not take high doses of myrrh for long periods. Avoid myrrh if you are pregnant or suffer from kidney disease.

Myrrh is a resin derived from small trees that grow near the Red Sea. Highly astringent, it has been valued in Chinese medicine since the seventh century as a styptic for wounds. Because of the resin's astringent, antiseptic, and anti-inflammatory effects, tinctures of myrrh are excellent for use in mouthwashes or gargles for sore throats. Myrrh has also been used against sores, hemorrhoids, arthritis pain, coughs, and indigestion. It is primarily used in tincture form, although it is also available as a powder. Myrrh is found in tinctures and salves sold to relieve mouth and throat irritations, gingivitis, wounds, coughs, colds, and bronchial congestion. It is also an ingredient in various preparations for indigestion and gas.

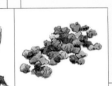

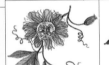

PASSION FLOWER
Passiflora incarnata

Active plant parts Flowers, fruiting tops of vine
Uses Insomnia, nervous tension and headache
Cautions Pregnant women should not take passion flower. Do not confuse with the ornamental blue passion flower, *P. caerulea*, which has toxic components.

Contrary to its name, this is not a substance to take along on a honeymoon. The herb is a calming sedative used to promote relaxation and sleep. The "passion" refers to the crucifixion of Jesus Christ: Jesuit priests in South America believed that they saw religious symbolism in the appearance of the flowers. Modern herbalists recommend the perennial vine's flowers and fruiting tops as a remedy for anxiety and as a mild sedative in cases of emotional upset, as well as for tension headaches, muscle and digestive spasms, and muscle tension caused by anxiety. Especially popular in Europe, passion flower is used in soothing herbal baths and taken dried and crushed in infusions and teas, in tinctures, as capsules or tablets, or combined with other herbs in over-the-counter sleep aids.

PEPPERMINT
Mentha piperita

Active plant parts Leaves
Uses Digestive tract problems, flatulence, bad breath, colic, stomach ulcers, nausea, sore throat
Cautions Peppermint tea may cause a choking sensation in babies.

Unknown to the ancients, peppermint is a hybrid of spearmint (*Mentha spicata*) and water mint (*M. aquatica*). A popular flavoring for toothpaste and candy, it was not cultivated commercially until the mid- to late 18th century. Eventually, it replaced spearmint as the herb of choice for relieving nausea and calming an upset stomach. Studies have shown that peppermint reduces muscle spasms in the digestive tract, especially those associated with irritable bowel syndrome. Research supports the value of enteric-coated peppermint-oil capsules for treating this ailment. Peppermint also has properties that aid the healing of stomach ulcers; it also helps to numb sore throats. Dried peppermint leaf is widely available and is found in teas, capsules, and tablets. Enteric-coated peppermint-oil capsules are available from a few sources in North America.

PERUVIAN BARK
Cinchona pubescens

Active plant parts Bark, root
Uses Fever, sore throat, leg cramps, arthritis, digestive complaints
Cautions Take only under the supervision of a physician. Pregnant women and people with peptic ulcers should not consume Peruvian bark. Excessive use may cause headache, rash, abdominal pain, deafness, and coma.

Those fond of the bitter aperitif Campari are familiar with the taste of Peruvian bark, or cinchona, the source of quinine. First noted by a Jesuit missionary to Peru in 1633, cinchona owes its fame to its antimalarial actions. (As a malaria remedy, it was replaced by synthetic chloroquine during World War I, but it underwent a revival in the 1960s, when the parasite that causes the disease developed a resistance to the synthetic pharmaceutical.) Modern herbalists advise the bark—sold as tablets, powders, and tinctures—for treating fever and arthritis, as an antispasmodic for muscle cramps, in gargles for sore throat, and as a bitter for digestive complaints.

PIPSISSEWA
Chimaphila umbellata

Active plant parts Leaves
Uses Urinary tract infections, kidney problems, rheumatism, gout, blisters and other skin conditions
Cautions No side effects have been documented.

The unusual name of this evergreen plant is derived from the Cree Indian word *pipsiskweu*, which means "it breaks into small pieces," a reference to the effect they thought it to have on kidney stones. Various North American Indian tribes employed pipsissewa to bring down fevers and tone the heart and kidneys. The mildly astringent and antiseptic leaves were used topically to soothe blisters, swellings, muscle aches, and eye irritations. White settlers, particularly in rural areas, took the leaf tea to relieve rheumatism and kidney and bladder problems. Although the tea does not break up kidney stones, its diuretic and antiseptic action can help relieve urinary tract infections, rheumatism, and gout. The bittersweet plant has also been used to flavor root beer.

PRICKLY ASH
Zanthoxylum americanum

Active plant parts Bark
Uses Toothache
Cautions Do not swallow the bark juice; it contains potentially toxic alkaloids. Do not use during pregnancy or lactation or while taking anticoagulant medication.

Prickly ash is represented by two species in North American folk medicine: *Zanthoxylum americanum*, or northern prickly ash, which grows in Quebec, Ontario, and the eastern U.S., and *Zanthoxylum clava-herculis*, or southern prickly ash, which is common in Arkansas and Texas. Both sport the prickly spines on their stems and ash-like leaves that give the plant its name. For medicinal purposes, the two species are considered interchangeable. Although the plant was used to reduce fevers and soothe rashes and joint pain, it was best known for relieving toothaches. Chewing the bark and packing the chewed mass around the aching tooth numbs the mouth and gums. Despite the lack of supporting evidence, it is still used to treat rheumatism. The bark is available in capsules or in a tincture.

PYGEUM
Prunus africana

Active plant parts Bark
Uses Enlarged prostate
Cautions Prostate problems must always be treated by a doctor.

For hundreds, possibly thousands, of years, pygeum has been cultivated in tropical Africa for its hard wood and medicinal bark. In the 1990s, as extracts of the bark became more popular in Europe, the large-scale commercial harvesting of the bark in Cameroon, Kenya, and other African countries came under scrutiny. As a result, the harvest and sale of the bark is regulated by an international treaty to ensure that the plant population does not become threatened. Traditionally used to treat problems of the urinary tract, pygeum is now widely prescribed in Europe to treat the inflammation associated with benign prostatic hyperplasia (BPH), or enlarged prostate. A diuretic and anti-inflammatory, it comes in capsules, tablets, and tinctures (often combined with other herbs). It may be sold as *Prunus africana*, *Pygeum africanum*, African cherry, or African plum.

SENECA ROOT
Polygala senega

Active plant parts Root
Uses Cough, chest congestion
Cautions Use only in limited doses. Taken internally, large amounts may cause stomach upset, vomiting, and diarrhea.

The Seneca Indians used poultices of this plant's yellow root to treat snakebites and promote milk production in cattle. Hence, the plant was also known as senega snakeroot, rattlesnake root, and milkwort. The settlers used the root as a remedy for a variety of ailments, including fever, pleurisy, rheumatism, and gout. In the 19th century, Philadelphia doctor John Barton recommended the root for dropsy, hives, and croup and admitted that he "sometimes treated patients almost entirely with Seneca." It was most effective when used as an expectorant to help relieve wheezing, coughs, and congestion, particularly in cases of asthma and bronchitis. Little used in North America today, the plant is a common ingredient in lozenges, cough syrups, and teas sold in Europe.

SUNDEW
Drosera spp.

Active plant parts Whole plant
Uses Coughs, asthma, bronchitis, skin conditions
Cautions No side effects have been documented.

The leaves of sundew (*Drosera rotundifolia*) and other species of this unusual plant family have sticky hairs that capture and digest insects. A tiny herb, sundew typically grows no taller than 15 cm (6 in.) and is usually found in bogs and wetland environments. Nevertheless, because the plant is threatened in parts of North America, only cultivated sundew (or products manufactured from it) should be used in home remedies. In folk tradition, sundew was taken as a tea or tincture to treat coughs (especially whooping cough), asthma, and bronchitis, as it still is today. Constituents of the herb have been found to have cough-suppressant and antispasmodic effects. In earlier days, the plant's antibacterial leaves were chopped and applied as a poultice to corns, warts, and sunburn.

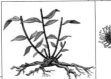

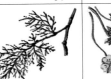

TEA TREE
Melaleuca alternifolia

Active plant parts Leaves
Uses Fungal infections, acne, warts, lice, cuts
Cautions The oil may irritate sensitive skin. The oil is nontoxic but should be used internally only under a doctor's supervision.

Native to Australia, tea tree has been used for centuries by the indigenous Aborigines to treat colds, skin problems, and fatigue. The tree was named by British naturalist Joseph Banks, who enjoyed a tea made from its leaves while exploring and mapping the east coast of Australia in the 18th century. After the therapeutic properties of the essential oil were researched in the 1920s, tea tree quickly became known for its topical antiseptic, antibacterial, and antifungal effects. Today the aromatic oil is still widely recognized as a natural remedy for fungal skin conditions, such as athlete's foot, ringworm, and vaginal yeast infections. It may also be effective in treating minor cuts and lice. Tea tree oil is sold as an essential oil, as a cream, and in many over-the-counter health products. When buying the essential oil, be sure that it is unadulterated.

TORMENTIL
Potentilla tormentilla

Active plant parts Rhizome
Uses Diarrhea, gingivitis, cuts and scrapes
Cautions Internal use may irritate the stomach. Do not use for more than three to four days at a time.

The rhizome of tormentil and other species of *Potentilla*, including erect cinquefoil (*P. erecta*), contains 15 to 20 percent tannic acid, which makes it a strong astringent. Named for its ability to ease any "torment" that afflicted the body, tormentil was used to stop bleeding, relieve diarrhea, and treat gastroenteritis and dysentery—all of which are conditions that can be helped by an astringent. The rootstock tincture may also prove effective as a mouthwash (used to soothe inflamed mucous membranes of the mouth and throat) and as a vaginal douche. In addition, extracts of the rhizome have shown antiviral and mild immunity-boosting potential. The reputed fever-reducing effect of tormentil tea, however, has not been validated. Both the dried herb and the rhizome, sometimes sold as cinquefoil, are commercially available in North America.

TURMERIC
Curcuma longa

Active plant part Rhizome
Uses Indigestion, liver problems, arthritis, sprains, skin conditions
Cautions Large doses may irritate the stomach. Internal use is contraindicated in cases of bile duct obstruction. Those with gallstones or ulcers should use only after consulting a doctor. Do not give to children under two years of age. Topical use may cause a rash.

Since ancient times, the powdered rhizome of turmeric has been used as both a culinary spice—it is an ingredient in curry powder—and an herbal medicine, chiefly to treat indigestion. In India and Asia, turmeric has been used for centuries to remedy countless ailments, ranging from bruises to blood clots. Today its possible benefits may be just as numerous. In the 1970s, studies of turmeric revealed cholesterol-reducing, antioxidant, and anticoagulant potential. It also stimulates the flow of bile and protects the liver. As an antibacterial, it fights the protozoan that causes dysentery. As a topical anti-inflammatory, it reduces arthritis swelling.

UVA URSI
Arctostaphylos uva-ursi

Active plant parts Leaves
Uses Kidney, bladder, and urinary tract infections
Cautions Internal use may irritate the stomach and cause nausea, vomiting, and convulsions. Do not use during pregnancy. Do not use for more than one week at a time without consulting a doctor.

Although bears love to eat the red berries of uva ursi (also known as bearberry), it is the plant's leaves that contain its healing potential. Uva ursi has been used for hundreds of years to treat kidney, bladder, and urinary tract disorders. Indians applied the leaves to skin rashes and sore muscles. Frontier settlers used them to treat hemorrhoids, "diseases of the urinary organs," and poison ivy. Used internally, uva ursi acts as an efficacious urinary antiseptic in the treatment of nephritis, cystitis, and urethritis. Its effectiveness, however, depends on the alkalinity of the urine, which can be achieved by consuming milk, tomatoes, potatoes, and fruit juices or taking 1 to 2 teaspoons of baking soda a day.

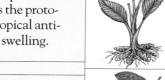

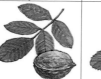

WALNUT
Juglans spp.

Active plant parts Leaves
Uses Skin rashes, fungal infections, cuts and abrasions, diarrhea
Cautions Excessive internal use may cause stomach irritation.

The dried leaves of the English walnut (*Juglans regia*) and black walnut (*J. nigra*), a North American species, have been used to treat such skin conditions as acne, eczema, and ulcers. In folk medicine, the leaves were also used internally to help remedy gastrointestinal irritations, expel worms, purify the blood, and ward off bedbugs. Although the leaves are little used in modern herbal medicine, their mildly antimicrobial and astringent effects can help heal skin rashes and minor cuts and scrapes. The leaves are also mildly antifungal and may be beneficial in treating such infections as athlete's foot and ringworm. Internally, walnut's astringency may help remedy diarrhea. The bark of some species of walnut, including butternut (*J. cinerea*), is also taken as a gentle purgative in cases of chronic constipation. The nuts themselves are said to help lower cholesterol.

WILD STRAWBERRY
Fragaria vesca

Active plant parts Leaves
Uses Diarrhea, sore throat
Cautions No side effects have been documented. Use of the leaf may cause allergic reactions in those hypersensitive to strawberries.

The leaves of wild strawberry are valued for their mild astringent and diuretic effects. Both the leaves and the fruit were believed to provide a "cooling effect" on the body and thus were used to relieve so-called hot ailments, including indigestion, tuberculosis, jaundice, and rheumatism. The fruit's juice was also applied to sunburn, skin rashes, and facial blemishes. Although the aromatic tea was used to treat these ailments, as well as gout and urinary tract disorders, it may be efficacious only in relieving diarrhea and sore throat. The tea's reputed potential to stimulate the appetite, improve circulation, and calm the nerves lacks scientific evidence—in fact, the tea is known more for its flavor than for its medicinal benefits. Although the fruit, too, lacks therapeutic value, it was often used by early settlers as a teeth whitener and mild laxative.

WILD YAM
Dioscorea villosa

Active plant part Rhizome
Uses Derivatives are used to treat menstrual cramps, muscle spasms, menopausal symptoms, rheumatism, and skin rashes.
Cautions Do not take during pregnancy.

A far cry from the sweet potato served up at dinner, the ill-flavored wild yam has garnered a lofty medicinal reputation. In the Americas, Indian women made preparations of the boiled rhizome to relieve menstrual and labor pain. Studies of species of *Dioscorea* in the 1930s and '40s led to the development of anti-inflammatory cortisones and many steroid drugs, including synthetic progesterone and the birth-control pill. Many drugs created to treat asthma, arthritis, high blood pressure, menstrual and menopausal discomforts, and skin rashes contain semi-synthetic derivatives made from a precursor compound (diosgenin) found in wild yam—but while these derivatives are highly active, diosgenin is not. For this reason, wild yam itself has no medicinal effect.

WORMWOOD
Artemisia absinthium

Active plant parts Leaves
Uses Skin inflammations
Cautions The U.S. FDA classifies the herb as "unsafe." Health Canada also has concerns about its safety. Use only in small doses and under a doctor's supervision. Children and pregnant women should avoid the herb entirely.

Wormwood's gray, bitter-tasting leaves were used to expel worms and stimulate digestion. Although its anthelmintic action has not been proven, wormwood, like many bitter herbs, is believed to strengthen weak digestion when taken in very small doses. Larger amounts are toxic, and internal use is inadvisable. Extracts of wormwood were used to make absinthe, a green liqueur that was popular—until it was outlawed—in the early 20th century. Absinthe produced a dream-like high and sometimes caused hallucinations and psychosis. Vincent van Gogh, who cut off his ear and mailed it to his beloved, may have been an absinthe addict.

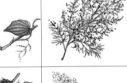

YELLOW DOCK
Rumex crispus

Active plant parts Rhizome, roots
Uses Constipation, anemia, skin conditions
Cautions Do not ingest the fresh leaves; they contain oxalic acid, which can cause kidney stones and gout. Use may cause nausea or dermatitis. Do not take during pregnancy or lactation.

Yellow dock was used to cleanse the blood, skin, liver, and bowels. The active principles of the root and rhizome, called anthraquinones, act as gentle laxatives, stimulate bile flow in the liver, and help to expel toxins efficiently from the body. In folk medicine, yellow dock was wrongly thought to "purify the blood" and remedy ailments that were once believed to be caused by the buildup of toxins in the blood—among them venereal disease, tuberculosis, and jaundice. Despite yellow dock's lack of efficacy for these conditions, its iron content is beneficial in the treatment of anemia, and today, as long ago, the herb's astringency and other cleansing effects are utilized to treat such skin conditions as boils. The leaves, once eaten as a spring tonic, are now known to be toxic when ingested.

YUCCA
Yucca spp.

Active plant parts Roots, leaves
Uses Arthritis, sprains
Cautions Small amounts cause no documented side effects. Long-term use may prevent the absorption of vitamins A, D, E, and K.

Many species of *Yucca*, including Mojave yucca (*Y. schidigera*) and the fabled Joshua tree (*Y. brevifolia*), flourish in the arid climate of the southwestern United States. The Indians used these desert plants to make food, rope, sandals, and baskets. Yucca root was also used in salves, poultices, and washes to treat skin inflammations, rheumatism, sprains, and dandruff. The roots contain anti-inflammatory saponins, which foam when shaken with water. On the frontier, pioneers used *Y. glauca* to make a lathering soap and named the plant soapweed. A 1975 study showed that yucca's saponins could reduce blood pressure and cholesterol levels, the frequency of migraines, and arthritis pain. However, the Arthritis Foundation in the U.S. challenged the study and warned that taking yucca for medicinal purposes should not replace treatment by a doctor.

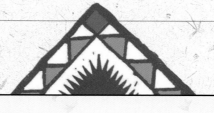

PREPARING HERBAL REMEDIES

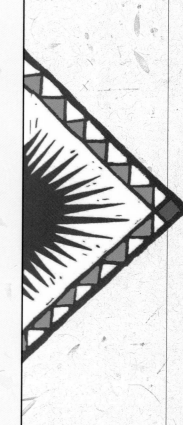

After a century-long absence, the herbs that were an everyday part of home medical care are back in force—this time in the form of commercial tablets and tinctures, capsules and tea bags, extracts and gels. But it's easier than you think to go back to basics and prepare traditional remedies yourself. The following 11 pages offer tips on harvesting and drying herbs, along with basic recipes for teas and decoctions, syrups and tinctures, lotions and oils. Poultices and plasters can be whipped up as needed, while homemade gargles and skin creams can be stored in the refrigerator for later use.

HARVESTING & DRYING

Herbs harvested from your garden can be used right away, or they may be dried. Drying helps to preserve the active principles and allows you to store the herbs for future use. If properly prepared and stored, some herbal preparations will retain their healing properties for up to a year; fresh herbs, on the other hand, last only a few days.

Leaves and Stems

Gather both annual and perennial herbs just before the plant flowers, when the active principles are most potent. Armed with an open basket and a sharp knife or clippers, harvest on a sunny day in mid-morning, after the dew has dried but before the wilting noontime heat descends. To avoid stunting the plants, cut no more than half the leaves from annuals, such as chamomile, and no more than a third from perennials, such as echinacea.

To prepare the herbs for drying, swish them in cool water to wash away dirt and debris. Gently pat dry, then either hang the plants upside down or place them on paper-towel-lined trays or nonmetal screens. Place them in a dark, well-ventilated spot where the temperature stays between 21°C and 32°C (70°F and 90°F).

Although drying times vary according to the weather and the type of plant, herbs usually dry in one to two weeks. For faster results, dry them in the oven—a method preferred for such tough-leaved plants as lovage. Arrange the herbs in single layers on trays and place in a 21°C to 35°C (70°F to 95°F) oven for 24 to 48 hours; leave the oven door ajar, and gauge the temperature with an oven thermometer. Leaves are ready to be stored when they feel brittle but are not so dry that they crumble. If you are using only the leaves, rub them off the stem onto a piece of paper. If you are using the stems, too, test them for dryness: they should break, not bend.

The bounty of medicinal herbs includes such standbys as chamomile, spearmint, sage, thyme, dandelion, and peppermint.

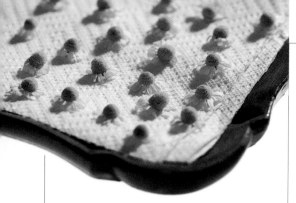

Dry flower heads on trays lined with paper towels or on nonmetal screens.

Flowers

Harvest herbs grown for their flowers just after they bloom. Remove dirt and insects from the flower heads by shaking them gently. To dry, either hang upside down by the stem or cut off the flower heads and place them on trays. If oven-drying, place the flower heads in a 27°C (80°F) oven until the petals rustle when touched.

Seeds

Seeds are ready to be harvested when they turn brown and the stalks start to wither (usually early fall). Secure a bunch of seed heads in a paper bag and hang it upside down in a place where the temperature does not exceed 35°C (95°F). When the seeds have dried (usually in a week), they will fall into the bag when you shake it. Dry them one more week before storing.

To dry seeds, cut about 15 cm (6 in.) of stalk with the seed head. Tie in bunches, then secure a paper bag over the heads.

Berries

Pick berries when they are just ripe, discarding any that are soft or show signs of mold or blight. Set them in a single layer on an oven-proof tray lined with paper towels. Preheat the oven to 32°C (90°F), then turn it off. Place the tray in the oven for two to three hours, leaving the oven door ajar. To finish drying, transfer the tray to a warm, dry space where the temperature does not exceed 35°C (95°F).

Roots

Although most roots can be dug up any time the ground is not frozen, fall is preferred. Separate the roots as needed and replant the remainder. Wash the roots well, chop, and arrange in a single layer on an oven-proof tray. Preheat the oven to 35°C (95°F), then turn off the heat and place the tray in the oven for two to three hours, leaving the door ajar. Transfer the roots to a warm place to finish drying. (This may take from three to five weeks, depending on the thickness of the roots and the humidity; properly dried roots snap when bent.) Since some roots reabsorb moisture, check them regularly after storing and discard any that are soft.

Storing

Before storing dried herbs, crumble leaves, stems, and flowers; bark, berries, and seeds should remain whole. Place in glass jars and close the lids tightly. Check for condensation over the next two weeks; if you see any moisture, place the plant matter on paper towels and dry in a warm place for another day or two.

Store dried plant matter in a cool, dark place for up to one year. Discard if any insects or molds appear.

Bark

Fall is the best time to collect most tree and shrub bark. Strip it from a branch (preferably one scheduled for pruning) instead of from the trunk. Wipe or dust off any insects or moss. Break or cut the bark into pieces 5 cm (2 in.) square or smaller. Spread the bark on a tray lined with paper towels and let dry for several weeks until the bark is easily snapped or, in the case of thick bark, chipped with a hammer.

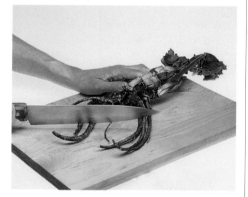

After washing roots thoroughly, chop them with a chef's knife into small pieces no more than 5 cm (2 in.) long; this will speed the drying process.

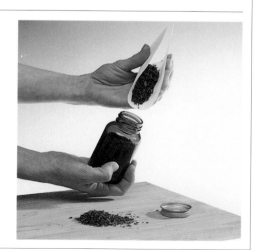

HERBAL TEAS

When it comes to herbal libations, the word "tea" has become a blanket term for what can be technically differentiated as teas, infusions, and decoctions. Infusions are typically stronger than teas, but both are made with soft plant parts: fresh or dried leaves, stems, or flowers. Decoctions are teas made with tougher plant parts—fresh or dried bark, berries, seeds, or roots—that usually require longer brewing.

*All **herbal libations,** such as this dandelion decoction, must be strained through a fine sieve or cheesecloth. For best results, make a fresh tea or decoction each day.*

Teas and Infusions

A tea is made with boiling water. An infusion, on the other hand, is made with water that has only just begun to boil, lessening the chances of the herb's volatile oils being lost to steam. To prepare either, warm a ceramic, glass, or stainless steel teapot by swishing a bit of boiling water in it, then pouring the water out. Using the amounts specified in the recipe, add the herb to the teapot. For a tea, pour boiling water over the herbs. Cover and let steep for 5 to 10 minutes, then strain through cheesecloth or a fine sieve. For an infusion, cover the herbs with just-boiled water and steep for 10 to 30 minutes before straining.

To make herbal tea bags, handy for traveling, place 1 to 2 teaspoons of the herb on a square of muslin, fold the muslin over the herb, and tie with string.

Decoctions

To make a decoction, spoon the specified amount of plant matter into a medium-size pan; avoid aluminum, copper, or iron pans, which may react chemically with the plant. Cover the plant matter with cold water, set the pan over medium heat, and simmer 15 to 30 minutes or for as long as the recipe directs. Strain through cheese-cloth or a fine sieve. As with teas and infusions, you may wish to add a touch of honey or sugar to improve the taste.

SYRUPS & TINCTURES

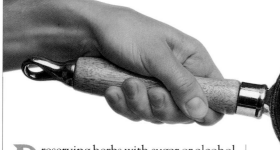

Preserving herbs with sugar or alcohol makes it possible to keep them for long periods. Syrups last for two months (longer if refrigerated), and tinctures keep for up to two years. Store them in a cool, dark place.

Syrups

Boiling herbal teas with sugar yields a homemade cough syrup or sore-throat soother. Choose teas with expectorant properties, such as licorice, elecampane, and thyme, or those with mucilage, such as slippery elm. Do not give syrup made with honey to a child under one year of age; honey may contain bacteria that can cause a serious reaction in infants.

BASIC HERBAL SYRUP

2 cups strong herbal tea
2 cups sugar or honey

Place the sugar in a saucepan. Bring the tea to a boil in another pan, then pour it over the sugar. Using a wooden spoon, stir the mixture over medium-low heat until the sugar is dissolved (about 10 minutes). Remove from the heat and let cool. Pour the thickened syrup into sterilized bottles, cork or cap tightly, and refrigerate.

Sterilize First!

Storage jars should always be sterilized, no matter what herbal preparation you make—including alcohol-based tinctures. Choose heat-proof bottles or jars, such as those used for jam. Cover the jars and any metal lids with water and boil them on top of the stove for at least 10 minutes; keep them hot until ready to use. (Do not boil rubber rings and lids with rubber rims; rinse them instead with hot water.) Alternatively, use a commercial sterilizing solution. Follow the directions on the label, then rinse the jars with freshly boiled water and dry in a hot oven. Do not try to sterilize containers in the microwave. Microwaves heat the food or liquid in a container, not the container itself.

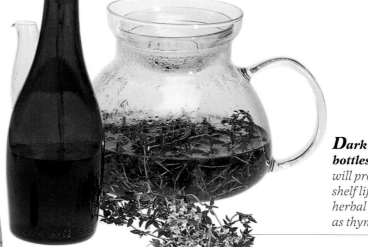

***Dark glass bottles** or jars will prolong the shelf life of such herbal preparations as thyme syrup.*

Tinctures

Tinctures, usually made by steeping herbs in alcohol, are a mainstay of the home herbal pharmacy. The alcohol not only has a preservative effect but also helps to extract the plant's active principles. Tinctures made with ethyl (drinkable) alcohol may be taken internally, but in much smaller doses than teas or infusions—a matter of drops, in fact. They can also be added to a plain sugar syrup in proportions of three parts syrup to one part tincture. Most herbalists advise using vodka in tinctures. Although brandy and rum will provide more flavor—desirable when trying to disguise the taste of unpalatable herbs—their lower proof lessens their preservative powers.

Nonalcoholic tinctures, suitable for children, pregnant women, and people with gastric inflammation, may be made with vinegar or glycerin. Neither substance, however, works as well as alcohol for preserving, and glycerin is weaker as a solvent. Moreover, both substances may alter the herb's chemical makeup.

Notes of Caution

◆ Do not make tinctures with rubbing (isopropyl) alcohol or wood (methyl) alcohol; these solvents are toxic if taken internally.

◆ When taking tinctures, pregnant women should reduce the amount of alcohol. Bring the water used to dilute the tincture to a near boil. The alcohol will evaporate in five minutes.

ETHYL ALCOHOL TINCTURE

Either dried or chopped fresh herbs are suitable for this recipe. Tinctures made with ethyl alcohol should always be diluted for internal use and can also be used externally, diluted or straight.

200 grams (7 oz) dried herb or 300 grams (10½ oz) fresh herb
1 liter (approximately 4 cups) vodka or other alcohol

Place all of the ingredients in a sterilized jar that can be capped tightly. Cap the jar, shake it well, and place in a dark, warm place for 10 to 14 days; shake it daily. Strain the liquid through a jelly bag, as shown below, squeezing out as much liquid as possible. (If you don't have a jelly bag, a piece of cheesecloth or muslin will do. A winepress, too, can be used.) Pour the preparation into sterilized dark bottles and stopper tightly. Cork stoppers are preferred: they will pop out if the mixture produces gases, thereby preventing the bottle from exploding. (Tinctures made with weak alcohol, such as wine, are more likely to produce gases.) If using a regular bottle cap, store the bottle in the refrigerator. The tincture should keep for up to two years.

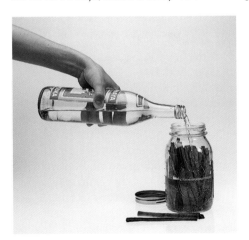

Step 1 *After placing the herbs in a sterilized jar, add ethyl alcohol to within 2.5 cm (1 in.) of the top. Shown here are cinnamon sticks combined with vodka.*

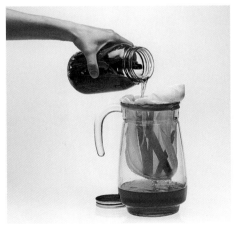

Step 2 *After the plant matter has been steeped and the jar has been shaken daily for 14 days, fit a sterilized pitcher with a jelly bag and strain the mixture.*

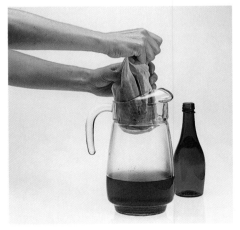

Step 3 *When the liquid has drained, wring out the residue until you have extracted as much liquid as possible. Store in a sterilized bottle.*

INFUSED OILS

The active principles of a plant can be extracted in oil, creating an herbal preparation that is suitable for direct application to the skin. Made by either hot or cold methods, these infused oils are less irritating than the plant's essential oil; for this reason, they are often used in massage. Infused oils keep for up to a year, although most tend to lose their potency after about six months.

Heat-Infused Oils

Heat-infused oils are made by simmering herbs in oil. Leafy herbs that lend themselves to this process include nettle and chickweed. Cayenne and other "hot" spices that are prized for use in massage oils work best when infused with heat. If you need only a small amount of oil, divide the following recipe as needed but keep the same proportions of oil to herb.

BASIC HEAT-INFUSED OIL

255 grams (9 oz) dried herb
or 510 grams (18 oz) fresh
chopped herb
3 cups olive, sunflower, almond,
or other pure vegetable oil

Combine the herbs and the oil in the top of a glass, stainless steel, or enamel double boiler set over boiling water. Simmer for two to three hours, then let cool. Pour the oil into a sterilized pitcher fitted with a jelly bag, then squeeze out as much of the liquid as possible. Pour the oil into sterilized dark bottles or jars and cap tightly. Store in a cool place out of direct sunlight.

Cold-Infused Oils

Step 1 Pour the oil over the herb. Shown here are lavender flowers, a popular choice for cold infusion. The resulting lavender oil makes a relaxing rub.

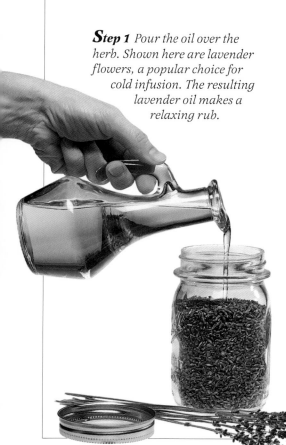

The preparation of cold-infused oils is similar to that for making "sun tea." It is the preferred method for extracting the active principles of flowers, such as those of St. Johnswort. Because olive oil is unlikely to become rancid, it is a good choice for use in cold infusions.

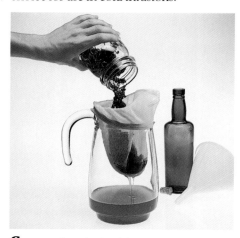

Step 2 After the herb has macerated, strain the mixture into a pitcher. Store the oil in a sterilized dark jar or bottle with a cork stopper.

BASIC COLD-INFUSED OIL

It is not necessary to chop the herbs used in cold-infused oils, but it helps to cut them into manageable pieces.

255 grams (9 oz) dried herb
or 510 grams (18 oz) fresh herb
3 cups olive, sunflower, almond,
or other pure vegetable oil

Pack the herbs into a clear, wide-mouthed glass jar. Add the oil. Cap the jar tightly and shake it well. Place the jar in a warm, sunny location and leave it undisturbed (except for the occasional shaking) for four to six weeks. To speed the process, bruise chopped herbs with a mortar and pestle before adding the oil. Bruised herbs will release their oils in one to two weeks.

When the mixture has macerated sufficiently and darkened in color, pour it into a jelly bag set in a clean pitcher or large jar, then wring out the bag to extract all the oil. Pour the oil into sterilized dark jars and cap tightly. For a stronger infusion, repeat the entire process, using the infused oil and new herbs.

POULTICES & COMPRESSES

Herbal poultices, plasters, and compresses are applied directly to the skin to relieve a variety of conditions, including headache, fever, bruises, and skin irritations.

Poultices and Plasters

Poultices are herb pastes used to ease aches, sprains, or broken bones. They also help draw out infection, as well as splinters and thorns. When the herbs are wrapped in gauze, which keeps them from touching the skin, the poultice is called a plaster; plasters are preferable when using such skin-irritating herbs as mustard. Both poultices and plasters can be made with fresh, powdered, or dried herbs.

Making a mustard plaster is simple. Mix one part mustard powder and two parts flour in a bowl, then add just enough water to make a paste. Spread the paste on a dishcloth, fold, and press it against the skin. Remove it if the skin becomes irritated.

FRESH-HERB POULTICE

Estimate the amount of fresh herbs needed to cover the injured area, allowing for their reduction in size when cooked. Place the herbs in a saucepan, cover with water, and simmer for 5 to 15 minutes or until the plant matter is very soft.

Drain the herbs in a colander, pressing out any remaining liquid. Spread the herb onto the affected area (the herb should be as hot as you can tolerate) and cover it with gauze. When the poultice cools, repeat the process. Placing plastic wrap or a hot-water bottle over the bandage will help hold in the heat. Leave the poultice on for up to three hours. If skin irritation occurs, remove the poultice immediately.

DRIED-HERB POULTICE

Powdered- or dried-herb poultices, suitable for bruises and other small injuries, are easier to make. Simply place the dried herb in a small bowl and stir in hot water or tea, a teaspoonful at a time, to make a paste. Then follow the procedure for applying a fresh-herb poultice.

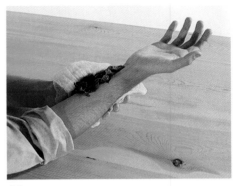

To apply a poultice, first rub vegetable oil on the skin; the oil makes removing the poultice easier. Hold the herbs in a large piece of gauze and place them directly on the affected area. Then bind the area with the gauze to hold the poultice in place. Shown here are raspberry leaves.

Compresses

Herbal compresses are moist cloths that have been saturated in herbal teas. They can be applied cold or hot, depending on the complaint: headaches and fevers generally respond well to cold, whereas bruises and sprains usually call for heat.

To make a compress, first prepare a tea, infusion, or decoction of an appropriate herb. (Alternatively, use a diluted tincture.) Dip a clean, soft cloth (a washcloth is ideal) into the liquid, wring out gently, fold, and place against the painful area. Secure with plastic wrap.

Apply for up to two hours as necessary. Refresh the compress as needed to maintain the proper temperature. The liquid keeps in the refrigerator for up to two days in a tightly closed, sterilized jar.

HEALING BALMS

For thousands of years, herbs have been used to make emollient substances that restore moisture, soothe rashes, and aid the healing of wounds. Most of these balms are made with vegetable or animal oils. A thickener, such as lanolin, is often used to create the desired consistency, and a hardener (usually beeswax) is added for firmness.

Because these preparations deteriorate relatively quickly, make them in small batches. You can prolong their shelf life by storing them in the refrigerator or by adding a preservative, such as glycerin. As with any homemade herbal preparation, spotlessly clean utensils and sterile storage jars are essential.

Ointments

Herbal ointments, which are made with fats or oils, keep therapeutic herbs in contact with the skin for long periods of time and protect damaged skin from inflammation and moisture. They can be made with a variety of fats and oils, depending on their intended use.

BASIC SALVE

Herbal salves help wounds and sores to heal. The easiest recipe is based on petroleum jelly, available at any drugstore.

> *140 grams (5 oz) minced fresh herb*
> *or 60 grams (2 oz) dried herb*
> *455 grams (16 oz) petroleum jelly*

Have ready a heat-proof glass pitcher or measuring cup with a jelly bag or cheesecloth tied to the rim. Melt the petroleum jelly in a double boiler. Add the herbs and simmer, stirring constantly, for 15 to 20 minutes. Pour the mixture into the jelly bag. Wearing protective gloves, wring the liquid from the bag into the pitcher, then quickly pour it into a wide-mouthed storage jar. Screw the lid on loosely, then tighten it once the ointment has cooled.

BEESWAX BALM

This spreadable, relatively nongreasy ointment is harder than the basic salve and won't melt in hot climates. It makes a good lip balm. Beeswax is available at natural-products stores and pharmacies.

> *⅔ cup (5 oz) vegetable oil*
> *½ cup (4 oz) beeswax*
> *130 grams (4½ oz) minced fresh herb*
> *or 50 grams (1¾ oz) dried herb*

Combine the oil and the beeswax in a double boiler and heat until the beeswax has melted. Add the herbs and simmer for one to two hours, stirring often. Strain the mixture through a jelly bag into a heat-proof glass pitcher and proceed as described in the Basic Salve recipe.

BASIC SKIN-RASH OINTMENT

This softer ointment is particularly useful for treating skin rashes of any kind. Herbs known to have rash-healing properties include burdock, yarrow, calendula, goldenseal, and witch hazel.

Test Your Skin

Allergic skin reactions are possible with all herb-based products. Before using any homemade topical preparation, apply a small amount to the inside of your forearm and wait 24 hours. If the skin reddens or itches, do not use the preparation.

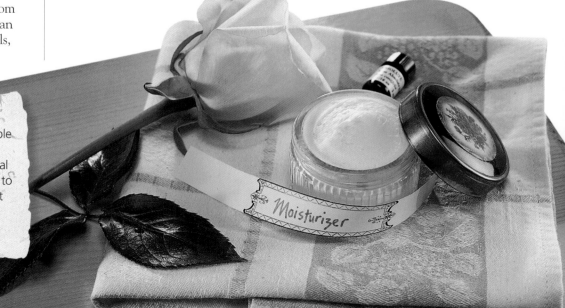

2 cups olive oil or heat-infused oil
¼ cup (2 oz) beeswax
115 grams (4 oz) dried herb
* or 310 grams (11 oz) fresh herb*

Heat the oil and the beeswax in a double boiler until the beeswax has melted. Add the herbs and simmer for one to two hours, stirring often. Cover and let sit in a warm place for several hours. Strain, then pour into a sterilized jar. Cover when cool.

Creams

Based on water, oil, and wax, skin creams penetrate the skin yet allow it to breathe, hence their use as moisturizers and cleansers. Prepare them with care: the oil and water will separate if proper emulsion does not take place. To avoid this, make sure that the ingredients are at the same temperature and add the water slowly.

Basic Cleansing Cream

Among the herbs to choose from are dandelion, linden flower, nettle, lavender, sage, thyme, and yarrow.

1 tablespoon beeswax
2 tablespoons lanolin
⅜ cup almond or olive oil
2 tablespoons herbal tea
* of choice*
2 drops essential oil of choice

Melt the beeswax and the lanolin in a double boiler. Warm the oil over low heat, then beat it into the mixture. Meanwhile, heat the herbal tea slightly, then take it off the heat. Using a wire whisk, beat it into the mixture, one teaspoonful at a time; the mixture should cool and thicken. Slowly whip in the essential oil. Spoon the mixture into a sterilized jar.

Lotions

Lotions are liquid solutions that are usually water-based, although alcohol or witch hazel may be used. They are good for everything from soothing dry skin to bathing inflamed body parts. Tinctures may be added to boost the cooling effect.

Basic Skin Lotion

Use a glass bowl and a wire whisk for best results. Herbs that are suitable for a soothing skin lotion include chamomile, calendula, and evening primrose.

⅓ cup strong herbal tea
⅓ cup or more of glycerin

Place the ingredients in a small mixing bowl. Beat with a wire whisk until the mixture is smooth and creamy. Pour into a sterilized glass bottle and cap tightly.

Dry-Skin Moisturizer

A moisturizer for dry skin is made in the same way as a cleansing cream, but it requires ingredients richer in fatty emollients, such as cocoa butter, avocado oil, and wheat germ oil. Herbs that contain mucilage are useful for dry skin; they include borage, plantain, mullein, and marsh mallow. Moisturizers are said to be most effective when applied to damp skin after bathing.

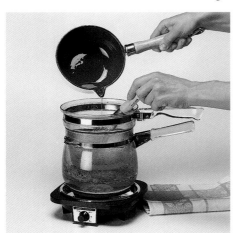

Step 1 *After melting the beeswax and the cocoa butter in a double boiler, use a wire whisk to incorporate the avocado and wheat germ oils. Remove from heat.*

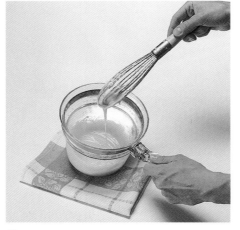

Step 2 *Whisk in the warmed herbal tea, one tablespoon at a time, until the mixture is cool. Then whisk in the essential oil before spooning into small jars.*

¼ cup beeswax
2 tablespoons cocoa butter
5 tablespoons avocado oil
½ teaspoon wheat germ oil
4 tablespoons herbal tea of choice
6 drops essential oil of choice

Melt the beeswax and the cocoa butter in a double boiler; stir until blended. Meanwhile, gently warm the avocado and wheat germ oils in a separate pan. Use a wire whisk to whip the warmed oils into the mixture in the double boiler; it should take on a creamy consistency. Remove from heat. Warm the herbal tea and beat it into the mixture until cool. Finally, whip in the essential oil. Spoon the moisturizer into sterile jars and close the lids tightly. Store in a cool place.

GARGLES & MOUTHWASHES

Many herbal teas make excellent gargles and mouthwashes, useful for soothing sore throats and easing the pain of canker sores and other mouth disorders. The herbs you use will depend on your complaint.

Astringent herbs, whose tannins tighten the mucous membranes and may temporarily relieve a tickle or a feeling of rawness in the throat, are among the most helpful. Herbs with a high mucilage content are also beneficial; the mucilage coats and protects irritated membranes. Tinctures, diluted at two teaspoons to one cup water, can also be used as gargles, rinses, and mouthwashes. (Tinctures should never be used straight.)

BASIC HERBAL GARGLE

Astringent, tannin-rich herbs include raspberry, blackberry, and white oak leaves or bark. Among herbs with a high mucilage content are horehound, hyssop, mullein, marsh mallow, plantain, slippery elm bark, and flaxseed.

1 teaspoon dried herb
  or 3 teaspoons chopped fresh herb
1 cup water

Place the herbs in a saucepan. In another pan or teapot, bring the water to a boil, then pour it over the herbs. Simmer for one to two minutes. Remove from heat and let steep for five minutes. Strain through cheesecloth or a fine sieve into sterilized jars. The gargle can be used three or four times a day.

HERBAL MOUTHWASH

The antiseptic properties and aromatic flavor of members of the mint family—notably peppermint, spearmint, catnip, and pennyroyal—are effective against bad breath. Other good choices include fennel, sage, and myrrh.

1 teaspoon dried herb
  or 3 teaspoons chopped fresh herb
1 cup water

Prepare as directed in the recipe for Basic Herbal Gargle. Mouthwashes can be used as often as desired.

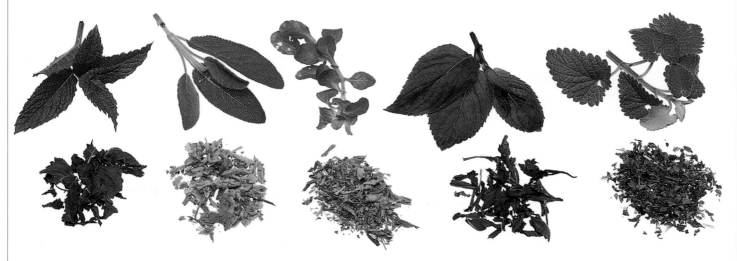

Spearmint, *shown fresh and dried, is often used to flavor chewing gum, and temporarily freshens the breath.*

Sage, *a fragrant member of the mint family, contains thujone, an antiseptic that kills oral bacteria.*

Pennyroyal *works well in mouthwashes because of its pleasant aroma, but do not ingest the oil, which is toxic.*

Peppermint, *popular as a flavoring for toothpastes, contains menthol, which temporarily masks bad breath.*

Catnip *tea, which has a pleasant flavor and is thought to be mildly sedative, can be used as a gargle or mouthwash.*

STEAM INHALATIONS

Two of the annoying symptoms of colds and allergies—a clogged nose and a tight chest—can often be relieved temporarily with one of Grandma's favorite remedies: steam inhalations. Inhaling steam increases the amount of fluid in the respiratory tract, which thins the mucus and makes it easier to expel. A few drops of an essential oil added to the water boosts the expectorant and congestion-clearing actions. The warmth and moisture of steam also have a soothing effect on irritated tissues.

BASIC HERBAL INHALATION

For use in steam inhalations, mint leaves and chamomile flowers are favored by herbalists. Thyme and marjoram may be added to enhance the expectorant effect.

Pine, rosemary, and eucalyptus oils are also popular choices.

*4 cups boiling water
5 to 10 drops
    essential oil of choice
Heat-proof bowl
    and large towel*

Pour boiling water into a heat-proof bowl and stir in essential oil. From a sitting position, bend over the bowl and quickly put the towel over your head to form a tent. Taking care not to get too close to the steam, breathe in the vapors for about 10 minutes. Repeat two or three times a day.

Note: Although it is safe to inhale the steam from water to which an essential oil has been added, the oils themselves

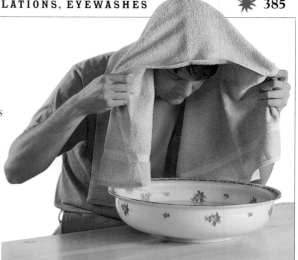

Steam inhalations *are soothing—and simple. Doctors recommend staying in a warm place for 30 minutes afterward to allow the respiratory system to adjust.*

should never be ingested. Asthmatics and pregnant women should consult their doctors before using inhalation therapy.

EYEWASHES

Homemade infusions can be used as an eyewash or in a compress to soothe mild eye irritations, such as eyestrain, itchy eyes, inflamed eyelids, conjunctivitis (pinkeye), and sties. Tinctures can also be used, but only in weak solutions made with no more than ½ to 1 teaspoon tincture to one cup of water. To prevent eyewashes from stinging, add a few grains of salt to the solution, to match the salinity of tears.

Note: Sterilizing equipment for eyewashes is extremely important. Sterilize your eyecup as directed on page 144.

BASIC HERBAL EYEWASH

Herbs that may offer some relief from sore or inflamed eyes include goldenseal, rose hips, chamomile, calendula, parsley, celandine, and red-raspberry leaf.

*1 to 2 teaspoons chopped herb
1 cup boiling water*

Place the herbs in a saucepan, add boiling water, and simmer for 15 minutes. Strain through a fine sieve into a sterilized jar, making sure that no debris passes through. Let cool. Store in the refrigerator. You may use the eyewash two or three times a day, for no longer than three weeks. To use the wash in a compress, soak a washcloth in the cooled liquid, wring it out, fold it, and place it over the eyelids.

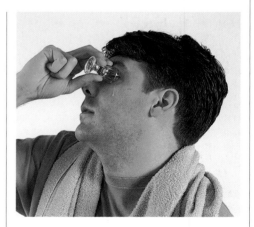

To use an eyewash, *pour the liquid into a sterilized eyecup. Place the cup against the affected eye, tilt the head back, and blink your eye several times.*

BUYER'S GUIDE

Today the shelves of most drugstores are jammed with a baffling array of herbal products, many promising better health or implying disease-curing powers. Unfortunately, not all of these products are effective—or even safe. Therefore, it is vital that you become an informed consumer before buying.

Herbs have a great range of effects on the body; these effects depend not only on the plant but also on your own physiology, lifestyle, and any medicines you may be taking. Some, like peppermint, require no more caution than obeying the rule of "moderation in all things"—even water can be dangerous if taken to excess. Others, like ginger, are more potent and should be used with more caution. Still others, such as ephedra, are as potent as regular drugs and should be treated as such. When no toxicological studies have been conducted on an herb, an elementary guide to its general safety is the extent and length of its historical and modern use. Such plants as slippery elm and ginseng would not have been utilized for centuries unless they were generally safe when taken in the proper doses. Still, it is incumbent on the consumer to learn all he can about herbs that were used mainly in the past or are very new to the scene.

Aside from variations in strength, differences in purity may also exist. Cases of contamination with toxic plants, such as belladonna, or with heavy metals, such as mercury, have been reported. In addition, a few imported remedies have been known to be adulterated with such synthetic drugs as corticosteroids and tran-quilizers, making it all the more important to buy from a reliable manufacturer.

Check the Label

But how do you judge the reliability of a manufacturer? For starters, look for its name and address on the product label. You may wish to write to or call the company to find out how long they have been in business, what kind of quality control measures are in force, how the herb's identity and potency are determined, which clinical tests have been conducted on the product, and whether the company is a member of any trade group, such as the American Herbal Products Association or the Canadian Health Food Association. These associations work in implementing current law and in developing guidelines for good manufacturing practices. (Be aware, however, that membership in such a trade group does not constitute an automatic guarantee of a company's reliability.)

Aside from the manufacturer's name and address, the product label should state

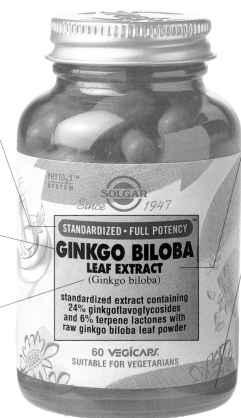

If a product is standardized, it offers an exact —and optimal— amount of the plant's active ingredient.

The common name of the plant is usually found in large letters.

The scientific name should also appear on the label. (In this case the scientific name is the same as the common name.)

A label should also identify the plant part— for example, leaf, root, or flower.

Look for an expiration date on the bottom of the bottle or elsewhere. Also check the label for an eight-digit General Product (GP) or Drug Identification Number (DIN)— indication of the product's approval for sale by Health Canada.

the common and scientific names of the plant, the plant part (leaf or root, for example), and the quantity of herb. It may also indicate whether the plant was cultivated or collected in the wild, an expiration date, and a batch or lot number. When buying a product that contains several different herbs, read the label carefully to determine whether the individual herbs are present in therapeutic amounts; in some cases, they are present in such low quantities that they lack any health benefits whatsoever.

Regulations

In recent years, a resurgence of interest in herbal medicine has led federal governments in both the United States and Canada to reevaluate their regulations about the sale of herbal remedies. In the United States, an anticipated move by the Food and Drug Administration to curtail the availability of herbs by classifying them as drugs led the U.S. Congress to pass the Dietary Supplement Health & Education Act (DSHEA) in 1994.

In Canada, the Food and Drugs Act defines herbal products as drugs if they are sold to "treat or prevent diseases or symptoms." An herbal remedy can be sold in Canada as a therapeutic product provided that it has undergone review by the federal government's Health Protection Branch. Health Canada issues a General Product (GP) or Drug Identification Number (DIN)—an eight-digit number preceded by GP or DIN—to a product that has been verified for its effectiveness and safety and has been approved for sale in Canada. When consumers are considering the purchase of an herbal remedy, they should look for a DIN on the front of the product label.

Even with these strictures, reading an herbal product's label may or may not give you the information you seek. Accordingly, it is important to find out—from a reliable source—the effects of an herb (including any potential side effects), before taking it. Moreover, not all manufacturers comply with these rules. Over the years, a number of manufacturers have made deceptive claims and sold products that have not been deemed safe by government authorities.

Nor can you necessarily expect reliable information from all physicians and pharmacists, many of whom have had little or no training in the use of herbal products. Fortunately, training programs for both groups of professionals are now in place in many parts of North America.

Where, then, do you turn? The best sources are herbal reference books from trusted publishers or experts; these should provide a balanced view of potential risks and benefits involved in using a particular herb. Avoid naive or promotional herbals, which often pass on misinformation and tout herbs as virtual panaceas.

Standardization Counts

Once you have researched an herb, another challenge presents itself: choosing from the many brands on the shelf. Is there really a difference among them? Frequently. It is a fact that not all plants of the same species contain the same amount of active principles. These levels can vary widely, depending on the conditions in which the plant was grown, harvested, dried, and stored. Herbs harvested from the wild are especially subject to variation in the strength and quantity of active principles. For this reason, it is possible for a consumer to unwittingly overdose or underdose on an herbal product made from potent botanicals.

Some manufacturers have resolved this problem by producing products that

Use Common Sense

Herbs can be potent medicine, and even the safest products must be used judiciously. Follow these general guidelines.

◆ Purchase from reliable sources.

◆ Do not exceed the recommended dosage without professional advice.

◆ Discontinue use if you notice any side effects.

◆ Store products in a cool, dry place out of the reach of children.

◆ Do not use most products after one year from date of purchase.

◆ Do not give botanicals to children or use them while pregnant or nursing unless under the advice of a qualified health-care practitioner.

◆ Use herbs as a treatment for serious health problems only under the advice and supervision of a qualified health-care practitioner.

◆ Ask your doctor or pharmacist about any possible interactions with prescription medications.

are standardized through high-quality cultivation methods or by chemical analysis, so that each unit of dosage provides optimum strength and efficacy. Nevertheless, the active principles of the vast majority of herbs marketed today are only partially known or even entirely unknown. If you choose to use products that have not been standardized and validated by scientific studies for safety and efficacy, you should attempt to learn even more about the herb and the manufacturer. Doing so will increase your chances of purchasing a safe, beneficial product.

GLOSSARY

ACTIVE PRINCIPLE A plant chemical that exerts a medicinal effect.

ADSORB To combine with irritant substances by adhesion.

ALTERATIVE Medicine that gradually and favorably alters the course of an ailment.

ANALGESIC A substance that provides temporary pain relief.

ANTHELMINTIC A medicine that expels parasitic worms, especially of the intestine.

ANTIBACTERIAL Destroying or inhibiting the growth of harmful bacteria, or an agent that does so.

ANTICOAGULANT A substance that inhibits blood clotting.

ANTI-INFLAMMATORY Controlling inflammation, or a substance that does so.

ANTIMICROBIAL Destroying or inhibiting the growth of microorganisms, or a substance that does so.

ANTIPYRETIC An agent that reduces fever.

ANTISCORBUTIC Preventing or counteracting scurvy, or an agent that does so.

ANTISEPTIC Preventing or stopping the growth of microorganisms that cause infection, or an agent that does so.

ANTISPASMODIC Calming nervous or muscular spasms, or an agent that does so.

ASTRINGENT Drawing together the soft tissues, such as skin or mucous membranes, or a substance that does so.

BITTER(S) A substance that stimulates the secretion of saliva and gastric juices.

CARCINOGEN A term applied to any substance capable of causing cancer.

CARMINATIVE A substance that removes gas from the gastrointestinal tract.

CATARRH Inflammation of the nose and other air passages, causing a discharge.

CATHARTIC A powerful purgative.

CHILBLAINS Painful, itchy swellings on the skin caused by exposure to cold.

COLITIS Inflammation of the colon, usually causing bloody diarrhea.

COUMARIN A lactone created during the glycoside-breakdown process in certain plants; acts as an anticoagulant.

COUNTERIRRITANT A substance that causes superficial inflammation in order to lessen the effects of inflammation of an underlying or adjacent area, or to distract from the pain of inflammation elsewhere.

DECOCTION An extract made by boiling plant bark, roots, berries, or seeds in water.

DEMULCENT A substance that soothes irritated mucous membranes.

DIAPHORETIC An agent that promotes sweating, often used to treat fever.

DISTILLATION The vaporization of a liquid mixture by heat, usually followed by separation of its components through collection of the vapor's condensation.

DIURETIC A substance that increases the flow of urine.

DYSENTERY An infectious disease characterized by severe diarrhea.

ECLECTIC(S) A system of herbal medicine developed in the U.S. in the 19th century; the physicians who subscribed to it.

EDEMA An abnormal accumulation of serum-like fluid in the body tissues.

EFFICACY The ability to produce an effect (*adj.*: efficacious).

EMETIC An agent that induces vomiting.

EMMENAGOGUE A substance that induces menstruation.

EMOLLIENT Something that softens and soothes the skin and mucous membranes.

ENTERIC-COATED Used to describe pills with a special coating that allows them to dissolve in the intestine, not the stomach.

ESSENTIAL OIL The volatile oil extracted from plants by means of steam distillation.

ETHNOBOTANY The plant lore of a race or people or the study of such lore.

EXFOLIATE To remove the surface of something, as skin, in layers or scales.

EXPECTORANT A substance that promotes the loosening and expelling of phlegm.

FEBRIFUGE An agent that reduces fever.

FLAVONOIDS Plant compounds with numerous structural categories (flavones, isoflavones, flavonols, etc.) and biological properties; many are plant pigments. *Example*: Silymarin, from milk thistle.

GENUS Botanically, a like group of plants within a family, made up of one or more species; first word in a plant's Latin name.

GLYCOSIDE An active plant constituent, of varying chemical structures, containing one or more sugar groups.

GRAVEL Sand-like particles in the kidneys and bladder, made of the same substance as kidney stones but usually passed in the urine without notice.

GRIPE A dated term for pinching, spasmodic intestinal pain.

HEMOSTATIC Controlling or stopping the flow of blood.

HEPATIC Having to do with the liver.

HERBAL A guidebook that describes plants and their medicinal properties.

HYPERTENSION High blood pressure.

HYPNOTIC An agent that induces sleep.

HYPOGLYCEMIA Low blood sugar.

HYPOTENSION Low blood pressure.

IMMUNOSTIMULANT An agent that boosts the activity of the immune system.

INFUSION A water-based preparation in which flowers, leaves, or stems are steeped in water that is not boiling.

INHALATION Infused steam that is inhaled in order to clear congestion or produce another therapeutic effect.

INTERMITTENT FEVER A regularly recurring fever, as in malaria.

LACTONE Any one of numerous organic oxides formed from a hydroxy acid. *Example:* The lactone within digitoxin, derived from digitalis, or foxglove.

LATEX Milky fluid produced by the cells of various seeds plants, such as milkweed.

LIQUID EXTRACT An aqueous or alcoholic extract, of varying strengths, of a plant. *Examples:* Tea, tincture.

MACERATE To soak an herb or other substance in order to soften or dissolve it.

MATERIA MEDICA A collective term for drugs and medicines of all kinds; Latin for "medical matter."

MUCILAGE A gelatinous plant substance made of complex sugar molecules.

MUCOUS MEMBRANE The lining of a body passage, such as the throat, that is protected by secretions of mucus.

NERVINE A tonic used to tone the nervous system or calm anxiety.

NEURALGIA Pain along a nerve.

OFFICIAL In the case of a medicine, sanctioned for medicinal use by virtue of being listed in a pharmacopeia.

PHARMACOGNOSY The study of the chemistry and medical applications of plant and animal products.

PHARMACOPEIA A book describing drugs, chemicals, and medicinal products; usually issued by an official authority and acknowledged as a standard reference.

PLACEBO A drug with no pharmacological activity, administered mainly for a psychological effect; often used as a control in clinical trials.

PLASTER A medicine wrapped in gauze or a cloth and applied to the skin.

POULTICE An herbal preparation usually applied hot to the affected area to relieve pain or swelling.

PRINCIPLE *See* Active principle.

PROSTAGLANDINS Hormone-like substances with a wide range of functions, including causing uterine contractions.

PULMONARY Relating to the lungs.

PURGATIVE A very strong laxative.

RENAL Relating to the kidneys.

RESIN A translucent, sticky substance secreted by such plants as conifer trees.

RHIZOME An underground plant stem.

RUBEFACIENT A substance that stimulates blood flow to the skin, producing redness.

SAPONIN A foaming agent found in certain plants; often used in medicines.

SESQUITERPENE Any of a class of terpenes; a derivative of such a terpene.

SIMPLE An herbal preparation or vegetable drug made of only one ingredient.

SOPORIFIC A medicine that induces sleep.

SPASMOLYTIC An agent that relieves muscle spasms.

SPECIES (*abbr.:* spp.) Botanically, a group of plants sharing at least one distinct trait; a unit of classification just below genus; the second word in a plant's Latin name.

STOMACHIC A substance that increases the activity of the stomach and relieves indigestion.

STYPTIC An agent that contracts the tissues; an astringent.

TANNIN Any of various soluble plant constituents that combine with proteins; tannins are often used in medicine for their astringent properties.

TERPENE Any of various hydrocarbons occurring in essential oils and resins.

THOMSONIAN(S) Follower(s) of Samuel Thomson, an early-19th-century herb doctor who spurned physicians.

TINCTURE A medicine prepared by macerating an herb in water or alcohol.

TINNITUS Ringing in the ears.

TONIC An agent (often a liquid) used to restore tone to the system or to individual organs; also used to refresh and invigorate.

VARIETY (*abbr.:* var.) Botanically, a distinct variation within a species, having a name of its own; often used interchangeably with "cultivar."

VASOCONSTRICTOR An agent that decreases the diameter of blood vessels.

VASODILATOR An agent that increases the diameter of blood vessels.

VOLATILE OIL An oil that vaporizes readily and is often obtained by distillation. Also called essential oil.

VULNERARY Useful in healing wounds; a vulnerary remedy.

WASH A liquid medicinal preparation for external use.

WEN An abnormal growth or cyst.

INDEX

An index entry followed immediately by a **boldface** page number refers to one of the 246 alphabetical entries or special features in the Herbal Remedies A-to-Z section or the Addendum. Illustrations are indicated by **boldface** page numbers within the listings.

E

F

G

N

Q - R

S

T

X - Y

Z

ACKNOWLEDGMENTS & CREDITS

SPECIAL APPRECIATION is extended to the following individuals and institutions for their generous assistance: Dr. Russell H. Anthony, Dr. Steve Beckstrom-Sternberg, Chanchal Cabrera, Coebler's Mill, Mary Lee Criner, Bob Duwe, Frontier Nursing Service, Frances Green, Gene Hale, Health Canada, Madalene Hill, Micheline Ho, Arvilla Payne-Jackson, Perry Keats, Peter J. Kool, Dr. Leo Lemonds, Lawrence E. Liberti, MSc, RPh, Manilaq Association Tribal Doctors Program, Ronald May, Medtech Laboratories, Inc., Dr. Ron Pelley, Betty Reed, Bruce K. Riggs, James St. Clair, Dr. Fred J. Smithcors, Tom Snyder, Dr. Vince Tokaney, Carl Totemeier, Dr. Arthur Tucker, William Woys Weaver, Willner Chemists, Honey Wilson, Lance Yamamoto.

COMMISSIONED ILLUSTRATIONS

Tom Edgerton	28, 58, 88, 118, 148, 178, 208, 238, 268, 298, 328, 358
Mick Ellison	56, 59
Steven Fuller	260
Ray Skibinski	290, 352, 361, 362, 363, 364, 365, 366, 367, 368, 369, 370, 371, 372, 373
Wendy Smith-Griswold	81, 140, 141, 294

PHOTOGRAPHY

Abbreviations

ANS	Academy of Natural Sciences, Philadelphia
CC	Colin Cooke
HI	The Hunt Institute for Botanical Documentation/ Carnegie Mellon University
WHC	William Helfand Collection, New York

Pages: 2 Corbis-Bettmann. **3** *Left* ANS; *right* ANS. **6** CC. **7** *Top left* CC; *bottom left* WHC; *top right* The LuEsther T. Mertz Library of the New York Botanical Garden; *bottom right* CC. **8** *Top left* Collection of Sam Taylor/Tony Sciarelli Photography; *bottom left* CC; *bottom right* Corbis-Bettmann. **9** *Top left and middle right* CC; *bottom right* ANS. **11** HI. **12** Bodleian Library, Oxford University. **13** *Top left* Corbis-Bettmann; *middle right and bottom* WHC. **14** Brown Brothers. **15** *Top* WHC; *bottom* CC. **18** Science Photo Library/Photo Researchers Inc. **20** CC. **21** CC. **22** The Granger Collection. **23** WHC. **24** *Left* Lloyd Library and Museum, Cincinnati, Ohio; *bottom* CC. **25** International Aloe Science Council. **26** *Border and spots* America Hurrah Archive, New York. **26** *Bottom left* CC; *bottom center* Corbis-Bettmann. **27** *Top, left and right* New York Public Library, Rare Books Division, Astor, Lenox and Tilden Foundations; *bottom* Historic Hudson Valley, Tarrytown, New York. **29** *Top right* Chris Tortora / Woodfin Camp & Associates; *all other images* Shaker Museum and Library, Old Chatham, New York. **30** *Left* Lloyd Library and Museum, Cincinnati, Ohio; *right* The Granger Collection. **31** *Bottom left* The Granger Collection; *right* Plate 26 from *Tibetan Medical Paintings*, published by Serindia Publications, London. **32** CC. **33** Corbis-Bettmann. **34** CC. **35** CC. **36** CC. **37** CC. **38** Combe Inc. **39** Corbis-Bettmann. **41** *Top left* WHC; *all others* CC. **42** Stock Montage. **43** Church & Dwight Co., Inc. **44** ANS. **45** ANS. **46** ANS. **47** L.L. Bean / Public Affairs Office. **48** CC. **49** *Left and right* Corbis-Bettmann. **50** Culver Pictures Inc. **51** Lloyd Library and Museum, Cincinnati, Ohio. **52** CC. **54** CC. **55** CC. **56** *Bottom left* Cranbrook Institute of Science / photograph courtesy of Chelsea House Publishers. **57** CC. **59** *Bottom left* Archive Photos; *center* Corbis-Bettmann; *top right* Richard Alexander Cooke. **60** CC. **61** CC. **62** ANS. **63** Lloyd Library and Museum, Cincinnati, Ohio. **64** CC. **66** ANS. **67** CC. **68** CC. **69** Lloyd Library and Museum, Cincinnati, Ohio. **70** ANS. **71** ANS. **72** CC. **73** Lloyd Library and Museum, Cincinnati, Ohio. **74** ANS. **75** Corbis-Bettmann. **76** ANS. **77** Lloyd Library and Museum, Cincinnati, Ohio. **78** ANS. **79** *Top* ANS; *bottom* from *The Tale of Peter Rabbit* by Beatrix Potter, © Frederick Warne & Co., 1902, 1987. Reproduced by kind permission of Frederick Warne & Co. **80** CC. **82** CC. **83** CC. **84** CC. **85** WHC. **86** *Left* The LuEsther T. Mertz Library of The New York Botanical Garden; *right* James McInnis. **87** *All objects* Photos by Richard S. Machmer. **89** *Top left and right* Courtesy, Winterthur Museum; *bottom left* Animals Animals / Earth Scenes, Photo by John A. Anderson; *bottom center* Derek Fell's Horticultural Picture Library; *bottom right* ANS. **90** ANS. **91** CC. **92** CC. **93** Corbis-Bettmann. **94** ANS. **95** Photo from *Shelf Life* by Jerry Jankowski © 1992, published by Chronicle Books, San Francisco, California. **96** ANS. **97** WHC. **98** *Top* Lloyd Library and Museum, Cincinnati, Ohio; *bottom* Corbis-Bettmann. **99** Lloyd Library and Museum, Cincinnati, Ohio. **100** CC. **102** WHC. **103** CC. **104** CC. **105** WHC. **106** ANS. **107** ANS. **108** *Top* Jules Selmes; *bottom* New York Public Library, Picture Collection. **109** Medpharm GmBHScientific. **110** *Left* ANS; *right* Photo by William Edwards / Image Bank. **111** Corbis-Bettmann. **112** Rice's Seed Company / Rose Selavy U.S.A. Inc. **113** CC. **114** CC. **115** *Top* Culver Pictures Inc.; *bottom* CC. **116** *Left* Photo © Steven Foster; *right* CC. **117** *Top left* Photo © Steven Foster; *top right and bottom* Don Dudenbostel / Museum of Appalachia. **119** *Left, right and bottom* Photos by Darryl Patton from his book *Tommie Bass: Herb Doctor of Shinbone Ridge*; *center* HI. **120** ANS. **121** Corbis-Bettmann. **122** Corbis-Bettmann. **124** ANS. **125** *Top* CC;. *bottom* WHC. **126** ANS. **127** New York Public Library, Picture Collection. **128** Photo © Steven Foster. **129** Photo by

Janeart / Image Bank. **130** CC. **132** CC. **133** CC. **134** CC. **135** ANS. **136** *Top* Corbis-Bettmann; *bottom* Lloyd Library and Museum, Cincinnati, Ohio **138** ANS. **139** ANS. **141** *Bottom* Ginger Hudson. **142** CC. **143** ANS. **144** CC. **145** Corbis-Bettmann. **146** *Top right* American College of Nurse Midwives; *top center and bottom* Corbis-Bettmann. **147** *Top and bottom* American College of Nurse Midwives. **149** *Top* CC; *bottom* National Library of Medicine, Bethesda, Maryland. **150** CC. **152** CC. **153** Painting by Grant Wood, "Farmer with Pigs," from Fruits of Iowa, 1932 Coe College Library, Cedar Rapids, Iowa, Photograph by George T. Henry. **154** ANS. **155** CC. **156** CC. **157** CC. **158** Lloyd Library and Museum, Cincinnati, Ohio. **159** Shaker Museum and Library, Old Chatham, New York. **160** Culver Pictures Inc. **161** *Top* WHC; *bottom* (3) David Murray. **162** ANS. **163** Photo © Steven Foster. **164** CC. **165** Corbis-Bettmann. **166** CC. **167** ANS. **168** CC. **169** Lloyd Library and Museum, Cincinnati, Ohio. **170** Gilroy Visitors Bureau, Gilroy, California. **171** CC. **172** ANS. **173** The Granger Collection. **174** *Left* ANS; *bottom* CC. **175** CC. **176** CC. **177** *Top* Painting by Nellie Mae Rowe courtesy of Judith Alexander; *bottom* CC. **179** *Top center and right* Arvilla Payne-Jackson; *bottom left* Animals Animals / Earth Scenes / © Richard Schiell; *bottom second from left* Photo © Steven Foster; *bottom center* CC; *bottom right* Animals Animals / Earth Scenes / © Ken Cole. **180** ANS. **181** WHC. **182** Corbis-Bettmann. **183** Corbis-Bettmann. **184** HI. **185** Corbis-Bettmann. **186** *Left* Corbis-Bettmann; *right* © The Stock Market/Owaki/Kulla, 1994. **187** CC. **188** The Granger Collection. **189** CC. **190** Norman Owen Tomalin / Bruce Coleman. **191** WHC. **192** Dave Nagel / Gamma Liaison. **193** CC. **195** CC. **196** *Left* CC; *top* Culver Pictures Inc. **197** *Bottom left* Culver Pictures Inc.; *right* Culver Pictures Inc. **198** *Left* ANS; *bottom right* CC. **199** CC. **200** HI. **201** Collection of Sam Taylor/Tony Sciarelli Photography **202** ANS. **203** ANS. **204** Corbis-Bettmann. **205** The Granger Collection. **206** Painting by George Rodrigue, "Doc Moses, Cajun Traiteur," Rodrigue Gallery, New Orleans, Louisiana. **207** *All* Vermillionville Folklife Plantation, Photography by David J. Breaux Visual Communications. **209** *Top right and center* Photography by David J. Breaux Visual Communications; *bottom left* CC. **210** CC. **211** *Top* Corbis-Bettmann. **211** *Bottom* New York Public Library, Picture Collection. **212** *Top* CC; *bottom* Corbis-Bettmann **213** Corbis-Bettmann. **214** ANS. **215** *Top* Corbis-Bettmann; *bottom* CC. **216** CC. **218** *Left* ANS; *bottom* CC. **219** HI. **220** Lloyd Library and Museum, Cincinnati, Ohio. **221** CC. **222** ANS. **223** *Top* CC; *bottom left* WHC. **224** Corbis-Bettmann **225** Photo © Steven Foster. **226** ANS. **227** ANS. **228** ANS. **229** HI. **230** ANS. **231** Lloyd Library and Museum, Cincinnati, Ohio. **232** WHC. **233** Photo by Michael Molkenthin. **234** CC. **235** WHC. **236** *Border, spots* CC; *top right* Joe Graham, Texas A & M University, Kingsville Library Archives; *bottom left* Tex-Mex Curios, Inc. **237** *Spot* CC; *bottom* CC. **239** *Top center, bottom left and right* CC; *top right* Tex-Mex Curios, Inc. **240** CC. **241** ANS. **242** Culver Pictures Inc. **243** ANS. **244** WHC. **245** CC. **246** *Left* HI; *bottom* CC. **247** CC. **248** ANS. **249** Photo © Steven Foster. **250** *Center* WHC; *right* Photo © Steven Foster. **251** ANS. **252** CC. **253** Lloyd Library and Museum, Cincinnati, Ohio. **254** Lloyd Library and Museum, Cincinnati, Ohio. **255** CC. **256** ANS. **257** CC. **258** ANS. **259** Lloyd Library and Museum, Cincinnati, Ohio. **260** *Top left* Stack's Coin Galleries, New York; *top center* The Granger Collection. **262** CC. **263** CC. **264** ANS. **265** *Top* Animals Animals / Earth Scenes / © John Pontier. **265** *Bottom left* Animals Animals / Earth Scenes / © Richard Kolar. **265** *Bottom right* Animals Animals / Earth Scenes / © Ted Levin. **266** *Border and left details* Weaving by Marilyn Paytianio / Jerry Jacka Photography; *right* CC. **267** *Center* Basketry by Elsie Holiday / Jerry Jacka Photography; *bottom left and right* Chris Roberts; *top* Wind Altar Prayer Board / Brooklyn Museum of Art 03.325.3776.1-4/Museum Expedition 1903, Museum Collection Fund. **269** *Left* The

Wheelwright Museum of the American Indian, Santa Fe, New Mexico; *right* Sandpainting by Art Etcitty / Jerry Jacka Photography; *bottom right* Carl Taylor / Jerry Jacka Photography. **270** ANS. **271** The Granger Collection. **272** Lloyd Library and Museum, Cincinnati, Ohio. **273** CC. **274** ANS. **275** ANS. **276–7** © Lois Ellen Frank. **278** ANS. **279** *Top* WHC; *bottom* Culver Pictures Inc. **280** CC. **281** ANS. **282** ANS. **283** ANS. **284** ANS. **285** CC. **286** ANS. **287** *Top right* Corbis-Bettmann; *bottom left* CC. **288** CC. **289** *Top left* Culver Pictures Inc.; *right* The Granger Collection. **290** ANS. **291** *Top left* Culver Pictures Inc.; *right* ANS. **292** ANS. **293** Ira Block / National Geographic Image Collection. **295** CC. **296** *Bottom* CC. **297** *Bottom left group* Stuhr Museum of the Prairie Pioneer, Grand Island, Nebraska; *bottom right* Oregon Historical Society, Neg. #OrHi 95673. **299** *Top* Dr. J. F. Smithcors; *bottom left and right* Dr. Leo Leroy Lemonds. **300** ANS. **301** WHC. **302** ANS. **303** CC. **304** CC. **305** Culver Pictures Inc. **306** ANS. **307** *Left* ANS; *right* Henry Thayer & Co. **308** Lloyd Library and Museum, Cincinnati, Ohio. **309** *Bottom left and right* HI; *center* J. E. Holbrook, from *North American Herpetology*, 1842, New York Public Library, Rare Books Division. **310** *Bottom left* HI; *all snake images* (4) J. E. Holbrook, from *North American Herpetology*, 1842, New York Public Library, Rare Books Division. **311** Jim Neel. **312** CC. **313** The Granger Collection. **314** Photo by Alvis Upitis / Image Bank **315** CC. **316** CC. **317** Corbis-Bettmann. **318** ANS. **319** Guy Marche / FPG. **320** Lloyd Library and Museum, Cincinnati, Ohio. **321** WHC. **322** CC. **323** ANS. **323** CC. **324** ANS. **325** *Left* Theodor DeBry / Mary Evans Picture Library, London; *center* Cat. 130497, Department of Anthropology, Smithsonian Institution. **326** *Border* PhotoDisk; *top right and bottom* Alaska on Madison Gallery, New York. **327** *Top and bottom left* (3) Alaska on Madison Gallery, New York; *bottom right* The Frances Greene Tribal Doctors Program at Manilaq Association and the family of Della Keats, Traditional Eskimo Healer. **329** *Top* Jesuit Oregon Province Archives, Gonzaga University, Spokane, Washington; *bottom* (4) Alaska on Madison Gallery, New York. **330** WHC. **332** CC. **333** Courtesy, Winterthur Museum. **334** CC. **335** The Advertising Archives Ltd., London. **336** ANS. **337** Culver Pictures Inc. **338** CC. **340** Lloyd Library and Museum, Cincinnati, Ohio. **341** CC. **343** The Granger Collection. **344** Animals Animals / Earth Scenes / © Zig Leszcynski. **345** Paul Geiger. **346** ANS. **347** ANS. **348** Lloyd Library and Museum, Cincinnati, Ohio **349** ANS. **350** ANS. **351** *Top* Photo © Steven Foster; *bottom* WHC. **352** WHC. **353** Bibliothèque Nationale, Paris. **354** ANS. **355** CC. **356** *Border* © Bob Abraham The Stock Market; *top* © Don Mason The Stock Market; *center* Ski Kwiatkowski. **357** June Gutmanis. **359** *Top right* ANS; *top left and bottom* (4) Photos © Steven Foster. **375** CC. **376** CC. **377** CC. **378** CC. **379** CC. **380** CC. **381** CC. **382** CC. **383** CC. **384** CC. **385** CC. **386** CC.